Also in the Variorum Collected Studies Series:

PEREGRINE HORDEN
Hospitals and Healing from Antiquity to the Later Middle Ages

G.E.R. LLOYD
Principles and Practices in Ancient Greek and Chinese Science

VERN L. BULLOUGH
Universities, Medicine and Science in the Medieval West

LUIS GARCÍA-BALLESTER (Eds Jon Arrizabalaga, Montserrat Cabré, Lluís Cifuentes, and Fernando Salmón)
Galen and Galenism
Theory and Medical Practice from Antiquity to the European Renaissance

LUIS GARCÍA-BALLESTER
Medicine in a Multicultural Society
Christian, Jewish and Muslim Practitioners in the Spanish Kingdoms, 1222–1610

DAVID L. COWEN
Pharmacopoeias and Related Literature in Britain and America, 1618–1847

ROGER FRENCH
Ancients and Moderns in the Medical Sciences
From Hippocrates to Harvey

JERRY STANNARD (Eds Katherine E. Stannard and Richard Kay)
Herbs and Herbalism in the Middle Ages and Renaissance

JERRY STANNARD (Eds Katherine E. Stannard and Richard Kay)
Pristina Medicamenta
Ancient and Medieval Medical Botany

DANIELLE JACQUART
La science médicale occidentale entre deux renaissances (XIIe s.–XVe s.)

JOHN M. RIDDLE
Quid pro quo
Studies in the History of Drugs

VARIORUM COLLECTED STUDIES SERIES

Pharmacy and Drug Lore in Antiquity

John Scarborough

Pharmacy and Drug Lore in Antiquity

Greece, Rome, Byzantium

Routledge
Taylor & Francis Group
LONDON AND NEW YORK

First published 2010 by Ashgate Publishing

Published 2016 by Routledge
2 Park Square, Milton Park, Abingdon, Oxon OX14 4RN
52 Vanderbilt Avenue, New York, NY 10017

Routledge is an imprint of the Taylor & Francis Group, an informa business

British Library Cataloguing in Publication Data
Scarborough, John.
Pharmacy and drug lore in antiquity : Greece, Rome, Byzantium.
– (Variorum collected studies series ; 904)
1. Pharmacy – Greece – History – To 1500. 2. Pharmacy – Rome. 3. Pharmacy – Byzantine Empire. 4. Botany, Medical – Greece – History – To 1500. 5. Botany, Medical – Rome. 6. Botany, Medical – Byzantine Empire.
I. Title II. Series
615.1'0938–dc22

ISBN 9780754659549 (hbk)

Library of Congress Control Number: 2009933508

ISBN 13: 978-0-7546-5954-9 (hbk)

VARIORUM COLLECTED STUDIES SERIES CS904

CONTENTS

This volume contains xxviii + 354 pages

PREFACE

As one of my former graduate students once remarked, "drugs are everywhere you look in Greek and Roman literature." So they are, and often the classical scholar either passes over such mentions as "irrelevant," or "too technical," thus reinforcing the separation – more like a wall – of the medical and other sciences from what are usually labeled the humanities. This almost rigid division is a most modern convention: even Charles Darwin was proud of his knowledge that might have stemmed from adolescent reading in Aristotle, Theophrastus, or Pliny the Elder, and until World War II, physicians and pharmacists frequently composed luminous histories of their professions, often in full command of the Greek and Latin texts that undergirded most sources ranging forward into the nineteenth century; other physicians penned some of the more memorable works of fiction in western literature, with Somerset Maugham and Conan Doyle often cited as examples of the multiply-talented and trained medical scientists who created lasting masterpieces, and Anton Chekhov's plays and short stories remain on anyone's canonical listings of Russian literature. Early nineteenth century schools of medicine in Europe and the United States generally required a background in the classical languages, but by about 1870, Greek had fallen by the wayside, and Latin gradually yielded its place of honor to the burgeoning fields of biology, chemistry, and physics. By the 1950s, few entered the profession knowing Latin, much less the classical origins of western medicine with its purported Hippocratic ideal. Occasionally, the better textbooks in biology, chemistry, and physics featured potted biographies of the Great Figures in the very short histories of these modern studies, and if a student was fortunate enough to have an instructor who understood how rapidly the theoretical notions have changed since the breakthrough research of Louis Pasteur, that student heard something of the ancient wisdom of an Aristotle, who had enunciated a principle that still holds in all of the sciences: our hypotheses will necessarily change the more facts are gathered.

Especially striking in the history of western medicine and pharmacy is the incredible durability of the Greco-Roman concepts of "how the body works," "what constitutes disease" (and health), fused into what early twentieth century physicians still called a Humoral Pathology. One can discern the beginnings of such ideas in the pure speculations of the Pre-Socratic philosophers, shortly to be augmented by further presumably practical applications of the theoretical Elements and Qualities into the operative functions of living things, from plants to people. By the fourth century BC, it had become intellectually fashionable (at least in Athens, southern Italy, and western Asia Minor) to assume *chyloi* ("liquids" thus "humors") likewise existed in plants and animals in the continual and cyclical process of life, from birth through senescence and death. The task of the physician became the restoration and maintenance of an ideal proportion (a *krasis*) of particularly essential humors (there long remained much disagreement about how many of them there were, and what they actually might be). A lengthy debate among philosophers and physicians eventually narrowed them down to four, and once Galen of Pergamon (AD 129–after 210) canonized the theory of *the* four humors as adapted from the Hippocratic tract *Nature of Man*, those four (blood, phlegm, black bile, yellow bile) retained their authoritative status well into the early twentieth century. Durable also was the understanding of how the universe consisted of four elements (air, water, fire, earth), only experimentally disproven by a famous demonstration by Antoine Lavoisier in 1783 that water was *not* an element, but two of them.

Farmers and others who made their livings on and from the land were the vast majority of citizens in the Greek *poleis*, the succeeding Hellenistic states, as well as the Roman Republic, Empire, and the continually evolving "later" Roman culture we call "Byzantine." What farmers, fishermen, and hunters knew was what most would know: agriculture, the seas and rivers that fed people living in the cities abutting them, and the world of wilderness that flanked every farm – all spoke of seasons; farmers measured them by weather-cycles spliced with rising and setting constellations, as they plowed, planted, weeded, harvested, stored, and consumed, beautifully resonated in the hexameters by Hesiod of Ascra (*fl. c.* 700 BC) in his *Works and Days*; millennial-ancient skills in fashioning nets, hooks, fishing spears, and multi-generational expertise in the catching of marine foodstuffs fused with what "parts" were edible (or not), varieties of sea and freshwater animals – from monk seals and sea urchins to the immense swarms of tuna that "ran" annually through the Aegean into the Black Sea – supplied most everyone with what today we like to think of as a "balanced diet," coupled with the ordinary consumption of olives and their precious oils, honey gathered from the beehives that dotted many of the temperate locales from Spain through the Levant, and the wines and beers quaffed from earliest times. Children grew up knowing not merely the planting and harvesting of wheat and barley but also the many varieties of uncultivated plants, how and where they grew, whether in season their fruits ("berries") were nourishing or dangerous, and the astonishing varieties of those smaller creatures whose life-cycles often paralleled the crops and wilderness botany likewise known from childhood. Those included beetles, grasshoppers, dipterids (flies, mosquitoes and their kin), the helicopter-like dragonflies clouding the surfaces of springtime lakes and ponds, and hundreds of others among the insects accompanied the wormy denizens with multiple legs, and the gossamer beauty of a dewy spider web with its nightly quota of encased insects sometimes evoked poetic metaphor. Snakes were everywhere, some harmless and certainly beneficial (rat and rodent control depended on them), others death-dealing, especially to children and the elderly.

Custom, legend, magic, and folklore enwreathed plants and animals, particularly the kinds that killed or others that brought relief from pain or gave cures from illnesses, with explanations often tendered through rituals, themselves tied to the cycles of seasons: *miasmata* came and went in an ironclad regularity reflected in "wet" and "dry" months, and if mists rose on wetlands and swamps, diseases also appeared as they thickened and dispersed when the air returned to a clarity frequently commemorated in poetry; fevers were definite illnesses (not symptoms), so that when the Hippocratic *Epidemics* were set down sometime in the late fifth or fourth centuries BC, some physicians recorded case histories of patients who presented recurrent fevers as diseases linked with seasons, and thereby could devise prognoses (usually rather gloomy). An anonymous author extended the notion of "good climate" engendering "good health," and the Hippocratic *Airs Waters Places* is a ringing argument for the salubrious natural settings that produced the "best people," an argument some modern students have labeled an early variety of medical anthropology. Once doctors and philosophers assumed a triplicate theory of a balancing of Elements, Qualities, and Humors, it was logical to presume that cures for ailments consisted of diets and drugs (as early as Homer known as *pharmaka*) that restored any imbalances: an "earthy, cold, wet, phlegmatic" disease displayed a "bad proportion" (*dyskrasia*) treated by foods and substances that were "fiery, hot, and dry;" and suggested *pharmaka* derived from plants had "faculties," "powers" or "properties" (*dynameis*) opposite the "powers" of the disease.

These "Hippocratic" theories were *not* held by most physicians or philosophers: in fact the pervasive and ordinary understandings of the natural world continued to be in terms of magic, botanical astrology, and the numberless kindred presumptions, first discerned in the three meanings of *pharmakon* as employed by Homer in the *Iliad* and *Odyssey*. "Drug" is but one of the basic concepts (and the poet is not interested in "how" it works), as is "magical spell," or "magical potion," neatly associated by the poet in the famous shape-shifting (men to pigs) performed by Circe on Odysseus' men, and our hero is protected by something called *moly*, a "magical shield" against Circe's wiles. And yet, side-by-side pharmaceutical magic was a hardheaded, agricultural sense of botany that provided occasional nomenclatures to specific kinds that caused specific actions on or in the body. When Theophrastus set down his herbal pharmacology and toxicology in Book IX of the *Historia plantarum*, his on-the-spot sources were the ever-present *rhizotomoi* ("rootcutters"). They were semi-professionals who dug up the roots, gathered seeds, stems, and leaves of the generally uncultivated species in the countryside, those particular kinds of plants known to have *dynameis* (soporifics, sudorifics, etc.), as well as those known to be poisonous (hemlock, mandrake, henbane, and others). On market days, the *rhizotomoi* hawked the roots and plant parts as *pharmaka*, and Theophrastus recorded the kinds offered for sale, as well as how they were collected, the seasons that marked the "maturity" of each, and the rigidly observed rituals through which occasional types were "safely" collected. The *rhizotomoi* intertwined field botany and farm lore with magic explanations and rituals of gathering pharmaceutically active plants, beliefs quite in keeping with the combination of the rational and superstitious so vividly delineated in Theophrastus' "Superstitious Man" in the *Characters*. Not too far distant are the spells, incantations, rituals, and curses displayed in the *Papyri Graecae Magicae*, which occasionally give unelaborated specific names for substances "as if anyone would know this."

Once the Linnaean system of botanical nomenclatures became widespread in the late eighteenth century and throughout the nineteenth century, field botanists identified the numerous species of pharmaceutically active plants enumerated by Theophrastus and Dioscorides of Anazarbus (*fl. c.* AD 70), whose *Materia medica* had become a standard reference for drug lore of all kinds from his own day through the eighteenth century.[1] By the end of the nineteenth century, pharmacognocists and phytochemists had delineated "active principles" in the species described by Theophrastus and Dioscorides,[2] and these data often became incorporated into the widespread and encyclopedic dispensatories characteristic of pharmacy before about 1950.[3] It was not, however, until the

---

[1] The sumptuous ten volumes of the *Flora Graeca* (1806–1840) remain a monument to the dogged determination, talents, skills (and wealth) of John Sibthorp (1758–96), Ferdinand Bauer (1760–1826), James Edward Smith (1759–1828), and John Lindley (1799–1865). Even though some of the locales in the *Flora Graeca* may not be precise and correct, the tomes reflect botanical distribution, taxonomies, and native utility long before modernization and urban sprawl blurred indigenous species, a "natural state" basically obliterated after World War II. See William T. Stearn, "From Theophrastus and Dioscorides to Sibthorp and Smith: the Background and Origin of the *Flora Graeca*," *Biological Journal of the Linnean Society*, 8 (1976), 285–98 with plates 1 and 2.

[2] Still to be superseded is the running commentary on Dioscorides' *Materia medica* by Berendes that accompanies his German translation, viz. J. Berendes, *Des Pedanios Dioskurides aus Anazarbos Arzneimittellehre in fünf Büchern* (Stuttgart: Ferdinand Enke, 1902; rptd Wiesbaden/ Schaan [Liechtenstein]: Sändig, 1983). In English, we now have the generally accurate translation by Lily Y. Beck as *Pedanius Dioscorides of Anazarbus De materia medica* (Hildesheim and New York: Olms-Weidmann, 2005), but notes are brief and concerned with species identification.

[3] E.g. the various editions of Horatio C. Wood and Charles H. LaWall, eds, *The Dispensatory of the United States of America*, 21st ed. (Philadelphia and London: J.B. Lippincott, 1926 [1792 double-columned pages]), 22nd ed. (1937 [1894 pages]), etc. Comparable and equally comprehensive were those in German, French, Italian, Spanish, etc., e.g. G. Frerichs, G. Arends, and H. Zörnig, eds, *Hagers Handbuch der Pharmacuetischen Praxis*, 2 vols (Berlin: Julius

growing importance of pharmacognosy in the practice of pharmacy – ironically coinciding with the near-disappearance of botanical drugs proffered by the giant industrial pharmaceutical companies – that the underlying assumptions of the ancient masters of drug lore became apparent,[4] and with the publication of John Riddle's *Dioscorides on Pharmacy and Medicine*,[5] one could speak of "drug affinities" as understood by our Greek, Roman, and Byzantine predecessors. Although controversial among traditional scholars,[6] Riddle's combination of Greek and Latin texts, with the latest pharmacognostic research findings as drawn from laboratories throughout the world, demonstrated how Theophrastus, Dioscorides, and others in antiquity classed their drugs according to "what they did" in or on the body. Much of the current "alternative medicine" and "natural medicine" as revived in many countries, especially in the European Union, is founded on the presumption that isolation of active principles in natural pharmaceuticals indicates a plant's utility,[7] *but* always in its multi-substance, multi-chemical action and reactions as found in nature.[8] Phytochemists, biochemists, plant physiologists, pharmacists, ethnobotanists, and pharmacognocists have produced a "natural medicine" that a Theophrastus or a Dioscorides would have comprehended in its broader scope, since a majority of

---

Springer, 1925); a reprint of 1938 appeared under Nazi auspices, and remained a standard reference throughout World War II, with prized copies employed for a half-century thereafter (my own copy comes from Cape Town, South Africa, where it was apparently used until recently as a basic work of reference by a German-speaking pharmacist).

[4] Standouts in English include the multi-edition *Pharmacognosy* by George Edward Trease and William Charles Evans, 11th ed. (London: Baillière Tindall, 1978), with the 14th ed. (1996) as William Charles Evans, *Trease and Evans' Pharmacognosy* (London and Philadelphia: W.B. Saunders). The 1st edition appeared in 1934.

[5] Austin: University of Texas Press, 1985. See also John M. Riddle, "The Medicines of Greco-Roman Antiquity as a Source of Medicines for Today," in Bart K. Holland, ed., *Prospecting for Drugs in Ancient and Medieval European Texts: A Scientific Approach* (Amsterdam: Harwood Academic, 1996), pp. 7–18.

[6] Not surprisingly when applied to the question of "effectiveness" of ancient contraceptives and abortifacients, always a politically and religiously laden topic. John M. Riddle, *Contraception and Abortion from the Ancient World to the Renaissance* (Cambridge, Mass., and London: Harvard University Press, 1992), and *Eve's Herbs: A History of Contraception and Abortion in the West* (same press, 1997). See the very perceptive and generally positive review of *Contraception and Abortion* by Paul T. Keyser in *Bryn Mawr Classical Review* 04.04.08.

[7] See esp. Max Wichtl, ed., *Herbal Drugs and Phytopharmaceuticals: A Handbook for Practice on a Scientific Basis*, 3rd ed., trans. from the 4th German edition by Josef A. Brinckmann and Michael P. Lindenmaier (Stuttgart and Boca Raton: Medpharm and CRC Press, 2004).

[8] Or as it is put regarding *Valerianae radix* in *ibid.*, p. 631, "...there is also evidence that the effectiveness of the total extract differs from that of the individual substances. Therefore, the general opinion in the practice of phytotherapy today is that the efficacy of valerian depends on the interplay between constituent groups rather than individual substances." This statement could apply to almost *all* "natural" drugs.

the better handbooks on medicinal plants are careful to describe how the "natural product" "acts" when prescribed in treatment of particular ailments.[9] Even with a continual hybridization, horticultural breeding for desirable characteristics, and re-distribution of species around the globe, one can – with some confidence – attribute specific physiological results to individual substances *within* the "natural" product. Of course, we assume that human physiology is basically the same as it was 2000 years ago, and we also assume that plant species in their broadest classifications exhibit similar phytochemical properties as they did among Greek, Roman, and Byzantine physicians and their patients.

The essays assembled in this collection are some of my investigations into the fascinating questions of how and why our Greek, Roman, and Byzantine forebears thought as they did about drugs and pharmaceuticals. By leading off with "The pharmacology of sacred plants, herbs, and roots" (I), I hope to suggest that whatever we might think about the biochemical or phytochemical properties of drugs, the ancients (and many folk medical practitioners to this day) explained "how drugs work" by means of what we call "magic," but this does not mean "superstition" or "irrationality" if one thinks of "magic" as simply part of nature, as indicated repeatedly by Homer, the anonymous authors of the spells in the *Papyri Graecae Magicae*, the ancient Hermetics, and many other texts from the full sweep of classical antiquity. There is, from the very beginnings of Greek civilization (and likely the ancient Near Eastern cultures that preceded), a grand mixture of the precisely empirical with the hoarily traditional and deeply emotive religious customs that almost always package individual and community responses to illness. "Medications for burns" (II) surveys how farm lore in cultures from ancient Egypt through the Byzantine Empire contributed a most practical understanding of fats, oils, and other oleaginous substances, and how such substances were commonly employed in the treatment of burns, one of the most ordinary injuries sustained in any era, including our own. "Hippocratic pharmacology" (III) indicates some of the botanical drugs recorded in several tracts in the Hippocratic *corpus*, and the likelihood that certain Aristotelian concepts infuse the theoretical notions of "how drugs work" and – again – how rural expertise fed medical practitioners with much of their own skills in the use and compounding the drugstuffs in the fourth century BC and perhaps later. "Theophrastus" (IV) sets out some of the comparative phytochemistry and medical botany one can discern in Book IX of the *Historia plantarum*,

[9] Among many: Ben-Erik van Wyk and Michael Wink, *Medicinal Plants of the World: An Illustrated Scientific Guide to Important Medicinal Plants and their Uses* (Pretoria: Briza, 2004); Ingrid and Peter Schönfelder, *Das neue Handbuch der Heilpflanzen: Botanik, Arzneidrogen, Wirkstoffe, Anwendungen* (Stuttgart: Franckh-Kosmos Verlag, 2004); Paul Schauenberg and Ferdinand Paris, *Guide des plantes médicinales* (Neuchâtel and Paris: Delachaux & Niestlé, 1977).

by identifying species and genera through modern nomenclatures, and why Theophrastus' *rhizotomoi* were the rural experts of the 4th century BC, and why Theophrastus chose to honor their knowledge within the templates of Peripatetic philosophy.[10] Toxicology is the focus of the two "Nicander" essays (V and VI), and here is the panoply of snakes, scorpions, spiders, insects, and myriapods that caused fear and loathing among Greek and Hellenistic farmers and city-slickers alike. Of interest is the widespread study by Aristotelian-styled natural historians of poisonous creatures in the Hellenistic centuries, and Nicander's *Theriaca* and *Alexipharmaca*, likely written at Pergamon before 130 BC, not only adapted the works of an Apollodorus (*fl. c.* 250 BC), but also the results of research performed by Attalus III.[11] The analysis is based on the Greek text established by Gow and Scholfield,[12] whose notes were inordinately helpful as guides into the comparative natural history, only superseded by the long desired collection of entomological data published by Beavis.[13] VII – XII take up Roman pharmacy from a number of angles: Dioscorides' lengthy account of opium is the basic text in VII, and I trust that we can leave behind the pernicious myth that Marcus Aurelius was a drug addict: he was *not*, as a careful analysis of Galen's relevant passages easily demonstrates; the Eastern commerce in drugs can explicate important aspects of Roman pharmaceuticals, as suggested in VIII, and Pliny the Elder's manners and methods of extraction of earlier Greek and Latin tracts on pharmacology indicate his usual enthusiastic sandwiching of sources, likely based on circulating handbooks of "inventors and their drugs," as detailed

---

[10] Recently, I have published a recast, "updated" account in my "Drugs and Drug Lore in the Time of Theophrastus: Folklore, Magic, Botany, Philosophy and the Rootcutters," *Acta Classica*, 49 (2006), 1–29; in some respects, this is a response to the perceptive critique of my 1978 essay by Anthony Preus, "Drugs and Psychic States in Theophrastus' *Historia plantarum* 9.8–20," in William W. Fortenbaugh and Robert W. Sharples, eds, *Theophrastean Studies On Natural Science, Physics and Metaphysics, Ethics, Religion, and Rhetoric* (New Brunswick and Oxford: Transaction Books, 1988), pp.76–99. And superseding all previous editions of Theophrastus' *Historia plantarum*, IX, is Suzanne Amigues, ed., trans., and extended commentaries, *Théophraste. Recherches sur les plantes*, Tome V: *Livre IX* (Paris: Les Belles Lettres, 2006 ["Budé" series]).

[11] As I argue in "Attalus III of Pergamon: Research Toxicologist," in Louise Cilliers, ed., *Asklepios: Studies on Ancient Medicine. Acta Classica Supplementum II* (Bloemfontein/Pretoria: Classical Association of South Africa, 2008), pp. 138–56.

[12] A.S.F. Gow and A.F. Scholfield, eds, with a translation and notes, *Nicander: The Poems and Poetical Fragments* (Cambridge: University Press, 1953). A revised text with commentaries has been published in the Budé series by Jean-Marie Jacques as *Nicandre Oeuvres*, II: *Les Thériaques. Fragments iologiques antérieurs à Nicandre* (Paris: Les Belles Lettres, 2002) and III: *Les Alexipharmaques. Lieux parallèles du livre XIII des Iatrica d'Aétius* (2007). Philologically, Jacques' edition solves many problems, but does not do justice to the natural history embedded in Nicander's two poems.

[13] Ian C. Beavis, *Insects and Other Invertebrates in Classical Antiquity* (Exeter: University of Exeter Press, 1988).

in IX; how Methodist physicians, in particular Soranus of Ephesus, employed drugs in increasingly harsh prescriptions (the "metasyncritic" method), forms X, and XI takes up Criton, Trajan's court physician and cosmetician, and would-be historian; Galen's always complicated and occasionally warped understanding of an earlier Greek (esp. "Hippocratic") and Hellenistic pharmacology receives comment in XII, and it seems clear enough that although Galen boasted of his deep mastery of pharmaceutical lore, with the exception of mineralogy, much of his drug lore is derivative. Finally, in XIII and XIV, are the Byzantine heritages, and in XIII there is a seriatim series of texts (some in translation) that show how Oribasius, Alexander of Tralles, Aetius of Amida, and Paul of Aegina were *not* parroting Dioscorides or Galen or any of the earlier texts in pharmacology, but rather streamlining, adapting, rearranging, and augmenting their sources; and it is especially important to note that each of the Byzantine writers – practicing physicians – offer a kind of commentary on the medical classics in reflection of their own practice: if Galen was wrong, he was wrong. And in XIV, one comes almost full circle, back to the farmers and woodsmen, who knew plants and animals in their natural settings: not only do the imaginary garden tracts indicate an ordinary knowledge of plants, but the tenth century *Geoponica* documents the practical and rural knowledge of insecticides, anesthetics, and presumably exotic foodstuffs quite in keeping with the millennial-old understandings of seasons, and the rhythms that defined the agricultural year. It should be of little surprise that mandrake roots and "apples" were known and used for exactly the same purposes as set out by Dioscorides 1000 years earlier.

After graduating from Baker University with double majors in History and Zoology, I spent a year as a student at the University of Kansas School of Medicine. As an undergraduate, any course marketed as "biological" gained my attention, and I became immersed in chemistry, botany, entomology, physiology, and comparative anatomy. At Baker, Ivan L. Boyd was a world expert on liverworts, and we spent a number of days on the banks of fern-infested streams in eastern Kansas, seeking these relatively rare bryophytes. At the same time, having had two years of Latin in what then was called Junior High School, I remained fascinated by languages and Roman history, and one of my minors (the other was chemistry) in college was German. At the University of Kansas, reforms were afoot in the curriculum of medical education, so that we were present at simple surgeries, accompanied famous professors of psychiatry and general medicine on their rounds, learning the nuances of diagnosis, prognosis, and therapies, as well as that unteachable art of how to ask a patient pertinent and seemingly neutral questions about symptoms of illness. L.R.C. Agnew delivered a series of guest lectures on the history of medicine in Scotland and England in the eighteenth and nineteenth centuries, and his occasional comments about the ancient heritages in near-modern practice set one to thinking about those historical underpinnings. Biochemistry in those days had just begun to reflect the double helix, and our major textbook had a mere two lines on the subject,[14] so that my independent research on how the eye perceived colors and shadows hypothesized about the rods and cones, and the physiological roles of fat-soluble vitamins, research that is rather "historical" in view of what current ophthalmology now knows about molecular structures and the always controversial nature of light. We learned anatomy the old-fashioned way, dissecting cadavers, and consigning to a proper burial the remnants of what once had been a thinking, living human being (unforgettable is one's first glimpse of the coal-black lump that was a smoker's lung). Attached to biochemistry were laboratory sessions on pharmacology in which we learned how the body's organs and tissues responded to drugs, responses attested by staining technologies seen under the microscope in histology. Obstetrics and gynecology formed part of our early medical education, and we occasionally witnessed births, carefully supervised by world-class obstetricians, and the guest lectures by parasitologists introduced us to medical entomology and the fears of testicular infestation by soldiers in the Pacific Theaters of World War II. Kansas in those days was famed for its innovative techniques in reconstructive plastic surgery, and surgeons shared in vivid slides how reaping machines on the western plains sometimes ripped dermis and deeper structures from inebriated or less-than-attentive farmers. A wonderful year, all told, but the Romans remained, and I decided to switch from medicine into ancient history and seek a PhD in Roman history, continue study of Greek, and write that book on Roman medicine the librarians at the Logan Clendening Library said they did not have. History of Medicine at Kansas had fallen on lean times, but the Clendening Library's splendid holdings (sorely lacking in pre-Renaissance texts) kept alive the older devotion by medical professors who wrote books about the long history of the profession, represented by Ralph Major's two volumes,[15] awarded each year to the winner of the still conducted history essay contest. My own "Galen of Pergamon" fetched an honorable mention.

---

[14] "The mechanism of self-duplication [in a molecule of DNA] is a more difficult problem Some insight into the mechanism of self-duplication is at hand. The Watson–Crick formulation of DNA structure states that each DNA molecule is a double-stranded helix in which the two strands are bound by hydrogen bonds between amino and keto groups on adjacent bases, adenine to thymine or guanine to cytosine." Abraham White, Philip Handler, Emil L. Smith, and DeWitt Stetten, Jr., *Principles of Biochemistry*, 2nd ed. (New York: McGraw-Hill, 1959), p. 614, with Fig. 9.3 (p. 192) of "Model of a proposed structure of deoxyribonucleic acid (DNA) showing a double helix, as suggested by Watson and Crick." In its 4th ed. (1968), *Principles* has greatly expanded the descriptives of DNA (pp. 193–200 and 649–60 [significantly titled as part of "Genetic Aspects of Metabolism"]), and in the 7th ed. (1983) in two volumes (Vol. I: *Principles of Biochemistry: General Aspects*; Vol. II: *Principles of Biochemistry: Mammalian Biochemistry*), Vol. I, part 4 (pp. 699–833) caries the title "Molecular Genetics."

[15] Ralph H. Major, *A History of Medicine*, 2 vols (Springfield, Illinois: C.C. Thomas, 1954).

So many fine mentors guided me that it becomes difficult to list them all. At the University of Denver, Allen Breck and Georg Barený fired their lectures and seminars with the panoramas of the Byzantine centuries and the complicated histories of medieval Hungary, the Czech lands, Poland, and Kiev Rus, and seminars in British history under the direction of Raymond Carey gave necessary skills in research, long before reliable photocopy machines and computer technologies. At the University of Pennsylvania, Michael Jameson's seminar on the Athenian Empire revealed how inscriptions can often supplement and correct the historical accounts (here mostly Thucydides) to gain a far better understanding than from written texts alone, and R.E.A. Palmer's instruction in Roman historiography (mostly Livy) showed why Latin is a nuance-packed language, eminently suited for law. At the University of Illinois, Chester G. Starr's magisterial knowledge of ancient and modern military history became an introduction into how armies and navies actually function, quite distant from romantic notions so popular among historical novelists, and Deno John Geanakoplos' seminars in Byzantium demonstrated a wealth of untapped texts, ranging from the early Byzantine medical encyclopedists to eye-witness accounts of the crusades and the final days of Constantinople in 1453; Raymond Stearns' expertise in Colonial American Science linked well with my primary interest in medical history, since the learned physicians almost always spoke in terms of humors, much as had their classical predecessors; John Heller's Greek classes incorporated texts that included Aristophanes, Plato, smatterings of Aristotle and Theophrastus, and many more, as well as the expected Aesop, Xenophon and the New Testament (only when I was a departing, former member of his classes, did John Heller shyly share that he was a widely known scholar in the Latin and Greek terminologies of the eighteenth century, especially of the *Species Plantarum* by Carl Linnaeus);[16] in Latin, John Bateman insisted that I learn to scan poetry, even though I was not particularly fond of Catullus; and by means of William Donovan's spritely classes in Greek and Roman archaeology came an introduction into the history and major sites of Italy and Greece, as well as indications of proper excavation procedures, which served me in good stead while I was a field archaeologist for a season in Jordan. That book I vowed to write seven years before at Kansas was published in 1969.[17]

Post-doctoral mentors added much as I continued to wrestle with questions of context and sources in Greek, Roman, and Byzantine medicine, and the '70s were a now-storied time of numerous, special seminars, conducted by the then-

---

[16] Ten essays (1945–78) collected and reprinted as John Lewis Heller, *Studies in Linnaean Method and Nomenclature* (Frankfurt am Main and New York: Peter Lang, 1983 [*Marburger Schriften zur Medizingeschichte* 7]).

[17] *Roman Medicine* (London and Ithaca, New York: Thames and Hudson, and Cornell University Press); rptd. 1976.

doyens in their particular fields. At the 1970 Institute of Greek Philosophy and Science, held at Colorado College, the seminars and lectures by David Furley, Benson Mates, Kenneth Dover, and Gregory Vlastos emphasized the interplay among philosophers, physicians, and students of nature, from the Pre-Socratics to the Roman Platonists and Byzantine commentaries; the 1972 Institute of Roman Law (Boalt Hall, University of California, Berkeley) featured seminars and lectures by the gracious and witty David Daube on "Protecting the Non-Tipper" as well as hundreds of other topics, from sessions on how to read legal Latin to essential problems in Roman water law, slave law, and questions of *status*; the 1972 Institute also was highlighted by lectures and seminars conducted by Reuven Yaron, who gave us a solid introduction into the legal systems of the ancient Near East; the Second Institute of Roman Law (1973) continued with David Daube's explications of such subjects as The Twelve Tables, the Praetor's Edict, and why Cato the Elder's farm lore linked securely with Roman land law, and we were honored to hear Peter Garnsey in guest lectures on how and why the Romans could think of justice as a two-tiered system, lectures based on his widely and warmly reviewed book on the topic.[18] And when Sir Ronald Syme sponsored an invitation for me to become a Visiting Fellow at Wolfson College, Oxford, in 1981, that time among the "dreaming spires" included my first chills in frequently and gently turning the pages of a manuscript (Arabic, Dioscorides) a millennium old at the Bodley Oriental, the recurrent hours with Sir Ronald as he ruminated on coinages and inscriptions, the habitual meetings with Alistair Crombie at Trinity who indulgently fielded my queries about texts and sources in medieval medicine, and many others scattered among the colleges set in this green island of books and scholars and libraries unmatched elsewhere. My twisting and winding paths from Baker University and medical school in Kansas, through fortuitous circumstances to learn from mentors of skill, occasional genius, and frequent kindness in Denver, Philadelphia, Champaign (Illinois), Colorado College, Berkeley, and Oxford, may illuminate why I approach ancient and Byzantine medicine and pharmacy as I do, and why I believe I have been extraordinarily lucky to be able to combine medicine and pharmacology with the Classics.

JOHN SCARBOROUGH

University of Wisconsin
Madison, Wisconsin
June 2009

---

[18] Peter Garnsey, *Social Status and Legal Privilege in the Roman Empire* (Oxford: Clarendon Press, 1970).

PUBLISHER'S NOTE

The articles in this volume, as in all others in the Variorum Collected Studies Series, have not been given a new, continuous pagination. In order to avoid confusion, and to facilitate their use where these same studies have been referred to elsewhere, the original pagination has been maintained wherever possible.

Each article has been given a Roman number in order of appearance, as listed in the Contents. This number is repeated on each page and is quoted in the index entries.

There is additional information relevant to the articles in the Addenda and Corrigenda section. Asterisks in the margins of the articles are to alert the reader to specific references in this section.

ACKNOWLEDGEMENTS

Grateful acknowledgement is made to the following institutions and publishers for their kind permission to reproduce the articles included in this volume: Oxford University Press (for article I); Elsevier, Amsterdam (II); Librairie Droz, Geneva (III, X); Springer Science and Business Media, Dordrecht (IV); the American Institute of the History of Pharmacy, Madison, WI (V, VI, VIII); Cambridge University Press (VII); the Royal Institution, London, and Oxford University Press (IX); University Press of America, Lanham, MD (XI); Franz Steiner Verlag, Stuttgart (XII); and Dumbarton Oaks Research Library and Collection, Washington D.C. (XIII, XIV).

ABBREVIATIONS AND SHORT TITLES

AbhKM *Abhandlungen für die Kunde des Morgenlandes*

Adams, *Vocabulary*

J.N. Adams, *The Latin Sexual Vocabulary*. London and Baltimore: Duckworth and Johns Hopkins University Press, 1982

Aetius, ed. Cornarius

Jan Cornarius, ed., and trans. [Latin], *Aetii Medici graeci contractae ex veteribus medicinæ Tetrabiblos, hoc est quaternio, id est libri universales quatuor sermones complectetes, ut sint in summa quatuor sermonum quaterniones, id est sermones XVI*. Basel: Froben, 1543

Aetius, ed. Kostomoiris

ΓΕΩΡΓΙΟΥ Α. ΚΩΣΤΟΜΟΙΡΟΥ, ed., *ΑΕΤΙΟΥ ΛΟΓΟΣ ΔΩΔΕΚΑΤΟΣ*. Paris: Librairie C. Klincksiek, 1892 [Bk. XII]

Aetius, ed. Olivieri

Alexander Olivieri, ed., *Aetii Amideni libri medicinales I–IV*. Leipzig and Berlin: Teubner, 1935 [*CMG* VIII 1]

Alexander Olivieri, ed., *Aetii Amideni libri medicinales V–VIII*. Berlin: "In Aedibus Academiae Litterarum" [Akademie Verlag], 1950 [*CMG* VIII 2]

Aetius, ed. Zervos

Skévos Zervòs, ed., *Aetii Sermo sextidecimus et ultimus. Erstens aus Handschriften veröffentlicht*. Leipzig: Verlag von Anton Mangkos, 1901 [Bk. XVI]

S. Zervos, ed., *'Αετίου 'Αμιδηνοῦ περὶ δακνόντων ζῴων καὶ ἰοβόλων ὄφεων, ἤτοι λόγος δέκατος τρίτος* [in]*'Αθηνᾶ*, 18 (1906), 241–302 [Bk. XIII]

Alexander of Tralles, ed. Puschmann

Theodor Puschmann, ed., and trans., *Alexander von Tralles*. Vienna: Wilhelm Braunmüller, 1878–1879; 2 vols; rptd Amsterdam: Adolf M. Hakkert, 1963

Alexander of Tralles, trans. Brunet

F. Brunet, trans., *Médecine et Thérapeutique Byzantines. Oeuvres Médicales d'Alexandre de Tralles*. Paris: Librairie Orientaliste Paul Geuthner, 1933–37; 4 vols

AHR *American Historical Review*

André, *Les noms*

Jacques André, *Les noms de plantes dans la Rome antique*. Paris: Les Belles Lettres, 1985

Anthimus, ed. Liechtenhan

Eduard Liechtenhan, ed. and trans. [German], *Anthimi De observatione ciborum ad Theodoricum regem Francorum epistula*. Berlin: "In Aedibus Academiae Scientiarum" [Akademie Verlag], 1963 [*CML* VIII 1]

ANRW *Aufstieg und Niedergang der römischen Welt*

Aristotle, *HA*, ed. Balme

D.M. Balme, ed., *Aristotle Historia animalium*, Vol. I: *Books I–X: Text*, prepared for publication by Allan Gotthelf. Cambridge and New York: Cambridge University Press, 2002. [also] D.M. Balme, ed., and trans., *Aristotle History of Animals, Books VII–X*, prepared for publication by Allan Gotthelf. Cambridge, Mass., and London: Harvard University Press, 1991 [*LCL*]

Aristotle, *HA*, trans. Thompson

D'Arcy Wentworth Thompson, trans., *The Works of Aristotle*, Vol. IV: *Historia animalium*. Oxford: Clarendon Press, 1910

Aristotle, *PN*, ed. Ross

David Ross, ed., *Aristotle. Parva Naturalia*. Oxford: Clarendon Press, 1955

[Ps.] Aristotle, *Prob.* trans. Forster
E.S. Forster, trans., *The Works of Aristotle*, Vol. VII: *Problemata*. Oxford: Clarendon Press, 1927
[Ps.] Aristotle, *Prob.* ed. and trans. Hett
W.S. Hett, ed. and trans., *Aristotle. Problems*. Cambridge Mass. and London: Harvard University Press and William Heinemann, 1936 [*LCL*]
BHM *Bulletin of the History of Medicine*
Boulos, *North Africa*
Loutfy Boulos, *Medicinal Plants of North Africa*. Algonac [Michigan]: Reference Publications, Inc., 1983
Caelius Aurelianus, ed. and trans. Drabkin
I.E. Drabkin, ed. and trans., *Caelius Aurelianus On Acute Diseases and On Chronic Diseases* Chicago: University of Chicago Press, 1950
Celsus, ed. Marx
Frideric Marx, ed., *A. Cornelii Celsi quae supersunt*. Leipzig and Berlin: B.G. Teubner, 1915 [*CML* I]
Celsus, ed. and trans. Spencer
W.G. Spencer, ed. and trans., *Celsus De medicina*. Cambridge Mass. and London: Harvard University Press and William Heinemann, 1935–38; 3 vols [*LCL*]
CCAG *Catalogus Codicum Astrologorum Graecorum*
CHG E. Oder and C. Hoppe, eds., *Corpus hippiatricorim Graecorum*. Leipzig and Berlin: B.G. Teubner, 1924–27; 2 vols; rptd Stuttgart: Teubner, 1971
CIL *Corpus Inscriptionum Latinarum*
CJ *Classical Journal*
CMG *Corpus Medicorum Graecorum*
CML *Corpus Medicorum Latinorum*
CQ *Classical Quarterly*
CTCM *Catalogus Translationum et Commentariorum: Mediaeval and Renaissance Latin Translations and Commentaries*
Delatte, *Anecdota*, II
A. Dellate, ed., *Anecdota Atheniensia et alia*, Tome II: *Textes relatifs à l'histoire des sciences*. Liége and Paris: Faculté de Philosophie et Lettres and Librairie E. Droz, 1939
Dietz
F.R. Dietz, ed., *Scholia in Hippocratem et Galenicum*. Königsberg: Gebrüder Bornträger, 1834; 2 vols; rptd as one vol. Amsterdam: Adolf M. Hakkert, 1966
Dioscorides, trans. Berendes
J. Berendes, trans., *Des Pedanios Dioskurides aus Anazarbos Arzneimittellehre*. Stuttgart: Ferdinand Enke, 1902; rptd Wiesbaden and Schaan [Liechstenstein]: Sändig, 1983
Dioscorides, "Preface" (trans. Scarborough and Nutton)
John Scarborough and Vivian Nutton, "The *Preface* of Dioscorides' *Materia Medica*: Introduction, Translation, Commentary," *TS*, n.s. 4 (1982), 187–227
Dioscorides, ed. Wellmann
Max Wellmann, ed., *Pedanii Dioscuridis Anazarbei De materia medica libri quinque*. Berlin: Weidmann, 1906–14; 3 vols; rptd 1958
DK (or) Diels-Kranz
Hermann Diels and Walther Kranz, eds and trans., *Die Fragmente der Vorsokratiker*, 6th ed. Berlin: Weidemann, 1954; 3 vols; rptd Dublin/Zürich: Weidmann, 1968
DSB *Dictionary of Scientific Biography*
Duke, *Herbs*
James A. Duke, *CRC Handbook of Medicinal Herbs*. Boca Raton: CRC Press, 1985
Duke, *GRAS Herbs*
James A. Duke, *Handbook of Phytochemical Constituents of GRAS Herbs and Other Economic Plants*. Boca Raton and London: CRC Press, 1992
Ermerins
F.Z. Ermerins, *Anecdota Medica Graeca e Codicibus MSS. Expromsit*. Berlin, 1840; rptd Amsterdam: Adolf M. Hakkert, 1963

Fabricius
Cajus Fabricius, *Galens Exzerpte aus älteren Pharmakologen*. Berlin: Walter de Gruyter, 1972
FGrHist
Felix Jacoby, ed., *Die Fragmente der griechischen Historiker*. Leiden: E.J. Brill, 1923–58; 3 vols in 16 parts
Galen, trans. Daremberg
Ch. Daremberg, trans., *Oeuvres anatomiques, physiologiques et médicales de Galien*. Paris: J.B. Baillière, 1854–56; 2 vols
Galen, ed. Kühn (or simply K.)
C.G. Kühn, ed., *Claudii Galeni Opera omnia*. Leipzig: Cnobloch, 1821–1833; 20 vols in 22 parts; rptd Hildesheim: Georg Olms, 1964–65; cited by vol. number + page
Galen, *De usu partium* (ed. Helmreich)
G. Helmreich, ed., *Galeni De usu partium libri XVII*. Leipzig and Berlin: B.G. Teubner, 1907–1909; 2 vols; rptd Amsterdam: Adolf. M. Hakkert, 1968
Galen, *Doctrines* (ed. and trans. De Lacy)
Philip De Lacy, ed., trans., comm., *Galen On the Doctrines of Hippocrates and Plato*. Berlin: Akademie Verlag, 1978–1984; 3 vols [*CMG* V 4, 1, 2]
Galen, *Natural Faculties* (ed. and trans. Brock)
Arthur John Brock, ed., and trans., *Galen On the Natural Faculties*. London: William Heinemann, 1916 [*LCL*]
Galen, *Parts* (trans. May)
Margaret Tallmadge May, trans., *Galen On the Usefulness of the Parts of the Body*. Ithaca, New York: Cornell University Press, 1968; 2 vols
Galen, *Procedures* (trans. Duckworth, Lyons, and Towers)
W.L.H. Duckworth, trans., *Galen On Anatomical Procedures: The Later Books*, ed. M.C. Lyons and B. Towers. Cambridge: Cambridge University Press, 1962
Galen, *Procedures* (ed. Simon)
Max Simon, ed. [Arabic] and trans., *Sieben Bücher Anatomie des Galens*. Leipzig: J.C. Hinrichs, 1906; 2 vols
Galen, *Procedures* (trans. Singer)
Charles Singer, trans., *Galen On Anatomical Procedures*. London: Oxford University Press for the Wellcome Historical Medical Museum, 1956
Galen, *Prognosis* (ed. and trans. Nutton)
Vivian Nutton, ed., trans., comm., *Galen On Prognosis*. Berlin: Akademie Verlag, 1979 [*CMG* V 8, 1]
Galen, *Scripta Minora*
J. Marquardt, I. Mueller, and G. Helmreich, eds, *Claudii Galeni Scripta minora*. Leipzig and Berlin: B.G. Teubner, 1884–93; 3 vols; rptd Amsterdam: Adolf M. Hakkert, 1967
GMPT
Hans Dieter Betz, ed., *The Greek Magical Papyri in Translation*, Vol. I. 1st ed. Chicago: University of Chicago Press, 1986; 2nd ed., 1992
Geoponica (ed. Beckh)
H. Beckh, ed., *Geoponica sive Cassiani Bassi scholastici De re rustica eclogae*. Leipzig and Berlin: B.G. Teubner, 1895; rptd Stuttgart: Teubner, 1994
Gurlt, *Geschichte*
E. Gurlt, *Geschichte der Chirurgie und ihrer Ausübung*, Vol. I. Berlin: August Hirschwald, 1898
Harig, *Intensität*
Georg Harig, *Bestimmung der Intensität im medizinischen System Galens*. Berlin: Akademie Verlag, 1974
Henderson, *Maculate Muse*
Jeffrey Hendeson, *The Maculate Muse. Obscene Language in Attic Comedy*, 2nd ed. New York and Oxford: Oxford University Press, 1991
Hill, *Botany*
Albert F. Hill, *Economic Botany*, 2nd ed. New York: McGraw-Hill, 1952

Hippocrates (ed. Joly)
Robert Joly, ed. and trans., *Hippocrate*, Tome XIII: *Des lieux dans l'homme. Du système des glandes. Des fistulas. Des hémorroïdes. De la vision. Des chairs. De la dentition.* Paris: Les Belles Lettres, 1978 [Budé]
Hippocrates (ed. and trans. Jones and Withington)
W.H.S. Jones and E.T. Withington, eds. and trans., *Hippocrates*. Cambridge, Mass. and London: Harvard University Press and William Heinemann, 1923–31; 4 vols [*LCL*]
Hippocrates (ed. and trans. Littré)
Émile Littré, ed. and trans., *Oeuvres complètes d'Hippocrate.* Paris: J.B. Baillière, 1839–61; 10 vols; rptd Amsterdam: Adolf M. Hakkert, 1973–82
Hippocrates (ed. and trans. Potter)
Paul Potter, ed., trans., and comm., *Hippokrates Über die Krankheiten III.* Berlin: Akademie Verlag, 1980 [*CMG* I 2, 3]
Hippocrates (ed. and trans. Potter and Smith)
Paul Potter and Wesley D. Smith, eds and trans., *Hippocrates*, Vols V–VIII. Cambridge, Mass.: Harvard University Press, 1988–95 [*LCL*]
Hippocrates (ed. and trans. Smith)
Wesley D. Smith, ed. and trans., with an Introduction, *Hippocrates. Pseudepigraphic Writings. Letters – Embassy – Speech from the Altar – Decree.* Leiden and New York: E.J. Brill, 1990 [*Studies in Ancient Medicine*, Vol. 2]
Hunger, "Medizin"
Herbert Hunger, "Medizin" in *Die hochsprachliche profane Literatur der Byzantiner*, 2 vols Munich: Beck, 1978; Vol. II, pp. 287–320
Ideler
Julius Ludovicus Ideler, ed., *Physici et medici graeci minores.* Berlin, 1841–1842; 2 vols rptd as one vol. Amsterdam: Adolf M. Hakkert, 1963
Ilberg, *Schriftstellerei*
Johannes Ilberg, *Über die Schriftstellerei des Klaudios Galenos*. Darmstadt: Wissenschaftliche Buchgesellschaft, 1974; rpts of articles that appeared in *Rheinisches Museum für Philologie*, N.F. 44 (1889), 207–37; 47 (1892), 489–514; 51 (1896), 165–96; and 52 (1897), 591–623
JHB *Journal of the History of Biology*
JHM *Journal of the History of Medicine and Allied Sciences*
JHS *Journal of Hellenic Studies*
JRS *Journal of Roman Studies*
K. = Galen (ed. Kühn): see Galen
Lange, ed., *Chemistry*
Norbert Adolph Lange, ed., *Handbook of Chemistry. A Reference Volume for all requiring ready access to chemical and physical data used in laboratory work and manufacturing.* Sandusky, Ohio: Handbook Publishers, Inc., 1946
Langslow, *Medical Latin*
D.R. Langslow, *Medical Latin in the Roman Empire.* Oxford and New York: Oxford University Press, 2000
LCL *Loeb Classical Library*
Löw, *Flora*
Immanuel Löw, *Die Flora der Juden*. Vienna, 1928–1934; 4 vols; rptd Hildesheim: Georg Olms, 1967
Löw, *Pflanzennamen*
Immanuel Löw, *Aramæische Pflanzennamen*. Leipzig: Wilhelm Engelmann, 1881
LSJ
Henry George Liddell and Robert Scott, rev. Henry Stuart Jones and Roderick McKenzie, *A Greek–English Lexicon*, 9th ed. (1940), with revised supplement. Oxford: Clarendon Press, 1996

Maggiulli, *Nomenclatura*
Gigliola Maggiulli, *Nomenclatura Micologica Latina*. Genoa: Università di Genova Facoltà di Lettera, Istituto di Filologia Classica e Medievale, 1977
Majno, *Healing Hand*
Guido Majno, *The Healing Hand. Man and Wound in the Ancient World*. Cambridge, Mass.: Harvard University Press, 1975
Martindale, ed. Todd
R.G. Todd, ed., *Extra Pharmacopoeia Martindale*, 25th ed. London: The Pharmaceutical Press, 1967
Martindale, ed. Reynolds
James E.F. Reynolds, assisted by Anne B. Prasad, eds, *Martindale: The Extra Pharmacopoeia*, 28th ed. London: The Pharmaceutical Press, 1982
Martindale, ed. Parfitt
Kathleen Parfitt, ed., *Martindale: The Complete Drug Reference*, 32nd ed. London and Taunton, Mass.: The Pharmaceutical Press and World Color Book Services, 1999
Merck Index, ed. Stecher
Paul G. Stecher, ed., *The Merck Index: An Encyclopedia of Chemicals and Drugs*, 8th ed. Rahway, New Jersey: Merck & Co., 1968
Merck Index, ed. O'Neil
Maryadele J. O'Neil, ed., *The Merck Index: An Encyclopedia of Chemicals, Drugs, and Biologicals*, 13th ed. Whitehouse Station, New Jersey: Merck & Co., 2001
Meyer, *Botanik*
Ernst H.F. Meyer, *Geschichte der Botanik*. Königsberg: Gebrüder Bornträger 1854–57; 4 vols; rptd Amsterdam: A. Asher & Co., 1965
Nicander (ed. and trans. Gow and Scholfield)
A.S.F. Gow and A.F. Scholfield, eds, and trans., with notes, *Nicander: The Poems and Poetical Fragments*. Cambridge: Cambridge University Press, 1953
NTM *Schriftenreihe für Geschichte der Naturwissenschaften, Technik and Medizin*
Nutton, *Democedes*
Vivian Nutton, *From Democedes to Harvey: Studies in the History of Medicine*. London: Variorum Reprints, 1988 (Collected Studies Series CS277)
Nutton, ed., *Problems*
Vivian Nutton, ed., *Galen. Problems and Prospects. A Collection of Papers submitted at the 1979 Cambridge Conference*. London: Wellcome Institute for the History of Medicine, 1981
Oribasius (ed. Bussemaker, Daremberg, and Molinier)
U. Cats Bussemaker and Ch. Daremberg, eds, and trans., *Oeuvres d'Oribase*. Paris: J.B. Baillière, 1851–76; 6 vols [Vol. VI: A. Molinier, ed. *Anciennes traductions latines de la synopsis et des euporistes*]
Oribasius (ed. Raeder)
Johannes Reader, ed., *Oribasii Collectionum medicarum reliquiae*. Leipzig and Berlin: B.G. Teubner, 1928–33; 4 vols; rptd Amsterdam: Adolf M. Hakkert, 1964 [*CMG* VI 1, 1 – VI 2, 2]
Johannes Raeder, ed., *Oribasii Synopsis ad Eustathium. Libri ad Eunapium*. Leipzig and Berlin: B.G. Teubner, 1936; rptd Amsterdam: Adolf M. Hakkert, 1964 [*CMG* VI 3]
Pahlow, *Heilpflanzen*
M. Pahlow, *Das große Buch der Heilpflanzen*. Munich: Gräfe und Unzer, 1979; 5th ed. 1982
Paul of Aegina (ed. Heiberg)
I.L. Heiberg, ed., *Paulus Aegenita*. Berlin and Leipzig: B.G. Teubner, 1921–24 [*CMG* IX 1 and 2]
Paul of Aegina (trans. Adams)
Francis Adams, trans., *The Seven Books of Paulus Aegineta...with a Commentary Embracing a Complete View of the Knowledge Possessed by the Greeks, Romans, and Arabians on All Subjects Connected with Medicine and Surgery*. London: The Sydenham Society, 1844–47; 3 vols
PGM Karl Preisendanz, ed., *Papyri Graecae Magicae: Die griechischen Zauberpapyri*, 2nd ed., Albert Hinrichs. Stuttgart: B.G. Teubner, 1973–74; 2 vols; papyri usually cited by "collection" and line number

PH *Pharmacy in History*
Polunin, *Flowers of Europe*
Oleg Polunin, *Flowers of Europe*. London and New York: Oxford University Press, 1969
Polunin, *Flowers of Greece*
Oleg Polunin, *Flowers of Greece and the Balkans*. Oxford and New York: Oxford University Press, 1980
Polunin and Everard, *Trees*
Oleg Polunin, *Trees and Bushes of Europe,* with Drawings by Barbara Everard. London and New York: Oxford University Press, 1976
Polunin and Smythies, *South-West Europe*
Oleg Polunin and B.E. Smythies, *Flowers of South-West Europe*. London and New York: Oxford University Press, 1973
RE *Paulys Realencyclopädie der classischen Altertumswissenschaft*
REB *Revue des Études byzantines*
Riddle, *Dioscorides*
John M. Riddle, *Dioscorides on Pharmacy and Medicine*. Austin: University of Texas Press, 1985
Riddle, *Latin Dioscorides*
John M. Riddle, "Dioscorides" in F. Edward Cranz and Paul Oskar Kristeller, eds, *CTCM*, Vol. IV (Washington, D.C.: Catholic University Press of America, 1980), pp. 1–143
Riddle, *Studies*
John M. Riddle, *Quid pro quo: Studies in the History of Drugs*. Gower House/Hampshire and Brookfield, Vermont: Ashgate, 1992 (Variorum Collected Studies Series CS367)
Rufus (ed. Daremberg and Ruelle)
Ch. Daremberg and Ch. Émile Ruelle, eds and trans., *Oeuvres de Rufus d'Éphèse*. Paris: J.B. Baillière, 1879; rptd Amsterdam: Adolf M. Hakkert, 1963
Rufus (ed. Gärtner)
Hans Gärtner, ed., trans., and comm., *Rufus von Ephesos. Die Fragen des Arztes an den Kranken*. Berlin: Akademie Verlag, 1962 [*CMG* supplementum IV]
Rufus (ed. Sideras)
Alexander Sideras, ed., trans., comm., *Rufus von Ephesos Über die Nieren- und Blasenleiden.* Berlin: Akademie Verlag, 1977 [*CMG* III 1]
SA *Sudhoffs Archiv*
Sarton, *Introduction*, I
George Sarton, *Introduction to the History of Science*, Vol. I: *From Homer to Omar Khayyam.* Baltimore: Williams and Wilkins for the Carnegie Institution of Washington, 1927
SB Heidelberg
Sitzungsberichte der Akademie der Wissenschaften, Heidelberg, Philos.-hist. Klasse
Scarborough, *Medicine*
John Scarborough, *Roman Medicine*. London and Ithaca, New York: Thames and Hudson and Cornell University Press, 1969; rptd 1976
Scarborough, "Nicander II"
John Scarborough, "Nicander's Toxicology, II: Spiders, Scorpions, Insects and Myriapods," *PH*, 21 (1979), 3–34 and 73–92
Schauenberg and Paris, *Guide*
Paul Schauenberg and Ferdinand Paris, *Guide des plantes médicinales*, 3rd ed. rév. & augm. Neuchâtel and Paris: Delachaux & Niestlé, 1977
Scribonius Largus (ed. Helmreich)
G. Helmreich, ed., *Scribonii Largi Conpositiones*. Leipzig and Berlin: B.G. Teubner, 1887
Scribonius Largus (ed. Sconocchia)
Sergio Sconocchia, ed., *Scribonii Largi Compositiones.* Leipzig: B.G. Teubner, 1983
Sezgin, *Geschichte* III
Fuat Sezgin, *Geschichte des arabischen Shriftsttums*, Vol. III: *Medizin – Pharmazie – Zoologie – Tierheilkunde*. Leiden: E.J. Brill, 1970

Soranus (ed. Ilberg)
J. Ilberg, ed., *Sorani Gynaeciorum libri IV. De signis fracturarum. De fasciis. Vita Hippocratis secundum Soranum*. Leipzig and Berlin: B.G. Teubner, 1927 [*CMG* IV]
Soranus (trans. Temkin)
Owsei Temkin, trans. *Soranus' Gynecology*. Baltimore: Johns Hopkins University Press, 1956
Suda (ed. Adler)
Ada Adler, ed., *Suidae Lexicon*. Leipzig and Berlin: B.G. Teubner, 1928–38; 5 vols; rptd Stuttgart: Teubner, 1971
TAPA *Transactions of the American Philological Association*
Temkin, *Double Face of Janus*
Owsei Temkin, *The Double Face of Janus and Other Essays on the History of Medicine*. Baltimore: Johns Hopkins University Press, 1977
Temkin, *Galenism*
Owsei Temkin, *Galenism*. Ithaca, New York: Cornell University Press, 1973
Theophrastus (ed. Wimmer)
Frideric Wimmer, ed., *Theophrasti Eresii opera, quae supersunt, omnia*. Paris: Didot, 1866; rptd Frankfurt am Main: Minerva GmbH, 1964
Theophrastus, *HP*
Theophrastus, *Inquiry into Plants* or *Historia plantarum*
Till, *Arzneikunde*
Walter C. Till, *Die Arzneikunde der Kopten*. Berlin: Akademie Verlag, 1951
Trease and Evans, *Pharmacognosy*
George Edward Trease and William Charles Evans, *Pharmacognosy*, 11th ed. London: Baillière Tindall, 1978; William Charles Evans, *Trease and Evans' Pharmacognosy*, 14th ed. London and Philadelphia: W.B. Saunders, 1996
TS *Transactions and Studies of the College of Physicians of Philadelphia*
Ullmann, *Medizin*
Manfred Ullmann, *Die Medizin im Islam*. Leiden: E.J. Brill, 1970
Usher, *Plants*
George Usher, *A Dictionary of Plants Used by Man*. London: Constable, 1974
Wood and LaWall
Horatio C. Wood, Jr., and Charles H. La Wall, eds, *The Dispensatory of the United States of America*, 22nd ed. Philadelphia and London: J.B. Lippencott, 1927
ZDMG *Zeitschrift der Deutschen Morgenländischen Gesellschaft*

I

The Pharmacology of Sacred Plants, Herbs, and Roots

Greek botany produced the landmark *Inquiry into Plants* by Theophrastus of Eresus (c. 370–288 B.C.),[1] and this work stands as one of the most remarkable documents of the Peripatetic school.[2] Along with his *Causes of Plants,*[3] Theophrastus' *Inquiry* set a pattern followed in Western botany until the invention of a sexual parts nomenclature by Linnaeus in the eighteenth century.[4] Yet, although morphology dominates Theophrastus' *Inquiry,* one finds at the end of the tract an account of herbal lore, the first such work on herbal pharmacy to survive in Greek.[5] The *Inquiry* was set down by about 300 B.C. and reflects the standards of Aristotle and his general ἱστορίαι, in which data were gathered and organized into particular subjects of knowledge, for instance, a history of medicine by Meno,[6] numerous histories of city constitutions (of which only one survives, the famous *Constitution of the Athenians*),[7] and so on.

Book IX of Theophrastus' *Inquiry* from time to time employs "facts" that come from folk medicine sources, generally labeled the ῥιζοτόμοι;[8] these were a semiprofessional class of "rootcutters" who had their own standards of knowledge and whose folklore about various roots and herbs mirror the deepest traditions of Greek "inquiry" on several, simultaneously applied levels from pure "magic" to utter rationalism. This mixture of assumptions about plants observed in book IX of the *Inquiry into Plants* has caused some modern scholars great discomfort as they attempt to "explain" the irrational elements, while preserving the basic format of Theophrastus' presumably "scientific" gathering of data about herbs and drugs made from plants.[9]

In some respects, this medley of approaches need not be dissected, since the multicombination of views—whether described as magical or religious or rational—had been characteristic of Greek thought since the days of Homer.[10] The amalgamation of the rational with the irrational regarding herbs and drugs received an initial form in the *Iliad* and *Odyssey,* a form that would remain rather typical of Greek thinking on drug lore from Homeric Greece through the later centuries when the *Papyri Graecae Magicae* were composed. Quite seriously, Herophilus could say that "drugs are the hands of the gods,"[11] a significant quotation when one considers that the man who reputedly made this statement was one of the famous medical researchers at the Ptolemaic Museum in the 270s and 260s B.C.;[12] moreover it is Galen of Pergamon (129–after 210 A.D.) who embeds Herophilus' phrase in a consideration of drugs, apparently with tacit approval. Thus the blend of the rational with the divine would also be characteristic of the so-called scientific levels of Greco-Roman pharmacy, while even such as Dioscorides (fl. c. 65 A.D.) and Galen sought to "explain" drug action within intellectual patterns of natural theory that evolved gradually from pre-Socratic philosophy.

THE INITIAL INTELLECTUAL CONTEXT: HOMER'S "ILIAD" AND "ODYSSEY"

Even though there is some evidence to suggest a carryover into Homeric times of Mycenaean practices in drug lore,[13] it is in the Homeric epics that one first discerns a clear idea of a "drug" among the Greeks, represented in its broadest meaning by *φάρμακον*. Standing alone, the word means "magic" or "charm" or "enchantment," but eight adjectives used by Homer divide *φάρμακον* into variations of effects, ranging from the extremely harmful (a poison) to very beneficial (a remedy).[14] The contrast in effects of *φάρμακα* is well illustrated in a single episode from the *Odyssey*.[15] Circe has agreed to change Odysseus' men back into their proper forms, and she administers *φάρμακον ἄλλο* for this purpose,[16] as contrasted to the *φάρμακον οὐλόμενον* that had changed them into swine.[17] The "other drug" (or "spell," here) is for benefit, whereas the "evil drug" previously given has turned men into pigs. Homer, of course, is not interested in speaking about the actual substances that might be part of either *φάρμακον* but only about their effects. Circe herself is one of the first figures in Western literature to represent a skilled sorceress, and her talents include manipulation of the poisons and remedies, known apparently from mythic and folk traditions.[18] Yet her craft is powerless against a *φάρμακον* that Homer calls *μῶλυ*,[19] described as having a black root and a "flower like milk,"[20] that protects the hero against Circe's wiles as she "prepared . . . a potion (*κυκεών*) in a cup of gold . . . and put in it a drug (*φάρμακον*) with evil intent in her heart."[21] Μῶλυ is a gift to Odysseus from Hermes, and the poet notes that this is what the gods call it,[22] but that the root is difficult for mortals to dig up.[23] Homer does not say *how* the herb (if that is what *μῶλυ* is)[24] protects Odysseus, and one learns neither whether the hero drank it in a countermeasure before his meeting with the sorceress or chewed the root nor anything substantive that might show how Odysseus' shield against Circe's *φάρμακον* in the *κυκεών* was achieved.

Although Homer does not specify the particulars of his drug lore, it would not be completely accurate to characterize these veiled lines about *φάρμακα* as simply magical.[25] Lloyd suggests that there is a combination of divine and nondivine assumption in the *φύσις* of the *μῶλυ* that Hermes showed Odysseus,[26] and another interpretation of this passage argues that this early use of *φύσις* means a thing's "appearance."[27] A further level of meaning may be gleaned if one also assumes a primary sense of *growth*, "the natural form being thought of as the result of growth."[28] These may be more sophisticated analyses than the poet ever intended, but coupled with the vague generalities about healing and harmful substances are clear indications of an ongoing inquiry into such matters, albeit rather muffled. In the *Odyssey* one reads of a drug that "quiets all pains and quarrels," a beneficial drug that comes from Egypt, where the land brings forth many φάρμακα, both good and ill "when they are mixed."[29] The poet adds that Egypt is a country where every man is a physician, "learned above the rest of mankind."[30] The beneficial drug from Egypt is probably the opium poppy, mentioned in the *Iliad* as a plant that "bows its head to one side [and] in a garden is heavy with its fruit and the spring rains."[31] *Fruit* appears to be poetic license for the "poppy juice" as it drips from the head when harvested by slitting,[32] and the ripe opium poppies are indeed slit for their valuable exudations in the spring.[33] This is solid information interwoven by the poet into his episode about Gorgythion's death from an arrow shot by Teucer, and it can be argued that those who were listening to the poet's song[34] would have known what the pain-killing drug from Egypt actually might be. Poets and playwrights certainly must make allusions to substances with which their audiences would be familiar, and it seems reasonable to suppose that Greek listeners of the eighth or seventh centuries B.C. were acquainted with the powers and properties of the opium poppy (*Papaver somniferum* L.), which had already enjoyed a long history in ancient drug lore[35] and would continue to do so.

Homer couches his account of mixing opium with wine in a context of god-delivered and god-derived powers and knowledge,[36] and it is again a woman (Helen, daughter of Zeus) who possesses this specialized skill, making a link with the drug and sexual sorcery recorded of Circe.[37] Yet even though Homer emphasizes a mythological setting of treacherous females who "know" the plants and drugs, modern scholars are ill advised in presuming that the lore of drugs and poisons is used exclusively by women, in spite of the perpetuation by males of this quasi-mythology in texts ranging as widely as Sophocles, Seneca, and Petronius: anonymous gathering of pharmacological data, especially those of magical importance, has both male and female antecedents.[38] Moreover, Homer specifies a geographic origin for his drug, indicating something more than purely mythical explanation or a complete dependence upon the well-known tales he fused into the *Iliad* and *Odyssey*. Some modern scholars may be right as they connect the myths of Greek antiquity with a more generalized and universal mythology as revealed by sexual themes and similar motifs,[39] but Homer designates too many specific plants for one to assume a totally mythical context. Curiously enough, *Papaver somniferum* originated in Asia Minor,[40] so that the poet would be speaking of a "local" plant, even though the drug allegedly came from Egypt. Importantly, the episode of Hermes's gift of a φάρμακον to Odysseus is one of the rare examples of the appearance of magic in the Homeric poems.

In its broader setting, the "profession" of medicine is mentioned with some respect by Homer, and it is significant that those who are knowledgeable of matters medical and herbal were among the few traveling, skilled craftsmen (δημιουργοί) made welcome in the settlements of Homer's world, perhaps a reflection of a continuous and gradual infiltration of medical and herbal lore from the Near East and Egypt, as argued by Burkert.[41] If correct, Burkert's hypothesis may indicate why later Greek medicine—especially among the Hippocratic physicians—remained tied to a long-standing custom of being a "family trade," in which specifics of the medical craft descended through the generations by means of elders imparting skills to the youths of the family. Δημιουργός is the term for "physician" as late as Plato and the Hippocratic *Ancient Medicine*,[42] but δημιουργός had become the word applied to a less-than-expert medical man if Aristotle's famous distinction between δημιουργοί and ἀρχιτεκτονικοί[43] records an aspect of this hoary tradition going back into Homeric Greece. The semilegendary Epimenides, a ῥιζοτόμος ("rootcutter") and traveling purifier a century before Socrates and Plato[44] is probably typical of the δημιουργοί in the sixth and fifth centuries B.C., and the common presence of such practitioners may have induced Plato to observe how Homeric medicine failed to consider internal diseases or ailments,[45] not to speak of the medical theories assumed for regimen and specific treatments. Later writers provide similar observations.[46] Celsus (*Med.*, proem. 3) gives a typical description of just what Homeric medicine and pharmacy was: "They only treated wounds with the knife and with drugs."[47] *Medicamenta* were part of this earliest form of medical care, as far as later Greek and Roman writers were concerned, but the aspect that Celsus terms (from his Greek sources) διαιτητική came only "after greater attention was paid to literary discipline,"[48] by which (he explains) he means the rise of Greek philosophy and philosophers. And since *vulneribus ferro mederi* was common in Homeric times, "the knowledge of anatomy evidenced in the poems is almost as sophisticated as that in the Hippocratic writings, and indeed anywhere before the serious study of anatomy in the Hellenistic period."[49]

One can conclude that Homer's warriors and the itinerant δημιουργοί might have reasonable knowledge of anatomy as it would be appropriate for the treatment of wounds, but there is something faulty in the "doxographical" approach to the Homeric poems. Searching for verbal carryovers that can be specified in later Greek literature falsifies the living quality of the Greek in Homer's poems, although the language of epic generally is conservative and archaic and tends to be dignified. Onians has aptly observed that early Greek was marvelously fluid in description of thought, intelligence, and consciousness,[50] and it becomes somewhat futile to chase identities of plants in the *Iliad* and *Odyssey*, unless there is particular evidence (internal or external) supporting special nomenclature. Reading, for example, "onion" or "garlic" or "snowdrop"[51] for Homer's μῶλυ is founded simply on the presumption that later Greek sources record an earlier meaning or that specific antidotes can be matched with specific poisons (snowdrop to counteract stramonium, for example) when there is no evidence in the texts that such identities were assumed. In fact, what Plato, Celsus, and Galen say about early medical and pharmacological thinking, as revealed in the Homeric epics, suggests a lack of concern regarding "naming" things except in association with deities, events, or repeated epithets. In later Greek botany and pharmacy, the characteristic use of particular nomenclatures would find full expression after the rise of philosophy and philosophers—to paraphrase Celsus.

All cultures have basic assumptions about health and disease,[52] so that one can presume Homer's Greek world had appropriate concepts that included "how drugs worked." In contrast to the exorcism displayed in many worldwide systems of treatment,[53] Homeric medicine and drug lore do not exhibit an "expelling" function, although occasional chants might be added after soothing medicines were applied to wounds.[54] One can argue that since the "causes" of the wounds and fractures mentioned by Homer are obvious, there would be little need to assume divine or pseudodivine forces to explain the nature of these manifest injuries; but commonly occurring fevers, headaches, and like "diseases" ("symptoms" in modern diagnostics) probably required religious expertise to ascertain their causes and thereby to prescribe treatments. If Homeric medicines did not perform an "expelling" role, there must have been other fundamental actions assumed for drugs, explanations for "how drugs work." If Smith is correct, early Greek medicine and pharmacy combine theurgy (in its widest sense of supernatural or divine agencies in both diseases and their treatments) with the practical application of drugs,[55] foreshadowing later abstractions so common in medicophilosophical thought in later Greek medicine. Theurgy remained fundamental throughout Greek history even after the accession of Christianity,[56] and theurgy continued to exist side by side with other "medical intervention" systems. Early Greek theurgy and theurgic medicine and drug lore had no specific concepts about what a disease would be "in advance of an attack," unlike other theurgic approaches that supposed invading spirits (among a number of agents) against which theurgic medicine and pharmacy might be directed.[57] Homer's poems depict gods and goddesses acting on and through "natural" forces. Thus, on Smith's hypothesis, Homeric theurgic medicine and pharmacology would presume "natural causes" for illnesses but would also use supernatural powers as a portion of the "explanation" of how and why the disease came into being. Homeric similes give only the top layer of assumptions about how man is related to the life of other things generally, and Homer's comparisons between men and stalks of wheat, leaves, and animals are familiar. Underneath such similes is a series of primary concepts about man and his growth, maturity, and withering, processes analogous to those observed among plants and in an everyday manner in agriculture.

Homer's *Iliad* and *Odyssey* supply plain evidence, in early Greek intellectual contexts, of concepts about the workings of drugs; and by employing certain adjectives to focus these concepts[58] Homer "explains" how "good drugs" or "bad drugs" might function. Also there *is* an ideal environment, a place where good health is normal and where *φάρμακα* apparently would be neither feared nor used for cures: this is the Elysian Plain, where Menelaus will go instead of dying, and in this perfect setting there are no harsh weather patterns. To the Elysian Plain continually blows Zephyros' breeze, always "to revive men."[59] Weather magic and medical skills seem intimately joined by Homer, a connection also observed in the Homeric *Hymn to Pythian Apollo* (lines 189–94) and especially in Empedocles (Frag. 101 Wright = Frag. 111 DK): "You will learn drugs [*φάρμακα*] for ailments and for help against old age. . . . You will check the force of tireless winds, which sweep over the land destroying fields with their blasts, . . . you will bring back restorative breezes, . . . you will bring out of Hades the life-force of a dead man."[60] Homeric imagery (certainly echoed by Empedocles) suggests how drugs are compounded from elements of divinity—as is revealed in commonly known myths—and then are fused by means of an ever-present lore of agriculture, providing an essential context for hearers of the poems.

FROM HOMER TO THEOPHRASTUS

Even as one leaves the era of the Homeric epic, one notes that there is much disagreement about what *should* be accepted as knowledge of plants and herbs, particularly in regard to basic farm lore itself. Hesiod most assuredly knows practical botany, but except for some carefully sarcastic lines about asphodel and mallow as foods available to the poorest of peasants,[61] the poet from Ascra (fl. c. 700 B.C.) has little to say about presumed properties of plants, being apparently far more concerned with customs and superstitions associated with sex and general purification.[62] Lloyd notices the diverse opinions held by experienced farmers,[63] and Hesiod grumbles about these contradictory notions as they apply to the planting season, when "one man praises one day, another another,"[64] in spite of the presumably objective evidence signaled by the rising and setting of various stars and constellations.

Murky as is the evidence for pre-Theophrastean concern about plants and their properties, some of the various bits of texts and traditions that do survive firmly indicate not only an interest but also a continual debate on several simultaneous and intertwined levels, which incorporated the wide swath of Greek thinking on magic and agriculture, plants and herbal remedies, religious customs and the world of nature. Argument began early about the "nature" of plants in relationship to other forms of life, and when Aristotle (*De An.* 410b22) mentions the faulty theories of the Orphics on how plants breathe ("Orpheus," Frag. 11 DK), he shows how very old this debate was. Speculation began quite early about the *φάρμακον* used by Medea to lull the guardian reptile of the golden fleece, and the lost poems of the semi-legendary, pre-Homeric Musaeus may have stated that Medea used a *φάρμακον* with *ἄρκευθος* (*Juniperus oxycedrus* L., the prickly juniper),[65] a tradition faithfully reproduced many centuries later in the *Argonautica* by Apollonius of Rhodes.[66] There are hints that Musaeus composed poems specifically on the healing properties of plants, suggested by Theophrastus' *Inquiry into Plants* (IX.19.2), where Musaeus[67] and Hesiod[68] are cited as authorities on the magical properties of *τριπόλιον* (probably *Aster tripolium* L., the sea aster or sea starwort):[69] "[It is] useful for every good treatment, [and] they dig it up at night, pitching a tent there." Pindar (*Pyth.* III.51–53) says that the traditional medical treatments of Asclepius consisted of incantations (*ἐπῳδαί*), surgery, soothing drinks or potions, and amuletic drugs (*φάρμακα περιάπτειν*), perhaps in reflection of medicine's venerated and dual methods (drugs and surgery), with the addition of magical herbs that could be hung or worn appropriately. The combination of incantations, potions, amulets of herbs, and surgery as the assumed ideal of medical practice in Pindar has no trace of discomfort or conflicting feelings; one can presume that all four approaches to medicine and the lore of herbs existed in the Greek world of Pindar's time (518–438 B.C.) without too much notice, even though there would be certain practioners who would argue against supernatural explanations for disease (as in the Hippocratic *Sacred Disease*) or against the excessive influence of philosophical theory in medicine (as in the Hippocratic *Ancient Medicine*).

Athenian playwrights have unwittingly left clear indications that there was an ordinarily accepted "common knowledge" of drugs and herbal remedies in the fifth century B.C. and that such pharmaceutical lore was generally accepted simultaneously in both magicolegendary and empirical-practical ways. Playwrights, whether of tragedy or comedy, must use allusions readily comprehended by their audiences, so that mentions of herbs or drugs in the plays can be presumed to be understood by Athenians who sat through the productions, staged in honor of Dionysus. Two examples will be illustrative: a fragment from the lost *Rhizotomoi* (*Rootcutters*) by Sophocles, and puns and allusions made on particular herbal contraceptives by Aristophanes in his *Peace* and *Lysistrata*.

Among the many proofs adduced by Macrobius (fl. 430 A.D.)[70] in his *Saturnalia* to demonstrate Vergil as the complete rhetorician is Vergil's command of the details of Greek literature and the underpinnings of beliefs that produced Greek tragedy. Macrobius argues that Vergil's Dido is modeled after Sophocles' Medea in the *Rhizotomoi* (*Rootcutters*), and Macrobius quotes *Aeneid*, IV.513 to introduce his evidence for Vergil's borrowing of Sophoclean imagery:

> Herbs she had gathered, cut by moonlight with a bronze knife
> Poisonous herbs all rank with juices of black venom.[71]

Macrobius then writes that Medea in Sophocles' *Rhizotomoi* is presented "cutting poisonous herbs with her face turned away lest she perish from the strength of their noxious aromas, then pouring the herbs' juice into bronze jars, the herbs themselves being cut with bronze sickles."[72] Macrobius next quotes two passages from Sophocles' lost *Rhizotomoi:*

> [Medea] receives the juice whitely clouded, oozing from the cutting, while she averts her eyes from her hand; she receives the juice in bronze jars.
>
> These bark baskets shield and hide the ends of the roots that [Medea] cut with bronze sickles while she was naked, shrieking and wild-eyed.[73]

Apart from the ceremonial use of bronze implements and the fearful caution displayed in the gathering of this mysterious root sap, these opaque passages relate some important details: the sap is a milky or cloudy white, and the herb is particularly valued for its root. It is probable that these two quotations by Macrobius from Sophocles' *Rhizotomoi* are from the *parodos* of the play, introducing Medea in her "professional function" of harvesting herbs for magical purposes. Yet there is just enough information in these lines to suggest that the Athenian audience might be familiar with the plant and its poisonous odors, produced when its roots were severed. Local drugsellers (*φαρμακοπῶλαι*) and rootcutters (*ῥιζοτόμοι*) who plied their trades in Attica a century after Sophocles would relate *their* cautions when they cut the roots of *θαψία* (*Thapsia garganica* L., the so-called deadly carrot): one should not stand to the windward while cutting *θαψία* roots, and as a precaution one should anoint oneself with oil to prevent swelling and blistering from the *θαψία* odors and exudations.[74] *Θαψία*, with its black-barked root and white interior (the sap is milky),[75] was put in the "dangerous class" of roots,[76] alongside hemlock (*Conium maculatum* L.), as a matter of ordinary knowledge simply because it was so very common as a wild plant in Attica and particularly dangerous to cattle brought in from other disticts of Greece.[77] Perhaps Athenians sitting through the performance of Sophocles' *Rhizotomoi* would have nodded in recognition at the chorus of rootcutters and also sensed personal connections with Medea's roots and magical implements, connections in their turn interlocked with the legends of Circe and Medea as well as the farmers' lore about the "deadly carrot."

In the Homeric *Hymn to Demeter* (line 209), one reads that the goddess willingly drinks a potion (*κυκεών*) made by mixing meal, water, and pennyroyal (*γλήχων* [also βλήχων]-*Mentha pulegium* L.). Pennyroyal apparently retained its quasi-mythical associations with the functions of birthing and nursing the newborn for many centuries, as attested by Soranus' recommendation of its strong, sweetish odor (somewhere between peppermint and camphor) in the delivery chamber.[78] Yet this tight link between pennyroyal and "female functions" has another aspect than the simply magical or legendary, neatly given precision by puns in Aristophanes' *Lysistrata* (line 89) and *Peace* (line 712). In *Lysistrata*, one chuckles at the nicely obscene pun on βλήχων,[79] but the *Peace* line provides a vivid allusion to a woman's sexual attractiveness, with the suggestion of κυκεῶνα βληχωνίαν ("pennyroyal potion") as a remedy for too "much fruit."[80] Aristophanes is not emphasizing pennyroyal's venerated associations with Demeter (although Athenians would certainly appreciate those traditions) but rather the well-known fact that pennyroyal quaffed in solution prevented pregnancies—a most useful detail in the folk traditions of the day, since a prostitute, or "flute girl," stayed in business only as long as she did not become pregnant.[81] The playwright assumes that everyone in the audience (both men and women) would know pennyroyal by sight in the fields and also would know the "ordinary use" for the "pennyroyal potion" by women—or the allusions and puns on the name of the herb would not have gained laughter from the mixed audience.

Pennyroyal's reputation as a female contraceptive and abortifacient is verified in the Hippocratic writers,[82] Dioscorides,[83] and Galen.[84] One may presume that the pharmaceutical details on the effects of pennyroyal solutions or pessaries, as they are listed in Hippocratic writings, are extracts gathered from midwives' oral traditions or (perhaps more relevantly) from an ever-present prostitutes' lore. Aside from folkloristic connections with aphrodisiacs generally,[85] pennyroyal's pharmaceutical properties (as understood by modern pharmacognosy) confirm antiquity's basic empirical observations.[86] Until quite recently pennyroyal and its extract, the ketone pulegone, was commonly employed as an emmenagogue and as an abortifacient. Generally called "pennyroyal oil" or "*pulegium* oil," this extract acts as a mild irritant to the kidneys and bladder in excretion and reflexly stimulates uterine contractions. Contrasted to the "pennyroyal potion" of Greek antiquity, with its aparently nontoxic action, the modern extract of pennyroyal oil exhibits very poisonous effects. Convulsions result from as little as four milliliters.[87] Pennyroyal oil contains not less than 85 percent pulegone, while the natural extract gained from the dried leaves and flowering tops of *Mentha pulegium, Mentha longifolia* (L.) and *Hedeoma pulegioides* (L.) Pers. (US sp.) has about 1 percent of the volatile oil, along with tannin and bitter principles.[88] The ancient preparation apparently served well in its intended use, and its urinary effects were observed in conjunction with the action of κανθαρίς (the aphrodisiac today called "Spanish fly").[89] Aristophanes' puns certainly reflect a "common knowledge" of pennyroyal among the citizens of fifth-century-B.C. Athens, and one also receives a brief glimpse of the technical expertise of midwives and call girls as they plied their trades in the same era. That men as well as women would be presumed aware of what the "pennyroyal potion" was supposed to do suggests how common this particular herb was and also that the use of "sexual drugs" (whether magical or not) was not the particular knowledge of women alone.

THEOPHRASTUS AND BOTANICAL FOLKLORE

Homer's *μῶλυ* was to later Greeks an averter of drugs and witchcraft,[90] something that had the power to ward off noxious effects, a substance termed an *ἀλεξιφάρμακον*. In his *Inquiry into Plants*, Theophrastus offers an opinion as to why squill (*Urginea maritima* Baker) should be a good *ἀλεξητήριον* (averter): he suggests that because plants that grow from bulbs are very long-lived (his phrase can be rendered as something like "tenacious of life"), they are thus suited to be planted in front of the entrance to a house where the squill "fends off trouble (*δήλησις*) that threatens the dwelling."[91] Theophrastus is *not* saying squill actually does what "it is said" (*λέγεται*) to do (ward off spells from a house), but he is attempting to explain why many in his culture might believe squill has such powers and properties, carefully linked by Theophrastus to its property in being able (*δύναται*) to aid the storage of other fruits and vegetables: "If the stalk of the fruit of the pomegranate [*ῥόα-Punica granatum* L.] is set in squill," it will keep for a long time; and even when hung, squill bulbs 'live' for a long period, as do many bulbous plants. Elsewhere, Theophrastus records instances in which squill becomes part of a purification ritual. A superstitious man has chanced to see a statue of Hecate wreathed in garlic at one of the countryside altars set at forks in the road, and he rushes home to hire priestesses, who carry squill (bulbs?) around to cleanse him.[92] Parker believes this is part of an ancient tradition of "blood purification,"[93] and one notes how the stereotypical superstitious person employs several plants in an ordinary day, using a leaf of the *δάφνη* (the sweet bay, *Laurus nobilis* L.) carefully chewed in the early morning (a "sacred bay"),[94] and how he will purchase myrtle (*μύρσινη-Myrtus communis* L.) and frankincense (*λιβανωτός-Boswellia* spp.) every fourth and seventh day of the month for sacrifices to the Hermaphrodites.[95] Again, Theophrastus carefully depicts folkloristic practices without necessarily condemning them (although the stereotypes in his *Characters* generally bring laughter at the extreme antics portrayed), and the underlying questions posed by the skilled botanist are significant: Why are *these* particular plants associated with religious or magical practices and how can they be related to known properties (*δυνάμεις*) of herbs and herbal drugs, especially as understood in agricultural lore?

Squill is a particularly apt example of the mixture in the Greek mind of practical botany, magicoreligious rituals of great antiquity, and precise knowledge of pharmacological and medical utility.[96] The first-known mention of squill is in a fragment of an elegiac poem by Theognis (fl. c. 544 B.C.), and this small bit establishes that squill was widely understood in its botanical and agricultural context for its pungent properties: "Neither a rose nor a hyacinth grows on a squill."[97] A close second, in terms of earliest mention of squill in Greek, is in one of the scrappy remnants of the poems of Hipponax (fl. 540–537 B.C.), and the two lines show immediately a close link between the use of squill and the religious practice of expelling a scapegoat (*φαρμακός*) to cleanse a community of perceived impurities or pollution: "Pelting him in the meadow and beating / With twigs and squills like unto a scapegoat."[98] The brutality of this use of a *φαρμακός* to cleanse a diseased city is summarized by a late Byzantine polymath, John Tzetzes (fl. c. 1130), who describes how a *φαρ-*

μακός was selected and sacrificed in "ancient times."[99] Significantly, Tzetzes cites Hipponax as "describing the custom best,"[100] although most of the data in Tzetzes' account are unattributed: "After hitting [the *φαρμακός*] seven times on the penis with squills and [branches] of wild figs and other uncultivated [plants], in the end they [sacrificed the *φαρμακός*] in a fire burning wood of wild trees."[101]

Squill and certain other herbs (for example, the so-called chaste tree [*Vitex agnus castus* L.])[102] are given special significance in the Greek custom of choosing a *φαρμακός* to rid a community of plague or pestilence or a household of its sense of hunger (perhaps a carryover from the hoary fear of famine as suggested by the term *βούλιμος*). Tzetzes labels his account as one of *κάθαρμα* (ritual cleansing); but squill as an acrid cultivar and widely known herbal remedy for coughs, asthma, and *ἀλεξιφάρμακον* when "hung whole in front of entrances [to houses]"[103] is closely intertwined with the concept of the *φαρμακός*, an obvious analogue of *φάρμακον*, first noted as a "poison" or "beneficial drug" or "spell" in the Homeric epics. It is, however, not until hellenistic Greek, that the ancient *φαρμακός* "scapegoat," (accented on the final syllable) was wedded to a second meaning, namely, "poisoner," "sorceror," or "magician" (accented on the initial syllable),[104] quite probably a revival of the Homeric sense, much as Theophrastus wrestles with defining plants with "medicinal properties,"[105] as contrasted to ordinary plants.[106] Squill, as Theophrastus acknowledges, has peculiar properties (*δυνάμεις*) that span the range from the purely pharmacologic to venerated folkloristic practices, mirrored partially in his spoof of the superstitious man in *The Characters*. As Stannard has noted, squill attained such widespread use that there was a variety called "squill of Epimenides,"[107] identified as French sparrow grass (*Ornithogalum pyrenaicum* L.) by Hort and his sources.[108] If the tradition preserved in Apuleius reflects historical fact,[109] Epimenides was a magician or student of magic (a magus), and according to Theophrastus' normal custom of not naming living authorities,[110] Epimenides probably lived and "gathered roots and herbs"[111] quite some time before Theophrastus' century.[112] Epimenides' "cleansing" activities were intimately associated with "squill," although several herbs were called by that name in Greek.[113] One may also note the reappearance of the very ancient and very muted Near Eastern ties with the magicoreligious association of squill, as Lucian pokes fun at the "Chaldean" practice of "cleansing with torches and squills."[114] One ascertains the survival of various forms of purification rites employing squill at least as late as the second century A.D. in the eastern Roman Empire, and the unattributed sources among John Tzetzes' "the ancients" may include texts from Roman and Byzantine times,[115] as well as his cited names and quoted lines from Hipponax and Lycophron of much earlier Greek centuries. The properties of squill were highly esteemed for their powers of *κάθαρμα* throughout a millennium among Greeks and Romans. "It is tempting," writes Parker, ". . . to see [squill] as the vegetable equivalent of an animal, the impure puppy, a dishonourable plant appropriately used in a ritual applied to polluted persons."[116] Parker, however, admits difficulty with such an interpretation of the symbolism of a plant like squill, because there were so many possible uses,[117] from pure rituals in magicoreligious observances to straightforward herbal lore and pharmacology.

Theophrastus is well aware of the quandary in describing a plant that had both traditional and sacred uses and also a history of employment as a drug among herbalists and physicians. His morphological botany could be secured by close and patient observation,[118] but some other method than either pharmacology or botany was necessary to depict squill—and similar plants—as they were comprehended by the varying practitioners in the Greek world of c. 300 B.C. Not surprisingly, Theophrastus meets this problem within the structure and format of book IX of his *Inquiry into Plants,* the part of the treatise that considers plants of "medical utility," as well as important questions as to sources of information about such plants.[119]

Theophrastus begins his *Inquiry* (IX.18) by writing, "As has been noted, there are roots and shrubs that have many powers (*δυνάμεις*) affecting not only living bodies but also bodies without life (*τὰ ἄψυχα*)," and his first example is an *ἄκανθα* (probably gum arabic), which, "as they say" (λέγουσι), thickens water when put into it. His second example is the root of marsh mallow (*ἄλθαια-Althaea officinalis* L.), which has the same property if it is shredded into a container of water and allowed to stand in open air; but one identifies marsh mallow by its similarity with mallow (*μαλάχη*-either *Malva rotundifolia* L., or *Malva sylvestris* L.), and Theophrastus describes differences between the two species in terms of their leaves, stalks, flowers, seeds, and roots. Then follows the medical employment of *ἄλθαια*: "They employ (*χρῶνται*) marsh mallow for fractures, and in sweet wine for coughs, and in olive oil for open ulcers [or wounds]." The pharmacology implied by Theophrastus is the property of marsh mallow to make a glue when mixed with water (similar to the gum arabic), a property acting on a "lifeless body," in turn rendering it useful in the treatment of fractures.[120] The choice of marsh mallow seems deliberate, rather than simply one gum-producing plant selected from many examples: *ἀλθαίνω* is a common verb (heal),[121] and the noun *ἄλθεξις* as "healing" or "cure" appears in both the Hippocratic *Fractures* and Nicander's coinage as *ἀλθεστήρια* (healing remedies).[122] Theophrastus' deft connection of medicinally useful plants with their effects on nonliving things has thus been precisely laid down, beginning with roots and shrubs that have various properties, spanning a range from straightforward drugs that act in living patients to the plants that have powers to affect nonliving matter. By this simple technique of association Theophrastus is able to proceed from herbal remedies to plants that have other effects and uses, including those of magicoreligious and sacred importance. His manner of consideration, however, is carefully paced step by step as he advances from plants affecting nonliving matter through plants that act in or on animals other than human beings[123] to those that affect both "body and intellect [or soul]."[124] Parenthetically, Theophrastus precedes his "body and intellect" plants with, "And legends are concocted not without reason."

Inquiry into Plants IX.18.3–11, takes up the subject of fertility and antifertility herbs, the curiosa of aphrodisiacs and anaphrodisiacs. Most importantly, however, Theophrastus notes that his first instance of a plant that has *both* aphrodisiac properties (*ὄρχις*, lit. "testicle," probably early purple orchid, *Orchis mascula* [L.] L., from which a drink called salep is made from the macerated tubers[125]) has "leaves like a squill,"[126] indicating immediately how the botanist is investigating such plants, which are firmly linked to sacred ceremonies well known to his readers.

Ὄρχις is also an excellent example of the intermeshing of a common "doctrine of sympathy" or—more loosely—the "doctrine of signatures,"[127] which Greek and Roman herbal lore continually interwove with more empirical pharmacological observations. Much as Theophrastus employs the ordinary name *testicle* for the double-propertied *Orchis mascula* (and he does so without any hint of self-contradiction or of the insertion of dissonant facts), so also one recalls Theophrastus' connections between the quasi-religious practice of planting squill to avert spells on a house and his concept of long-lived squill bulbs (VII.13.4), and one can thereby sense also the numerous but unstated folkloristic and magicoreligious customs that hover in the shadows of *Inquiry* IX.18.3–11. Preus argues that any effect such plants would have regarding conception or contraception would be expressed by the modern term *psychosomatic,*[128] but the application of any modernisms to Theophrastus' delicately skilled arguments and attempts to document pharmacological properties of sacred plants and herbs does the injustice of inserting presentism. Moreover, except for a direct reference to an otherwise unknown Aristophilus of Plataea (called a "drugseller," φαρμακοπώλης), who said he "had some [drugs] that could engender greater potency as well as eliminating it completely,"[129] almost all of the data in *Inquiry* IX.18.3–11 are qualified by "it is claimed," "are said," "it is said," "if this account is true," and "they say," phrases that delineate Theophrastus' manner of simply recording what he has heard, without necessarily approving or denying the purported facts. He does state his basic acceptance, however, that such things and effects are quite possible, with "It is paradoxical, as I have said, that opposite effects result from a single nature [φύσις]; but it is not paradoxical that such properties [δυνάμεις] exist."[130] Implicitly he has admitted the possibility of traditional claims for sacred plants like squill, but Theophrastus firmly rejects generally (ὅλως) the assertions made for ἀλεξιφάρμακα that might be worn as charms or attached to a house.[131] Exceptions could perhaps be allowed for sacred herbs; but if they are unsanctioned by hallowed magicoreligious traditions of either a public or private nature, Theophrastus is unwilling to entertain possible effects from herbs simply said to be powerful.[132]

The majority of *Inquiry* IX is taken up not with considerations of claims for plants that are magical, semioccult, or plants that have religious connections, but with a careful analysis of medicinal properties of somewhat less than sixty major herbs and herbal remedies.[133] Yet Theophrastus' main source of information for such plants are the ῥιζοτόμοι, a professional group of herbalists who collected medicinal roots and herbs, selling them at country fairs, hawking their virtues for pains and ailments of many kinds; added to the ῥιζοτόμοι as sources of data on herbs are the φαρμακοπῶλαι (drug vendors), who also touted their products in the venerated manner of folk medicine to country and city dwellers alike.[134] *Inquiry* IX.8.5–8 shows rather vividly these sources of Theophrastus' data and how he sorted out useful facts from the merely mythical: the drug vendors and rootcutters suggest that one should cut roots only while standing to the windward, especially in the case of θαψία (the deadly carrot, *Thapsia garganica* L.),[135] and that one should coat one's body with oil before trying to dig up or cut the roots. Furthermore, the herbalist has to exercise caution while gathering the fruit of the wild rose (probably the rose hips): these must be collected while the individual stands to the windward, because picking the rose hips could harm one's eyes. Theophrastus does not dismiss these assertions as "old wives' tales," but comments that there is some credence to be placed in them because of the properties (δυνάμεις) of these plants, which tend to be harmful, seizing "as they say" like a fire and burning. Digging hellebore[136] for a long time causes dizziness, and the ῥιζοτόμοι advise one to eat garlic beforehand and to quaff some undiluted wine. Theophrastus honors such reports from the rootcutters, but he derides other procedures espoused by the rootcutters as "far-fetched and irrelevant," including the practice of digging up peonies at night to avoid being seen by woodpeckers (this may cause the loss of an herbalist's eyesight) or the stipulation that one should beware of the buzzard (*Buteo* spp.) while cutting a κενταυρίς (probably *Centarium umbellatum* Gilib., the feverwort or centaury) or that while cutting the All-Heal (πάνακες) of Asclepius, one should make an offering "in its place" of fruits and baked meal. Theophrastus writes that "praying while cutting is perhaps reasónable, but the additions to this caution are ridiculous," showing he is carefully separating the patently superstititious from the empirically reasonable or from particular customs that have long-standing magicoreligious associations. One should not, however, be misled into thinking that Theophrastus advocates a medical botany bereft of magic and religion or an herbalism forsaking its ancient agricultural and sacred heritages: he says to accept rootcutters' and farmers' tales at face value and then to test them both with the logic of empiricism as well as field collection of plants, ascertaining those practices that, in effect, "make sense."

Theophrastus' grudging ambivalence about hoary rituals and his apparently reluctant piety suggest how murky are the differences in Greek antiquity between magic and religion as well as between the presumably "objective" observations gathered by farmers and those customary deferences of homage to the venerated powers of certain plants. Edelstein rightly recognizes the "specific problem of pharmacology in connection with the efficacy of plants"[137] but then proceeds to argue that Greek and Roman views are neatly categorized into a tripartite division. First the properties of medicinal plants (and by logical extension, the causes of diseases) are marked by purely "scientific" and empirical observations, seeing "in plants nothing but natural powers."[138] Second, since Nature is divine, plants and drugs derived from them are divine, which can be fitted within a class of traditional religion of a deistic character, an "interpretation which accepts the divinity of the plants because of the divinity of the intellect in the human being who applies them."[139] Third, Edelstein scornfully derides "magical belief . . . sorcery and such nonsense. . . . All the great pharmacologists rejected those things. Andreas and Pamphylus [*sic*] and [those who accepted magic] constituted a small minority; they were scholars rather than physicians; they were antiquaries. These men were isolated as were those who believed in the demonic character of diseases."[140] Somehow Edelstein has chosen to ignore the grand and opaque jumble of opinions characteristic of his "great pharmacologists," including many authors represented in the Hippocratic corpus, Theophrastus, Dioscorides, Soranus, Rufus, and Galen. Edelstein seems to be aware of the artificial and imposed manner of his precise categories of "pharmacological thinking" in classical antiquity, since he slithers into a supporting argument that begins, "But all the pharmacologists, nay almost all the physicians, believed in sympathetic remedies."[141] In turn this "proves" the rarity of pure empiricism and pure magic in ancient pharmacy, proof that collapses when one reads the admixture of scorn and praise by Galen for amulets and medical astrology,[142] the quotation of local customs attached to various herbs by Dioscorides,[143] or the painstaking evidence of botanical lore sandwiched with magicoreligious observances as assembled by Theophrastus. One cannot—as Edelstein does—dismiss medical magic as "found only in the magical papyri which contain not the knowledge of physicians but prescriptions of folklore"[144] any more than one can assert truthfully that Pliny the Elder is a "superstitious layman"[145] without carefully qualifying what this might mean among Roman aristocrats in the early Roman Empire.

Edelstein's "rationalistic supernaturalism"[146] unwittingly signals why almost all pharmaceutical texts in classical antiquity—from Homer and Theophrastus to Galen and the *Papyri Graecae Magicae*—encompass aspects of magic, empiricism in its strictest sense, religion as understood in its context of historical observation, and the constant shifting and mingling with one another of these three broad approaches. Sometimes there is the clear imprint of philosophy as *it* wrestled with definitions and attempted clarity, and sometimes witchcraft is incorporated as a meaningful part of man's investigation into the world of nature and its mysteries. To call some drugs "divine remedies" or "sacred stuff,"[147] as does Galen in his *Compound Drugs according to Place in the Body,* says no more and no less than that this particular substance acts in a godlike manner. Quite openly, Galen (quoting Asclepiades) can write that certain drugs have the "property (δύναμις) of Asclepius,"[148] not too distant from common, modern perceptions of aspirin and sulfonamides as "wonder drugs." Not comprehending molecular chemistry or the physiology of drug action does not make one a "superstitious layman."

DEFINITIONS, HERBS, AND THEIR PROPERTIES: GRECO-ROMAN INTERPRETATIONS

Theophrastus urges his readers to honor only certain of the magicoreligious traditions attached to a few plants, but once he has discarded fully rank superstitions as explanations for how some plants "work" as drugs, he attempts to fuse the data of the ῥιζοτόμοι with a curiously muddled definition of an "herb." He is clearly uneasy regarding the specifics of an "herb" or an "herbal remedy" as provided by his oral and written sources, and the description of πόαι (herbs) includes substances that have "medicinal powers" (φαρμακώδεις δυνάμεις), comprising "juice" (χυλισμός), "fruits" (καρποί), "leaves" (φύλλα), and "roots" (ῥίζα), because the "rootcutters term an 'herb' certain of the medicinals,"[149] and an "herb" consists of one or all of these parts. Theophrastus' hesitant definition of *herb* may have been borrowed directly from the ῥιζοτόμοι, or perhaps from the medicobotanical works of Diocles of Carystos,[150] or Theophrastus may have invented it himself. The ῥιζοτόμοι certainly had given him a basis for this definition, because they did not call all roots "herbs" but only roots from a group of medicinal plants or healing parts of certain plants.[151] Theophrastus continues to display his uncertainty as he writes that such δυνάμεις (probably now a mix of "powers" and "properties") of medicinal roots are distinguished from the δυνάμεις of roots generally. Thereby the "roots" that are medicinal include all four parts of the plant, especially the leaves, as the ῥιζοτόμοι themselves say. Consequently, "herbs" are all four parts, not merely the roots.[152]

By attempting to impose the morphological approach as he struggles with the basic question of how one distinguishes an "herb" from other plants, Theophrastus has provided a particularly unsatisfactory substitute for the answer to the question of "how drugs work," especially in view of the firm answers given in traditional superstitions and some religious connotations. In his listing of the herbs that follows in *Inquiry* IX one must link his brief descriptions of drug action with previous morphologies of plants that form almost all of *Inquiry* I–VIII. It is significant that Theophrastus does not employ the theory of elements and qualities to explain "how drugs work," as does the Pseudo-Aristotelian *Problems:* "The [substance] that according to its own nature, is not overcome by the body's heat and that enters the veins, and because of its excess heat or cold [is not concocted]: this is the φύσις of a drug."[153] The unknown author has grappled rather well with the basic questions of delineating a theory to explain drugs and their actions, as contrasted to foods or plant derivatives without noted pharmacological properties. There seems, oddly enough, a better awareness in the philosophical speculation regarding plants by the author of *Problems* than in the murky groping toward a morphological definition of *herb* by Theophrastus. It is not surprising that many scholars have assumed that book IX of *Inquiry into Plants* is a later addition by unknown medical botanists, a hypothesis disproven by the manuscripts.[154]

Toxic substances were reasonably understood by the second century B.C., as suggested by the difficult poems of Nicander of Colophon (fl. c. 140 B.C.), the *Theriaca* and *Alexipharmaca*.[155] Nicander borrowed heavily from an earlier Greek toxicologist named Apollodorus,[156] who, in turn, may have inherited his concepts from Diocles of Carystos. Again agricultural lore shows vividly in Nicander's semiplagiarism of details on the black widow spider, various cobras, wasps, large centipedes, and millipedes,[157] as well as in his description of what one did to administer an antidote for an excessive consumption of the famous aphrodisiac made from blister beetles.[158] Greek pharmacy had a good botanical morphology from Theophrastus, a rough taxonomy of plants derived from folklore, some medical entomology and toxicology as recorded by Nicander, and a mass of details on herbs and herbal concoctions as revealed in the Hippocratic tracts on women's ailments.[159] An organizing principle, however, appeared in none of these authors regarding "how drugs worked," even though Theophrastus' basic botany was superb. In classical antiquity, pharmacy and toxicology remained aspects of medical practice that occasionally purloined venerated superstitions or religious customs or that with leaps of uncertainty adapted and adopted facets of philosophical physical theory (especially the concepts of elements, qualities, and humors) to account for observed actions of drugs. As Riddle has remarked, at the very least Greco-Roman pharmaceutical theory included the firm notion of a "drug poison,"[160] first discerned in Homer's poems. Most physicians and pharmacologists, however, sought to reject divine explanations for drugs and their effectiveness, and those of the so-called Hippocratic persuasion were sometimes emphatic in dismissing *both* the magicoreligious and philosophic interpretations,[161] leaving either a jumble of empirical observations or a strange and quixotic denial of the efficacy of any drugs. Folk medicine, however, continued to carry on with its venerated assumptions, and even when Dioscorides of Anazarbus (fl. c. 65 A.D.) was able to produce his magnificent summary of drugs in the famous *Materia Medica,*[162] he acknowledges quite frequently the staying power of numerous folk traditions linked with particular pharmaceuticals.

Dioscorides is a watershed in the development of Greco-Roman pharmacy, and his masterpiece of compression, *Materia Medica,* brilliantly demonstrates the efforts of a skilled physician and astute medical botanist to bring order out of the chaos that characterized drug lore up to his own day. As a young man, Dioscorides probably studied herbs and herbal pharmacology with resident experts in Tarsus,[163] and there is just sufficient evidence to indicate that he spent a portion of his mature medical practice in the context of a Roman legion.[164] Most importantly, however, Dioscorides went about the business of testing herbs and drugs with a precision that would be noteworthy in any century[165] and invented an entirely fresh method of classifying drugs by what they did or did not do when given to a patient—a system called by Riddle, "drug affinity."[166] The prevailing medical theories in the early Roman Empire were generally linked in some way with a debased form of "medical atomism,"[167] and in the remarkable preface to his *Materia Medica* Dioscorides flatly rejects this and all other philosophic explanations of drugs when he writes, "They have not measured the activities of drugs experimentally, and in their vain prating about causation they have explained the action of an individual drug by differences among particles, as well as confusing one drug for another."[168] At the same time, he says he has checked "what was universally accepted in the written records and [made] inquiries of natives in each botanical region."[169]

At the conclusion of his discussion of black hellebore (*Helleborus niger* L.),[170] Dioscorides furnishes a typical example of how he treats long-lived religious or quasi-superstitious customs connected to herbs. His farmer-informants have told him that if one plants vines close to the root of the hellebore, the wine from such grapes will make an excellent purgative, and Dioscorides adds, "they sprinkle it [the wine] around houses thinking it to be a purification (*καθάρσιος*) from defilement [in a religious sense]"; moreover, when his informants dig up the hellebore, they stand facing the sunrise and pray to Apollo and Asclepius, watching all the while for an eagle (*ἀετός*) in flight as an evil omen, since "the bird engenders death should it see the digging of the hellebore; at any rate, it has to be dug up very quickly, since drowsiness is caused from its exuded vapors." Dioscorides merely acknowledges the belief that black hellebore was sacred to a god[171] by describing a series of steps taken by his informants when they dig up the root, passing rapidly to a clear, natural reason why such religious customs and precautions became accretions upon this particular medicinal root. Since Dioscorides mentions hellebore's association with an apparently ancient rite of purification, it is probable that the plant had some local history of use in such rituals (no locale is specified), quite reminiscent of the widespread employment of squill.[172] Perhaps herbs like squill and the hellebores were early considered sacred plants due to their heavy pungency, especially when they were cut or bruised, much as Dioscorides notes the "exuded vapors" (*ἀποφοραί*) from the cut hellebore roots. Parker's comments on the corollaries of using the hellebores (there are two main types: a "white" and a "black") in the medical and mythological treatment of madness,[173] said to have been invented by Melampus for the daughters of Proetus, are pointed and relevant,[174] although Hippocratic physicians strove to perceive insanity quite apart from divine causes, as one reads in the eloquent presentation by the author of the Hippocratic *Sacred Disease*,[175] very often cited as *the* Greek medical work that provided the seedbed for medical approaches in the West. Dioscorides, however, carefully limits his account of black hellebore to verified uses in terms of his "drug affinity" system, uses that are pharmacological and classed by pharmacognostic means.[176]

As brilliant as was Dioscorides' new classification method for drugs, later writers on pharmacology chose to revert to other systems, alphabetizing plants and drugs in place of Dioscorides' precise groupings according to physiological action. Although Dioscorides' collected data were incorporated into almost all future tracts on pharmacy in the West until the Renaissance, those data were rearranged according to the predilections of later writers, including the polymathic and enormously influential Galen of Pergamon (129–after 210 A.D.).[177] Galen's drug lore is a gigantic potpourri of herbs, animal products, written sources quoted verbatim, and quasi-legendary and pseudofolkloristic facts all compacted into three separate systems of organization, as he attempted to bring some sort of harmony into the chaos of pharmaceutical data as he found them in the second century.[178] In spite of some oddly informal sources of pharmaceutical information, such as one Orion the Groom,[179] Galen's drug lore became a model for later Byzantine encyclopedists,[180] who took the explicit humoral theory (borrowed directly from the Hippocratic *Nature of Man*)[181] as the major explanation of "how drugs worked." Except for certain compound recipes, which had their own venerated pedigrees,[182] the "drugs-by-degrees" classification, as evolved from Galen through successive Byzantine medical writers to Paul of Aegina (fl. c. 640 A.D. in Egypt), was based on the ancient notions of humors and qualities, an outlook that dominated Western pharmacy until the mid-nineteenth century. Later Roman and Byzantine pharmacy and pharmacology refined Greco-Roman theory on drugs and occasionally added new substances, but there was always a powerful undercurrent of folk medicine displayed in cults to the saints in the Byzantine Empire,[183] as well as a tenacious survival of nonlearned conceptions about drugs.[184] Two aspects of how pharmacology was perceived for sacred plants are illustrated by pharmacological astrology and the widespread acceptance of magical properties exemplified by the formulas and doctrines of Thessalus of Tralles and the collection of texts in Greek, Coptic, and demotic known as the *Papyri Graecae Magicae*.

"HERMETIC" MEDICAL ASTROLOGY AND HERBAL PHARMACOLOGY

An important and often ignored facet of late hellenistic and Roman religion are the so-called Hermetic texts.[185] Having purported origins in particular revelations by a Hermes Trismegistus, Asclepius, and other pagan gods of Greco-Egyptian background, "Hermetic" medical revelations assume multiple aspects that attempt to reconcile several competing concepts of medicine and pharmacy, employing the device of an "archetypal" beginning. The "Hermetic" manner of medicine and pharmacology is sharply defined in an astrological-pharmaceutical text by a Thessalus, called *Powers of Herbs.*[186] The preface to Thessalus' *Powers of Herbs* was first published in the *Catalogus Codicum Astrologorum Graecorum*[187] and was simply called Thessalus' *Letter to Claudius* (or *Nero*). Publication of the full *Powers of Herbs* awaited proper collation of several Greek and Latin manuscripts, and the complete (and dual) texts were eventually published by Friedrich in 1968. In the preface (= *Letter*), Thessalus of Tralles informs the emperor about a revelation by Asclepius, earlier revealed to him by Hermes Trismegistus,[188] naming the herbs truly associated with the planets[189] and the signs of the zodiac.[190] The *Powers of Herbs* and its preface date to the reigns of Claudius and Nero (sometime between 41 and 68 A.D.),[191] and the preface precedes (in the *Catalogus* texts,) a tract on twelve plants linked to the twelve signs of the zodiac,[192] an exposition of seven planets associated with seven plants attributed to Thessalus of Tralles,[193] and a clipped treatise attributed to an "Alexander" that surveys the same seven plants. The *Catalogus* texts indicate the wealth of ancient works discussing plants and herbs and their relationships to the planets, the signs of the zodiac and the traditional three decans (10-degree units) into which each was divided, and plants linked with the "fifteen fixed stars."[194] Thessalus' preface (*Letter*) and the full text of his *Powers of Herbs* represent medical astrology and pharmacology, and there are many instances of Roman physicians and scientists who believed astrology was an important diagnostic tool: Galen's *Crisis Days* (III. 5–6)[195] indicates how astrology pinpoints both diagnosis and prognosis in diseases,[196] although his account is bereft of the mysticism permeating corollary "Hermetic" works.[197] If Galen thinks of medical astrology as a diagnostic technique, the so-called Hermetic writers believe that herbal and medical astrology are revelations, explaining why certain plants have healing powers and properties.

In place of Theophrastus' confusion, Dioscorides' brilliant but inapplicable "drug affinity" system, and Galen's basic uncertainty about classifications of drugs, authors in the Hermetic traditions could claim that their acceptance of divine power was an active manner of receiving it that thereby increased its strength, much as a person instructed by Poimandres can say he "has been invested with the power and instructed in the Nature of the Whole and in the Greatest Divinity."[198] Such herbal astrology is marked by a simplicity—a deceptive simplicity from the standpoint of modern pharmacology—illustrated by "A Plant of the Sun: Chicory," from Thessalus' *Powers of Herbs:*[199]

A Plant of the Sun: Chicory (*κιχώριον*)[200]

(1) First named among the plants of the sun is "heliotrope"; yet there are many kinds of "heliotropes," and of all these most efficacious[201] is the one called chicory. (2) Its juice mixed with oil of roses is an ointment.[202] (3) It is suitable for relieving heartburns,[203] and it releases tertians,[204] quartans, and intermittent fevers,[205] and mixed with an equal part of the oil of unripe olives, it stops headaches. (4) If someone looking toward the sunrise smears on the juice of the chicory, invoking the presence of the [god] Helios, and begs to give him praise, he will be most favored among all men on that day. (5) One prepares from the chicory's root little pills (*καταπότια*) for heartburns and disorders of the stomach, in

which the stomach is afflicted and will not accept foods, and for disorders of the stomach in which the stomach receives nourishment but does not promote digestion: downy woundwort,[206] 8 drachmas; saffron crocus,[207] 2 drachmas; Pontic honey, 14 drachmas; mastic flower,[208] 6 drachmas; ginger[root],[209] 4 drachmas; pepper,[210] 4 drachmas; Dead Sea bitumen/mineral pitch,[211] 2 drachmas; anise,[212] 4 drachmas; mastic gum/resin,[213] 4 drachmas; the root of the chicory, 24 drachmas; pound these ingredients in a mortar with very old mead (honey plus wine, *οἰνομέλι*)[214] and make lozenges of 1 drachma. Drink one with water for heartburns; drink one with the best wine for stomach ailments.

Parallels to Thessalus' recipe occur in Pliny, Columella, Dioscorides, Galen, the *Papyri Graecae Magicae,* and the Byzantine *Geoponica,*[215] but Thessalus' "chicory stimulant" seems unique among Roman prescriptions. Initially, the botany appears poor, with the "heliotrope" including the chicory; Thessalus, however, is not saying this is *the* heliotrope but rather that it belongs to a broad class of herbs "attracted to the sun," the literal meaning of the word. And excepting the self-anointing with chicory juice while invoking Helios, the recipe is a fairly straightforward listing of ingredients and preparation methods frequently encountered in the drug books of Galen and later Byzantine pharmacy. Moreover, folk medicine retains employment of mastic, anise, and chicory as stomach calmers, traditions backed to some extent by the physiological chemistry of the herbs. Thessalus' *Power of Herbs* encompasses a number of Greco-Roman pharmacological traditions, including the technical approaches seen in Dioscorides and Galen, as well as specifics of drugs and herbs found in the magical papyri. Hermetic astrological herb lore could claim it knew *why* such plants had pharmaceutical properties by their clear linkages to the divinities represented by constellations and planets (including the sun and moon) at various points in the zodiac. Festugière classes some of these texts of astrological herbalism according to which plants were associated with the sun, and he gives these plants separate status by means of determination of the contents of the list (categories labeled A, B, C, etc.).[216] For example Chicory is Festugière's type B, with a special listing of herbs for the moon, Saturn, Jupiter, Mars, Venus, and Mercury.[217]

The presence of pepper and ginger in Thessalus' *Powers of Herbs* shows that the text dates from the first half of the first century, on grounds independent of manuscript attribution. In full revival was a flourishing trade with Far Eastern markets,[218] and Dioscorides' *Materia Medica* shows fresh incorporation into the Roman pharmacopoeia of Indian, Malayan, and some Chinese spices.[219] Thessalus is well aware of good ingredients for his recipes, and there is a sophistication in *Powers of Herbs* reflecting formal drug lore of the day infused with the "Hermetic" assertions of special knowledge about herbal medicine. Such a pharmacology of sacred plants, organized along astrological lines, received a patina of acceptable "science" in the Roman Empire, although Roman law frowned upon the application of astrology to political ends.[220]

SACRED PLANTS IN THE MAGICAL PAPYRI

The Greek, Coptic, and demotic texts known as the *Papyri Graecae Magicae* mention over 450 plants, minerals, animal products, herbs, and other substances as presumably "pharmaceutically active" in the recorded spells, incantations, formulas, and imprecations. The texts in the collection are dated generally to Roman and Byzantine Egypt (c. 30 B.C.–c. 600 A.D.), but several instances of drug lore (e.g., the multiingredient incense called *κῦφι*) indicate a heritage going back many centuries, probably to dynastic Egypt. One cannot dismiss the documents contained in the *Papyri Graecae Magicae* as simply written forms of jumbled superstitions with a pseudopatina of Egyptian learning:[221] the *Papyri Graecae Magicae* have yielded a trove of insights on how Jew, Christian, and pagan perceived their world; and an important facet of our fresh understanding of these precious documents that emerge from beliefs of "common people" is the pharmacology of magical and sacred plants and drugs.

Ritual is essential for the Greco-Egyptian *ῥιζοτόμος* (here generally "herbalist"), much as suggested by Pfister in his basic essay on magical conceptions of plants,[222] a suggestion nicely illustrated by the following from the *Papyri Graecae Magicae:* "**Spell for picking a plant:** Use it before sunrise. *The spell to be spoken:* I am picking you, such and such a plant, with my five-fingered hand, I, NN, and I am bringing you home so that you may work for me for a certain purpose. I adjure you by the undefiled name of the god: if you pay no heed to me, the earth which produced you will no longer be watered as far as you are concerned—ever in life again, if I fail in this operation [then follow magical words]; fulfil for me the perfect charm."[223] One presumes the herbalist recited this spell as he went out to gather plants, and his work began before dawn, much as suggested in context by Thessalus of Tralles in *Powers of Herbs* and by Dioscorides when he mentions folk customs concerning certain powerful roots and their collection. Specifics followed by an herbalist come a little later in the magical papyri: "Among the Egyptians herbs are always obtained like this: the herbalist first purifies his own body, then sprinkles with natron and fumigates the herb with resin from a pine tree after carrying it around the place 3 times. Then after burning *κῦφι* and pouring the libation of milk as he prays, he pulls up the plant while invoking by name the daimon to whom the herb is being dedicated and calling upon him to be more effective for the use for which it is being acquired."[224] Natron and its use is very ancient, indeed,[225] and the full ritual includes burning pine resin and *κῦφι* and an offering of milk, each an aspect of hoary religious observances in many cultures, not only ancient Greek and Egyptian.[226] And, as the papyrus text continues, one soon comprehends that *all* herbs are sacred, since the invocation uttered at the moment of picking the plant is as follows: "You were sown by Kronos, you were conceived by Hera, you were maintained by Ammon, you were given birth by Isis, you were nourished by Zeus the god of rain, you were given growth by Helios and dew. You [are] the dew of all the gods, you [are] the heart of Hermes, you are the seed of all the primordial gods, you are the eye of Helios, you are the light of Selene, you are the zeal of Osiris, you are the beauty and glory of Ouranos, you are the soul of Osiris' daimon which revels in every place, you are the spirit of Ammon."[227] The invocation proceeds by naming a number of gods, goddesses, powers, and properties, thus assuring the herbalist of his sacred function as well as the primary acknowledgement of awe regarding the god-given properties of such plants. In many respects the act of collecting herbs is an act of worship, and the herbalist understands that the powers contained in these plants emerge from the divinity within each part collected (this is perhaps similar to the ῥιζοτόμοι and their definition of *herb* as recounted by Theophrastus) and that the plants conversion into "drugs" simply extends their powers for the kindly benefit of man.

With the natural awe in mind, as well as Betz's thought that "magic is the art that makes people who practice it feel better rather than worse,"[228] one may contemplate the pharmacology of a few representative texts from the magical papyri, for instance, this contraceptive recipe:

> **A contraceptive, the only one in the world:** take as many bittervetch seeds as you want for the number of years you wish to remain sterile. Steep them in the blood of a menstruating woman. Let them steep in her own genitals. And take a frog that is alive and throw the bittervetch seeds into its mouth so that the frog swallows them, and release the frog alive at the place where you captured him. And take a seed of henbane, steep it in mare's milk; and take the nasal mucus of a cow with grains of barley, put these into a [piece of] leather skin made from a fawn and on the outside bind it up with a mulehide skin, and attach it as an amulet during the waning of the moon [which is] in a female sign of the zodiac on a day of Kronos or Hermes. Mix in also with the barley grains cerumen from the ear of a mule.[229]

This contraceptive recipe certainly displays the typical ingredients expected in magical concoctions (nasal mucus, a mule's earwax, menstrual blood, etc.), but sandwiched within are two pharmacologically potent herbs, bittervetch (ὄροβος = *Vicia ervilia* [L.] Willd.) and henbane (the papyrus has ὑοσκύεμος as contrasted to the usual ὑοσκύαμος,[230] *Hyoscyamus niger*), both widely known in Greco-Roman pharmacy and in modern folk medicine and pharmacognosy. Dioscorides notes the use of the vetch in the treatment of skin diseases of several kinds[231] and gives warning regarding its ingestion since it engenders headaches, disturbs the bowels, and draws down blood in the urine. As Riddle notes,[232] vetch was used to treat cancer until the early nineteenth century, and active principles isolated from the herb include vicianin (a cyanogenetic glycoside), guanidine, and xanthine. Overdosage would resemble cyanide poisoning, much as Dioscorides suggests. Henbane is a rather poisonous plant from which hyoscyamine is obtained and was well known in classical antiquity as a drug that could cause madness or—as Dioscorides writes—"frenzies."[233] Preparations made from the henbane have atropinelike effects[234] and have some limited utility in modern therapeutics in the relief of spasms in the urinary tract. The scribe may indicate that the concoction is to be swallowed through the device of having the frog ingest the seeds (frogs and fertility were intimately linked in Egyptian and Greek lore),[235] but the basic function of the recipe is in its amuletic powers, a common approach as seen in the following text from the magical papyri. Yet muffled among the earwax, blood, milk, and nasal mucus is a record of the potency of two drugs, fully understood in the formal pharmacy of classical antiquity.

Even a short text from the magical papyri will yield numerous insights:

> Carried [with a magnetic] stone, or even spoken, [this verse] serves as a *contraceptive:* "Would that you be fated to be unborn and to die unmarried." Write this on a piece of new [papyrus] and tie it up with hairs of a mule.[236]

Apart from the quotation of Homer (*Il.* III.40), this small bit from late Roman or Byzantine Egypt does not appear to contain anything of particular interest until one

I

checks the ancient references on the "lodestone" in the context of obstetrics and gynecology. The scribe has compacted an enormous lore on magnetic stones and "women's problems" into a single line recommending the lodestone as an amulet, although the use of quasi-Homeric lines as spells is also very common in the magical papyri. The lodestone charm appears in the writings of Soranus of Ephesus (fl. c. 98–117 A.D.), whose *Gynecology* was the finest tract of its kind before the European Enlightenment. Soranus' mention of the lodestone amulet suggests how common such charms must have been in the first and second centuries, and he writes that some individuals believe "some things" are useful according to their "antipathy," for example the lodestone, the "Stone of Assius," the stomach curd from a rabbit, and "some other amulets to which we ourselves pay no heed. But one must not forbid their use: even if the amulet has no real effect, it will possibly gain a cheerful attitude in the woman"[237] being treated for uterine hemorrhage. Soranus thus provides a listing of some charm ingredients while disapproving them, even though his patients obviously valued them all. Moreover, the lodestone was deemed very useful in ancient medicine as a "blood assimilator," as recorded by Dioscorides,[238] Galen,[239] Pliny the Elder,[240] and the Byzantine compilation of farm lore, the *Geoponica*.[241] Similar in properties was the "Stone of Assius" (probably some kind of pumice), which was an effective styptic esteemed by Dioscorides and other Roman medical writers.[242] Physicians and pharmacologists thought the lodestone was useful in treatment for uterine bleeding and other similar ailments, and it appears the magical papyrus records a logical assumption by the common folk: one could, indeed, wear the saying on a lodestone, since the magnetite already had styptic and presumably divine powers to prevent bleeding; such logic would also proceed to the next step, which meant that a contraceptive power was likewise provided in the stone.

Herbs, drugs, medicinal minerals, animal products used as medicines, and insects appear frequently in varying contexts in the magical papyri.[243] Particularly fascinating is a "substitution list" of names of herbs and other substances given as "code names," as explained by the scribes:

> **Interpretations** which the temple scribes employed, from the holy writings, in translation. Because of the curiosity of the masses they [i.e., the scribes] inscribed the names of the herbs and other things which they employed on the statues of the gods, so that they [i.e., the masses], since they do not take precaution, might not practice magic, [being prevented] by the consequence of their misunderstanding. But we have collected the explanations [of these names] from many copies [of the sacred writings], all of them secret. *Here they are:*
>
> A snake's head: a leech
> A snake's "ball of thread": this means soapstone
> Blood of a snake: hematite
> A bone of an ibis: this is buckthorn
> Blood of a hyrax: truly of a hyrax
> "Tears" of a Hamadryas baboon: dill juice
> Crocodile dung: Ethiopian soil
> Blood of a Hamadryas baboon: blood of a spotted gecko
> Lion semen: human semen
> Blood of Hephaistos: wormwood
> Hairs of a Hamadryas baboon: dill seed

Semen of Hermes: dill
Blood of Ares: purslane
Blood of an eye: tamarisk gall
Blood from a shoulder: bear's breach
From the loins: camomile
A man's bile: turnip sap
A pig's tail: leopard's bane
A physician's bone: sandstone
Blood of Hestia: camomile
An eagle: wild garlic(?)
Blood of a goose: a mulberry tree's "milk"
Kronos' spice: piglet's milk
A lion's hairs: "tongue" of a turnip
Kronos' blood: . . . of cedar
Semen of Helios: white hellebore
Semen of Herakles: this is mustard-rocket
[A Titan's] blood: wild lettuce
Blood from a head: lupine
A bull's semen: egg of a blister beetle
A hawk's heart: heart of wormwood
Semen of Hephaistos: this is fleabane
Semen of Ammon: houseleek
Semen of Ares: clover
Fat from a head: spurge
From the belly: earth-apple
From the foot: houseleek.[244]

This list of "interpretations" is striking in what it tells us about divine names given to ordinary herbs—divine names that the scribes insist are not understood by "the masses." The preface to the listing also shows a professional pride by the unknown priests who "know the codes" and suggests that the practice of magic had adopted as part of its skills and techniques the lore of herbalism.

If the "interpretations" of *PGM* XII. 401–44, are intended to explain code names taken for granted by priests, scribes, and probably the common people, there are many more instances in the magical papyri in which substances are merely named without further ado, and some of these terms disguise multiingredient drugs. In four (probably five) different passages of the *Papyri Graecae Magicae* one reads of the use of something called κῦφι,[245] which is a very ancient Egyptian incense, ointment, and edible drug,[246] containing up to thirty-six ingredients, all pharmacologically active.[247] If formal sources in ancient and Byzantine pharmacy—for instance, Dioscorides, Oribasius, and Paul of Aegina—did not specify ingredients in the various formulas for κῦφι, we would be reduced to learned speculation regarding just what this "sacred incense of Egypt" *was*. The κῦφι recipes show a sophistication of drug compounding among the common folk and a close study of the historical evolution of κῦφι indicates a slow "improvement of the product" from dynastic Egypt through the seventh-century texts of Paul of Aegina. In itself, the history of κῦφι destroys an accepted mythology of modern medical historians, who assume ancient medicine and pharmacy developed to a certain point, then remained utterly static for countless centuries. If κῦφι originated from the magicomedicine and pharmaceutics of dynastic Egypt, it became not only a substance that would be part of a magical tradition but also a drug adapted into the pharmaceutics of learned medicine, suggested by the ten-ingredient *κῦφι* given by Dioscorides.[248] The magical papyri certainly take *κῦφι* "for granted," offering no detailed explanation of either the ingredients or its significance other than to imply its importance in such procedures as *The Bear-charm which accomplishes everything,*[249] in which *κῦφι* is one item in a list offered to the "Bear" (constellation).

The cacophony of competing claims, apologies, and vitriolic criticism of magicians and magic (including purported drug lore) in the second century is dramatically illustrated by a masterful diatribe of Hippolytus of Rome (c. 170–c. 236 A.D.). As part of an ongoing and antagonistic free-for-all among Christians and non-Christians alike, Hippolytus' rhetorical fury is directed, in part, at the blatant charlatanism displayed by the practitioners of magic who "offer the Egyptian magicians' incense called *κῦφι*,"[250] accompanied by loud and noisy manipulation of gawking crowds. Hippolytus knows his drugs and simulates deep anger at the degradation of herbalism he has observed, remarking that all of the hocus-pocus of invisible writing produced by the magicians of Rome is easily understood with the use of malachite, powdered galls, milk, fish sauce (*garum*), spurge (*τιθύμαλος*), and fig juice.[251] Hippolytus' feigned tirade against practicing magicians delineates how popular such professionals were in the early Roman Empire.

PHARMACOLOGY AND MAGICORELIGIOUS ASSUMPTIONS: SOME CONCLUSIONS

Recent research on occult doctrines and texts in the Renaissance has convincingly demonstrated that underneath the bland labels of *Hermeticism, magic, astrology, witchcraft,* and similar terms, there is an enormous mélange of views and practices, a hodgepodge of concepts often in open conflict with one another. Vickers writes that "the influence of the hermetic texts was small in comparison with that of the main occult sciences, and their presence in the Renaissance . . . makes for just one more syncretic ingredient in an already syncretic mixture."[252] A comparable pasticcio characterized Greco-Egyptian "Hermeticism," as indicated by Fowden in *The Egyptian Hermes;* and once Fowden has led us through the curiously interwoven, yet conflicting, documents of this ancient Hermeticism, a clear awareness emerges of the patchwork quality in thinking, even with such presumably unified subjects like herbalism.[253] An analogous miscellany characterizes the data in the magical papyri, the erudite authors on matters pharmacognostic like Dioscorides, and almost all other extant Greek and Roman texts—from poetry to philosophy—that take up or mention the myriad of different facts gleaned from folk customs presuming divine or magicomedical properties in plants and herbs.

Even with the evidence of continually shifting and fluctuating hybrids of assumptions about *φάρμακα*, which seem to wax and then fade into composite forms through the centuries, a few limited conclusions can be drawn. At first glance, the presence of women as "experts" in drug lore, as seen first in Homer, might suggest that such expertise emerged solely from the arcane knowledge of sex and birthing, perhaps guarded, if not hoarded, by females. To be sure, many of the rituals that festoon rootcutting and the gathering of herbs do traditionally incorporate women as the "main characters," but the generally cited evidence of poetry ignores the plentiful and contrary evidence of male expertise in aphrodisiacs and matters obstetric as found in such authors as Theophrastus. In certain respects, Greek and Roman men were as fond of creating fantasies about women as are modern males, so that when one notes the listing of men who were learned in sexual and erotic magic, as provided by Galen, one is also reminded of the male practioners of erotic bewitchments as they appear in the *Papyri Graecae Magicae*. Modern psychology also has demonstrated the strong presence of a generalized masculine fear of women, particularly in the basic consideration of sex, so that the student of ancient erotic magic may be forewarned not to accept the notion of a special feminine expertise in drugs.

Magicoreligious concepts about drugs may probably be linked with very old traditions ultimately stemming from the civilizations of the ancient Near East. The curious presence of the δημιουργός in the pages of Greek literature, from Homer to Aristotle, may indicate a survival, if not an infusion, of Assyrian or Babylonian medical customs; and further study of Egyptian texts of magicopharmacy and rituals associated with the prescribing of drugs most likely will demonstrate further links with the later practices of Greek medicine. At the very least, one must conclude that the magicoreligious documents of the Greeks, which contain data on potent herbs, have very apparent links with cultures and religions of the ancient Near East.

Greek and Roman perceptions of the basic causes of pharmaceutical properties—in particular those of plants—continually fused religious and empirical data; and the pattern of thought in its multiple levels on the actions of drugs, first enunciated by Homer, remained fairly consistent throughout the centuries of Greek, Roman, and Byzantine pharmacology. This pattern combined the conviction of divine powers of drugs—whether beneficial or deleterious—with deeply rooted observations gathered by farmers over hundreds of generations; and properties (δυνάμεις) attributed to varying φάρμακα quite frequently were amalgams of venerated rituals fused with carefully deduced pharmaceutical effects, for instance, the association of squill with purification ceremonies and its treatment in the *Materia Medica* of Dioscorides. The δυνάμεις of herbs and drugs could be viewed "rationally" through magicoreligious means, by one who also assumed the basic divinity of the world at large (and therefore of the men and the plants that lived in that world) or accepted explanations of botanical astrology. All these and other approaches touched on above were quite acceptable to most thinkers in classical antiquity so that Edelstein is almost certainly incorrect to argue the utter rarity of pure magic or pure empiricism in ancient pharmacy and medicine. Even as Theophrastus muddles his definition of "herb" thanks to the folk customs of his oral sources, the ῥιζοτόμοι, he not only applies the precepts of Aristotelian morphology to his herbal botany but also acknowledges the prevalence of a belief in sympathetic pharmacology, a "doctrine of signatures" applied to orchid bulbs, a belief paralleled in spells of the *Papyri Graecae Magicae* that note the efficacy of "mule products" as contraceptives.

Theophrastus' painstaking considerations of religious and folkloristic practices concerning plants and herbal preparations provide priceless details about the so-called unlettered levels of Greek society as they conceived herbal medicine and its functions. The magical papyri, in spite of priestly attempts to restrict knowledge of herbal lore, show quite vividly the ordinary and sophisticated command of drug compounding by the common people, a command not surprising in view of their usual rural upbringing. They would know the plants from childhood, and they would also know the appropriate magicoreligious connotations and their proper interpretations. Drugs were indeed "the hands of the gods."

Notes

1. O. Regenbogen, "Theophrastos," in *RE* Suppl. VII (1940), 1354–1562 (esp. 1453–79: botany). John Scarborough, "Theophrastus on Herbals and Herbal Remedies," *Journal of the History of Biology* 11 (1978): 353–85. G. E. R. Lloyd, "Theophrastus, the Hippocratics, and the Root-Cutters," in *Science, Folklore and Ideology: Studies in the Life Sciences in Ancient Greece* (Cambridge, 1983), 119–35. Almost all plants are identified according to international systematics in botany, with the usual abbreviations of authors' names (e.g., L. for Carl von Linnaeus [1707–1778]). The Latin binomials employed sometimes also contain indications of priorities. For instance "L" sometimes appears as "[L]," indicating that Linnaeus was the original author of a name, revised by some more modern botanist, whose naming had been accepted by the international community of botanists, who, in turn, wished to retain Linnaeus' priority, even with the "new" name. One can gain insight into the formation of modern botanical names by consulting William T. Stearn, *Botanical Latin*, 2d ed. (Newton Abbot, England, 1973). A standard listing of priorities and author's names for plants is the *Draft Index of Author Abbreviations Compiled at the Herbarium, Royal Botanic Gardens Kew* (London, 1984), followed faithfully by D. J. Mabberley, *The Plant-Book* (Cambridge, 1987). Numerous botanical equivalents are conveniently provided in George Usher's *Dictionary of Plants Used by Man* (London, 1974) and Oleg Polunin's *Flowers of Europe* (London, 1969) and *Flowers of Greece and the Balkans* (Oxford, 1980). Various "flora," however, differ as to which binomials are listed for particular genera and species, so that nonbotanists often become confused regarding the "real" name. See the lists "Floras and Handbooks" and "Periodicals" in Mabberley, *Plant-Book*, pp. 637–49.

2. Theophrastus' *Inquiry into Plants* is frequently cited by its Latinized title, *Historia plantarum* or simply *HP;* the most commonly used Greek text of *Inquiry* is that edited and translated in two volumes by Arthur Hort in the Loeb Classical Library (London, 1916). Victorian prudery, however, caused Hort to omit certain passages from both the Greek text and English translation (viz., *Inquiry*, IX.18.3–11 on ὄρχις as an aphrodisiac and other plants as anaphrodisiacs; see also nn. 124–32 below), so that one must still employ F. Wimmer, ed., *Theophrasti Eresii Opera* (Paris, 1866; rpt. Frankfurt, 1964) for the complete Greek text. (*Inquiry*, IX.18.3–11 = Wimmer, pp. 159–61, with Latin translation). An English translation of these "missing lines" was published as Chalmers L. Gemmil, "The Missing Passage in Hort's Translation of Theophrastus," *Bulletin of the New York Academy of Medicine* 49 (1973): 127–29 (a spare translation with no commentary). One must also be extremely wary of accepting many of the proposed nomenclatures for plants as listed in the "Index of Plants" of the Hort edition. The identifications and binomial names were provided by William Thiselton-Dyer, and many are no more than wildly inappropriate guesses. Unfortunately, many of these false nomenclatures have entered *LSJ*, where they mislead novitiates unacquainted with Thiselton-Dyer's less-than-skilled botany. Far better are the nomenclatures in the *Oxford Latin Dictionary*, and best are listings in Jacques André, *Les noms de plantes dans la Rome antique* (Paris, 1985); useful among older lexicons are A. Carnoy, *Dictionnaire*

étymologique des noms grecs de plantes (Louvain, 1959) and R. Strömberg, *Griechische Pflanzennamen* (Göteborg, 1940). Had John Raven of Cambridge been able to complete and publish his projected *History of Botany in Ancient Greece* before his death in 1980, we might, indeed, have a reliable guide to the plant lore in English. Colleagues were treated to a foretaste of the study in Raven's 1976 Gray Lectures, with the subject on "Plants and Plant Lore in Ancient Greece." Nick Jardine, "Ancient Greek Botany," in *John Raven by his Friends* ed. John Lipscomb and R. W. David [Bath, 1981; privately printed], 88–90) writes the following about one aspect of the 1976 Gray Lectures: "Throughout the lectures John succeeded in communicating a specific enthusiasm, an enthusiasm which gave life to all his interests, classical, philosophical and botanical, the enthusiasm of the hunt. Sometimes the quarry was a person. In the opening lecture the hapless Sir William Thiselton-Dyer, F. R. S., successor to Hooker in the directorate of Kew, and author of the diagnoses of plant names that enliven the standard Greek dictionary, Liddell and Scott, is hunted down. With unholy glee the superficiality of his scholarship and the absurdity of his diagnoses are gently but remorselessly exposed" (p. 89).

3. Books I and II only of *Causes* have appeared in the Loeb series: *Theophrastus "De Causis Plantarum"* ed. and trans. Benedict Einarson and G. K. K. Link (Cambridge, Mass., 1976); for the remainder (*Causes*, III-VI) cf. Wimmer (see n. 2), 218–319.

4. On Theophrastus as a botanist, see Ernst H. F. Meyer, *Geschichte der Botanik,* (Königsberg, 1854–57; rpt. Amsterdam, 1965), I:146–88; A. G. Morton, *History of Botanical Science* (London, 1981), 29–43; and Edward Lee Greene, *Landmarks of Botanical History*, ed. Frank N. Egerton (Stanford, 1983) I:128–211.

5. Scarborough, "Theophrastus" (see n. 1), 353–55.

6. W. H. S. Jones, *The Medical Writings of Anonymus Londinensis* (Cambridge, 1947; rpt. Amsterdam, 1968), 5–8.

7. Exhaustively, P. J. Rhodes, *A Commentary on the Aristotelian Athenaion Politeia* (Oxford, 1981).

8. Scarborough, "Theophrastus" (see n. 1), 354–55, 359–60. Lloyd, *Ideology* (see n. 1), 120–22. Greene (see n. 4), I.120–27.

9. Very common in the modern literature is the use of some "school" of psychology or psychiatry, and studies are replete with "psychosexual" or "psychosomatic" explanations—as if the ancient Greeks thought in terms identical to those of modern Freudians, Jungians, Piaget, or even Eric Berne. Sometimes, however, ancient Greek drug lore becomes part of a debased structural anthropology in modern scholarship, especially prominent in works by followers of Claude Lévi-Strauss, e.g., Marcel Detienne, *The Gardens of Adonis: Spices in Greek Mythology*, trans. Janet Lloyd (London, 1977). See my review and comments on Detienne's book in *Classical Journal* 76 (1981): 175–78.

10. Two books stand out in this respect, whose authors attempt to interpret early Greek thinking in ancient terms, not modern ones: Richard Broxton Onians, *The Origins of European Thought* (Cambridge, 1951) and Robert Parker, *Miasma: Pollution and Purification in Early Greek Religion* (Oxford, 1983).

11. Quoted in Galen, *Compound Drugs According to Place of Ailment* VI.8 (in C. G. Kühn, ed., *Galeni Opera Omnia* [Leipzig, 1821–33], XII:966).

12. P. M. Fraser, *Ptolemaic Alexandria* (Oxford, 1972), I:348–57.

13. Cynthia Wright Shelmerdine, *The Perfume Industry of Mycenaean Pylos* (Göteborg, 1985), 123–30.

14. *Od.* X.394, *οὐλόμενον*; II.329, *θυμοφθόρον*; I.261, *ἀνδροφόνον* (viz. *φάρμακον ἀνδροφόνον διζήμενος, ὄφρα οἱ εἴη / ἰοὺς χρεχρίεσθαι*); *Il.* XXII.94 and *Od.*X.213, *κακόν*; *Od.* IV.230, *λυγρόν* [cf. X.236]; IV.229 and X.287, *ἐσθλόν*; *Il.* V.401 and 900, *ὀδυνήφατα φάρμακα*; and IV.218, *ἤπιον*.

15. X.391–94.

16. *Od.* X.392.

17. *Od.* X.394.

18. One may observe how these stories degenerated as they were passed along over the centuries, e.g. Pliny, (*HN* XXV.10–12) says that the "origin of botany" was closely aligned with pure magic, and he notes that Medea and Circe were early investigators of plants—and that Orpheus was the first writer on the subject of botany. His reflections on the topic, from the vantage point of the "enlightened" first century, are instructive of the differences between Homeric Greece and Pliny's Roman intellectual world eight hundred years later: *Durat tamen tradita persuasio in magna parte vulgi veneficiis et herbis id cogi eamque unam feminarum scientiam praevalere* (XXV.10). The old "folk traditions" remained strong. Further degeneration of the Circe legend appears in Ael. *On Animals* I.54, in which the sorceress kills merely by touch. By the time Augustine wrote his *City of God,* folklore was current in Italy that women (esp. women who ran inns) gave drugs along with cheese to travelers and thereby changed their guests into beasts of burden; August., *City of God,* XVIII.18; cf. Apul., *Golden Ass* (*Metamorphoses*) III.24, and *Apologia* (*De Magia*), 31 (*Apuleius,* ed. R. Helm, vol. II. [Leipzig, 1972], 36–37).

19. *Od.* X.305.

20. *Od.* X.304: *ῥίζῃ μὲν μέλαν ἔσκε, γάλακτι δὲ εἴκελον ἄνθος.*

21. *Od.* X.316–17.

22. *Od.* X.305.

23. *Od.* X.305–06.

24. In some later Greek texts, *μῶλυ* means "garlic," viz., *Allium sativum.*, e.g., Theophr., *Inquiry into Plants,* IX.15.7; the Hippocratic *Nature of Women* 85 (*Oeuvres complètes d'Hippocrate* ed. E. Littré [Paris, 1839–61], VII:406); and Diosc. *Mat. Med.* III.47 (*Pedanii Dioscuridis Anazarbei "De Materia Medica,"* ed. M. Wellmann, [Berlin, 1906–14], II:60). E. Steier, "Moly," *RE,* vol. XVI (Stuttgart, 1933), cols. 29–33. Jerry Stannard, "The Plant Called Moly," *Osiris* 14 (1962): 254–307, esp. 255–56. G. M. Germani, "Ulisee, Circe, e l'erba moly nella tradizione Omerica e nella realità poetica," *Rassegna di clinica, terapia, e scienze affini* 14 [1934]: 168–172) offers mandrake (*Mandragora officinarum*), which can be rejected; likewise the identification of Homer's *μῶλυ* as black hellebore (*Helleborus niger*) is merely fanciful, e.g., in Oswald Schmiedeberg, *Über die Pharmaka in der Ilias und Odyssee* (Strassburg, 1918), 25–29, esp. 27. Cf. Carnoy, *Dictionnaire* (see n. 2), 180. Robert Graves (*The Greek Myths* [Harmondsworth, 1955], II:367) offers "wild cyclamen" after rejecting John Tzetzes' guess of "wild rue."

25. As does Walter Artelt, *Studien zur Geschichte der Begriffe, "Heilmittel," und "Gift"* (Leipzig, 1937; rpt. Darmstadt, 1966), 38–46, with minor modifications.

26. G. E. R. Lloyd, *Magic Reason and Experience: Studies in the Origins and Development of Greek Science* (Cambridge, 1979), 31.

27. D. Holwerda, ΦΥΣΙΣ (Groningen, 1955), 63.

28. Lloyd, *Magic* (see n. 26), 31, n. 106.

29. *Od.* IV.220–30. This seems to be the earliest reference to compound *φάρμακα* in the Greek world.

30. *Od.* IV.231–32; cf. Hdt. II.84.

31. *Il.* VIII.306–7.

32. Diosc. *Mat. Med.* IV.64.1 (Wellmann [see n. 24], II:218–19) and IV.64.7 (ibid., p. 221).

33. George Edward Trease and William Charles Evans, *Pharmacognosy,* 11th ed. (London, 1978), 570; Albert F. Hill, *Economic Botany,* 2d ed. (New York, 1952), 260; Varro E. Tyler, Lynn R. Brady, and James E. Robbers, *Pharmacognosy,* 8th ed. (Philadelphia, 1981), 226–27.

34. viz., *Od.* IV.220–32.

35. Guido Majno, *The Healing Hand: Man and Wound in the Ancient World* (Cambridge, Mass., 1975), 108–11; and A. Lucas, *Ancient Egyptian Materials and Industries*, 3d ed. (London, 1948), 401 (on poppy seed oil).

36. *Od*. IV.219–34.

37. *Od*. X.391–94; cf. *Il*., XI.638–41 (and slightly earlier in line 623): Hecamede mixes a potion (κυκεών) for Nestor and his companions; the potion consisted of Pramnian wine, grated goat's cheese, and white barley meal. Delatte argues that this name was attached to the ritual drinking and initiations at Eleusis; see Armand Delatte, *Le Cycéon: Breuvage rituel des mystères d'Éleusis* (Paris, 1955); see also A. Delatte, *Herbarius* (Liège, 1938), 1–6 for women in legendary roles as drug compounders.

38. Macrob. *Sat*. V.19.9–10 (quotations from Sophocles' lost play, *Rootcutters*); Sen. *Medea*, passim, but esp. 705–70; Petron. *Sat*. 137–38; and Lloyd, *Science* (see n. 1), 76–79 for women as sources of medical information. But almost all of the names of "herbalists" and experts on folk medicines (including matters of sexual nature), as given by Theophrastus, Pliny, Galen, and Athenaeus are those of men, not women. Friedrich Pfister, in "Pflanzenaberglaube," *RE*, XIX, pt. 2 (1938), 1446–56, esp. 1448–49.

39. E.g., C. G. Jung, "Commentary on the Visions of Zosimus," in *Alchemical Studies*, trans. R. F. C. Hull (Princeton, 1967), 66–108, esp. 99 on Circe; Jolande Jacobi, "Symbols in an Individual Analysis" in *Man and His Symbols*, ed. C. G. Jung (London, 1964), 272–303, esp. 283: ("The pig is closely associated with dirty sexuality [Circe . . . changed the men who desired her into swine]"); Wolfgang Lederer, *The Fear of Women* (New York, 1968), 35 ("Odysseus . . . refused to yield to Circe's advances on the grounds that his vigor would be impaired"), 57 ("Passive innocence of the dangerous woman is far less common than her active destructiveness" [with the example of Circe]), and 126 (Circe as a death goddess). Cf. Robert Graves, *The White Goddess* (New York, 1966), 448–49; idem, *Greek Myths* (see n. 24), I.177, with sources. Lederer and Graves provide a full panoply of references to the vast literature in comparative mythology, anthropology, and psychoanalytic theory.

40. Trease and Evans, *Pharmacognosy* (see n. 33), 569; Tyler et al., *Pharmacognosy* (see n. 33), 225–26.

41. W. Burkert, "Itinerant Diviners and Magicians: A Neglected Element in Cultural Contacts," in *The Greek Renaissance in the Eighth Century* B.C., ed. R. Hägg (Stockholm, 1983), 115–20 and idem; *Die orientalisierende Epoche in der griechischen Religion und Literatur*, SBHeidelberg (Heidelberg, 1984), no. 1, 43–48. One may argue that a "familial control" over sacred drug lore could explain why Polydamnia is called the daughter of Thon, but Theophrastus (*Inquiry into Plants*, IX.15.1) expresses his basic skepticism regarding these tales.

42. Pl. *Symp*. 186d. The Hippocratic *Ancient Medicine*, I.11 (*Hippocrates*, ed. W. H. S. Jones [London, 1923–31], I:12).

43. Arist. *Pol*. 1282a3: "'Physician' [ἰατρός] is both the ordinary practitioner [δημιουργός] and the master of the art of medicine [ἀρχιτεκτονικός]."

44. See nn. 107–13.

45. esp. Pl. *Resp*. 406a, 408a and *Ion* 538c.

46. E.g., esp., Celsus, *Med*. proem 3 and Galen, *Thrasyb*. 33 (ed. G. Helmreich, in *Claudii Galeni Pergameni Scripta Minora* [Leipzig, 1884–93], III:78) after quoting *Od*. IV.230–31.

47. *Sed vulneribus tantummodo ferro et medicamentis mederi*.

48. Celsus, *Med*. proem 9, with 6.

49. Wesley D. Smith, "Physiology in the Homeric Poems," *TAPA* 97 (1966): 547–56, esp. 547.

50. Onians, *Origins* (see n. 10), 13–65.

51. Andreas Plaitakis and Roger C. Duvoisin, "Homer's Moly Identified As *Galanthus*

I

nivalis L.: Physiologic Antidote to Stramonium Poisoning," *Clinical Neuropharmacology* 6 (1983): 1–5. Cf. suggestions in the references in n. 24 above.

52. See, e.g., Clifford Geertz, "Curing, Sorcery, and Magic in a Javanese Town" in *Culture, Disease, and Healing*, ed. David Landy (New York, 1977), 146–54.

53. E.g., Melford E. Spiro, "The Exorcist," in *Burmese Supernaturalism* (Englewood Cliffs, N.J., 1967), 230–45.

54. *Il.* IV.189–219; V.401–2, 889–90; XI.828–47; *Od.* XIX.457.

55. Wesley D. Smith, "So-Called Possession in Pre-Christian Greece," *TAPA* 96 (1965): 403–26.

56. Onians, *Origins* (see n. 10), 489–90.

57. Among many examples, see Klaus Stopp, "Medicinal Plants of the Mt. Hagen People (Mbowamb) in New Guinea," *Economic Botany* 17 (1963): 16–22 and, generally, John Mitchell Watt, "Magic and Witchcraft in Relation to Plants and Folk Medicine," in *Plants in the Development of Modern Medicine*, ed. Tony Swain (Cambridge, Mass., 1972), 67–102.

58. See n. 14.

59. *Od.* IV.568. Cf. *Il.* V.795, X.575, and XIII.84.

60. M. R. Wright, *Empedocles: The Extant Fragments* (New Haven, 1981), 261, frag. 101 (= frag. 111 DK), as adapted and slightly altered from Wright's translation. The text (apud Diog. Laert. VIII.59), as edited by Wright (p. 133), is basically identical to that provided by Diels-Kranz, *Fragmente* I:353–54. "Drugs" as a translation of *φάρμακα* is more fitting than Wright's "remedies" and certainly less restrictive than the "Gifte" of Diels-Kranz.

61. Hes. *Works and Days* 41. (*Hesiod: Works and Days*, ed. M. L. West [Oxford, 1978], 153, commentary).

62. West on *Hesiod, Works and Days* 733–734. Cf. Plut. *Mor., Dinner of the Seven Wise Men*, 157D–158B for Hesiod as learned in medicine. The debate over the "magic food," *ἄλιμον*, occupied much learned discussion in antiquity: Walter Burkert, *Lore and Science in Ancient Pythagoreanism*, trans. Edwin L. Minar, Jr. (Cambridge, Mass., 1972), 151 with n. 174; to Burkert's list of refs. on *ἄλιμον* one can add Porph., *Life of Pythagoras* 34 (*Porphyre: Vie de Pythagore. Lettre à Marcella*, ed. Edouard des Places [Paris, 1982], 52), which gives a twelve-ingredient formula for *ἄλιμον*, including poppy seeds, squill, asphodel, and honey.

63. Lloyd, *Ideology* (see n. 1), 119–20.

64. Hesiod, *Works and Days* 824.

65. *Scholia to Apollonius of Rhodes* IV.156 (= Musaeus frag. 2 DK). *Juniperus oxycedrus* yields a distillation of the heartwood, an oil called Oil of Cade, used in the Middle East as an antiseptic and as an external parasite killer; see George Usher, *Dictionary of Plants Used by Man* (London, 1974), 329.

66. Apollonius of Rhodes, *Voyage of the Argo*, IV.156–58.

67. Musaeus frag. 19 DK.

68. R. Merkelbach and M. L. West, eds., *Fragmenta Hesiodea* (Oxford, 1967), p. 173, frag. 349 in "Fragmenta dubia."

69. Dioscorides IV.132 (Wellmann [see n. 24], II:277) not surprisingly retains some of the folklore about *τριπόλιον*, writing that "it is written that the flower changes its color three times a day." Dioscorides recommends its white root, mixed in two drachmas of wine, as a diuretic and that the root is "cut into antidotes." In southern European folk medicine, the root of *Aster tripolium* has been used to cure eye diseases. Oleg Polunin, *Flowers of Europe* (Oxford, 1969), no. 1365 (p. 427 with plate 142).

70. Alan Cameron, "The Date and Identity of Macrobius," *JRS* 56 (1966): 25–38.

71. Verg. *Aen.* IV.513–14; trans. C. Day Lewis, *The Aeneid of Virgil* (Oxford, 1952), 96.

72. Macrob. *Sat.* V.19.9 (*Macrobius*, ed. J. Willis [Leipzig, 1970], I:326).

73. Macrob. *Sat.* V.19.10 (= Soph. frag. 534 Pearson).

74. Theophr., *Inquiry into Plants* IX.8.5; Scarborough, "Theophrastus" (see n. 1), 359. Dioscorides IV.153.2 (Wellmann [see n. 24], II:298–99).

75. John Gerarde, *The Herball or Generall Historie of Plantes,* vol. 2 (London, 1633), p. 1030.

76. Theophr., *Inquiry into Plants,* IX.8.3.

77. Theophr., *Inquiry into Plants* IX.20.3. Apparently, Athenian cows were immune to its poisonous properties.

78. Soranus, *Gynecology,* II.2.2 (*Sorani Gynaeciorum,* ed. J. Ilberg Corpus Medicorum Graecorum [Leipzig, 1927], p. 51). Soranus flourished in the reign of Trajan (98–117 A.D.).

79. Jeffrey Henderson, *The Maculate Muse* (New Haven, 1975), 135: "Pubic hair is almost always conceived in agricultural terms as a flowering growth . . . . Pennyroyal is jokingly used by Lysistrata . . . to refer to the Boeotian girl's neatly dipilitated campus muliebris, with a clever reference to the smooth, fertile plains of that region . . . with neatly trimmed pennyroyal plots."

80. Ibid., 186 with n. 137. The pennyroyal potion is prescribed for too much *ὀπώρα* (fruit or sex). Apparently, pennyroyal was hawked in the city along with reed mats, eels, and the like. Aristoph. *Ach.* 861, 869, and 874.

81. John Scarborough, *Facets of Hellenic Life* (Boston, 1976), 179–85; idem, "Nicander's Toxicology," pt. II, "Spiders, Scorpions, Insects, and Myriapods," *Pharmacy in History* 21 (1979): 3–34 and 73–92 (esp. 74–75 with nn. 240–246 and 249–254).

82. E.g., *Nature of Woman* 32 (*Oeuvres complètes d'Hippocrate,* ed. E. Littré [Paris, 1839–61], 8:364) among many refs; see X:751 for index entries for *pouliot.*

83. Dioscorides III,31.1 (Wellmann [see n. 24], II:40).

84. Gal. *Properties and Mixtures of Simples* VI.3.7 (Kühn [see n. 11] 11:857). Cf. Gal. *Treatment by Venesection* 18 (Kühn, 11:304); trans. Peter Brain, *Galen on Bloodletting* (Cambridge, 1986), p. 93.

85. E. Steier, "Minze," *RE, XV.*2 (1931), 2020–28, esp. 2027–28. Nic. *Alex.* 128–29, links pennyroyal with the infamous aphrodisiac called "Spanish fly," made from the elytra (wing covers) of blister beetles; see Scarborough, "Nicander's Toxicology," pt. II (see n. 81), 73–74.

86. A. Tschirch (*Handbuch der Pharmakognosie,* vol. II, pt. 2 [Leipzig, 1917], 1107–08) summarizes the literature to the early twentieth century.

87. R. G. Todd, ed., *Extra Pharmacopoeia Martindale,* 25th ed. (London, 1967), 1544.

88. Malcolm Stuart, ed., *The Encyclopedia of Herbs and Herbalism* (London, 1979), 223–24. Cf. Trease and Evans, *Pharmacognosy* (see n. 33), 412–14 and R. D. Mann, *Modern Drug Use* (Boston, 1984), 138.

89. Gal. *Properties and Mixtures of Simples* III.23 (Kühn [see n. 11], XI:609); John Scarborough, "Some Beetles in Pliny's *Natural History,*" *Coleopterists Bulletin* 31 (1977): 293–96.

90. E. Rohde, *Psyche,* 2d ed., trans. W. B. Hillis (London, 1925), 198, n. 95; J. Murr, *Die Pflanzenwelt in der griechischen Mythologie* (Innsbruck, 1890), 31–35 and 104–6.

91. Theophr., *Inquiry into Plants* VII.13.4.

92. Theophr., *Characters* XVI.14.

93. Parker, *Miasma* (see n. 10), 307.

94. Theophr., *Characters* XVI.2.

95. Theophr., *Characters* XVI.10.

96. Jerry Stannard, "Squill in Ancient and Medieval Materia Medica, with Special Reference to its Employment for Dropsy," *Bulletin of the New York Academy of Medicine* 50 (1974): 684–713.

97. Theogn. 537 (in *Elegy and Iambus,* ed. J. M. Edmonds [London, 1931], I:292).

98. Hipponax frag. 48 in *Herodes, Cercidas, and the Greek Choliambic Poets,* ed. A. D. Knox (London, 1961; pt. 2 of vol. entitled *Theophrastus: Characters,* ed. J. M. Edmonds) 34) as translated by Knox.

99. John Tzetzes, *Chiliades* V.726–61 (*Ioannis Tzetzes Historiarum variarum Chiliades,* ed. T. Kiessling, [Leipzig, 1826], 185–86).

100. John Tzetzes, *Chiliades* 5.743 (Kiessling, p. 185). Although modern scholars debate the reliability of later compilations regarding the *φαρμακός* rituals, one may certainly trust the main lines (squill and its importance) in summaries by such as John Tzetzes. See Jan Bremmer, "Scapegoat Rituals in Ancient Greece," *HSCP* 87 (1983): 299–320. Bremmer's arguments, however, that all such plants are symbolic (e.g., esp. 302–13: such herbs had no "fruit," and thereby justified the brutal treatment of "nonfruitful" or "marginal" persons) ignores the plentiful evidence of squills and their use in medicine and herbal remedies.

101. John Tzetzes, *Chiliades* 734–36 (Kiessling, p. 185).

102. Ἄγνος, as in Plut. *Mor., Table Talk* 693F, in which we learn that at Chaeronea a slave is beaten with branches of the *Vitex agnus castus* to drive away a "great hunger" termed *βούλιμος*. The "honey" of *Vitex agnus castus* was famed in antiquity for its use as a wound healer (Arist., *HA* 627a7–9), and the fruit of the "tree" (*Vitex agnus castus* is more of a bush) was valued as an emmenagogue, contraceptive, and sedative; see Diosc. *Mat. Med.* I.103.1–2 (Wellmann [see n. 24], 1:95). Traditionally, the leaves and fruit ("Monks' peppers") are sexual suppressants. Usher (see n. 65), 602. Stuart, *Herbs* (see n. 88), 282–83. Walter H. Lewis and Memory P. F. Elvin-Lewis, *Medical Botany* (New York, 1977), 322.

103. Diosc. *Mat. Med.* II.171.3 (Wellmann [see n. 24], I:239).

104. *Septuagint: Exod.* VII.11 and *Malach.* III:5.

105. Theophr., *Inquiry into Plants,* VIII.1.

106. Scarborough, "Theophrastus" (see n. 1), 356–57.

107. Stannard, "Squill" (see n. 96), 689.

108. Theophr. *Inquiry into Plants* VII.12.1; Hort (see n. 2), II:477 s.v.

109. Apul., *Apol.* 27 (Helm [see n. 18], 31).

110. Einarson, Introduction to *De Causis Plantarum* (see n. 3), xix-xx.

111. Diog. Laert. *Lives of the Eminent Philosophers: Epimenides* I.112.

112. The texts give contradictory evidence: Pl., *Laws* I.642d4 indicates a floruit of c. 500 B.C.; Arist., *Constitution of the Athenians* 1 points to a floruit of c. 600 B.C.. See commentary by Rhodes (see n. 7), 81–82.

113. Stannard, "Squill" (see n. 96), 687–89.

114. Lucian, *Menippus, or Descent into Hell* 7. Cf. E. Steier, "Skilla," *RE* Suppl. III.1 (1927), 522–26, esp. 524.

115. E.g., *Geoponica* XV.1.6–7 (*Geoponica,* ed. H. Beckh [Leipzig, 1895], 432).

116. Parker, *Miasma* (see n. 10), 231–32.

117. Ibid., 232.

118. Theophr., *Inquiry into Plants* I.6.7–9; I.10.7; II.5.5; VII.2.2; VII.4.12; VII.9.4; and VII.13.1–7.

119. Scarborough, "Theophrastus" (see n. 1), 355–60.

120. In folk medicine, both the common mallow, *Malva rotundifolia* L., and high mallow, *Malva sylvestris* L., retain their usefulness; the dried leaves of both species contain mucilage and tannin, making them quite suitable for preparations to treat inflamed tissues and coughs. A decoction of the flowers (*Flores malvae*) is employed for gargling and as a mouthwash. Usher (see n. 65), 375; Todd, *Martindale* (see n. 87), 1533.

121. Lycoph. *Alex.* 582. Nic. *Ther.* 496 and 587; Nic. *Alex.* 112.

122. The Hippocratic *Fractures,* X.3 (*Hippocrates,* ed. E. T. Withington [see n. 42], III.120–21); Nic. *Ther.* 493.

123. Theophr., *Inquiry into Plants* IX.18.2.

124. Ibid. 3. With οὐ μόνον τῶν σωματικῶν ἀλλὰ καὶ τῶν τῆς ψυχῆς, the Greek text in Hort's edition breaks off, presumably due to its offensive content—offensive to a squeakily prudish mind of the late Victorian era (the omitted passages contain only the mildest references to aphrodisiacs and a single, rather bland notice of an "Indian drug" that promotes multiple erections in the male). Sarton rightly comments that "Such prudishness in a scientific book is truly shocking." George Sarton, *A History of Science*, vol. I (Cambridge, Mass., 1959), 555, n. 96. See also above, n. 2.

125. Polunin, *Flowers of Europe* (see n. 69), 577 no. 1894. Todd, *Martindale* (see n. 87), 81.

126. Theophr., *Inquiry into Plants* IX.18.3 (Wimmer [see n. 2], 160).

127. Jerry Stannard, "Medicinal Plants and Folk Remedies in Pliny, *Historia Naturalis*," *History and Philosophy of the Life Sciences* 4 (1982): 3–23, esp. 14–15, with refs. to sources and secondary works.

128. Anthony Preus, "Drugs and Psychic States in Theophrastus' *Historia Plantarum* 9.8–20," in *Theophrastean Studies*, ed. W. W. Fortenbaugh and R. W. Sharples, Rutgers University Studies in Classical Humanities 3 (New Brunswick, 1988), 76–99.

129. Theophr., *Inquiry* IX.18.4 (Wimmer [see n. 2], 160).

130. Ibid.

131. Theophr., *Inquiry* IX.19.2–4.

132. The pharmacological effects of squill (*Urginea maritima* Baker) are fairly well understood. It has a digitalislike action on the heart, and in small amounts is employed occasionally as an expectorant. The outer scales are removed from the bulb. In Europe, a powdered form of rat poison is manufactured from squill. It contains not less than 70 percent alcohol[60%]-soluble extractive, as well as goodly percentages of scillarin A and scillarin B (A is a pure crystalline glycoside; B a mixture of glycosides). Todd, *Martindale* (see n. 87), 692. Trease and Evans, *Pharmacognosy* (see n. 33), 504–6. G. Baumgarten and W. Förster, *Die Herzwiksamen Glykoside* (Leipzig, 1963), 70–75.

133. John Scarborough, *Pharmacy's Ancient Heritage: Theophrastus, Nicander and Dioscorides* (Lexington, Ky., 1985), 19–20.

134. Ibid., 6, and Scarborough, "Theophrastus" (see n. 1), 355–59.

135. See nn. 74–77.

136. Theophr., *Inquiry into Plants* IX.8.6. The particular hellebore (white or black) is not distinguished.

137. Ludwig Edelstein, "Greek Medicine in Its Relation to Religion and Magic," in Owsei Temkin and C. Lilian Temkin, eds., *Ancient Medicine: Selected Papers of Ludwig Edelstein* (Baltimore, 1967), 205–46 (quotation from p. 230); orig. *Bulletin of the History of Medicine* 5 (1937): 201–46.

138. Ibid.

139. Ibid., 231.

140. Ibid., 231–32.

141. Ibid., 232.

142. John Scarborough, *Roman Medicine* (London, 1969), 119–20.

143. John M. Riddle, *Dioscorides on Pharmacy and Medicine* (Austin, 1985): 14–24.

144. Edelstein, "Magic," in *Ancient Medicine* (see n. 137), 232, n. 88.

145. Ibid., 230.

146. Ibid., 231.

147. Gal., *Compound Drugs According to Place in the Body* VIII.2 (Kühn [see n. 11], 13:126), quoting from the works of Andromachus on remedies for upset stomach.

148. Gal., *Compound Drugs According to Kind* VII.6 (Kühn, XIII:986).

149. Theophr., *Inquiry into Plants* IX.8.1.

150. Scarborough, "Theophrastus" (see n. 1), 355–56 with nn. 10–17.

151. Theophr., *Inquiry into Plants* IX.8.2.

152. Scarborough, "Theophrastus" (see n. 1), 356–57 with texts.

153. Pseudo-Aristotle, *Problems*, 864b9–12; John Scarborough, "Theoretical Assumptions in Hippocratic Pharmacology," in *Formes de pensées dans la collection hippocratique: Actes du IVe Colloque international hippocratique Lausanne . . . 1981*, ed. F. Lasserre and P. Mudry (Geneva, 1983), 307–25, esp. the section 'Aristotelian Drug Theory' with nn. 7–28.

154. Benedict Einarson, "The Manuscripts of Theophrastus' *Historia Plantarum*," *CP* 71 (1976): 67–76, esp. 68–69 with the readings from manuscript U*; Scarborough, "Theophrastus" (see n. 1), 353–54, with summary of contrary views.

155. John Scarborough, "Nicander's Toxicology", pt. I, "Snakes," *Pharmacy in History* 19 (1977): 3–23 and pt. 2, "Spiders, Scorpions, Insects, and Myriapods," 21 (1979): 3–34, 73–92.

156. Max Wellmann, "Das älteste Kräuterbuch der Griechen," in *Festgabe für Franz Susemihl* (Leipzig, 1898): 1–31 and idem, "Apollodoros" [no. 69], in *RE*, I.2 (1894), 2895.

157. John Scarborough, "Nicander, *Theriaca*, 811," *CP* 75 (1980): 138–40.

158. Scarborough, "Beetles" (see n. 89), 293–96; idem, "Nicander's Toxicology", pt. II (see n. 81), 73–78.

159. See, e.g., the Hippocratic *Diseases of Women* I.75–79 (Littré [see n. 24], VIII:162–99).

160. Riddle, *Dioscorides* (see n. 143), 137–38.

161. See esp. the Hippocratic *Ancient Medicine* as contrasted with the Hippocratic *Nature of Man*.

162. See n. 24.

163. John Scarborough and Vivian Nutton, "The *Preface* of Dioscorides' *Materia Medica:* Introduction, Translation, Commentary," *Transactions and Studies of the College of Physicians of Philadelphia* n.s. 4 (1982): 187–227 (esp. 192–194).

164. Ibid., 213–17; Riddle, *Dioscorides* (see n. 143), 2–4.

165. Scarborough, *Pharmacy's Ancient Heritage* (see n. 133), 63–65, 72–76 on silphium; Scarborough and Nutton, "*Preface*" (see n. 163), 199–202.

166. Riddle, *Dioscorides* (see n. 143), 94–131.

167. John Scarborough, "The Drug Lore of Asclepiades of Bithynia," *Pharmacy in History* 17 (1975): 43–57; Scarborough and Nutton, "*Preface*" (see n. 163): 206–8.

168. Dios. *Mat. Med.* 2, Preface (Wellmann [see n. 24], 1:2); translation from Scarborough and Nutton, "*Preface*" (see n. 163), 196.

169. Ibid., 5 (Wellmann [see n. 24], 1:3); translation from Scarborough and Nutton, "*Preface*" (see n. 163), 196.

170. Diosc. *Mat. Med.* IV.162.4 (Wellman [see n. 24], II:308–9).

171. Most likely to Zeus, through the eagle, but "the mythology of the eagle baffles analysis"; D'Arcy W. Thompson, *A Glossary of Greek Birds* (Oxford, 1936), 12.

172. See above pp. 348–52 with notes 91–117.

173. Parker, *Miasma* (see n. 10), 215–216.

174. But cf. Bennett Simon, *Mind and Madness in Ancient Greece* (Ithaca, N.Y., 1978), 218–19, 226, and 229.

175. See esp. *Sacred Disease*, II-IV (Jones, *Hippocrates* [see n. 42], III:140–51). One passage suggests the tone and approach of the writer: "My own view is that those who first attributed a sacred character to this malady were like the magicians, purifiers, charlatans and quacks of our own day, men who claim great piety and superior knowledge" (*Sacred Disease* II.1–5; trans. Jones, p. 141). Black hellebore is specifically prescribed by a Hippocratic physician in treatment of delirium accompanied by visual hallucinations in the *On Internal Diseases* 48 (Littré [see n. 24], VII:284–89, esp. 286–87). See also Owsei Temkin, *The*

Falling Sickness, 2d ed. (Baltimore, 1971), 68, 73, 76, 79, and 162 on later uses of hellebores in treatment of epilepsies.

176. Riddle, *Dioscorides* (see n. 143), 124, no. 162 in table 8, with refs. Cf. Scarborough, "Theophrastus" (see n. 1), 361–62.

177. The research of Vivian Nutton has proven the traditional dates for Galen (130–200 A.D.) wrong. Vivian Nutton, "The Chronology of Galen's Early Career," *CQ* 23 (1973): 158–71; idem, "Galen in the Eyes of His Contemporaries," *Bulletin of the History of Medicine* 58 (1984): 315–24.

178. John Scarborough, "Early Byzantine Pharmacology," in *Symposium on Byzantine Medicine*, ed. John Scarborough, Dumbarton Oaks Papers 38 (Washington, D.C., 1985), 213–32 (esp. the section "Galen's Pharmacy," 215–21).

179. Vivian Nutton, "The Drug Trade in Antiquity," *Journal of the Royal Society of Medicine* 78 (1985): 138–45 (see esp. 145). A similar characteristic is observed in the drug recipes of Criton, a major source for Galen's drug lore. John Scarborough, "Criton, Physician to Trajan: Historian and Pharmacist," in *The Craft of the Ancient Historian: Essays in Honor of Chester G. Starr*, ed. John W. Eadie and Josiah Ober (Lanham, Md., 1985), 387–405 (see esp. 394–97).

180. Scarborough, "Byzantine Pharmacology" (see n. 178), 215–16.

181. See, esp., *Nature of Man* IV–V (Jones, *Hippocrates* [see n. 42], IV:10–15).

182. E.g., the Egyptian compound-ingredient incense called *κῦφι*; Scarborough, "Byzantine Pharmacology" (see n. 178), 229–32.

183. See, e.g., Michael J. Harstad, "Saints, Drugs, and Surgery: Byzantine Therapeutics for Breast Diseases," *Pharmacy in History* 28 (1986): 175–80.

184. Gary Vikan, "Art, Medicine, and Magic in Early Byzantium," in *Byzantine Medicine*, ed. Scarborough (see n. 178), 65–86.

185. John Scarborough, "Hermetic and Related Texts in Classical Antiquity," in I. Merkal and A. G. Debus, eds., *Hermeticism and the Renaissance: Intellectual History and the Occult in Early Modern Europe* (Cranbury, N.J., 1988), 19–44.

186. Hans-Viet Friedrich, ed., *Thessalos von Tralles: griechisch und lateinisch* (Meisenheim am Glan, 1968). The most recent discussion of Thessalus in his "Egyptian" and "Hermetic" setting is Garth Fowden, *The Egyptian Hermes* (Cambridge, 1986), 161–65.

187. P. Boudreaux, ed., *Catalogus Codicum Astrologorum Graecorum*, vol. VIII, *Codicum Parisinorum*, pt. 3 (Brussels, 1912), 132–65 ("Excerpta ex codice 41" [Paris. gr. 2256]).

188. A. J. Festugière, *Hermétisme et mystique païenne* (Paris, 1967) for a French translation of parts of the *Letter*.

189. A. J. Festugière, *La Révélation d'Hermès Trismégiste*, vol. I, *L'Astrologie et les sciences occultes* (Paris, 1950), 150.

190. Friedrich, *Thessalos* (see n. 186), 43.

191. R. Reitzenstein, *Die hellenistischen Mysterienreligionen*, 3d ed. (Leipzig, 1927), 127–28.

192. Boudreaux, *Catalogus* (see n. 187), 139–51.

193. Ibid., 153–63; but cf. Pfister, "Pflanzenaberglaube" (see n. 38), 1452.

194. Festugière, *Révélation* (see n. 189), 137–86.

195. Galen (Kühn [see n. 11]), IX:903–13.

196. Scarborough, *Roman Medicine* (see n. 142), 120.

197. Cf. Ptol. *Tetrab.* III.12 (*Ptolemy: Tetrabiblos*, ed. and trans. F. E. Robbins [London, 1940], 316–33).

198. *Poimandres* I.27 (*Corpus Hermeticum*, ed. A. D. Nock and A.-J. Festugière, vol. I [Paris, 1946], 16).

199. *Powers of Herbs* II.1 (Friedrich [see n. 186], 199 and 203.

200. *Cichorium intybus* Cf. Theophr., *Inquiry into Plants* VII.7.1; Diosc. *Mat. Med.*

II.132 (Wellmann [see n. 24], 1:205–6); Pliny, *Natural History* XIX.129, XX.73, and XXI.88; *Geoponica* XII.28 (Beckh [see n. 115], 375–76): from Didymus; Columella, *Agriculture*, XI.3.27 and XII.9.2.

201. Apparently "as a drug." Diosc. *Mat. Med.* I.98 (Wellmann [see n. 24], 1:89).

202. Cf. Diosc. *Mat. Med.* I.99 (Wellmann [see n. 24], 1:90–91).

203. Cf. Galen (Kühn [see n. 11]), VI:604 VIII:343.

204. Cf. *PGM* XXXIII.

205. Ibid., and *PGM* VII.211–12.

206. *Stachys germanica L.;* Diosc. *Mat. Med.* III.106 (Wellmann [see n. 24], II:118); Pliny, *Natural History* XXIV.136.

207. *Crocus sativus L.;* Diosc. *Mat. Med.* I.26 (Wellmann [see n. 24], I:29–31).

208. *Pistacia lentiscus L.;* Theophrastus, *Inquiry into Plants* IX.1.2.

209. *Zingiber officinale* Rosc.; Diosc. *Mat. Med.* II.160 (Wellmann [see n. 24], I:226).

210. *Piper nigrum L.;* Diosc. *Mat. Med.* II.159 (Wellmann [see n. 24], I:224–26).

211. This is the famous *ἄσφαλτος*; Diosc.*Mat. Med.* I.73 (Wellmann [see n. 24], I:72–73).

212. Here *γλυκάνισον* = *ἄννησον*, which is *Pimpinella anisum L.; Scholia on Theocritus*, VII.63d (*Scholia in Theocritum Vetera* , ed. C. Wendel [Leipzig, 1914; rpt. Stuttgart, 1967], 95).

213. Made from *Pistacia lentiscus L.;* (see n. 208).

214. Cf. Diosc. *Mat. Med.* V.8 (Wellmann [see n. 24], III:12).

215. Parallel texts listed in n. 200.

216. Festugière, *Révélation* (see n. 189), 146–60.

217. Ibid., 150–52.

218. John Scarborough, "Roman Pharmacy and the Eastern Drug Trade," *Pharmacy in History* 24 (1982): 135–43.

219. Ibid., 137, with nn. 20–31.

220. Frederick H. Cramer, *Astrology in Roman Law and Politics* (Philadelphia, 1954), 232–83 (on drugs and magic, see pp. 276–78). See also the chapter "Astrologers, Diviners, and Prophets," in R. MacMullen, *Enemies of the Roman Order* (Cambridge, Mass., 1967), 128–162.

221. See *PGM*. The magical tracts in Greek and Coptic (with occasional and clipped commentary) of the Preisendanz texts, have recently been restudied and translated into English by a team of scholars under the general direction of Hans Dieter Betz; added to the Greek and Coptic texts of the Preisendanz collection are important translations (by Janet H. Johnson) of demotic magical papyri; the first volume of translations of the *PGM* has been published as Hans Dieter Betz, ed., *The Greek Magical Papyri in Translation*, vol. I, *Texts* (Chicago, 1986) [= *GMPT*]. Volume II will be indexes to the English translations as well as the Greek and Coptic texts.

222. Pfister, "Pflanzenaberglaube" (see n. 38).

223. *PGM* IV.286–95, trans. E. N. O'Neil in *GMPT* (see n. 221), 1:43.

224. *PGM* IV.2967–75, trans. E. N. O'Neil in *GMPT* (see n. 221), 1:95.

225. Packets of natron were placed in Egyptian mummies from about 2000 B.C. "Natron" is a compound of sodium carbonate and sodium bicarbonate and, mixed with fats, forms sodium soaps; Majno, *Healing Hand* (see n. 35), 131–36. Resins were also essential in Egyptian mummification; ibid., 137–38.

226. J. G. Frazer, *The Golden Bough*, vol. IV, *Adonis Attis Osiris*, 2nd ed. (London, 1907), 74–75 on milk, 221–22, 231–33, and 340–43 on pine cones, etc.

227. *PGM* IV.2979–89, trans. E. N. O'Neil (with some clipped commentary) in *GMPT* (see n. 221), 1:95.

228. Betz, Introduction to *GMPT* (see n. 221) 1:xlviii.

229. *PGM* XXXVI.320–32, trans. John Scarborough in *GMPT* (see n. 221) 1:277.

230. Diosc. *Mat. Med.* IV.68 (Wellmann [see n. 24], II:224).

231. Diosc. *Mat. Med.* II.108 (Wellmann [see n. 24], I:182).

232. Riddle, *Dioscorides* (see n. 143), 57.

233. Diosc. *Mat. Med.* IV.68.2 (Wellmann [see n. 24], II:225).

234. Todd, *Martindale* (see n. 87), 170–71.

235. *PGM* XXXVI.324, n. 40 in *GMPT* (see n.221) 1: 277.

236. *PGM* XXIIa.11–14, trans. John Scarborough in *GMPT* (see n. 221) 1:260.

237. Soranus, *Gynecology*, III.42.3 (Ilberg [see n.78], 121).

238. Diosc. *Mat. Med.* V.126 and 130 (Wellmann [see n. 24], III:94–95 and 96–97).

239. Gal., *Mixtures and Properties of Simples* IX.11 (Kühn [see n.11], XII:204).

240. Pliny, *Natural History* XXVI.127.

241. *Geoponica* XV.1.28 (Beckh [see n.115] 435).

242. Dioscorides V.124 (Wellmann [see n. 24], III:92); Gal., *Mixtures and Properties of Simples* IX.9 (Kühn [see n. 11], XII:202); Celsus, *Med.* V.7. Pliny, *Natural History*, XXXVI.131.

243. When published, *GMPT* vol. II (see n. 221) will contain separate indexes of plants, animals, etc.

244. *PGM* XII.401–44, trans. H. D. Betz and John Scarborough (with some clipped commentary) in *GMPT*, (see n. 221), 1:167–69.

245. *PGM* IV.1313 ("priestly Egyptian incense" as trans. W. C. Grese in *GMPT* [see n. 221], 1:63); as *PGM* IV.2971 (see n. 224); *PGM* V.221 (transliterated by E. N. O'Neil as *kyphi* [*GMPT* I:204]); *PGM* VII.538 ("sacred incense" as trans. R. F. Hock [*GMPT* I:133]); and *PGM* VII.873 ("lunar ointment" as trans. E. N. O'Neil [*GMPT* I:141]).

246. G. Ebers, "Ein Kyphirecept aus dem Papyros Ebers," *Zeitschrift für ägyptische Sprache und Altertumskunde* 12 (1874): 106–11. Scarborough, "Byzantine Pharmacology" (see n. 178), 231.

247. Full discussion and identification of ingredients in a twenty-eight-substance formula in Scarborough, "Byzantine Pharmacology" (see n. 178), 230–32.

248. Diosc. *Mat. Med.* I.25 (Wellmann [see n. 24], I:28–29); translated, with ingredients identified, in Scarborough, "Byzantine Pharmacology" (see n. 178), 230.

249. *PGM* IV.1275–1322, trans. W. C. Grese in *GMPT* [see n.221], 62–63).

250. Hippol. *Refutation of all Heresies* IV.28 (*Origenis Philosophumena sive Omnium Haeresium Refutatio*, ed. E. Miller, Patrologiae Graecae, vol. XVI, pt. 3 [Paris, 1863], col. 3090). The *Refutation*, formerly attributed to Origen, is now firmly among the works of Hippolytus; F. L. Cross, ed., *Oxford Dictionary of the Christian Church* (London, 1957), 641–42.

251. Hippol. *Refutation* IV.28 (Miller, cols. 3090–91).

252. Brian Vickers, Introduction to *Occult and Scientific Mentalities in the Renaissance*, ed. Brian Vickers (Cambridge, 1984), 1–55, esp. 3, following Charles Schmitt.

253. Fowden, *Egyptian Hermes* (see n. 186), 79 with n. 19, 162–65, 168.

II

On Medications for Burns in Classical Antiquity

Once the use of fire was incorporated into man's daily life, accidental burns were inevitable. Methods of treatment for such injuries were as necessary in antiquity as they are in modern times. Mankind has engaged in a search for soothing and healing medicines throughout history.

Treatment for injuries from fire was sought even in the earliest human settlement. Although there is no direct evidence that particular drugs and pharmaceuticals were employed, there is circumstantial proof that herbs were valued by Neanderthal man in Iraq as early as 60,000 B.C.[1] Thus, an important aspect of man's early attempts at medical practice was understanding the utility of plants.[2]

Plant and animal products have been traditionally selected for treatment of burns. Oils and "oily" substances, including vegetable and animal fats, were recognized early as useful medicaments. By the time documentation of technique appears in medical texts, there are records of traditions rooted deep in the prehistoric past.

Of signal interest are the various gums and resins employed against burns in the pharmaceutical writings of ancient Egypt. These inordinately puzzling medical texts from Pharaonic Egypt suggest the beginnings of customs in burn treatment that later appear in the drug lore of Greece, Rome, and early Byzantium.

Unless otherwise noted, all translations are by the author of the present essay.

BURN MEDICATIONS IN ANCIENT EGYPT

Burn treatments are featured in the famous Ebers Papyrus of about 1500 B.C.,[3] and modern readers can sample these arcane prescriptions in a fairly reliable German rendition.[4] The identification of substances mentioned is subject to ardent debate among scholars specializing in the languages of ancient Egypt, but agreement prevails as to the interpretation of the beginning of Ebers Papyrus, 482: "The Beginning of the [Section] on Drugs for a Burn," followed by "What one makes against [a burn] on the first day: put on it black mud (*ʿmʿ.t*).[5] The Ebers Papyrus, 482, thus gives a sequential series of treatments, depending on when the *swnw* ("priest-physician") applied the "drugs" to the burn. The text can also be interpreted to mean that treatments were supposed to continue for five days after the *swnw* first saw the patient. "What one does on the second day: cook the dung of a calf, mix it with *srm.t ḫpr.t* (probably "yeast"), [and] apply it [to the burn]," continues Ebers Papyrus, 482. Only on the third day of treatment are specific pharmaceuticals as understood in modern pharmacology applied.

> What one makes on the third day: *ʿꜣgj.t* (probably "resin" or "gum-resin") of the acacia (*Acacia arabica* Willd.) dried; mix in *šʿ.t* (a "paste") of barley; cook (or boil) *ḏꜣr.t* (colocynth, *Citrillus colocynthus* [L.] Schrad.); put in fat (or oil); bind [the burn] with it.

This article was published in *Clinics in Plastic Surgery*, Vol. 10, No. 4 (1983), pp. 603–610.

> What one makes on the fourth day: wax (viz. beeswax); fat (viz. suet) from a cow; boil a [piece of fresh] papyrus with beans; make a paste; bind [the burn] with it.
>
> What one makes on the fifth day: a colocynth; red ochre (viz. hematite, Fe_2O_3), one [measure]; [?]-part of a leaf, one [measure]; to be mixed with copper [fragments]; bind [the burn] with it.[6]

Von Deines and colleagues believe that these prescriptions were specific for burns resulting from direct exposure to an open flame, as contrasted with repeated burn injuries, which have different recipes for treatment.[7]

As Majno has emphasized, the modern student of ancient Egyptian medicine must never forget that what constituted "pharmacy" for the Egyptians was very different from later Greek notions, and certainly vastly dissimilar to modern ideas of the actions of drugs based on biochemical or physiologic principles.[8] This ancient Egyptian concept is nicely illustrated in Ebers Papyrus, 499:

> One more incantation for a burn on the first day: "Your son Horus has burned himself in the desert." "Is there any water here?" "There is no water here." "Water is in my mouth, a Nile is between my thighs, I have come to extinguish the fire." "Flow out, burn!" Say this over the milk of a woman who has given birth to a boy. Gum; a hair of a ram; apply to the burn.[9]

Therefore, even though we may be able to identify specific substances used by the Egyptians in their treatment of burns (e.g., honey, myrrh, opium poppy, terebinth resin, and various other medicinals),[10] we have little understanding of the rationale behind the prescriptions of the Egyptian *swnw*. Ghalioungui, Sigerist, and others[11] have investigated the practice of ancient Egyptian medicine in light of modern knowledge, but careful study of the texts leaves the modern medical historian with many questions unanswered. The theory and practice of Egyptian medicine remain unclear. One is forced, therefore, into a narrow conclusion concerning Egyptian burn treatments: a number of herbs and medicinals were indeed employed—and some even seem reasonable when viewed in the light of modern pharmacology;[12] but Egyptians "understood" such "drug actions" through complicated magical or religious assumptions, poorly comprehended by medical historians. We may find that better understanding will emerge when medical history admits the existence of a number of "systems" of medicine within a given culture, much as suggested by the anthropological models used by Lloyd for explanation of the beginnings of early Greek medicine and science.[13]

BURN TREATMENT IN GREEK MEDICINE

The ancient Greek notions of medical practice bear some similarity to present day ideas. Greek thinking produced the logical speculations of the Nature Philosophers in the seventh and sixth centuries B.C.[14] In their quest to explain how "things came to be" and how "things passed away," they laid the foundations of medical theories that were accorded recognition by the fifth century B.C.

Medical theory was built on the tripartite base of elements, qualities, and humors. The elements of earth, air, fire, and water served as the building blocks of the universe. This category included all living things. Qualities—the wet, the dry, the hot, the cold—characterized the elements as they were perceived by the senses. The humors—if one presumes only four, as did the author of the Hippocratic *Nature of Man*[15]—were blood, phlegm, black bile, and yellow bile. The make-up of human beings was defined as an ideal "blending" (Greek *krasis*) of elements, qualities, and the humors. Human disease was determined by an imbalance of elements, qualities, and humors. The task of a physician (Greek *iatros*) was first to diagnose the imbalance, then to render a prognosis, and finally to prescribe drugs (*pharmaka*) that would promote the restoration of the ideal *krasis*. Each *pharmakon* had its own characteristics or properties (*dynameis*) in terms of the elements and qualities, and it could be matched with the illness the *iatros* sought to correct.[16]

The earliest mention of treatment of burns by Greek physicians is the Hippocratic *corpus*. Scholars generally agree that although Hippocrates of Cos (*fl.* 430–400 B.C.) was well known by physicians in the late fifth century B.C.,[17] no specific writings attributed to him exist in the collection of Greek medical tracts which, as a whole, were given his name.[18] This Hippocratic *corpus* contains works on all aspects of medical practice—sometimes one contradicting another. They place emphasis on regimen, medical theory, and dietetics, and also include some crisp case histories such as the rightly famous *Epidemics* I and III, information on diagnostics, pharmacology, surgery, and some anatomy.[19]

Savants resident at the Ptolemaic Museum and Library at Alexandria in Egypt probably compiled the collection we call the Hippocratic *corpus* about 200 B.C. or somewhat later.[20] The various tracts in the *corpus* often show Greek medical thinking at its best. Many facets of the Hippocratic collection bear the marks of philosophical reasoning,[21] and pharmacology is liberally mixed with theory in many separate treatises, written by unknown writers from the fifth century through perhaps the second century B.C. A particular chapter in the Hippocratic *On Wounds* considers burn treatment, and it shows how the Greek *iatros* of the fourth and third centuries B.C. went about prescribing medications for burns:

> Regarding a Burn (*Peri pyrikaustou*). One ought to boil tender sucker-shoots of the holly oak (*Quercus ilex* L.), the bark being rather thick and green; cut it up into small pieces [and] add white wine; boil over a slow fire until it becomes the proper thickness for a salve; also [one can] prepare this with water. Another [recipe] which does not sting: use as a salve old pig's fat by itself; melt the pig's fat together with the root of the squill (*Urginea maritima* [L.] Baker), which has been split [in half], and apply it to the burn with a bandage; and on the next day, one should wet it down (i.e., "foment" it with this "warm" lotion). Another: melt old pig's fat and beeswax and mix with oil and frankincense (*libanōtos: Boswellia carteri* Birdw.) and shavings (*ichthyēmata*, lit. "fish-scales") of a lilly (*lōtos*: probably *Lotus corniculatus* L., bird's-foot trefoil, or fellbloom; possibly *Nymphaea* spp., water lily) [rhizome], and *miltos* (red chalk; reddle; a hematite + clays, Fe_2O_3), and spread this on the burn as an ointment. Boil the leaves of a cuckoo pint (prob. *Arum maculatum* L.) in wine and oil, and apply as a bandage. Still another: anoint [the burn] with old pig's fat, [and] then rub in roots of asphodel (*Asphodelus ramosus* L.) which have been pounded in wine and triturated. Still another: melt old pig's fat, mix with pine-resin and bitumen (*asphalatos*); smear this on a piece of linen cloth, warm it before a fire, [and] apply as a bandage.[22]

This short section of the Hippocratic *Wounds*, with its specific recipes for burn treatment, presents only 13 basic ingredients if one counts the wine, oil, and beeswax. The salves and ointments compounded by the unknown author are either emollient such as the animal and vegetable fats and oils, or detergent and astringent like the holly oak and the squill.

The author of the Hippocratic *Wounds* is not the first to record these various remedies and plants: Hesiod first noted *Quercus ilex* in about 700 B.C.,[23] as did Theophrastus in about 300 B.C.[24] Asphodel first appears in Hesiod's *Works and Days*, 41, and the flower has a lengthy history in Greco-Roman botany and herbal lore, starting with the works of Aristotle (*d.* 322 B.C.) and Theophrastus through Theocritus (*c.* 300–260 B.C. in Alexandria), Crateuas (physician to Mithridates VI of Pontus [111–64 B.C.]), and Dioscorides of Anazarbus (fl. c. A.D. 65).[25] Reddle is cited by numerous authors before our Hippocratic writer, and among them are Herodotus (c. 484–430 B.C.) and Aristophanes (c. 450–385 B.C.), and, later, Dioscorides.[26] Arum had been noted by Aristotle and Theophrastus and is given its honored place as a medicinal plant by Dioscorides and Pseudo-Dioscorides.[27] The author of the Hippocratic *Wounds* is probably the recipient not only of formal medical theory, perhaps explaining the "why" of his pharmacology, but also of a long and venerated folk medical tradition, acknowledged as supremely important in herbal medicine by Theophrastus in the ninth book of the fundamental *Historia Plantarum*.[28] Beeswax and hematite, burn treatments first mentioned in the Ebers Papyrus, are also cited by the author of the Hippocratic *On Wounds*, but each society used these materials in their own, unique fashion.

BURN MEDICATIONS IN EARLY ROMAN IMPERIAL MEDICINE

One of the most remarkable works in the history of ancient medicine is the *De medicina* by Cornelius Celsus (fl. in the reign of Tiberius [A.D. 14–37]). Argument rages among specialists concerning Celsus's professional status as a *medicus* ("physician"), but whether he was a practicing doctor or not,[29] Celsus's elegant and precise Latin tract is an important statement of sane, sensible, and well-founded medical practice in the early Roman Empire.[30] He clearly had read much, considered many medical theories of Greek origin, and made sound judgments of his own regarding the art of medicine as it existed in his own time. Among the many topics discussed in *De medicina* is the consideration of pharmaceuticals. Suggested here are herbs and concoctions for the treatment of burns:

> [Burns] are best treated by the leaves either of the lily (prob. *Lilum candidum* L., white lily) or of dog's tongue (*lingua canina*, prob. = Greek *cynoglōssos*, *Cynoglossum officinale* L.), or of the beet (*Beta* spp.), boiled in old wine and oil. Any of these substances, once applied [to the burn] promotes healing. But the course of treatment can be divided as follows: first a phase of moderately caustic (*exedentia*) and suppressant [ointments] both to keep blisters from forming and to roughen the skin; secondly, a phase of soothing salves to induce healing. Included in the first phase is lentil-meal with honey, or myrrh (*Commiphora* spp.) with wine, or Cimolian Earth (cimolite, a

hydrous silicate of aluminum, $2Al_2O_3 \cdot 9SiO_2 \cdot 6H_2O$, like kaolin, but which can be reddish), pounded with frankincense (*Boswellia* spp.) bark (*cum turis cortice*) and mixed with water, and when it is necessary to use it, diluted with vinegar. The second phase of medicines includes anything "fatty" (*lipara*, perhaps "oily"), but the most suitable is an [application] that contains lead dross and an egg yolk. There is also another treatment of burns: while there is inflammation, one leaves the lentil-meal and honey placed on the burn; when the inflammation has subsided, one applies [wheat] meal mixed with rue (*ruta; Ruta graveolens* L.), or with leek (*Allium porrum* L.), or with horehound (*Marrubium vulgare* L.), until the crusts fall off; then one applies bitter vetch (*Vicia ervilia* [L.] Willd.) mixed with honey, or iris-oil ('orris-butter' from *Iris florentina* L., or *I. germanica* L.), or terebinth-resin (viz. 'turpentine' or 'Chian turpentine' from *Pistacia terebinthus* L.) until the wound (*ulcus*) is clean; last one applies a dry strip of linen (*siccum linamentum*).[31]

Celsus derived many of his prescriptions from Greek sources, and there is good reason to assume that those he lists for burns also come from this tradition. He also suggested the use of Italian recipes.

Most of the detailed pharmacology from the Hellenistic era (323–30 B.C.) has been lost, but occasionally one may find lost sources by examination of quotations in extant texts. In the case of *De medicina*, V, 27. 13A, the occurrence of the *lingua canina* is unusual, and a quotation by the fourth century A.D. physician Oribasius shows that *cynoglōssos* (= *lingua canina*) was first used in a pharmaceutical prescription by Zopyrus of Alexandria, a surgeon and pharmacologist of the first century B.C.[32]

Celsus's drug lore on burn treatment has been enriched with the introduction of several new herbs into the prescriptions. A comparison of the list of treatments in *On Wounds*, 22 with those offered in *De medicina* suggests that burn medications became increasingly sophisticated from the time of Hippocratic pharmacology to the first century of the Roman Empire. Similarly, the number of species employed in herbal medicine increased in the period between Theophrastus' *Historia Plantarium*, IX, and his *On Odors*, and the publication of Dioscorides' *Materia Medica* in approximately A.D. 65. Ancient drug lore, much as Dioscorides stated explicitly in the Preface of the *Materia Medica*,[33] was continually improved through constant testing in the natural laboratory of living patients.

Roman medicine also relied on native folk traditions, as is well illustrated by Pliny the Elder's marvelous farrago, the *Natural History* (published in A.D. 77). A sampling of Pliny's suggestions for burn treatment—culled from hundreds of sources, both Greek and Latin—will show the grand mixture of the sensible and silly that characterizes the raw material of folk medicine in any age.

Burns are healed by plantain (*Plantago* spp.), and by bearwort (or inula, or a spikenard: *arction* = Greek *arktion;* probably *Inula candida* [L.] Cass., or *I. conyza* DC) so well that scarring (*cicatrix*) does not occur. The leaves of the bearwort are boiled in water and pounded, and are smeared on [the burn], as are the roots of the sowbread (*cyclaminos* = Greek *kyklaminos*, either *Cyclamen hederifolium* Aiton, or *C. graecum* Link, "Greek cyclamen") with the houseleek (*aizoum* = Greek *aeizōon, Sempervivum tectorum* L.) as well as that [part of] the plant St. John's wort (*hypericum* = Greek *hyperikon*, probably *Hypericum triquetrifolium* Turra) which I have termed *corissum* (probably = "stem").[34]

For the treatment of burns, bear's fat with the roots of lilies [is employed], as is the dried dung of the wild boar, ashes of pig-bristles made from plasterer's brushes and pounded up with pig's fat; [also used for burns] is the ash of the pastern-bone of an ox mixed with beeswax, the bile of a bull, the dung of a hare, but the dung of she-goats is said to heal burns without scarring (*sine cicatrice*). The best paste (viz. glue: *glutinum*) is from the ears and genitals of bulls, and there is no better remedy for burns; but no remedy is adulterated more often, decoctions (viz. boilings) being produced from just about any old skins and even from shoes. The best glue is from Rhodes, which is used by painters and doctors.[35]

For burns, ashes of a dog's head are employed in treatments as are the ashes of dormice mixed in oil, the dung of sheep mixed with beeswax, and the ashes of burned snails are so excellent for burns that no scar is apparent [after the burn has healed]. The fat of a snake is also employed, and the ash of pigeon droppings, applied with oil.[36]

Burns are healed by the ashes of a sea- or river-crab mixed in oil; for scalds from boiling water, fish-glue (*ichthyocolla*) and the ashes of frogs [are healing].[37]

The modern dermatologist may chortle at the dungs prescribed, but one should recall that classical pharmacology regularly esteemed dungs, as is noted in the works of Dioscorides and Galen. Animal manure continued to be employed in the treatment of burns well into the European Renaissance. Such lore from Greco-Roman pharmacy had been passed along by the Byzantine medical writers, including the sagacious Paul of Aegina (*fl.* in Alexandria *c.* A.D. 630–640).

Of interest to the modern pharmacognocist is the list of herbs in Pliny, *Natural History*, XXVI, 129: here are plantain, bearwort, sowbread, the houseleek, and a St. John's wort, all of which can be found mentioned in earlier Greek sources.[38] In fact, as Max Wellmann has demonstrated,[39] Pliny and Dioscorides often derived their medical and pharmaceutical data from a common source, Sextius Niger, an apparently skilled herbalist whose work was done a generation before Dioscorides, confirming that Niger worked during the same time as Celsus.

The great Dioscorides did not devote a specific section in the *Materia Medica* to medications for burns; he organized his drug lore on a system of what might be called "drug affinity."[40] His prescriptions for burn salves and applications are thus scattered throughout the five books of the *Materia Medica.* The remedies of Dioscorides were noted by almost all subsequent writers on the topic,[41] including Galen and the early Byzantine medical encyclopedists such as Paul of Aegina, who lived during the early seventh century. After the writings of Dioscorides, very few new drugs were added to the stock of Greco-Roman pharmacy, so that most medical authors who followed him, even Galen, cited materials used earlier and reworked them into various formulas or simply copied in toto large swatches of existing recipe collections.[42]

LATE ROMAN AND EARLY BYZANTINE BURN TREATMENT

Although the medical notables of the centuries between Dioscorides and Pliny and Paul of Aegina had much to say about drugs for the treatment of burns and skin ailments,* Paul presents the best summary. He offers the best recommendations for medications against burns in the early seventh century, which were later used by Arab physicians[43] and, until the seventeenth century, by most trained doctors in the West. Thus Paul of Aegina, IV, 11, "On Burns" (*Pros ta pyrikauta*, perhaps more accurately rendered "On the Parts [of the body] that Have Been Burned") functions as a concise compendium of burn medications and their efficacy as used in Greco-Roman pharmacy. Much is taken as known to the reader in Paul's account, especially the underlying "theory of degrees" for drugs, which had been proposed somewhat crudely by Galen,[44] and refined, streamlined, and summarized by later writers on pharmacology, especially by Aetius of Amida in the early sixth century.[45] One also needs to recall that late Roman and early Byzantine medicine was distinguished by a cleavage between the "medicine of the lecture hall" and the "medicine of the people," seen in the carefully drafted encyclopedias of Aetius and Paul as contrasted with the disorderly empirical statements set down by Alexander of Tralles (*fl.* in the reign of Justinian [A.D. 527–565]).[46] Paul is the quintessential student of the best medical authorities in Greek and Roman medicine; yet he also displays that peculiar quality of genius that so marked early Byzantine adaptations and precise extractions of the classical past, well known from the production of the *Digest* of Roman law by Justinian.[47] Paul's summary of burn treatments is thereby a distillation of Greco-Roman thinking on the topic, and represents the best of the time-tested remedies.

Parts [of the body] which have been burned need moderately cleansing drugs rather than [drugs] which are clearly hot or cold. Thus Chian Earth, Cimolian Earth, Cretan Earth (all forms of hydrous silicates of aluminum), and every kind of light earth being applied with vinegar are not too sharp, or when they are mixed with water, are excellent [treatments] and prevent the formation of blisters. And a complete raw egg quickly laid on with soft wool cools moderately and dries soothingly. Also smear the burn with black ink, or with frankincense (*Boswellia* spp.), or lay on a plaster of boiled lentil (*Ervum* spp.) made smooth, or a plaster of bitter vetch (*orobos: Vicia ervilia* [L.] Willd.). For scaldings from hot water—before blisters appear—pour on [the burn] frequently [the] brine of pickled olives, and plaster on the pickled olives themselves [pounded] with barley-meal; or pound cleavable alum (probably a form of potash alum, $KAl(SO_4)_2{\cdot}12H_2O$) with vinegar and rub it into [the scald]; or smear it with bull's bile, dissolved in a great quantity of water; or pour on it wood-ash lye mixed with garum or brine; or pound the bulbs of lilies (*krinon: Lilium candidum* L.), or hyacinths (probably the bluebell, *Scilla bifolia* L., or possibly *Hyacinthus orientalis* L.), or narcissus (*Narcissus* spp.) with oil of roses (*Rosa gallica* L.), and having made the trituration glutinous, smear it on [the burn]. And Marcellus† provides this recipe: smear a rag with honey, wrap it around some barley-kernels, and burn it [all], and take 8 drachmai of the ashes [with] 4 drachmai of white lead (*psimythion*: cerussite; $PbCO_3$; lead carbonate), 8 drachmai of butter, 16 drachmai of beeswax, 16 drachmai of goat-fat, [and] 16 drachmai of rose-oil. For parts [of the body] burned previously, apply as a plaster pounded

*Aretaeus of Cappadocia, Rufus of Ephesus, and Soranus of Ephesus, all of the early second century A.D.; Galen (A.D. 129—probably after A.D. 210); Oribasius, physician to Julian the Apostate (A.D. 361–363); Alexander of Tralles (*fl.* in the reign of Justinian, A.D. 527–565); and Aetius of Amida (*fl.* also in the reign of Justinian).

†This may be the Marcellus (*fl.* in the reign of Nero [A.D. 54–68] quoted by Galen (ed. Kuhn), XIV, 459.

Sicilian sumach (*Rhus coriaria* L.), barley-meal, and vinegar; or mix quicklime (*konios asbestos*; CaO)[48] with a wax-salve and placing it on a piece of linen, and apply it [to the burn]. And the medicine called "The Sphairion" (? perhaps an oak-gall)[49] is useful for these matters. Plaster parts [of the body] which are [burned deeply and] ulcerated with ground horehound (*prasion: Marrubium vulgare* L.); or plaster pounded purselane (*Portulaca oleracea* L.) with barley-meal; or place pigeon-droppings on a linen rag, burn it, mix the ashes with oil, and employ it [on the burn]. A marvellous drug (*thaumaston pharmakon*) is also [the] bark of a pine (*Pinus* or *Larix* spp.) or Corsican pine (*Pinus laricio* L.), or dried maidenhair fern (*Adiantum capillus-veneris* L.) made into a smooth paste, or the burned leaves of myrtle (*Myrtus communis* L.) which are ground [and] dusted on [the burn]. And each of these [ingredients] is well placed with a wax-salve (viz. cerate). And a good drug (*agathon pharmakon*) is pounded root of red alkanet (*Anchusa tinctoria* L.) 4 ounkiai, 9 ounkiai of white wax, 18 ounkiai of rose-oil, and through white lead (*psimythion*) with a little [portion] of stag marrow.[50]

Paul's offering includes ingredients culled from a number of earlier sources: Galen gives the essential information on the lye made from ashes of wood[51] and as an aside provides some interesting information on the common use of a liquid soap made from this substance. Garum was a highly esteemed but terribly bitter fish sauce that was used in Roman culinary arts and also served as a caustic application.[52] The bluebell, narcissus, and rose featured prominently in Dioscorides, as were sumach, horehound, purselane, Corsican pine, the maidenhair-fern, myrtle and alkanet.[53] Heraclides of Tarentum (first century B.C.) quoted by Galen provides information about quicklime;[54] white lead had been known since the time of Theophrastus.[55] *Sphairion*, which probably translates as "oak-gall," is taken from a reading in the Greek of Theophrastus.[56] Vinegar, wine, water, honey, dungs, bull-bile, olive oil, wax and wax-salve, animal fat, lentils, wheat meal and barley meal, various animal ashes, the bitter vetch, frankincense, eggs, and the "Earths" have survived as valuable constituents of burn remedies as compared with the recipes from Hippocrates and early imperial Rome, which have been discarded.

Emollients, detergents, and astringents comprise the basic ingredients of early Byzantine burn treatments, as they did in Hippocratic pharmacology. Indeed, the application of many of these herbs was sensibly prescribed. A large number of species contained a fair amount of tannin or tannic acid whose astringent properties were beneficial to burns. Other remedies such as frankincense, myrrh, wine, and vinegar exerted an antibacterial effect, while honey served to dry the wound to promote healing.

Relying on powers of observation and willingness to experiment, the peoples of classical antiquity devised many remedies for burns. Certainly not all treatments were efficacious but we must nonetheless look with admiration upon the accomplishments of those who worked almost twenty centuries ago.

FOOTNOTES

1. Solecki, 880–881
2. Lloyd, *Magic*, 17–18. Evans-Pritchard, 183.
3. Sigerist, 333–334. Bryan, passim.
4. Von Deines, Grapow, and Westendorff, IV, 1, 214–221.
5. *Ibid.*, 214.
6. *Ibid.*
7. *Ibid.*, 216–220.
8. Majno, 125.
9. Von Deines, Grapow, and Westendorff, IV, 1, 215.
10. *Ibid.*, 216–221. *Cf.* Sigerist, 340–345.
11. Ghalioungui, 139–149. Sigerist, 267–373. Majno, 69–140. Lefebvre, passim.
12. Majno, 111–125.
13. Lloyd, *Magic*, 16–19.
14. Lloyd, *Polarity*, 74–76. Adkins, 91–109. Onians, 13–92. Kirk and Raven, 232–235 and 320–361.
15. Hippocrates, IV, 1–4 (ed. Jones).
16. Scarborough, "Theoretical Assumptions," 281–284. Harig, 223–230.
17. Plato, *Phaedrus*, 270 C-D.
18. Lloyd, "Hippocratic Question," 189–190. *cf.* Smith, 60–63.
19. See esp. Littré's edition (with French trans.) and the edition of Jones and Withington (with English trans.).
20. Fraser, I, 346.
21. Scarborough, "Theoretical Assumptions," 290–293.
22. The Hippocratic *On Wounds*, 22 (ed. Littré, VI, 426–428).
23. Hesiod, *Works and Days*, 436.
24. Theophrastus, *Historia Plantarum*, III, 16. 1; III, 6. 4.
25. Aristotle, *Historia Animalium*, 627a8. Theophrastus, *Historia Plantarum*, I, 10. 7 and VII, 13. 2. Theocritus, VII, 68. Crateuas, Frg. 5 (ed. Wellmann). Dioscorides, II, 169.
26. Herodotus, IV, 91 and VII, 69. Aristophanes, *Ecclesiazusae*, 378. Dioscorides, V, 96.
27. Aristotle, *Historia Animalium*, 600b11. Theophrastus, *Historia Plantarum*, I, 6. 10. Pseudo-Dioscorides, II, 167.
28. Scarborough, "Theophrastus," 359–360.
29. Daube, 41–42.
30. Scarborough, *Roman Medicine*, 59–63.
31. Celsus, V, 27. 13A-B (ed. Marx, p. 235).
32. Oribasius, *Medical Collection*, XIV, 62. 1 (ed. Raeder, II, p. 231).
33. Scarborough and Nutton, 195–196.

34. Pliny, *Natural History,* XXVI, 129 (ed. Jones, VII, p. 362).
35. Pliny, *Natural History,* XXVIII, 235–236 (ed. Jones, VIII, pp. 158 and 160).
36. Pliny, *Natural History,* XXX, 109 (ed. Jones, VIII, p. 348).
37. Pliny, *Natural History,* XXXII, 119 (ed. Jones, VIII, p. 536).
38. esp. Dioscorides.
39. Wellmann, "Sextius Niger," 530–569. Stannard, 420–425.
40. Riddle, 119–122.
41. Dioscorides, V, 152–160.
42. Fabricius, 180–205.
43. *E.g.* al-Kindī, 120 and 125: ninth century A.D.
44. Galen, *Elements According to Hippocrates.* I, 9 (ed. Kühn, I, 485); *Commentary on Hippocrates' On the Nature of Man,* I, 7 (ed. Mewaldt, p. 22); *Simples,* I, 8; III, 13; and V, 1 (ed. Kühn, XI, 397, 573, and 704–706).
45. Aetius, I preface (ed. Olivieri, pp. 17–30).
46. Puschmann, passim. Brunet, passim.
47. Honoré, 257–286. Roby, xxii-xxviii.
48. Galen, XII, 958 (ed. Kühn).
49. Theophrastus, *Historia Plantarum,* III, 7. 4.
50. Paul of Aegina, IV, 11 (ed. Heiberg, I, p. 331).
51. Galen, XIII, 569 (ed. Kühn).
52. Curtis, 232–240.
53. Dioscorides, IV, 62 (bluebell); IV, 158 (narcissus); I, 108 (sumach); III, 105 (horehound); II, 124 (purselane); I, 69 (Corsican pine); IV, 135 (maidenhairfern); I, 39 (myrtle); IV, 23 (alkanet).
54. Galen, XII, 958 (ed. Kühn).
55. Theophrastus, *On Stones,* 56. Dioscorides, V, 88.
56. Theophrastus, *Historia Plantarum,* III, 7.4.

REFERENCES

PRIMARY TEXTS (Greek, Latin, Egyptian, Arabic):

Aetius of Amida: Olivieri, Alexander (ed.): *Aetii Amideni Libri Medicinales I-IV.* Leipzig, B. G. Teubner, 1935 (*Corpus Medicorum Graecorum* VIII 1). Greek text only.

Alexander of Tralles: (a) Brunet, F.: *Médecine et thérapeutique byzantines. Oeuvres médicales d'Alexandre de Tralles.* Paris, Paul Geuthner, 1933–1937; 4 vols. Volume, I: Introduction to Byzantine medicine; Vols. II–IV: Fench translation of the works of Alexander of Tralles. *(b)* Puschmann, Theodor (ed. and trans.): *Alexander von Tralles.* Vienna, 1878–1879; rptd. Amsterdam, Adolf M. Hakkert, 1963; 2 vols. Greek text and German translation.

Aristophanes: Bickley Rogers, Benjamin (ed. and trans.): *Aristophanes* Volume III: *The Lysistrata. The Thesmophoriazusae. The Ecclesiazusae. The Plutus.* Cambridge, Massachusetts: Harvard University Press, 1924. Greek Text and English translation (Loeb Classical Library, No. 180).

Aristotle: (a) Peck, A. L. (ed. and trans.): *Aristotle: Historia Animalium.* 2 vols. to date. Cambridge, Maasachusetts, Harvard University Press, 1965–1970. Greek text and English translation through *HA,* 581a. (Loeb Classical Library, Nos. 437–438). *(b)* Thompson, D'Arcy Wentworth (trans.): *The Works of Aristotle.* Volume IV: *Historia Animalium.* Oxford, Clarendon Press, 1910. English translation only.

Celsus: (a) Marx, F. (ed.): *A. Cornelii Celsi quae supersunt.* Leipzig, B. G. Teubner, 1915 (*Corpus Medicorum Latinorum* I). Latin text only. *(b)* Spencer, W. G. (ed. and trans.): *Celsus: De medicina.* 3 vols. Cambridge, Massachusetts, Harvard University Press, 1935–1938. Latin text and English translation.

Crateuas: Wellmann, Max (ed.): *Crateuae et Sextii Nigri Fragmenta.* In *Pedanii Dioscuridis Anazarbei De Materia Medica.* Volume III. Berlin, Weidmann, 1914, pp. 139–148. Greek text only.

Dioscorides and Pseudo-Dioscorides: Wellmann, Max (ed.): *Pedanii Dioscuridis Anazarbei De Materia Medica.* 3 vols. Berlin, Weidmann, 1906–1914; rptd. 1958. Greek text only. Pseudo-Dioscorides edited as *RV.*

Egyptian Medical Texts; (a) Hildegard von Deines, Hermann Grapow, and Wolfhart Westendorf (eds. and trans.): *Übersetzung der medizinischen Texte.* 2 vols. Berlin, Akademie-Verlag, 1958 (*Grundriss der Medizin der alten Ägypter,* IV 1 and 2). German translation and occasional transliterations of the Egyptian texts. *(b)* Hildegard von Deines and Hermann Grapow, *Wörterbuch der ägyptischen Drogennamen.* Berlin, Akademie-Verlag, 1959 (*Grundriss der Medizin der alten Ägypter* VI). The "dictionary." Egyptian transliterations.

Galen: (a) Kühn, C. G. (ed.): *Claudii Galeni Opera omnia.* 20 vols. in 22. Leipzig, Cnoblichius, 1821–1833; rptd. Hildesheim, Georg Olms, 1964–1965. Greek texts with Latin translations. *(b)* Mewaldt, J. (ed.): *Galeni In Hippocratis De natura hominis.* Leipzig, B. G. Teubner, 1914 (in *Corpus Medicorum Graecorum* V 9, 1). Greek text only.

Herodotus: Godley, A. D. (ed. and trans.): *Herodotus.* 4 vols. Cambridge, Massachusetts, Harvard University Press, 1920–1925. Greek text and English translation (Loeb Classical Library).

Hesiod: Evelyn-White, Hugh G. (ed. and trans.): *Hesiod. The Homeric Hymns and Homerica.* Cambridge, Massachusetts, Harvard University Press, 1914. Greek text and English translation (Loeb Classical Library).

Hippocrates: (*a*) Littré, E. (ed. and trans.): *Oeuvres complètes d'Hippocrate.* Paris, 1839–1861; rptd. Amsterdam, Adolf M. Hakkert, 1973–1982. 10 vols. Greek text with French translation. (*b*) Jones, W. H. S., and Withington, E. T. (eds. and trans.): *Hippocrates.* 4 vols. Cambridge, Massachusetts, Harvard University Press, 1923–1931. Greek texts with English translation (Loeb Classical Library).

al-Kindī: Levey, Martin (trans.): *The Medical Formulary or Aqrābādhīn of al-Kindī.* Madison, Wisconsin, University of Wisconsin Press, 1966. Facsimiles of Arabic text with English translation and commentary.

Oribasius: Raeder, J. (ed.): *Oribasii Collectionum Medicarum reliquiae.* 4 vols. Leipzig, B. G. Teubner, 1928–1933 (*Corpus Medicorum Graecorum* VI 1, 1–2). Greek text only.

Paul of Aegina: Heiberg, I. L. (ed.): *Paulis Aegineta.* 2 vols. Leipzig, B. G. Teubner, 1921–1924 (*Corpus Medicorum Graecorum* IX 1–2). Greek text only.

Plato: Fowler, Harold North: *Plato: Euthyphro. Apology. Crito. Phaedo. Phaedrus.* Cambridge, Massachusetts, Harvard University Press, 1914. Greek text with English translation (Loeb Classical Library).

Pliny: (*a*) Mayhoff, C., and Ian, L. (eds.): *C. Plini Secundi Naturalis historiae.* 6 vols. Leipzig, Teubner, 1865–1898. Latin text only. (*b*) Rackham, H., Jones, W. H. S., and Eichholz, D. E. (eds. and trans.): *Pliny: Natural History.* 10 vols. Cambridge, Massachusetts, Harvard University Press, 1938–1962. Latin text with English translation (Loeb Classical Library).

Pre-Socratic Philosophers: *(a)* Diels, Hermann, and Kranz, Walther (eds. and trans.): *Die Fragmente der Vorsokratiker*. Edition 6. 3 vols. Berlin, Weidmann, 1954. Greek texts with German translation. *(b)* Kirk, G. S., and Raven, J. E. (eds., trans. [selections], commentary).: *The Presocratic Philosophers*. Cambridge, University Press, 1960. Selected Greek texts with English translations and commentaries.

Theocritus: Gow, A. S. F. (ed., trans., with commentary): *Theocritus*. Edition 2. 2 vols. Cambridge, University Press, 1952. Greek text with English translation and detailed commentary.

Theophrastus: (a) Hort, Arthur (ed. and trans.): *Theophrástus: Enquiry into Plants and Minor Works On Odours and Weather Signs*. 2 vols. Cambridge, Massachusetts, Harvard University Press, 1916. Greek text with English translation (Loeb Classical Library). *(b)* Eichholz D. E. (ed., trans., and commentary): *Theophrastus: De lapidibus*. Oxford, Clarendon Press, 1965. Greek text, with translation and detailed commentary on Theophrastus' *On Stones*.

SECONDARY LITERATURE

Adkins, A. W. H.: From the Many to the One. Ithaca, New York, Cornell University Press, 1970.

Bryan, Cyril P.: Ancient Egyptian Medicine: The Papyrus Ebers. London, 1930; rptd. Chicago, Ares Press, 1974.

Curtis, Robert I.: In defense of Garum. Classical Journal, *78*:232–240, 1983.

Daube, David.: The mediocrity of Celsus. Classical Journal, *70*:41–42, 1974.

Evans-Pritchard, E. E.: Witchcraft, Oracles and Magic among the Azande. Oxford, Clarendon Press, 1937.

Fabricius, Cajus: *Galens Exzerpte aus älteren Pharmakologen*. Berlin, Walter de Gruyter, 1972.

Fraser, P. M.: Ptolemaic Alexandria. 3 vols. Oxford, Clarendon Press, 1972.

Ghalioungui, Paul: The House of Life (Per Ankh): Magic and Medical Science in Ancient Egypt. Edition 2. Amsterdam, B. M. Israël, 1973.

Harig, G.: Anfänge der theoretischen Pharmakologie im Corpus Hippocraticum. *In* Grmek, M. D. (ed.): Hippocratica: Actes du Colloque hippocratique de Paris 1978. Paris, Editions CNRS, 1980, 223–246.

Honoré, Tony: Tribonian. Ithaca, New York, Cornell Uni versity Press, 1978.

Lefebvre, G. Essai sur la médecine Egyptienne de l'époque Pharaonique. Paris, Presses Universitaires de France, 1956.

Lloyd, G. E. R.: The Hippocratic question. Classical Quarterly, 25:171–192, 1975.

Lloyd, G. E. R.: Magic, Reason and Experience. Studies in the Origins and Development of Greek Science. Cambridge, University Press, 1979.

Lloyd, G. E. R.: Polarity and Analogy. Two Types of Argumentation in Early Greek Thought. Cambridge, University Press, 1966.

Majno, Guido: The Healing Hand. Man and Wound in the Ancient World. Cambridge, Massachusetts, Harvard University Press, 1975.

Onians, Richard Broxton: The Origins of European Thought. Cambridge, University Press, 1951.

Riddle, John M.: Dioscorides. *In* Gillispie C. C. (ed.): Dictionary of Scientific Biography. Volume 4. New York, Scribner's, 1971, 119–123.

Roby, Henry John: An Introduction to the Study of Justinian's Digest. Cambridge, University Press, 1886.

Scarborough, John: Roman Medicine. Ithaca, New York, Cornell University Press, 1969; rptd. 1976.

Scarborough, John: Theophrastus on herbals and herbal remedies. Journal of the History of Biology, *11*:358–385, 1978.

Scarborough, John: Theoretical assumptions in Hippocratic pharmacology. *In* Lasserre, F., and Mudry, P. (eds.): Actes du Colloque hippocratique de Lausanne 1981. Lausanne, Université, 1983, pages 275–293.

Scarborough, John, and Nutton, Vivian: The Preface of Dioscorides' *Materia Medica:* Introduction, Translation, Commentary. Transactions and Studies of the College of Physicians of Philadelphia, *4*:187–227, 1982.

Sigerist, Henry E.: A History of Medicine. Volume 1: Primitive and Archaic Medicine, New York, Oxford University Press, 1951.

Smith, Wesley D.: The Hippocratic Tradition. Ithaca, New York, Cornell University Press, 1945.

Solecki, Ralph S.: Shanidar IV, A Neanderthal flower burial in northern Iraq. Science, *190*:880–881, 1975.

Stannard, Jerry: Pliny and Roman botany. Isis, *56*:420–425, 1965.

Wellmann, Max: Sextius Niger. Eine Quellenuntersuchung zu Dioskorides. Hermes, *24*:530–569, 1889.

III

THEORETICAL ASSUMPTIONS IN HIPPOCRATIC PHARMACOLOGY

Prefatory Remarks

Early in the history of man, the special properties of certain plants and other substances had been recognized for their medicinal qualities. One may assume that such qualities were regarded as part of the realm of "magic" (however defined)[1], but as early as Neanderthal Man in northern Iraq about 60,000 years ago, there were known herbs used for their healing powers[2]. Drugs and herbs of various kinds were an integral portion of the medical systems of ancient Mesopotamia[3], as well as the flourishing practice of a particular sort of medicine in ancient Egypt[4], although modern students remain baffled by how ancient Egyptians "explained" actions of their pharmaceuticals—if they sought answers to such questions. Any connections between the medical approaches of the ancient Near Eastern cultures, and the emergence of Greek medicine,

[1] G.E.R. Lloyd, *Magic, Reason and Experience* (Cambridge, 1979), 40-41, 44-45, and 150. Galen, *Compounding Drugs According to Place [on the Body]*, VI, 8 (ed. Kühn, XII, 966), quoting Herophilus, remarks that "drugs are the hands of the gods".

[2] Ralph S. Solecki, *Shanidar IV, a Neanderthal Flower Burial in Northern Iraq*, Science, 190 (1975), 880-881.

[3] See esp. R. Labat, *La pharmacopée au service de la piété (Tablette assyrienne inédite)*, Semitica, 3 (1950), 1-18; J.V.K. Wilson, *The Nimrud Wine Lists* (London, 1972), 74-76; several works by R. Campbell Thompson, including *The Assyrian Herbal* (London, 1924), *On the Chemistry of Ancient Assyrians* (London, 1925), and *A Dictionary of Assyrian Chemistry and Geology* (London, 1936); A. Leo Oppenheim, *Ancient Mesopotamia* (Chicago, 1964), 289-305 [with bibliographical reffs.]; Henry E. Sigerist, *A History of Medicine*, Vol. I: *Primitive and Archaic Medicine* (New York, 1951), 409-425 [with bibliographical reffs.]; and Guido Majno, *The Healing Hand: Man and Wound in the Ancient World* (Cambridge, Mass., 1975), 61-64.

[4] Paul Ghalioungui, *The House of Life (Per Ankh): Magic and Medical Science in Ancient Egypt*, 2nd ed. (Amsterdam, 1973), 139-149; Majno, *Healing Hand*, 108-124.

must remain in the category of speculation[5], but once we observe Hippocratic medicine in its developed form by the fifth and fourth centuries B.C., it is well equipped with pharmacology. Particularly prominent in the pharmacy and the pharmacodynamics of Hippocratic therapeutics are the common herbs of Asia Minor and the Near East, which can be paralleled with earlier botanicals in Mesopotamia and Egypt, but Greek physicians had added something new with a curious and insistent clarity: a theory of how drugs "worked". Like many other facets of Hippocratic medicine, the origins of pharmaceutical theory are to be found, at least in part, in the context of Greek philosophy, and the application of certain precepts of philosophical thinking to pharmacodynamics[6].

Aristotelian Drug Theory: A Backdrop for Hippocratic Pharmacology

In the Pseudo-Aristotelian *Problems*, one finds a valiant attempt at least to pose good questions concerning the actions of drugs, called *pharmaka* in Greek, a term that carried several nuances, ranging from "beneficial effect" to "poison"[7]. In the *Problems*, the author asks the all-important "why" about drugs: why do some drugs relax the stomach and not the bladder, and others the bladder and not the stomach? Is it true

[5] Georg Harig and Jutta Kollesch, *Neue Tendenzen in der Forschung zur Geschichte der antiken Medizin und Wissenschaft*, Philologus, 121 (1977), 114-136. Connectedness can be admitted, but evidence does not permit final statements on the matter as presumed in J.B. de C.M. Saunders, *The Transitions from Ancient Egyptian to Greek Medicine* (Lawrence, Kansas, 1963), and R.O. Steuer and J.B. de C.M. Saunders, *Ancient Egyptian and Cnidian Medicine* (Berkeley, 1959).

[6] This view is in contrast with that of Georg Harig, *Anfänge der theoretischen Pharmakologie im Corpus Hippocraticum*, in *Hippocratica: Actes du Colloque hippocratique de Paris* (4-9 septembre 1978), ed. M.D. Grmek (Paris, 1980), 223-245, esp. 235-236. It should be added, however, that Harig's study is an excellent beginning to the study of the almost untapped resources of Hippocratic pharmacology, and his idea of "Primary" and "Secondary" qualities as they are perceived for *pharmaka* has great merit, and is most attractive as an "operating thesis" at this stage of the modern study of ancient pharmacy. Harig has also argued for this view of pharmaceuticals in his excellent *Bestimmung der Intensität im medizinischen System Galens* (Berlin, 1974). Harig, *Anfänge*, 223-225, provides the basic bibliography of works on Hippocratic pharmacology. One may profitably contrast Harig's view with the clear links assembled by Lloyd, *Magic*, 44-45, but the connections include far more than simply philosophy.

[7] Φάρμακον as "poison": Thucydides, II, 48; Plato, *Phaedo*, 115a. Φάρμακον as "beneficial drug": Homer, *Iliad*, IV, 218 and V, 401; *Odyssey*, IV, 230, and X, 394; Soranus, *Gynecology*, IV, 38. 4 (ed. J. Ilberg [*CMG* IV, 1927], p. 151); and Galen, *Hygiene*, IV, 5. 12 (ed. K. Koch [*CMG* V 4, 2, 1923], p. 117). Φάρμακον as "magic potion" or "spell": Homer, *Odyssey*, IV, 220. Φάρμακον as "dye" or "color": Herodotus, I, 98. Φάρμακον as "chemical reagent": Otto Lagerkrantz, ed., *Papyrus Graecus Holmiensis: Recepte für Silber, Steine und Purpur* (Uppsala/Leipzig, 1913), XIII, line 45 (p. 23) and XXII, line 10 (p. 34). Φάρμαξις as "treatment of metals": Plutarch, *Moralia: Oracles at Delphi*, 395B [bronze]. Φάρμαξις as "medical treatment": Plato, *Philebus*, 46a. Φάρμακος as "scapegoat": Aristophanes, *Frogs*, 733.

that anything which is naturally moist and full of water, if it has the properties of a drug, relaxes the bladder[8]? Having posed his questions, the writer attempts to answer them: "It is in the bladder that the unconcocted moisture settles... the bladder is a receptacle for any moisture not concocted by the stomach... such moisture does not remain there but passes away without undergoing or causing any change[9]." Then the writer introduces a fundamental concept, the Theory of Elements, which will help "explain why" such drugs act as they do: "... anything which is of the nature of earth, if it has the properties of a drug, relaxes the stomach. For it is to the stomach that anything of an earthy nature is carried, so that, if it has any motive power *[kinētikon]*, it causes a disturbance in the stomach[10]". Important in the milieu of Peripatetic thinking, and thus to the author of *Problems*, is the notion of "power" *(dynamis)*[11], which can be well rendered as "property" as it applies to pharmaceuticals[12].

It may be argued that these theoretical foundations for Greek pharmacology emerged with the Hippocratic writers[13], but in the Hippocratic *corpus*, one finds assumptions of theories, yet little that qualifies as definition and development of drug theory[14]. By contrast, there are indications in several works of the Aristotelian *corpus*[15], particularly the *Problems*, that show decisions to state some pharmacological conclusions, based upon empirical evidence as well as upon certain assumptions about *dynameis* of the Elements. Moreover, once the author of *Problems* has incorporated the Elements in his theory of pharmacology, he then

---

[8] (Pseudo) Aristotle, *Problems*, 863b29-33.

[9] *Problems*, 863b34-35.

[10] *Problems*, 863b35-36 – 864a1-2.

[11] Δύναμις as "elementary force," viz. heat, cold, etc.: Aristotle, *Parts of Animals*, 646a14 and 650a5. Cf. the Hippocratic *Ancient Medicine*, 16. Δύναμις as "power" or "faculty": Aristotle, *Politics*, 1309a35.

[12] This is particularly the case in Theophrastus, *Historia Plantarum, e.g.* VIII, 11.1. *Historia Plantarum*, IX, is also especially illuminating in this respect. See John Scarborough, *Theophrastus on Herbals and Herbal Remedies*, Journal of the History of Biology, 11 (1978), 353-385.

[13] Harig, *Anfänge der theoretischen Pharmakologie*, in *Actes du Colloque hippocratique de Paris 1978* (Paris, 1980), 226-229. But some scholars believe that Aristotle was heavily influenced by Hippocratic medicine, *e.g.* W. Jaeger, *Aristotle's Use of Medicine as a Model of Method in his Ethics*, Journal of Hellenic Studies, 77 (1957), 54-61, and A. Preus, *Science and Philosophy in Aristotle's Biological Works* (Hildesheim/New York, 1975), 26-27 with nn. 72-81, although Preus recognizes Aristotle's use with "easy confidence information gained from the medical tradition and perhaps from personal contact with medical men (his father had been a doctor)" [p. 27].

[14] Harig, *Anfänge* passim, would argue that the "theory" is that of "primary" and "secondary" qualities. One can, of course, make note that Hippocratic pharmacy sought reliable dosages, terms in botanical recipes, and practical proportion in measuring various ingredients in compound medicines. Julius Berendes, *Das Apothekenwesen* (Stuttgart, 1907; rptd. Hildesheim, 1967), 30-32.

[15] Esp. *Historia Animalium*, 594a24 and 612a3-34 (observations of animals and their "instinctive" use of curative plants); *Metaphysics*, 1015a25; *Eudemian Ethics*, 1227a19-20; *Nichomachaean Ethics*, 1137a24-26; *Physics*, 195a1-2 (= *Metaphysics*, 1013b1-2).

proceeds to further definitions that specify particular actions of drugs. It is as if we are looking at a "blueprint" for drug theory here in the *Problems*, a series of assumptions taken for granted by later physicians from the Hippocratics through Galen and the later Byzantine medical writers.

Specific drugs are cited as the author of *Problems* refines his theory of drug action. It is known that *helleboros*[16] effects the upper digestive tract, while other *pharmaka*, like *thapsias ho opos*[17] and *elatērion*[18], have an effect on both upper and lower parts of the gastrointestinal system, while such herbs as *skammōnia*[19] affect only the lower bowels. The explanation proffered is the notion of Qualities, known from a long history in Greek philosophy going back to Anaxagoras[20]. The writer says that those drugs which have power over the stomach are either hot or cold, and those that

---

[16] Simply ἐλλέβορος in *Problems*, 864a4. Theophrastus, *Historia Plantarum*, IX, 9. 2, has two kinds, a "black hellebore" and a "white hellebore," suggesting the information available to the author of *Problems* was not as detailed. Since *Problems*, 864a4, says that ἐλλέβορος is used as an emetic, one may presume that this is the "white" hellebore (*Veratrum album* L.), commonly used as an emetic, according to Dioscorides, IV, 148 (ed. Wellmann). An alkaloid, cevadine, is contained in the root, and is still employed in veterinary medicine (as part of a mixture called veratrine) as an emetic for pigs and cattle. Scarborough, *Theophrastus*, Journal of the History of Biology, 11 (1978), 361-362. The Hippocratic writers generally have a clear notion of the actions of both hellebores (*Veratrum album* L., and *Helleboros niger* L), as numerous references indicate (Littré, X, 628-630 [index reffs.]).

[17] "The juice of θαψία" (*Problems*, 864a6), probably the *Thapsia garganica* L., known as the "deadly carrot" to Greek pharmacology. Dioscorides, IV, 153. Theophrastus, *Historia Plantarum*, IX, 9. 1 and 6. Pliny, *Natural History*, XIII, 124. This often tall perennial (from 30 to 250 cm.) has large, yellowish umbels and a distinctive fruit, oblong or elliptic, notched at the base and apex and is equipped with conspicuous lateral wings, 3 to 6 mm. broad. The root yields a resin (esp. in Spain, viz. the "Spanish turpethroot") employed in making plasters. The chemistry of *T. garganica* seems not to have been investigated. See John Scarborough, *Nicander's Toxicology, I: Snakes*, Pharmacy in History, 19 (1977), 3-23 esp. 11 [*T. garganica*].

[18] *Problems*, 864a5, simply has ἐλατήριον, which could be the "squirting cucumber" (*Ecballium elaterium* A. Rich): Theophrastus, *Historia Plantarum*, IV, 5. 1, and Dioscorides, IV, 150, in addition to the Hippocratic *Barren Women*, 238 (Littré, VIII, 443), or the drug made from the plant, as in Theophrastus, *Historia Plantarum*, IX, 9. 4. The name in Greek means "driver", which said graphically what this drug could do to the bowels. Scarborough, *Theophrastus*, Journal of the History of Biology, 11 (1978), 366. *E. elaterium* remains part of folk medicine, and the vines are cultivated, with the juice of the unripe fruits used as a purgative.

[19] *Problems*, 864a4: σκαμμωνία, which is probably the scammony (*Convolvulus scammonia* L.), also mentioned in Theophrastus, *Historia Plantarum*, IX, 20. 5, and Dioscorides, IV, 170, as well as Nicander, *Alexipharmaca*, 565. Greek and Roman physicians valued scammony as a purgative, and it continued to be used until quite recently. Its chemistry explains why it was valued for so long: constituents include starch, ipuranol, a reducing sugar, a methylesculetin, dihydroxycinnamic acid, and resin (8-13%). In the folk medicine of the Near East, the resin ("Levant Scammony Resin", "Levant Scammony", and other names) remains in use as a cathartic, and it causes the evacuation of large quantities of water. Sometimes the dried root is exported from Syria and Turkey. Scarborough, *Theophrastus*, 383.

[20] Cf. Aristotle, *Metaphysics*, 1083a11; *Physics*, 187a32 and 187b6-8; *Categories*, 8b26; *Nichomachaean Ethics*, 1173a15; the Hippocratic *On Fleshes*, 2 (Littré, VIII, 584 = R. Joly, ed., in *Hippocrate*, Tome XIII [Paris, 1978], 188), and *Nature of Man*, 5. See esp. G.E.R. Lloyd, *The Hot and the Cold, the Dry and the Wet in Greek Philosophy*, Journal of Hellenic

are characterized by heat are carried into the upper body once these *pharmaka* have entered the upper digestive tract, especially the stomach. The function of such hot drugs, so the author continues, is to melt anything in the upper body which is alien to them (viz. the *pharmaka*). If the *pharmakon* is too strong, it then takes the products of melting back down into the stomach, thus producing much heat and engendering much breath, which in turn, checks the effects of the drug and causes vomiting. Cold drugs, oppositely, since they are heavier, descend into the lower digestive tract, where they pass into ducts which lead into the upper body, and thence perform similar actions as the hot drugs. Drugs which do both are a combination of hot and cold, or as the author writes, "possess both qualities and are a mixture of hot and cold, and are the compound drugs now made by physicians[21]".

Once our author has Elements and Qualities in his theory of drug action, he then proceeds to ask further questions about particular sorts of qualities[22]. He notes that some drugs have a purging effect, while others that surpass them in bitterness and astringency do not have this effect. It would appear, so the writer says by way of a corollary question, that such Qualities (here perhaps also rendered "properties" as it shades into what *dynameis* do) result, not so much from Qualities *per se*, but because the drugs in question have not been "concocted"[23]. Here the writer is reflecting a puzzling and often-observed phenomenon in drug-therapy: why some substances are "foods" while others are "drugs", while others combine the properties of foods and drugs. In some respects the explanation provided by the author of *Problems* is unwieldy, but singularly satisfying; he is, of course, attempting a firm definition of "drug".

Anything which is excessively hot or cold, even though it might be small in bulk or quantity (*onkoi*, or "minute particles")[24], would overcome the "natural heat of the animal"[25], and being easily dissolved by the two parts of the digestive tract, would thereby act as drugs. Thus such substances *are* drugs. The drugs pass to the veins by the same ducts as do foods, but the drugs are not concocted, so that they overcome the natural heat of the animal, rather than being overcome by it, and thus pass through the system, carrying with them any obstruction, and the process is labelled purging, or "cleaning" *(katharsis)*[26]. Thus such materials as

Studies, 84 (1964), 92-106; S. Sambursky, *The Physical World of Late Antiquity* (London, 1962), 34-44; and W.K.C. Guthrie, *History of Greek Philosophy*, Vol. II (Cambridge, 1965), 286.

[21] *Problems*, 864ª19-23.

[22] *Problems*, 864ª24-37.

[23] *Problems*, 864ª28: ἄπεπτα.

[24] H.B. Gottschalk, *Heraclides of Pontus* (Oxford, 1980), 37-57. John Scarborough, *The Drug Lore of Asclepiades of Bithynia*, Pharmacy in History, 17 (1975), 43-57.

[25] *Problems*, 864ª29-30.

[26] *Problems*, 864ª34: κάθαρσις.

metals—copper and silver, and the like—ought to make good drugs, since they are not concocted easily by the body. Some foods, namely oil, milk, and honey, can act as purgatives, but do so because of their bulk when prescribed as purges: the body, so to speak, has an excess of milk, which cannot be concocted and thereby acts as a purge, and therefore, no food is a drug, since it acts like a drug only from its quantity, not from a particular property (here *dynamis*)[27]. Moreover, drugs have certain obvious characteristics—astringency, bitterness, and an unpleasant smell—which define them as opposites of foods, and foods become concocted and come to be part of the body, which drugs do not. Thus the author's conclusion: "The [substance] which, according to its own nature, is not overcome [by the body's heat] and which enters the veins, and because of its excess heat or cold [is not concocted]: this is the *physis* of a drug[28]."

Hippocratic Writers and Drug Theory

The authors of the various tracts of the Hippocratic *corpus* indeed reflect the notion of how Elements aid in determining the nature of the numerous *pharmaka* known and employed, but a greater sophistication concerning the properties of drugs characterizes the drug therapy of the Hippocratic physician, as contrasted with the occasionally awkward and self-defined drug theory in the pseudo-Aristotelian *Problems*. In terms of foods, Hippocratic authors do mirror the commonly-held notion that some foods act like drugs, while most foods do not, but the medical implications of that overall notion has developed into a clear idea of dietetics[29], as well as the application of sound diet in aiding the patient's recovery from an illness. Both treatment by opposites and treatment by similars are carried through by the Hippocratic physician[30], who seems to have understood the definition of "drug" and "food" much as is stated in the pseudo-Aristotelian *Problems*. Other factors, however, have been added to the basic drug theory set down by Aristotle and his students, especially in regard to the 200-odd plants employed by the pharmacy in the full scope of the Hippocratic *corpus*. Part of the Hippocratic physician's underlying assumptions about how drugs "worked" would be the primary Elements as seen in pseudo-Aristotle and elsewhere, but the

---

[27] *Problems*, 864b5: οὐδὲ γὰρ διὰ δύναμιν καθαίρει.

[28] *Problems*, 864b9-12.

[29] See esp. I.M. Lonie, *A Structural Pattern in Greek Dietetics and the Early History of Greek Medicine*, Medical History, 21 (1977), 235-260.

[30] Walter Artelt, *Studien zur Geschichte der Begriffe "Heilmittel" und "Gift"* (Leipzig, 1937; rptd. Darmstadt, 1968), 56, with nn. 8-9.

Hippocratic doctor has a primary goal in the restoration of a balance *(krasis)* in the patient's body through the application of drugs[31].

There is ample evidence in the *corpus* for the notion of Elements accompanied by Qualities, but apparently the Hippocratic physician believed that these two facets of a theory of how drugs worked were insufficient to explain particular drug actions in the human body. Hippocratic pharmacodynamics noted that *krasis* of the Elements would be a necessary goal, as would a *krasis* of Qualities, but Hippocratic pharmacology has added a third theoretical aspect: the *krasis* of Humors, which were presumed to be particular and specific to human beings in terms of medical treatment[32]. Little emphasis is placed on the *krasis* of the Qualities, except that the Hot, Cold, Wet, and Dry are assumed, much as are the four basic Elements of Fire, Air, Water, and Earth. It is, indeed, rather curious that none of the Hippocratic writers seems to have attempted a definition of "what a drug is" in the manner of the pseudo-Aristotelian *Problems*, but a delineating characteristic of drug therapy in the Hippocratic *corpus* is an absence of baldly-stated theory, and the assumption by the writers that such an underlying theory would be obvious and self-evident, given the manner in which the drugs were applied and used in illness.

A dual theory thus becomes typical of Hippocratic pharmacology, and drugs were used with the assumption of a restoration of a *krasis*, particularly of Elements and Humors. Each drug was presumed to have particular properties in terms of this dual theory, and the etiology of a specific disease, once diagnosed, would determine particular types of drug therapeutics. An example taken at random illustrates the general principles. In *On Regimen,* II, 54, one notes that the drug called *thymos* heats and dries[33], and would be very suitable for the restoration of *krasis* in a disease in which there was an excess of phlegm, presumed to be wet and cold. The *thymos* would, by its nature, expell the excess of phlegm, and

---

[31] For a summary of some of these points, see Jerry Stannard, *Hippocratic Pharmacology,* Bulletin of the History of Medicine, 35 (1961), 497-518.

[32] Karl Deichgräber, *Hippokrates De humoribus in der Geschichte der griechischen Medizin* (Wiesbaden, 1972), 20-27 [this work probably not directly linked with the Pseudo-Aristotelian *Problems*, but possibly with Diocles of Carystos].

[33] *On Regimen*, II, 54 (Littré, VI, 560 = R. Joly, ed., *Hippocrate: Du régime*, II, 54. 6 [Paris, 1967], p. 53), also notes that θύμον is a good bowel purge and diuretic, as well as having properties to expel phlegm: θύμον θερμόν, διαχωρεῖ καὶ οὐρᾶται, ἄγει δὲ φλεγματώδεα. The plant is most likely *Thymus capitatus* Hoffm. and Link., the so-called Conehead or Cretan thyme. Cf. Dioscorides, III, 36; Theophrastus, *Historia Plantarum*, VI, 2. 3; and Aristotle, *Historia Animalium*, $626^{b}21$. Most species in *Thymus* (including the common *T. vulgaris* L., "thyme," and *T. serpyllum* L., "creeping thyme") have an essential oil that contains thymol, which continues to be used as a linament, as well as a stimulant and for the relief of stomach upsets; the dried leaves are widely used as a condiment in flavoring meat dishes. Thymol has antiseptic properties: Majno, *Healing Hand*, 218-219, with reffs. Harig, *Anfänge*, 241, has θύμον as part of his list of simples assigned with "primary qualities"; Harig identifies the plant as *Satureja thymbra* L.

would be the "drug of choice" in this case. The Hippocratic writer does not tell us *why* the *thymos* would expel the unnecessary phlegm, but the comparison of this passage (as well as many others in the *corpus*) with an assumed theory of Elements, Humors, and to some degree of Qualities, as laid down in the works of Aristotle and his school, suggests that the theory of drug-action laid down in *Problems* is taken for granted. There is certainly no agreement about the *number* of Humors, but Humors *per se* were almost continually evoked[34].

Some Illustrations of Pharmacology in the Hippocratic corpus

In a study of limited scope, concentrating upon the background of theoretical pharmacy and pharmacology, only a few examples can be offered to illustrate the mode of understanding and use of drugs in many tracts in the *corpus*, but some particulars will also suggest that there was no basic uniformity among the Hippocratic writers concerning assumed theories of pharmacology. One notes that Humors and Elements are prominent, and that Qualities are assumed without much elaboration. In *Diseases* III, one reads a carefully prescribed set of treatments for various types of *pleuritis* (probably pleurisy)[35], which the author likens in some ways to *phrenitis*. The format of these pharmaceutical treatments takes the well-known sequence of the "if-then" formula, and one reads that if the patient receives care on the first or second day after the attack, and if the bowel movement has been clean and easy with but a little bile, then the physician is to administer a clyster (enema) using *thapsia*[36]. But if the patient is bilious, then the doctor should administer a good cholagogue, while if the expectoration is not bilious, one should not give such a drug since, as the author puts it, "the expectorant would not have the power to produce upward"[37], and the patient would suffer from labored breathing or suffocation by the seventh or ninth day; the corollaries with the pseudo-Aristotelian admonition about how the *dynamis* of a drug "overcomes" something in the body seem apparent. If, however, pain has occurred in the ribs and in the belly, the physician administers an enema (not specified), has the patient fast (time not specified), and then gives the

[34] C.R.S. Harris, *The Heart and the Vascular System in Ancient Greek Medicine* (Oxford, 1973), 74, and 216-217. E.D. Phillips, *Greek Medicine* (London, 1973), 48-52. Henry E. Sigerist, *A History of Medicine*, Vol. II: *Early Greek, Hindu and Persian Medicine* (New York, 1961), 318-325.

[35] *Diseases*, III, 16. 11-17 (ed. Paul Potter, *Hippokrates: Über die Krankheiten III* [Berlin, 1980; *CMG* I 2, 3], pp. 90-93 = Littré, VII, 148-150).

[36] *Diseases*, III, 16. 11 (ed. Potter, 90). See n. 17 above.

[37] *Diseases*, III, 16. 12 (ed. Potter, 90): Τὸ πτύσμα οὐ δυνήσεται ἄνω ἀνιέναι.

patient a drink containing *aristolochia*[38], *hyssōpos*[39], *kyminon*[40], *silphion*[41], *mēkōna leukē*[42] and *anthos chalkou*[43]. Why these *pharmaka*? All are astringents, suggesting that the Hippocratic physician is attempting to dry and heat in counteraction to the symptoms of pleurisy (the "symptoms", one should add, *were* the disease) signaled by pain in the belly and around the ribs, with the assumption that the pain would be caused by too much bile. The writer also says that "one ought to prepare these drugs before the first treatment[44], but that there are other things the doctor ought to do as well: "for the *dynamis* of the patient"[45], the physician should wash the patient's head with copious amounts of warm (hot?) water, and if a crisis occurs, then the physician treats spots with wet, heated bandages, afterwards rubbing with oil. But if the affections "descend like a storm"[46], the doctor should rest the patient with the following treatment so as not to make the condition worse: give boiled barley-water[47], thickened and sweetened with a little honey; after baths, give warm, sweet wine mixed with water in a small cup with a narrow opening; if coughing occurs, the patient is to drink and to spit up as much as possible "to be moist," so that the lung will be wetter and the coughs

---

[38] Ἀριστολοχία, a birthwort, *Aristolochia rotunda* L. Containing aristolochic acid, which is mildly toxic, this extract has been used as an aromatic bitter; in modern folk medicine in the Near East, *A. rotunda* (roots) are employed against intestinal worms, as a diuretic, and for the control of menstruation. Cf. Celsus, *De medicina*, V, 18. 7B; Galen, *Antidotes*, I, 14 (ed. Kühn, XIV, 82); Dioscorides, III, 4 (ed. Wellmann, Vol. II, pp. 6-8). Scarborough, *Nicander's Toxicology, I*, Pharmacy in History, 19 (1977), 11.

[39] Although the Greek ὕσσωπος would seem to suggest "hyssop", the plant is more likely one of the *Origanum* spp., esp. *O. vulgare* L., "sweet marjoram", or possibly *Majorana hortensis* Moench. Dioscorides, III, 25 (ed. Wellmann, Vol. II, pp. 35-36) notes that there are two kinds of ὕσσωπος: one grows in Cilicia, the other grows in gardens. Folk medicine uses decoctions of the leaves of *O. vulgare* as a mild anodyne, *e.g.* for toothaches.

[40] Κύμινον, *Cuminum cyminum* L., "cumin". In modern times, the seeds are used widely for flavoring, particularly in liqueurs, and as a constituent of curry powders. Cumin oil is used in perfumery (cumin oil is about 10% of the seeds). The plant contains pinene, dipentene, and cominic aldehyde, showing why modern veterinary medicine would still use the extract as an antispasmodic.

[41] Σίλφιον is one of the main "mystery plants" of classical pharmacology. Many guesses have been proposed, but most thus far have leaned toward a member of the onion or garlic family. A.C. Andrews, *The Silphium of the Ancients*, Isis, 33 (1941), 232-236. Scarborough, *Nicander's Toxicology, II: Spiders, Scorpions, Insects and Myriapods*, Pharmacy in History, 21 (1979), 3-34 and 73-92 [91 n. 369]. But it may be likely that the plant is an extinct species of the Asafoetida, related to *Ferula alliacea* Bois. of Iran, *F. assa-foetida* L. of eastern Iran and western Afghanistan. The coins of Greek Cyrene aid the solution by their stylized depictions of the plant, which was a major cash crop (though it only grew wild) for that city, before the plant's extinction. See E.S.G. Robinson, *Silphium*, in *Catalogue of the Greek Coins of Cyrenaica* (London, 1927), ccli-cclviii.

[42] This seems to be one of the poppies, perhaps another name for *Papaver somniferum* L., the major source of opium. Scarborough, *Theophrastus*, 370-373.

[43] Ἄνθος χαλκοῦ, "flowers of copper", a cuprous oxide. Potter, ed., *Diseases*, III, p. 128 (commentary).

[44] *Diseases*, III, 16. 13 (ed. Potter, 90).

[45] *Diseases*, III, 16. 13 (ed. Potter, 90): πρὸς δύναμιν.

[46] *Diseases*, III, 16. 13 (ed. Potter, 90): καταιγίζωσιν.

[47] *Diseases*, III, 16. 13 (ed. Potter, 90): πτισάνης χυλὸν κάθεφθον.

become fewer. Then the physician mixes the juice of a sweet or well wine-soaked *rhoie*[48] with a little goat's milk and honey, and this should be given to the patient in small amounts continuously during the day and through the night; sleep is to be prevented as much as possible so that the *katharsis* may be quick and complete.

The physician in *Diseases*, III, 16 is making several assumptions about his pharmacy and pharmacodynamics: he believes that the *dynamis* of the patient has to be guarded carefully, especially in light of the various astringent drugs that may be used (one notes that after the baths and after some warm wine, then the patient receives the juice of a pomegranate); he also thinks that a combination of astringents may prove to be more effective than single simples alone; he prescribes goat's milk and honey along with the pomegranate juice to bring about a *katharsis*, presuming—if the Aristotelian "blueprint" applies—that the foods in the compound will aid the cathartic effect by their presence as excess added to the *dynamis* of the pomegranate. The list of *pharmaka* in this short section of *Diseases* III is, in itself, suggestive of drug theory and some clear notion of pharmacodynamics that may have been inherited from folk medicine and then adapted into the dual theory that characterizes Hippocratic pharmacology as a whole.

The author of *Regimen in Health* appears to believe that the most valuable *pharmaka* are emetics and enemas[49]. Weather-theory is important, since the physician advises patients to use emetics in the six months of winter because these months are when the most phlegm is produced, and when diseases appear that attack the head and the body above the diaphragm. In the other six months of hot weather, the doctor advises the use of enemas because the weather is burning, the body is full of bile, which causes a heavy feeling in the groin and the knees and a "twisting of the bowels" (colic). Thus, in the summertime, the body has to be cooled, and the "humors that rise must be drawn downwards from these regions"[50]. Fat and moist patients are to receive enemas that are salty and thin, but those who are dry, lean, and weak, receive clysters that are greasy and thick. Oily or greasy enemas are to be made from milk, or water boiled with *erebinthoi*[51] or similar things, apparently other seedlike foodstuffs. On the other hand, the thin and salty clysters are made from brine and sea water.

---

[48] *Diseases*, III, 16. 13 (ed. Potter, 92): ῥοιή. This is the pomegranate, *Punica granatum* L. Harig, *Anfänge*, 242, lists ῥοιή among his "primary quality" drugs.

[49] *Regimen in Health*, V, 1-49 (ed. W.H.S. Jones in *Hippocrates*, Vol. IV [Cambridge, Mass., 1931; Loeb Classical Library], pp. 51-53).

[50] *Regimen in Health*, V, 10-12 (ed. Jones, 50; trans. Jones).

[51] *Regimen in Health*, V, 18 (ed. Jones, 50): ἐρέβινθος, *Cicer arietinum* L., the chickpea.

Regimen in Health also includes some interesting details on the preparation and use of emetics. One reads that the quantity of the emetic should be half a *cotyle*[52] of *hyssōpos* in a *chous*[53] of water, and if the patient actually consumed such an amount (about six pints, or 2.9 liters) he certainly would vomit. The writer of *Regimen in Health* says that one can make the mixture a little more palatable by pouring in some vinegar and adding a little salt: the patient is to drink the emetic slowly at first and then more quickly, apparently gulping it, "chugging" in the American idiom.

Again one is struck by the use of an excess of a mixture, in order to bring on a presumably desired result, and the use of foods as drugs may be a reflection of this author's reluctance to employ other, less well understood pharmaceuticals, which could have untoward effects quite undesirable. The author is apparently a physician, or perhaps a gymnastics expert[54], who believes in mild treatments, and the emetics and enemas he prescribes are gentle, with the possible exception of the *hyssōpos*: if the plant is one of the *Origanum* spp.[55], then the gentle action could be assumed, whereas if the plant mentioned here is true hyssop[56], then the effect on the patient would be a bit harsh. The modern observer is also struck by the almost total lack of theory in this section of *Regimen in Health*. Even the thought of "Humors" has to be assumed in translation, since the Greek text does not state this explicitly, although context would suggest that this is, indeed, what is meant. A vague notion of the Qualities and Elements seeps through, but the writer is far more interested in what might be called physiognomics[57], since his treatments are based upon "body-types", coupled with seasonal variations. *Pharmaka*, as such, play little role in the therapeutics of the author of *Regimen in Health.*

The *Diseases* III presents a careful and well-defined "if-then" pattern of pharmaceutical therapeutics, well ordered and with precise consideration and linkage with an overriding theory of *krasis* of Elements, Qualities, and Humors, particularly Elements and Humors. *Regimen in Health* represents an opposite tendency in the Hippocratic *corpus*, wherein the author has chosen not to emphasize either pharmaceuticals or the commonly-assumed theories of *krasis*, although the modern scholar can see aspects of those theories as the *Regimen in Health* presents a series of basic assumptions and admonitions on how a person is to stay healthy, using weather lore, physiognomics, and a few mild prescriptions for

---

52 This is about 1/2 pint or .27 liters.

53 Depending on various estimates, this is about 5 3/4 pints to 6 pints, or 2.9 liters to 3.2 liters.

54 Berendes, *Apothekenwesen*, 23-24.

55 See n. 39 above.

56 *Hyssopos officinalis* L.

57 See Elizabeth C. Evans, *Physiognomics in the Ancient World* (Philadelphia, 1969), esp. 17-28.

emetics and enemas, which would "free" or "cleanse" the body of excesses according to the season—a muted reflection of the theory of Balances of the Elements and Humors.

Conversely, when one considers the pharmacology of the Hippocratic *Wounds*, or the *Fistulas, Hemorrhoids, Diseases of Women*, and some other works in the *corpus*, there tumbles forth a veritable cacophony of drug lore, simples, occasional compounds, and numerous *pharmaka* used in almost every conceivable manner. It seems that the authors of these four tracts represent a contrary opinion among Hippocratic physicians, concerning *pharmaka*, than the viewpoint expressed in *Regimen in Health*. A modern observer might be tempted to call this tumbling pharmacology scattered and confused, at least at first glance, but careful analysis reveals that the writers of these four treatises have clear theories in mind regarding pharmaceuticals, and that there is a careful pattern of organization, quite similar to the "if-then" format of the pharmacotherapeutics in *Diseases* III. Some instances from *Wounds*, as well as a brief consideration of *Fistulas*, will serve to demonstrate the approaches to pharmacology in this type of Hippocratic tract.

The author of *Wounds*[58] favors a thin diet and mild treatment of recently contracted ulcers or wounds, and tells us that the general "drug of choice" for most wounds and ulcers is wine[59]—and recent research has confirmed the microbiological wisdom of this assertion[60]. The purpose of treatment is, of course, to bring the wound to suppuration as quickly as possible, and the writer notes that a wound becomes full of pus when the blood changes and takes on an excess of heat to become corrupt[61]. Wounds that are dry are closest to being "natural", so that the physician must do all he can to expell any "wet Humors" and restore the best, dry state. Bloody wounds are best treated—after the bleeding has ceased—with the application of dry sponges which are then wrapped in leaves and bound. Oil and emollients are generally not recommended. Purging, says the author, is good for those with wounds of the head, the belly, the joints, and those with wounds in danger of becoming gangrenous, or those wounds which require stitching up with sutures, but the wound is to be kept as dry as possible, using a sponge and assuming that summer is always better for prognosis in wounds than in the winter[62]. After considering other states of boils, wounds, spreading ulcers, deep wounds that have bone exposed, and the like[63], the author of *Wounds* comes to his

[58] *Ulcers* is the more "traditional" rendering of Περὶ ἑλκων into English; *Wounds* includes a greater variety of injuries in modern English than would *Ulcers*, hence the choice employed here.

[59] *Wounds*, 1 (Littré, VI, 400).

[60] Majno, *Healing Hand*, 186-188 with reffs.

[61] *Wounds*, 1 (ed. Littré, VI, 402).

[62] *Wounds*, 2 (ed. Littré, VI, 404).

[63] *Wounds*, 3-10 (ed. Littré, VI, 404-410).

pharmacology, the preparation of poultices, or as he writes, "poultices for swellings and inflammation of the parts surrounding the wound"[64]. Boiled *phlomos*[65], the raw leaves of the *triphyllon*[66], the boiled leaves of the *epipetron* and the *polion*[67], provide a suitable poultice if the wound needs cleansing, since, as the author says, "all these [drugs] have the power to cleanse"[68]. One can also prepare a good poultice by boiling the leaves of the *sykē*[69], the olive[70], and *prasion*[71], and another kind can be made by boiling the leaves of the fig, olive, agnus castus[72], and pomegranate (here *sidē*)[73]. The following can be used in their natural state:

---

[64] *Wounds*, 11 (ed. Littré, VI, 410).

[65] Φλόμος is probably *Verbascum sinuatum* L., a mullein. Cf. Theophrastus, *Historia Plantarum*, IX, 12. 3. Various spp. of *Verbascum* contain a mucilage, an essential oil, and saponosides.

[66] Τρίφυλλον is uncertain, although it may be *Trifolium fragiferum* L. (= *T. neglectum* Fisch. and Mey.), sometimes called "strawberry clover", often grown as fodder for livestock, particularly in wet soils.

[67] From the description of ἐπίμετρον in Theophrastus, *Historia Plantarum*, VII, 7. 4, ἐπίπετρον here in *Wounds*, 11, is probably *Sedum acre* L., the "yellow stonecrop" or "wall-pepper", long employed in folk medicine for its irritating properties; its chemistry includes alkaloids, esp. semadine, some glycosides, and mucilage. Modern folk medicine uses a decoction of the fresh leaves for local treatment of warts and corns, as well as for the promotion of wound healing, much as suggested here in *Wounds*, 11.

Πόλιον is probably *Teucrium polium* L., the "felty germander", given the description in Dioscorides, III, 110 (ed. Wellmann, Vol. II, pp. 121-122), which carefully distinguishes its white stems and grayish fuzziness. The plant is sometimes also called a "hulwort". Among spp. of *Teucrium, T. polium* seems to be the "preferred" variety in antiquity, since it is mentioned by Theophrastus, *Historia Plantarum*, I, 10. 4 and II, 8. 3 [in the consideration of insect-galls on plants], and VII, 10. 5 [where the "felty germander" is cited as illustrative of the difficulties in taxonomy of herbs, experienced by Theophrastus], as well as Apollodorus in Nicander, *Theriaca*, 64 and 583, showing the early entry of the plant into Greek herbal pharmacology. All. spp. of *Teucrium* contain high concentrations of tannin, bitter principles including picropulin, and at least two sugars (stachyose and raffinose). Modern herbal medicine uses the germander (esp. *T. chamaedrys*) as a tonic, choleretic, antiseptic, and diuretic, and an infusion of the plant aids the appetite and digestion, and eases the social problems of flatulence.

[68] *Wounds*, 11 (Littré, VI, 410): πάντα μὲν καὶ ταῦτα καθαίρει.

[69] Συκῆ is the common fig, *Ficus carica* L.

[70] The common olive (*Olea europaea* L.), ἡ ἐλαία, no longer exists generally in the wild state (botanists have designated the wild parent of the olive *Olea europaea* var. *oleaster* DC), although occasional "escapes" are observed. In addition to the well-known uses of olive oil (George Usher, *Dictionary of Plants Used by Man* [London, 1974], 421-422; M. Stuart, ed., *Encyclopedia of Herbs and Herbalism* [London, 1979], 229-230), the fresh leaves are sometimes employed as a weak astringent and antiseptic.

[71] Τὸ πράσιον is the "horehound", *Marrubium vulgare* L., containing marubiin as a bitter principle, as well as a volatile oil that have been used as a bitter tonic, expectorant, and diaphoretic. Scarborough, *Nicander's Toxicology, I*, Pharmacy in History, 19 (1977), 12.

[72] To ἄγνον is the "chaste tree" or the "Monk's pepper" (*Vitex agnus-castus* L.), long thought to be a powerful anaphrodisiac. Recent analytical research has discovered that the leaves contain a hormonal-like substance, which has been suggested as useful in the depression accompanying menopause. Scarborough, *Asclepiades*, Pharmacy in History, 17 (1975), 50; Stuart, *Herbs*, 282-283; W.A.R. Thompson, *Herbs that Heal* (New York, 1976), 157. The Hippocratic *Internal Diseases*, 30 (Littré, VII, 246) recommend the seeds of "Monk's pepper" in the treatment of affections of the spleen, and the plant appears in Dioscorides, I, 103, and in a garbled manner in Nicander, *Theriaca*, 71.

[73] Σίδη as opposed to the more usual ῥοιή.

malachē-leaves[74] pounded in wine, *pēganon*-leaves[75], and the leaves of *origanon chlōrēs*[76]. All of the above ingredients could also be used with boiled linseed[77], which has been pounded into a powder. If the physician thinks that a case of erysipelas[78] may overcome the wounds, he should apply *isatis*-leaves[79], pounded and put on raw along with the linseed (form not specified: perhaps powdered as in the previous line); or the linseed should be moistened with the juice of the *strychnos*[80], or of the *isatis*, and applied as a poultice. But if the wound is clean, and yet it and

---

[74] Ἡ μαλάχη is probably *Malva sylvestris* L., the "high mallow", which also appears in Theophrastus, VII, 7. 2, and Dioscorides, II, 118 [cod. F]. The plant has a mucilage, along with a volatile oil and tannin, making it ideal for herbal tea, and the chemistry explains why ancient pharmacy would value the mallow as a mild astringent, demulcent, and a drug with anti-inflammatory properties.

[75] Πήγανον is rue (*Ruta graveolens* L.), given high marks in many pharmacological sources from Greek and Roman antiquity, *e.g.* Nicander, *Theriaca*, 531, and Celsus, *De medicina*, V, 4; II, 31; III, 20. 4; IV, 27B; IV, 28. 2; as well as many references in Galen. Rue has rutin (rutoside; quercetin-3-rutinoside) still employed as a carminative and rubefaciant, as well as to reduce capillary fragility. Scarborough, *Nicander's Toxicology*, I, Pharmacy in History, 19 (1977), 11-12.

[76] It is uncertain exactly what "green marjoram" ὀρίγανον χλωρῆς might be, but it is possibly a variation, or an immature form of *Origanum vulgare* L., or *Majorana hortensis* Moench (= *Origanum majorana* L.). If so, it would possess the pharmacological properties of marjoram. See n. 39 above.

[77] Καρπὸν λίνου is the famous "flax-seed" or "linseed" from which is made the well-known oil. In modern veterinary practice, linseed oil is used as a laxative in large animals and in former time veterinarians employed the crushed seeds in a poultice for small animals, a practice that may have its origins in the "Hippocratic" sources of the Byzantine *Geoponica* (*Geoponica* [ed. Beckh], XVI, 20. 1 [p. 465-466]). In modern medicine, linseed oil has limited use as a topical demulcent and emollient. Scarborough, *Nicander's Toxicology, II*, Pharmacy in History, 21 (1979), 75-76 [with reffs., and details of the chemistry of linseed].

[78] Galen, *Method of Medicine*, XIV, 2 (ed. Kühn, X, 949) defines τὸ ἐρυσίπελας as "an inflammation of the liver, with swelling and fever", only part of the ancient description of the disease, in which skin eruptions that are sharply defined are accompanied by severe constitutional symptoms, viz. the Hippocratic *Ancient Medicine*, 19; *Prognostics*, 23; *Aphorisms*, V, 23; as well as Oribasius, XLV, 1. 3 [ed. Raeder, Vol. III, p. 160; *CMG* VI 2, 1]; and the Byzantine *Geoponica*, XII, 23. 5 [ed. Beckh, p. 372: parsley, or celery, made into a poultice with bread, cures erysipelas]. Modern medicine calls the affliction St. Anthony's Fire, or Rose, and describes it as an acute inflammatory disease of the skin caused by *Streptococcus erysipelas*.

[79] Commonly known as "woad" or "dyer's weed", ἴσατις is *Isatis tinctoria* L., one of the oldest sources of blue dye known to man. Dioscorides, II, 184, describes the extract as one of the finest styptics, a statement confirmed by the chemical properties of indigo (delta 2, 2'-bypseudoindoxyl; indigotin; indigo blue). The fermented leaves, and sometimes fresh leaves, remain useful as a vulnerary and styptic. A. Lubs, *The Chemistry of Synthetic Dyes* (New York, 1955), 551-576. R. Schweizer, *Künstliche organische Farbstoffe und ihre Zwischenprodukte* (Berlin, 1964), 320-334. The blue color does not develop until oxidation.

[80] Στρύχνος here in the Hippocratic *Wounds*, 11, is either the deadly nightshade (*Atropa belladonna* L.) or the thorn apple (*Datura stramonium* L.). Nicander, *Theriaca*, 74 and 878, also does not specify which variety, so that one may assume (from Nicander's jumbled data) that the undesignated plant is *Atropa belladonna*. Applied externally, the chemistry would suggest astringency. Scarborough, *Theophrastus*, Journal of the History of Biology, 11 (1978), 367.

the surrounding parts are inflamed, *phakoi*[81] are to be boiled in wine and then triturated very finely, then mixed with a little oil and applied as a poultice; or the leaves of the *kynosbatos*[82] can be boiled in water and then pounded into a fine powder and made into a poultice (but this particular recipe is more of a plaster than a poultice, since the author says to apply first a thin, clean piece of cloth, soaked in wine and oil, and then apparently to apply the white rose leaf powder)[83]. Another poultice consists of powdered linseed, mixed with wine and *sauridion* (= *kardamon*)[84]. And the last suggestion in this single section of the Hippocratic *Wounds* is to use linseed, agnus castus, and Melian alum[85] all macerated in vinegar to make the poultice.

In 21 lines of the Littré Greek text of *Wounds*, 11, there are 17 different substances prescribed for the making of poultices and one plaster for wounds. One characteristic of the *pharmaka* is clear enough: they are all dessicants, which would promote the "drying" of the wound desired by the writer who has defined his wound treatment as being dependent upon keeping the wound as dry as possible. Implicit throughout is the notion that *pharmaka* with properties of drying will promote healing in an ideal manner, and that the pus is blood which has become corrupted: drying drugs thus will bring back the *krasis* of the blood as it would normally be before the excess heat caused pus. The theory of Elements and Humors is implicit, with the notion of Qualities employed as a connection, and the various *dynameis* also hover in the background, since each *pharmakon* "acts" according to its drying nature. The 17 substances in *Wounds*, 11

[81] Lentils, *Lens esculenta* Moench (= *L. culinaris* = *Ervum lens*).

[82] This is probably the white rose, *Rosa sempervirens* L., which also appears in Theophrastus, *Historia Plantarum*, IX, 8. 5; Theocritus, V, 92; and Dioscorides, I, 94. Species in *Rosa* have high concentrations of Vitamin C (esp. the "rose hips"), nicotinamide, tannins, and pectins, making it quite suitable for use as a tonic, laxative, diuretic, astringent, and as part of a poultice to promote the healing of wounds.

[83] *Wounds*, 11 (Littré, VI, 410, lines 16-19).

[84] Apparently, σαυρίδιον is another name for κάρδαμον, which would make this the "garden cress" or "pepper grass" (*Lepidium sativum* L.), widely used as a salad plant and as an antiscorbutic. The seeds of *L. sativum* were eaten in antiquity like those of mustard.

[85] Generally called στυπτηρία in Greek, and *alumen* in the Roman medical sources, "alum" is the term that would apply to any one of a number of "astringent substances" which contained alum (*e.g.* "potash alum", $KAl(SO_4)_2.12H_20$, or "ammonium alum", $(NH_4)Al(SO_4)_2.12H_20$), or various combinations of ferrous sulfates ($FeSO_4 \cdot 7H_20$) with manganese, magnesium, aluminum, or silicon. Thus the famous "alum earths" of the Hippocratic writers, Celsus, Pliny, and Galen, the "Melian Earth" (silicate of aluminum) as well as "Lemnian Earth" (silicates and sulfates of aluminum, magnesia, and iron), "Eretrian Earth" (hydrated silicate of aluminum, streaked by iron and/or copper), as well as a number of other "earths" valued for their styptic powers. Used for their blood-clotting properties, "alums" were also used in Greek and Roman therapeutics to clean wounds, induce scarring, treat dysentery, prepare salves (esp. the famous collyria, or "eye salves") and—as here in the Hippocratic, *Wounds*, 11—to aid the healing of ulcerative forms. See esp. Dioscorides, V, 106, and Pliny, *Natural History*, XXV, 183-191, as well as Galen, *Mixtures and Properties of Simples*, IX, 2 (ed. Kühn, XII, 169-174). Melian Earth also appears in Celsus, VI, 19, and Dioscorides, V, 106. 1-2 (ed. Wellmann, Vol. III, pp. 75-76).

are carefully selected, and each has a history of use in Greek folk medicine that can be paralleled in earlier Greek sources (including Theophrastus, if one accepts the assumption that the composition of the *Historia Plantarum* preceded the compilation of data in the Hippocratic *Wounds*)[86].

The Hippocratic *Wounds* displays an enormous wealth of simples and compound drugs, all assumed to have this carefully defined drying, but not heating, power. In *Wounds*, 12, we read of a complicated preparation of a poultice for "old" ulcers and wounds that begins with the pounding of white unripened grapes in a mortar of red bronze (or copper), and passing the juice through a strainer and exposing the juice to the sun for a day and then covering it over at night so as not to be contaminated by the dew (apparently to keep as many of the wet Humors as possible from the mixture); one is supposed to pound the grapes throughout the day, so that the preparation may take up as many of the powers of the copper as possible, and then one exposes the juice to the sun for as long as is necessary to thicken it into the consistency of honey; then one puts this thickened juice into another bronze vessel, previously used for the boiling of turpentine resin[87], and now one is to boil the resin in wine until *that* mixture becomes like hard honey, etc.[88]. When the recipe is completed, one has a compound poultice that contains honey, myrrh[89], wine, frankincense[90], *natron*[91], flowers of copper, all to be boiled for three days. Another recipe in *Wounds*, 12 contains ox bile[92], honey, white wine, lotus

---

[86] See Scarborough, *Theophrastus*, Journal of the History of Biology, 11 (1978), 353-385 passim; it would appear that Theophrastus is beginning an attempt to define "herb" as distinct from other plants, but his taxonomic methods seem to cause confusion.

[87] Ῥητίνη τερμινθίνη could also simply be "turpentine", as apparently used by Diocles, Frg. 140 (ed. M. Wellmann [1901], p. 176); derived from *Pistachia terebinthus* L., the "resin" or turpentine (known as Chian turpentine) could be effectively used as a counterirritant.

[88] *Wounds*, 12 (Littré, VI, 412).

[89] Very common in Greek pharmacy, σμύρνα is one of the numerous spp. in *Commiphora*, with the greatest probability of the "myrrh" in Greek pharmacy being either *C. myrrha* (Nees.) Engl., or *C. abyssinica* (Berg.) Engl. Both species could have been part of the flourishing trade running from the coasts of Arabia up the Red Sea into Ptolemaic Egypt. Scarborough, *Asclepiades*, Pharmacy in History, 17 (1975), 47. See also Nigel Groom, *Frankincense and Myrrh* (London, 1981), 96-120, and Majno, *Healing Hand*, 208-218. As Majno demonstrates, myrrh had several antiseptic and bactericidal properties.

[90] Again fairly common in Greek pharmacy, λιβανωτός is *Boswellia carteri* Birdw. The gum, olibanum, is extracted from the trunk. Groom, *Frankincense and Myrrh*, 96-120. Majno, *Healing Hand*, 219, demonstrates the bacteriostatic properties of frankincense.

[91] Chemically, natron is a mixture of sodium carbonate and bicarbonate, with sodium sulphate and common salt as impurities, and the "best kind" came from Egypt. Majno, *Healing Hand*, 133. The most complete account of natron to be found in English, in the all-important context of Egyptian archaeology, is A. Lucas, *Ancient Egyptian Materials and Industries*, 3rd ed. (London, 1948), 297-347.

[92] *Wounds*, 12 (Littré, VI, 412, line 22): χολὴ βοὸς ξηρή.

shavings[93], frankincense, myrrh, saffron[94], and the flowers of copper. Six *more* recipes follow[95].

The Hippocratic *Wounds* is certainly not the only tract in the *corpus* that displays a manifest knowledge of botanicals and the long tradition of herbal lore that is applied to the treatment of ailments. One may also cite the *Fistulas*[96], perhaps a continuation of *Wounds*, as another example of the Hippocratic physician's employment of *pharmaka* with clear objects in mind. The healing of fistulas, so the author says, is promoted by using *tithymallos*[97], myrrh, a sitz-bath followed by the application of a pessary made from *strychnos*, goose fat[98], *chrysocolla*[99], white wax[100], as well as a poultice of boiled garlic[101]—among dozens of other medicines[102]. *Hemorrhoids* likewise contains many medicinal substances used in treatment[103], as does the *Diseases of Women*[104], and the modern observer is struck by the careful ordering in accordance with the underlying dual

---

93 *Wounds*, 12 (Littré, VI, 414, line 1): ἐν αὐτῷ λωτοῦ τορνεύματα.

94 *Crocus sativus* L., saffron, also appears in Theophrastus, *Historia Plantarum*, IV, 3. 1, and Dioscorides, I, 26, and in addition to its venerated, watersoluble yellow dye, the plant contains a bitter glycoside, picrocrocin, and an essential oil. 100,000 flowers produce 1 kg. of saffron. Usher, *Plants*, 183.

95 *Wounds*, 12 (Littré, VI, 414-416).

96 Ed. R. Joly in *Hippocrate* Tome XIII (Paris, 1978), pp. 137-145.

97 *Fistulas*, II, 2 (ed. Joly, p. 139). This would be one of the various species of spurges in the genus *Euphorbia*. Dioscorides, IV, 164, lists seven different kinds. In this enormous genus (over 2000 species), there is chemical variation from the deadly poisonous to the mildly laxative.

98 *Fistulas*, VII, 4 (ed. Joly, p. 142, line 15).

99 *Fistulas*, VII, 4 (ed. Joly, p. 142, line 16). This is a copper silicate of a bright blue-green color, with decidedly bactericidal properties. Majno, *Healing Hand*, 113-115.

100 *Fistulas*, VII, 4 (ed. Joly, p. 142, line 16): καὶ κηρὸν λευκόν. This is "beeswax", as shown by Theocritus, I, 27. By Galen's time, the "white wax" used in medicinals was commonly called "Etruscan wax" (Galen, *Compounding Drugs According to Kind*, I, 12 [ed. Kühn, XIII, 411]). Cf. Dioscorides, I, 70.

101 *Fistulas*, VII, 4 (ed. Joly, p. 142, lines 18-19). This is the common *Allium sativum* L.

102 In addition to giving his reasoning for the cause of strangury (*Fistulas*, VIII [ed. Joly, p. 142, lines 23-29: the bladder is heated from the rectum, and phlegm is attracted by the heat, and the inflammation results]), the author suggests the following for the treatment of prolapsed rectum: after using a soft sponge, anoint the prolapsus with a snail, and tie the patient's hands together and suspend him [upside down?], and the rectum will return to its normal position. If that does not work, then the physician is to fashion a belt for his hips with a cloth attached behind; then with a sponge moistened with lotus scrapings and hot water, one moistens the anus and positions the cloth between the legs, fastening it at the navel (*Fistulas*, IX, 1 [ed. Joly, p. 143]). Other treatments including washing out the rectum with burnt lees of wine, the juice of a myrtle, and applying a poultice made from powdered maiden-hair (*Fistulas*, IX, 2 [ed. Joly, p. 143]. With blood discharges, pharmaceuticals for treatment include a copper oxide, cypress-scrapings, cedar oil, turpentine—all in equal parts applied as a poultice, with thick wax applied to the external areas. Another poultice consists of silphium (only the best kind!) scrapings (*Fistulas*, IX, 3 [ed. Joly, p. 143[]), but one could also use a pomegranate peel soaked in hot water, powdered alum in white wine, honey and vermillion (*Fistulas*, IX, 4 [ed. Joly, pp. 143-144]), etc. One treatment is of special interest: a poultice made from pounded hemlock seeds and white wine (*Fistulas*, IX, 6 [ed. Joly, p. 144]).

103 Ed. R. Joly in *Hippocrate* Tome XIII (Paris, 1978), pp. 146-150.

104 Ed. E. Littré in Vol. VIII of *Œuvres complètes d'Hippocrate*, pp. 10-407.

theory of Elements and Humors whenever *pharmaka* are prescribed. Moreover, the apparent chaos in the prescriptions themselves dissolves if the Greek texts are studied carefully. Such painstaking care is in gross contrast to one of the other famous sources for Greek pharmacy and toxicology, Nicander's *Theriaca* and *Alexipharmaca*[105], in which drugs and herbs are jumbled together with touches of whimsy and obvious ignorance for the sake of obtaining a correct scansion. Of course, the basic taxonomy of plants, including some herbs, had been worked out by Theophrastus in the *Historia Plantarum*[106], and the Hippocratic physician almost certainly was aware of some advanced studies in botany, much as Dioscorides would later reflect some bits and pieces of Theophrastus[107], even though the great botanist would not be cited by name.

Some Preliminary Conclusions

Not only do the Hippocratic physicians exercise extreme care with their selection of *pharmaka* in terms of the dual theory, but they also have accepted the worth of herbal medicine and its hoary experience of "testing" drugs, as it would be stated two centuries later by Dioscorides[108]. Much as Theophrastus in the *Historia Plantarum*, Book IX, had gradually begun to accept the data of the rootcutters as he attempted some definitions of what were "herbs" and what were not[109], so too the Hippocratic physicians have fashioned a pharmacology in light of herbal medicine combined with an explicit and implicit triple theory of Elements, Qualities, and Humors, perhaps on the basis of some definitions extant in the pseudo-Aristotelian *Problems*, but with a continual emphasis upon Elements and Humors, as well as particular properties of *pharmaka*. Whether or not the Hippocratic physician consciously recalled Aristotelian drug theory, it is certainly clear that Hippocratic medicine had incorporated a vast number of the venerated uses of the herbs, minerals, and animal products that were known in Greek history

[105] Ed. and trans. with commentary by A.S.F. Gow and A.F. Scholfield, *Nicander: The Poems and Poetical Fragments* (Cambridge, 1953). Scarborough, *Nicander's Toxicology, I*, Pharmacy in History, 19 (1977), 3-23, and *Nicander's Toxicology, II*, Pharmacy in History, 21 (1979), 3-34 and 73-92 passim.

[106] O. Regenbogen, *Theophrastos*, RE, Suppl. VII (Stuttgart, 1940), 1354-1562 [1435-1479].

[107] H. Stadler, *Theophrast und Dioscorides*, in *Wilhelm von Christ zum sechzigsten Geburtstag* (Munich, 1891, Abhandlungen aus dem Gebiet der klassischen Altertums-Wissenschaft), 176-187, and Max Wellmann, *Das älteste Kräuterbuch der Griechen*, Festgabe für Franz Susemihl (Leipzig, 1898), 1-31.

[108] Dioscorides, [Preface], 1 and 5 (ed. Wellmann, Vol. I, pp. 1 and 3).

[109] Theophrastus, *Historia Plantarum*, IX, 8. 1-2. Scarborough, *Theophrastus*, Journal of the History of Biology, 11 (1978), 356-357.

long before the rise of "rational" medicine[110]. It is, one may say in conclusion, to the great credit of some of the Hippocratic writers that they recognized the value of many of these prescriptions, expunged of any superstitious content[111], a value that modern pharmaceutics has in some respects only begun to rediscover.

[110] Especially revealed in J.H. Dierbach, *Die Arzneimittel des Hippokrates* (Heidelberg, 1824; rptd. Hildesheim, 1969); this work has not been superseded.

[111] At least this was an ideal to be followed, according to Ludwig Edelstein, *Greek Medicine in its Relation to Religion and Magic*, Bulletin of the History of Medicine, 5 (1937), 201-246 = rptd. in O. and C.L. Temkin, eds., *Ancient Medicine: Selected Papers of Ludwig Edelstein* (Baltimore, 1967), 205-246 [esp. 230-232].

IV

Theophrastus on Herbals and Herbal Remedies

Theophrastus of Eresos (c. 370-288/85 B.C.) was the outstanding student of Aristotle, and is famed in the history of Western literature for his lampooning *Characters*, as well as numerous treatises on botany, petrology, and other subjects in natural history.[1] Best known is the *Historia Plantarum*, which formed the base for all succeeding studies of plant lore and classification until the Linnaean system.[2] Taking Aristotle's methodologies, illustrated in the *Historia Animalium, De Partibus Animalium*, and other zoological works, Theophrastus produced a botanical guide that displayed the best in the Peripatetic approaches to the world of nature.

There is some controversy over the authenticity of *Historia Plantarum*, IX, in which herbs and herbals appear. It is argued that there may be some genuine "Theophrastean" matter in Book IX, but that an unknown *rhizotomos* ("root-cutter") was the author.[3] In a recent survey of herbal documents, Stannard remains uncertain about Book IX, and his conclusion that "Book IX of Theophrastus' *History of Plants* ... is possibly spurious"[4] is typical of most essays touching on the subject. The problem is centered on the topics in Book IX, which seem at variance with the remainder of the treatise, but Einarson has shown that the best witnesses in the MS tradition do include Book IX.[5] Further-

1. The best summary is O. Regenbogen, "Theophrastos," *Real-Encyclopädie der classichen Altertumswissenschaft* suppl. VII (Stuttgart, 1940), cols. 1354-1562 (1435-1479: botany); this work is hereafter cited as *RE*.

2. The first edition of Carl Linnaeus's *Species Plantarum* appeared in 1753. A two-volume facsimile edition has been published (London: The Ray Society, 1957-1959), with extremely useful introductions and appendices by John L. Heller and W. T. Stearn. See also John L. Heller, "The Early History of Binomial Nomenclature," *Huntia, 1* (1964), 33-70.

3. Hugo Bretzl, *Botanische Forschungen des Alexanderzuges* (Leipzig: Teubner, 1903), p. 366 and n. 24.

4. Jerry Stannard, "The Herbal as a Medical Document," *Bull. Hist. Med., 43* (1969), 213.

5. Benedict Einarson, "The Manuscripts of Theophrastus' *Historia Plantarum*," *Class. Phil., 71* (1976), 67-76, esp. 68-69 with U*.

more many doubts about the textual contents of Book IX result from the state of corruption, interpolation, and omission in the MSS, especially those sections after IX, 18.

According to the usual definition of "herbal," Book IX of the *Historia Plantarum* would not qualify as one in *isolation* from the remainder of the work. Descriptions of the various plants are detailed in the main body of the treatise, while their medical properties are singled out in Book IX. But if Book IX is taken together with the previous descriptions, – it does fall under the definition given by Lawrence: "a book on plants of real or alleged medicinal properties, which describes the appearance of those plants, and provides information on their medicinal importance and use."[6] Book IX qualifies as an herbal; in fact it is the earliest herbal in Greek that has come down almost complete.

In the introduction to his edition of Theophrastus's *De Lapidibus*, Eichholz writes, "Theophrastus . . . mentions the medical properties of no earths, and of only one stone . . . Similarly, he excluded pharmacology from his treatise on plants."[7] Likewise, one reads in the standard *Kremers and Urdang's History of Pharmacy* that Theophrastus "was primarily a botanist," and that Dioscorides was "the first to deal with medical botany."[8] Whatever one may believe about the authenticity of Book IX of the *Historia Plantarum*, there is ample evidence in the rest of the work, and in *De Causis Plantarum*, that attests to Theophrastus's great interest in medicinals, and plant medicinals in particular. Omitting *Historia Plantarum* IX from consideration of the Theophrastean *corpus* does grave injustice to the history of ancient botany and ancient pharmacy: here are medicinals, derived from plants – and one animal. Moreover, Theophrastus assimilated much information from the writings of Diocles of Carystos (fl. in the time of Aristotle, 384-322 B.C.),[9] a

6. George H. M. Lawrence, "Herbals: Their History and Significance," in *History of Botany* (Los Angeles: University of California Press, 1965), p. 3; quoted in Stannard, "Herbal," p. 213.

7. D. E. Eichholz, ed., *Theophrastus: De Lapidibus* (Oxford: Clarendon Press, 1965), p. 7 and n. 2.

8. Glenn Sonnedecker, rev., *Kremers and Urdang's History of Pharmacy*, 3rd ed. (Philadelphia: Lippincott, 1963), p. 15.

9. Werner Jaeger, *Diokles von Karystos* (Berlin: De Gruyter, 1963), esp. pp. 114-123. Fragments of lost Theophrastean writings suggest a deep interest in medicine and pharmacology. Regenbogen, "Theophrastos," cols. 1426-1434, esp. col. 1427, nr. 3. F. Wimmer, ed., *Theophrasti Eresii: Opera* (Paris: Didot, 1866, reprint of Teubner, ed., 1854-1862), collects a number of fragments (incomplete) that illustrate this diversity of interest. Two examples among many will serve to demonstrate the "medical" aspects. Frag. 117 (Wimmer, p. 445) is from

physician who lived in Athens, and this puts Theophrastus in context with some of the important developments in Greek medicine and anatomy. Diocles was not one of the local *rhizotomoi* ("root-cutters"),[10] but a doctor who left a reputation for dissection and medical investigation of all kinds.[11] The list of Diocles' works is wide-ranging, and includes those on drugs.

Theophrastus tells us that he has procured much information from the *pharmacopōlai* ("drug-vendors") and *rhizotomoi,*[12] but Wellmann has shown that some basic medical data in *Historia Plantarum* IX came from the works of Diocles.[13] Theophrastus and Dioscorides,[14] as well as Apollodorus/Nicander,[15] used Diocles' materials on plants as medicinals. A number of fragments, collected by Wellmann,[16] clearly indicate Diocles' abilities; several of these fragments prove that Diocles' observa-

---

Athenaeus, X, 429b, on how Theophrastus records (in an untitled work) that Miletus had a custom that women drink water, but no wine; earlier the fragment records that one suffered death for drinking unmixed wine if he did so without a doctor's prescription to effect a cure. Frag. 178 (Wimmer, p. 461) is from Theophrastus's *Biting and Venomous Animals* and *Animals That Live in Holes* (the electric ray fish) = Athenaeus, VII, 314b-c. Galen (ed. C. G. Kühn), VI, 190 = K. Koch, ed., *Galeni De Santitate Tuenda* (Leipzig: Teubner, 1923 [*Corpus Medicorum Graecorum*, V, 4. 2]), III, 5.2-3 (Koch, p. 84), says that Theophrastus wrote a book (possibly titled *On Fatigue*) wherein gymnastics and medicine were combined.

10. M. Wellmann, *Die Fragmente der sikilischen Ärzte Akron, Philistion und des Diokles von Karystos* (Berlin: Weidmann, 1901), pp. 117-207 (fragments), as contrasted with the statement in *Kremers and Urdang's History of Pharmacy*, p. 15.

11. Wellmann, *Fragmente*, p. 117 (list of titles).

12. *Historia Plantarum*, IX, 8 passim; 11.7 and 9; 15.2; 16.3; 18.3 and 10; 20.4; henceforth this work is cited as *HP*.

13. Max Wellmann, "Das älteste Kräuterbuch der Griechen," in *Festgabe für Franz Susemihl* (Leipzig: Teubner, 1898), pp. 1-31, esp. pp. 22-31.

14. Theophrastus, *On Perspiration* (ed. Wimmer, pp. 403-408 [frag. 9]), p. 403, (2), 35-42; and p. 407 (30), 44-46. Wellmann, *Fragmente*, pp. 87-88. Wellmann, "Kräuterbuch," pp. 20-22, shows the common source from Diocles in Nicander and Dioscorides.

15. It is quite clear that Nicander had no competence in the subject matter of the two extant poems, *Theriaca* and *Alexipharmaca*; he borrowed (and mangled) the data in the works of Apollodorus (fl. sometime in the third century B.C.), who, in turn had borrowed some of the materials from the works of Diocles. M. Wellmann, "Apollodoros," *RE*, I, pt. 2 (Stuttgart, 1894), nr. 69, col. 2895. Franz Susemihl, *Geschichte der griechischen Litteratur in der Alexandrinerzeit*, 2 vols. (Leipzig: Teubner, 1891-1892), I, 784-785. John Scarborough, "Nicander's Toxicology, I: Snakes," *Pharm. Hist.*, *19* (1977), 3-23.

16. Wellmann, *Fragmente*, p. 117.

tions on pharmacology and plant medicinals were embedded in Theophrastus's works, especially Book IX of *Historia Plantarum.*[17]

Diocles' and Theophrastus's herbals, however, are far simpler than the multisubstance remedies that would be preserved by Nicander, Dioscorides, Galen, and later writers in Greek and Roman pharmacology. Moreover, Theophrastus seems uncertain about the definition of "herbal" as his sources of information had given it to him. Implicitly, silphium, frankincense, and myrrh do not form part of Theophrastus's medicinals,[18] although he does give myrrh as part of one of the few multisubstance remedies in the short *On Odors* (35). Once he has given his description of frankincense and myrrh, he attempts a definition of herbs (*poai*), which will include juices (*opoi*) not described previously.[19] These will be those substances which have "medical powers,"[20] and will comprise "extracted juice" (*chylismos*), "fruits" (*karpoi*), "leaves" (*phylla*), and "roots" (*rhiza*), because the *rhizotomoi* call "herbs medicinals,"[21] and they consist of these parts. This hesitant definition of "herb" may have been borrowed from Diocles or the *rhizotomoi*, but Theophrastus may have invented it on his own. The *rhizotomoi* had given him a piece of his basic information, because the *rhizotomoi* do not call all their roots herbs, but only those from the class of medicinals, or healing plants, or healing parts of certain plants.[22] Theophrastus still seems uncertain of his definition, because he continues by distinguishing those potencies (or "powers" [*dynameis*]) of roots which are general from those *dynameis* in roots which have use in healing or medicinals (*pharmakōdeis*). Thus roots which are medicinal include all four parts of the plant, especially the leaves, as root-cutters themselves say; consequently, "herbs" are all four parts, not just the roots.[23] Theoprastus gives full credit to the *rhizotomoi* and their imprecise descriptions, but he attempts to put some kind of label on their empirical

17. Ibid., nr. 150 (p. 191, from *Rootcutters*): *Scholia on Theriaca*, 628, compared with Nicander, *Theriaca*, 628, Dioscorides, *Materia Medica* (ed. M. Wellmann), III, 31 and 49, and Theophrastus, *HP*, IX, 11.1. nr. 152 (pp. 191-192, from *Rootcutters*): Erotian, *s.v.* *σησαμοειδές* (120, 6 Kl.) with Dioscorides, IV, 149, Rufus in Oribasius, II, 109, Strabo, IX, 418, and Theophrastus, *HP*, IX, 9.2. See also nrs. 156, 160, and 166 (the last from Theophrastus, *On Stones*).

18. *HP*, IX, 1 and 4.

19. Ibid., 8.1.

20. Ibid., *φαρμακώδεις δύναμεις.*

21. Ibid., *καλοῦσι γὰρ καὶ πόαν ἔνια τῶν φαρμακωδῶν οἱ ῥιζοτόμοι.*

22. Ibid., 8.2.

23. Ibid., *τῶν δὲ ῥιζῶν πλείους μὲν εἰσιν αἱ δύναμεις καὶ πρὸς πλείω.*

notions. What follow are "herbs," and only a few "herbals": plants are listed with only an occasional combination with other plants; yet his "herbs" are "herbals," because the medicinal properties of each plant are assumed to act singularly, most often with water, honey, and olive oil.

Lists of beneficial and harmful plants and extracts are as old as civilization, and the *Syriac Book of Medicines* suggests, as one example, how such listings became jumbled together over millennia.[24] Budge quotes from the Assyrian Kuyûnjik Collection a description of how Sennacherib (705-681 B.C.) "planted . . . all the herbs of the land of Khatti,"[25] and shows how many of these early prescriptions became embedded in later compilations that came to include Greek and Roman authors.[26] Among the Greeks is Diocles of Carystos,[27] along with a host of other authorities, both very ancient and quite recent.[28] Contained in the *Syriac Book of Medicines* are many folk traditions, side by side with the conclusions of the best Greek and Roman doctors and pharmacologists. So also Theophrastus has inherited a long history of empirical observation, which he records in Book IX of *Historia Plantarum*, but he puts these notions about "herbs" into the Peripatetic framework and classification system, which had served so well in the first eight books of *Historia Plantarum*, as well as in *De Causis Plantarum*. Each herb that is listed in Book IX meets his definition of "medicinal," as he has set it down in IX, 8.1 and 2, and sometimes that definition will lead Theophrastus to include nonbotanical matter.

Unlike the muddled nomenclature of snakes,[29] spiders, certain minerals,[30] insects, and other animals that might be employed in medicine, or that might be mentioned in the Greek texts of medicine and pharmacology, plant nomenclature is slightly more assured. A multitude of names was applied to poisonous snakes, for example, while plant names

24. E. A. Wallis Budge, ed. and trans., *Syrian Anatomy, Pathology, and Therapeutics, or "The Book of Medicines,"* 2 vols. (London: Oxford University Press, 1913).

25. Ibid., I, cxlviii.

26. The list includes Asclepiades of Bithynia, Galen, Hippocrates, Diocles, and several others.

27. *Syrian Anatomy*, I, 19-20 (Syriac text) and II, 18-19 (translation). Wellmann, *Fragmente*, could not include this Syriac fragment in his collection.

28. *Syrian Anatomy*, I, clxix-clxxi (summary of prescriptions that have association with famous physicians).

29. Scarborough, "Nicander's Toxicology," pp. 3-23.

30. John Scarborough, "The Drug Lore of Asclepiades of Bithynia," *Pharm. Hist.*, *17* (1975), 43-57 (49: *nitron*; 53-54: Sal Ammoniac).

in Theophrastus, Nicander, Dioscorides, Galen, and others have some consistency that helps in modern identification. Specific plants had names recognized throughout the Greek world, and where there is doubt, modern Greek sometimes preserves an essential word or core that helps key modern nomenclature.[31] Once a plant is keyed, one may determine through modern biochemistry and pharmacology if the substance had beneficial or harmful effects. Quite often, empirical observation as recorded by Theophrastus or Diocles is correct, although the manner of description fits the Peripatetic mold.[32]

In keeping with the traditions of Greek agriculture, as well as the structure of the entire *Historia Plantarum,*[33] Theophrastus describes how these useful medicinals will be gathered: by season and by method. The best juices are collected in the summer, while the most useful roots are gathered at the time of the wheat harvest (spring) or after the rising of Arcturus (autumn), when the plants "have lost their leaves or fruit."[34] Part of the method of gathering juices includes the part of the plant: stalk, root, and head. Juices from the stalks come from most plants, examples being wild lettuce and spurge. Theophrastus provides no examples for the class of "root-juices," perhaps in keeping with his previous definition of the "root" as the "whole" plant. The poppy (*mēkōn*) yields it juice from the head, the only plant so treated.[35] Subsumed under method of collection, following season and parts, are the actual procedures used in collecting: incisions, bruising, and cutting. Those plants with an abundance of juice have their sap collected into jars or vessels made for the purpose; probably Theophrastus implies this method for those plants that yield juice from their stalks. Those plants having little sap from the stalks had their juice absorbed into a ball of wool, as with *thridakinē* (*Lactuca scariola* L., "wild lettuce").[36] In the bruise method, the plants were cut down, water was poured over them, the fluid was strained, and the sediment retained.[37] This was the method

31. R. M. Dawkins, "The Semantics of Greek Names for Plants," *J. Hellenic Stud., 56* (1936), 1-11.

32. Pseudo-Aristotle, *Problems*, I, esp. 41, is a good parallel example.

33. Theophrastus valued – and named – the following agricultural writers: Chartodras, Androtion, and Satyrus. See note 142, below.

34. *HP*, IX, 8.2. *Cf.* Hesiod, *Works and Days*, 248.

35. *HP*, IX, 8.2.

36. *HP*, VII, 6.2 ("wild" lettuce). Theophrastus recognized several types of "wild lettuce" (*HP*, VII, 4.1 and 5). Θρῖδαξ (*Lactuca sativa* L.) is "lettuce" (*HP*, VII, 4.2 and 9).

37. *HP*, IX, 8.3, with Dioscorides, III, 7.

employed with the "roots" of hemlock (*kōnion*), which were thought to be more potent than the fruit,[38] and with *thapsia* (*Thapsia garganica* L., "deadly carrot").[39] In the cutting method, there was no variety, except in the seasons, either summer or autumn; hellebore is given as the example: the slender lower roots were taken, because the thick upper ones were considered useless.[40] Theophrastus does not distinguish which *helleboros* he means in this passage.

Before Theophrastus begins to list his "herbals," he prefaces the listing with some statements of the *pharmakopōlai* ("drug-vendors") and the *rhizotomoi*. This section (*Historia Plantarum*, IX, 8.5-8) illustrates quite vividly Theophrastus's sources of information, other than Diocles. The drug-vendors and root-cutters advise that one should cut roots only when standing to the windward, especially for *thapsia*; furthermore, one should oil his body first, before cutting the roots. The rest of IX, 8.5-8 is filled with more popular notions, folklore attending the occupations of root-cutting and drug-pandering.[41] These sources of information fit Theophrastus's ideas of gathering empirical knowledge, and he was interested "in things which are called fairy-tales by earlier thinkers."[42] He labeled these ideas as probably less than reliable, but included them because they had yet to be tested and apparently were useful to the *rhizotomoi* and *pharmacopōlai* in their work. That "use" can be placed within the doctrines of sympathy, which seemed to gain popularity in the fourth century B.C.,[43] and which moved the perception of *pharmaka* back into the pesudo-divine context they had had in Homer.[44] If Edelstein's contention is correct, *pharmaka* had been divested of their "magical" and "divine" nature in the Greek writings from c. 700 B.C. to the time of Theophrastus.[45] The new age of wide-ranging military ventures, and of new knowledge from the "far" East, was an age that seemed more willing to attribute multiple meanings and

38. *Cf.* Rufus in Oribasius, VII, 26.125, and Archigenes, Ibid., VIII, 2.30.

39. *HP*, IX, 8.3. Cf. IV, 153 (Θάψια). Dioscorides, IV, 153.2, notes that one had best dig it up only when there is no wind, because the root gives blisters. Cf. Pseudo-Aristotle, *Problems*, I, 41 [864a6].

40. *HP*, IX, 8.4: *φάσιν*.

41. *HP*, IX, 8.5-8.

42. Ludwig Edelstein, "Greek Medicine in Its Relation to Religion and Magic," *Bull. Hist. Med.*, *5* (1937), 201-246; reprinted in Owsei and C. Lilian Temkin, eds., *Ancient Medicine: Selected Papers of Ludwig Edelstein* (Baltimore: Johns Hopkins Press, 1967), pp. 205-246.

43. Pseudo-Aristotle, *Problems*, 886a24. Theophrastus, *On Odors*, 63.

44. *Odyssey*, IV, 230, among many references.

45. Edelstein, "Greek Medicine," pp. 233-235.

powers to *pharmaka*. Much later, Galen would reflect this change,[46] as does Pseudo-Aristotle in *Problems*,[47] probably set down in the generation of Theophrastus. Thus Theophrastus's herbs emerge from a wider context than simply the observations of Diocles: the root-cutters and drug-sellers are assumed to have information that would help provide full description and analysis of the plants. Their medical properties seem not to have been appreciated before Diocles and Theophrastus (the Hippocratic tradition avoids any "sympathetic" description of plants and derived drugs),[48] and *Historia Plantarum* IX is exactly the place one would expect to find plant medicinals.

Mandragoras (Mandrake [*Atropa mandragora* L., or *M. officinalis* L.; U.S. sp. *Podophyllum peltatum* L.])[49] is the first herb on Theophrastus's list (IX, 9.1). Its leaf is to be mixed with barley meal to make a poultice, and is beneficial on wounds. The root, scraped and soaked in vinegar, is deemed useful for erysipelas; also the root(?) is used as a remedy for gout, as a sleep inducer, for "potions" (*philtra*), and is given in "wine or vinegar." One prepares the root by cutting it into little balls (like radishes),[50] stringing them over new wine, and then hanging them over a fire to be smoked.[51]

Mandragoras is in Dioscorides,[52] Galen,[53] and Oribasius,[54] but not in Nicander. Similar to Theophrastus's "sleep inducer" is Galen's "pain killer."[55] The active principles in mandrake are podophyllotoxin, as well as picropodophyllin, and several peltatins. Medically, the effect of mandrake is quite similar to that of stramonium (*Datura stramonium* L.) and belladonna (*Atropa belladonna* L.), and produces lethargy. In modern times, mandrake is employed as an antispasmodic for dogs in veterinary practice, but is no longer recommended as a cathartic in

46. John Scarborough, *Roman Medicine* (London: Thames and Hudson, 1969), pp. 135 and 216, nn. 78-83 (astrology).

47. See note 43, above.

48. Edelstein, "Greek Medicine," p. 234.

49. It is unlikely that this is the Indian podophyllum (*Podophyllum emodi* Wall.), from the Himalaya Mountains and Kashmir.

50. Cf. *HP*, IX, 12.1.

51. Cf. Dioscorides, III, 7; IV, 75; and V, 71. *HP*, IX, 8.8.

52. Esp. IV, 75.

53. XI, 751 and 767, among many references.

54. Oribasius, XI, M.3 (cf. Dioscorides, IV, 75); J. Raeder, ed., *Oribasii Collectionum Medicarum Reliquiae*, 4 vols. (Leipzig: Teubner, 1928-1933 [*Corpus Medicorum Graecorum*, VI, 1, 2]), II, 119-120 (= XI, M.3).

55. Galen, X, 816 (= *Method of Medicine*, XII, 1): *ἐν τοῖς καλουμένοις ἀνωδύνοις φαρμάκοις*, among which is listed *μανδραγόρου ῥίζης*.

general medicine. Theophrastus's sources knew that the pain from gout would be alleviated with a mandrake "potion," but any beneficial effects in the treatment of erysipelas would come from the mild antibiotic action of wine or vinegar (if applied externally) against Group A hemolytic streptococci. Possibly the mandrake drink would have helped victims of erysipelas who had developed secondary symptoms.

Next comes *helleboros* (IX, 9.2), with a very cryptic summary that says simply "both the root and fruit are useful" as a purge. Shortly (IX, 10.1-3), Theophrastus adds a little more about *helleboros*, noting that there are two kinds, black and white; black is fatal to horses; white is eaten by sheep and thereby purged; white *helleboros* grows in the vineyards of Elea, and is used there to make a very diuretic wine. In IX, 14.1-4, we read that *Helleboros* (its "prepared" name is *sēsamōdē*)[56] keeps a long time, almost infinitely without losing its effectiveness, and in IX, 8.4, *helleboros* appears as part of the general description of "root-cutting."[57] By contrast, Diocorides has a lengthy description,[58] replete with superstitions, and Galen mentions *helleboros* as emerging from the Hippocratic writings,[59] as well as from the books of Archigenes.[60] It is curious that Theophrastus gives such short shrift to *helleboros*, unless he intends not to speak at length about those plants known to be deleterious. A related oddity is Nicander's omission of *helleboros* in both the *Theriaca* and *Alexipharmaca*; again this may be due to the influence of Diocles' original work, employed by Apollodorus, and in turn purloined by Nicander.[61]

Black *helleboros* is *Helleboros niger* L., and white *helleboros* is *Veratrum album* L. (U.S. sp. *Veratrum viride*, Ait., "green hellobore"). An alkaloid, cevadine, is contained in the root, which is also part of what is known as veratrine mixture, gained from the seeds of *Schoenocaulon officinale* (Lindl.) A. Gray. No longer used as an anodyne counterirritant, cevadine extract (as part of veratrine) is used in veterinary

56. Dioscorides, IV, 162.1: *καὶ ἐν Ἀντικύρᾳ σησαμοειδές, χρώμενοι πρὸς τὰς καθάρσεις αὐτῷ.*

57. See *HP*, IV, 5.1; VI, 2.9, for description; *De Causis Plantarum* (ed. Wimmer), VI, 13.4, for general qualities. See also *HP*, IX, 15.5 (Arcadia).

58. Dioscorides, IV, 148; 149; and 162. Virgil, *Georgics*, III, 451. See Elfriede Abbe, *The Plants of Virgil's Georgics* (Ithaca: Cornell University Press, 1965), pp. 49-50.

59. Galen, XI, 874 = *Blendings and Dynameis of Simple Medicines*, VI, 5.9.

60. Galen, XVI, 124 (Archigenes); XIV, 761 (antidote for hellebore); XIX, 739 and 744 ("black" hellebore); XIX, 744 ("white" hellebore); among many references.

61. Scarborough, "Nicander's Toxicology," pp. 3-23.

medicine as an emetic for pigs and cattle. Theophrastus does not specify what he means by "purge," but an administration of hellebore would promote heavy vomiting. Theophrastus's sources knew the dangers of hellebore, illustrated in an anecdote about a drug-vendor and a shepherd (IX, 17.1). A *Pharmakopōlēs* was impressing many by his ability to eat without harm "one or two roots" of hellebore, when a local shepherd came up and ate *all* the drug-vendor's supply without ill-effect. One could, therefore, build up a resistance to hellebore (any shepherd knew this), and the incident destroyed the drug-seller's reputation. Furthermore, Theophrastus adds that Thrasyas (otherwise unknown) could consume hellebore without harm, and that a certain Eudemus of Chios could drink hellebore and survive, because he had an "aid."[62] This turns out to be pumice (*kissēris*). It appears that toxicology had not emerged as a separate series of observations, except incidentally.[63] It is clear, however,that Theophrastus was aware that hellebore was quite toxic.

Following the clipped notice about hellebore, the same section (IX, 9.1) has a listing of uses for *panakes* (probably "all heal"). This passage seems badly corrupted, and any firm identification of the plant must await a critical text.[64] Perhaps of the *Valerium* spp., or *Ferulago*, the fruit was useful in treating miscarriage, as well as micturation problems (*tas dysourias*). Other references in Dioscorides (I, 6), Rufus in Oribasius (VIII, 24.6), and the Hippocratic *Aphorisms* (III, 31) do not help key the plant, because other suggestions are made for urination problems. The juice of the *panakes* also is useful in treating miscarriage, for sprains, the voice, and "for the ears." The root is beneficial for other problems of women (unspecified),[65] and for flatulence in beasts of burden.[66] Lastly, *panakes* is useful in making perfume (as in *Historia Plantarium*, IX, 7.2). One might hope that the further listing of *panakes* in IX, 11.1-4 would help to key either the full list of four "kinds" or the specific species. The *panakes* in IX, 9.2, is now called "Syrian,"

62. *HP*, IX, 17.3: ἡ βοήθεια.

63. Scarborough, "Nicander's Toxicology," pp. 3-7.

64. Sir Arthur Hort, ed. and trans., *Theophrastus: Enquiry into Plants*, 2 vols. (London: Heinemann, 1916 [Loeb Classical Library]), II, 468, states *Ferulago galbanifera*.

65. Πάνακες in the Hippocratic *corpus* (ed. E. Littré), VIII, 387, is recommended in treatment for displacement of the uterus; Littré thinks the plant is *Echinophora tenuifolia*. Soranus, *Gynecology* (ed. J. Ilberg [Leipzig: Teubner, 1927; *Corpus Medicorum Graecorum*, IV]), I, 19.62: πάνακος ῥίζης is a contraceptive.

66. This seems to be an echo of Aristotle, *Historia Animalium*, 604a12: πρὸς ὑποζυγίων φύσας.

and in IX, 11.1-3, we get three more "kinds:" "Chaeronean," *panakes* of Asclepius, and *panakes* of Heracles. "Chaeronean" may be from the *Inula* spp., and Theophrastus writes that this plant is most effective against the bites of spiders, snakes, and other reptiles. One gives "Chaeronean" in the following ways: in wine, in olive oil (smearing the wound), in a plaster, in vinegar, and with honey (for tumors: *phymatōn*). Nicander, *Theriaca*, 130, 223, and 826, and Oppian, *Cynegetica*, III, 439, allude to the snakebite, but the type of *panakes* (Nicander, *Theriaca*, 565) is quite different. The third on Theophrastus's list of *panakes* is the *panakes* of Asclepius (IX, 11.2), which appears in Nicander, *Theriaca*, 685, as *panakes Phlegyēion.*[67] Perhaps this is one of the *Ferula* spp., and Theophrastus says to scrape the leaf and stem (which taste salty: *halykōdē*) into an unnamed drink for benefit against snakebite. There are other uses: mix it with honey for disorders of the spleen, when blood accumulates around it; pound it up (root? leaf?) with olive oil, and anoint the head to cure headache; take scrapings in wine for stomachache; sprinkle it on a "wet" or "running" wound (*tōn helkōn tōn men hygrōn*) in hot wine (wash the wound first); apply a plaster of it, soaked in wine, for dry wounds. Again the major benefit would come from the lightly antibiotic qualities of wine, or from a similar effect in the honey mixture.[68]

The fourth *panakes* (*Historia Plantarum*, IX, 11.3) can be keyed, thanks to a reference in Dioscorides (III, 48.1). This is the *panakes* of Heracles, from which – so Dioscorides tells us – is extracted *opopanax*. Opopanax is a fetid gum resin, obtained from the roots of *opopanax Chironium* (L.) Koch, a yellow-flowered umbelliferous plant that resembles the parsnip;[69] opopanax was formerly used in perfumes and soaps.

67. *ἄγρει καὶ πάνακες φλεγυήιον, ὅ ῥά τε πρῶτος/Παιήων* Μέλανος *ποταμοῦ παρὰ χεῖλος ἄμεβξεν.* A. S. F. Gow and A. F. Scholfield, *Nicander* (Cambridge: Cambridge University Press, 1953), p. 234, identify the plant as *Echinophora tenuifolia*. See Dioscorides, III, 49.

68. On wine as an antiseptic, see Guido Majno, *The Healing Hand: Man and Wound in the Ancient World* (Cambridge, Mass.: Harvard University Press, 1975), p. 187: "The antiseptic power of wine is no myth ... Recent studies ... pin down the mechanism to the anthocyanes, a subgroup in the large group of polyphenols present in wine." Majno gives bibliographical data in nn. 255-260, p. 498. On honey, see ibid., p. 117: "Honey is antibacterial for several reasons. The most obvious is a simple concentration effect: being extremely hypertonic, it draws water from the bacterial cells, causing them to shrivel and die." References are in nn. 184-197, p. 484.

69. Cf. Celsus, V, 18.5, and Galen, XIII, 341 (recipe with opopanax). See Scarborough, "Asclepiades," p. 53.

Theophrastus says that this particular kind of *panakes* tastes bitter and smells like frankincense. It has two uses, plus an unusual third: first, one can drink it with wine to soothe stomach pains; second, mixed with honey, it helps heal dry wounds, and wet ones are helped by the substance alone. The third use not only is unusual, but proves also that *Historia Plantarum* IX stands solidly within Aristotelianism. Heracles's *panakes* is also beneficial for epilepsy, but it must be mixed "with the curd of a seal (*phōkēs pitua*)," in the proportion of one to four. *Pitua* = *tamisos*,[70] which means that Theophrastus is recommending the rennet from a seal for epilepsy. There are parallels in other authors: Nicander, *Theriaca*, 577, recommends the curd (*tamisos*) of a rabbit or stag as part of an antidote for snakebite, and Nicander, *Alexipharmaca*, 68, uses *puetia* instead of *tamisos*; Dioscorides, II, 75, recommends *pitua* of a rabbit, along with the curd of horses, deer, and other animals – the best being that of a seal – for epilepsy. Not much of this would make much sense, were it not for the scholiast's remarks on *Theriaca*, 577.[71] High-quality cheese was made with curds of various animals (used as a coagulant), and cheese fanciers could tell exactly what animal by the odor. Slightly useful against snake venom (the calcium),[72] *tamisos/pitua* would have small benefit for victims of the "sacred disease."[73]

The choice of a seal by Theophrastus is significant. It is the only animal he mentions in *Historia Plantarum* IX, and the seal was a particularly puzzling animal to Aristotle before him. Aristotle had dissected seals and bats to see why they were "merely quadrupeds badly formed."[74] He had determined that seal kidneys resembled those of an ox, that seals had no gall bladder,[75] did not breathe sea water, bore their young

70. Erotian, *s.v.* *τάμισος*.

71. *Scholia on Theriaca*, 577 (ed. A. Crugnola [Milan: Instituto Editoriale Cisalpino, 1971], p. 220). Also *Scholia on Theocritus*, VII, 16 (ed. F. Dübner [Paris: Didot, 1870(?)], p. 52): *τάμισος δὲ ἡ πυτία εἴρηται παρὰ τὸ θαμίζειν, ὅ ἐστι πυκνοῦν τὸ γάλα περὶ αὐτὸ στρεφόμενον. ἢ παρὰ τὸ ταμείων αξιοῦσθαι δὶα τὴν χῆσιν.*

72. G. L. McGrew and B. D. Johnson, "*In Vivo* Effects of Selected *Crotalus* Venoms on Serum Magnesium and Calcium," in A. de Vries and E. Kochva, eds., *Toxins of Animal and Plant Origin* (New York: Gordon and Breach, 1973), III, 1039-1054. E. R. Trethewie, "The Pharmacology and Toxicology of the Venoms of Snakes of Australia and Oceania," in W. Bücherl et. al., eds., *Venomous Animals and Their Venoms* (New York: Academic Press, 1971), II, 79-101, esp. 88. Scarborough, "Nicander's Toxicology," n. 135.

73. Owsei Temkin, *The Falling Sickness*, 2nd ed. (Baltimore: Johns Hopkins Press, 1971), pp. 22, 79.

74. Aristotle, *Progression of Animals*, XIX, 10 (714b10).

75. Aristotle, *Parts of Animals*, III, 9 (671b4-6), IV, 2 (676b28-30).

alive, produced a chorion, had bones like cartilage,[76] and had no external ears.[77] Last, Aristotle said that seals vomited up their curds when they were caught, and the *pitua* was medically useful for epileptics.[78] Theophrastus picked the seal as that animal which would give beneficial curd, most probably because Aristotle, his mentor, attached such importance to it in his study of animals. Likewise, this choice appears in Dioscorides, a fact which may be another instance of the long-range impact of Diocles.[79] At the very least, *Historia Plantarum* IX, 11.3, indicates the heritage of Aristotle, easily seen in *Progression of Animals*, *Parts of Animals*, and other works. The species is the monk seal (*Monachus monachus* Herm.), the same species that appears in *Odyssey*, IV, 404 and 451. Now a rarity, the monk seal was quite common during classical antiquity in the Mediterranean and Black Seas; it presently occurs only around Rhodes, Corsica, and Cape Caliacra (on the coast of Bulgaria).[80]

Returning to ordinary herbs, Theophrastus quickly lists *kyklaminos* (*Historia Plantarum*, IX, 9.3), *sikuos ho agrios* (IX, 9.4), and *chamaidrys* (IX, 9.5). *Kyklaminos* is the cyclamen, or "sow bread" (*Cyclamen europaeum* L.), from which is extracted cyclamin (triacetyloleandromycin), employed in modern medicine as an antibacterial, emetic, purgative, and hemolytic agent. Generally, cyclamen is a low, primulaceous herb in the *Cyclamen* spp. with tuberous rootstocks and nodding white, purple, pink, or red flowers with reflexed petals. Having written (VII, 9.4) that the root has bark, Theophrastus says (IX, 9.3) that the root is beneficial for running wounds, and mixed with honey is a good wound dressing.[81] Indeed, with the mild antibiotic character of honey added to the cyclamen, this dressing would be quite beneficial. Also the root

76. Aristotle, *Historia Animalium*, VI, 11 (566b27-567a15).

77. Aristotle, *Generation of Animals*, V, 2.24-29 (781b24-29); same as *Parts of Animals*, II, 12.21-24 (657a21-24).

78. Pseudo-Aristotle, *Marvelous Things Heard*, 77 (835b32-34).

79. Dioscorides, II, 75; see notes 9 and 17, above.

80. Two other species of the monk seal–rare–occur in the West Indies (*M. tropicalis*) and Hawaii (*M. schauinslandi*). Otto Keller, *Die antike Tierwelt*, 2 vols. (Leipzig, 1909; reprinted Hildesheim, 1963), I, 407-408, collects a few references. See also B. Mursalogu, "Occurrence of the Monk Seal on the Turkish Coasts," *J. Mammology, 45* (1964), 316-317; A. van Wijngaarden, "The Mediterranean Monk Seal," *Oryx, 6* (1962), 270-273; Judith E. King, "The Monk Seals (Genus *Monachus*)," *Bull. Brit. Mus.* (Nat. Hist.) *Zool., 5* (1956), 201-256. There is a summary in Noel Simon and Paul Geroudet, *Last Survivors* (New York: World Publishing Co., 1970), pp. 258-262.

81. See note 68, above.

can be used as a pessary for women, a reference that forms part of a suppository recipe in Soranus, *Gynecology*, III, 6.32 (Ilberg). The root is good as a charm to promote rapid childbirth; the charm is in little balls, made from the ashes of the root steeped in wine.[82] The juice of the cyclamen is good for "head purges" poured in (the nostrils?) mixed with honey.[83]

Sikuos ho agrios is labeled "squirting" or "wild" cucumber (*Ecballium elaterium* L.),[84] and Theophrastus says that the root is used to treat white leprosy and mange in sheep; the juice extracted was called *elatērion* ("the driver").[85] Related species, like the colocynth (*Citrullus colocynthis* Schrad.) contain albuminoids, pectin, and colocynthin, formerly used as a drastic purgative, and as a purgative for dogs and pigs in veterinary medicine. The Greek *elatērion* states what the extract can do to the bowels.

Chamaidrys is germander (or English treacle, or wood garlic: *Teucrium scordium* L.), which Theophrastus says is used for wounds, fractures, and wounds that seem to be spreading (the leaves, pounded up in olive oil); the fruit functions as a bile purge, and is beneficial for treating ulcers of the eye.[86] The fresh herb has a garlicky odor and a sharp, bitter taste. It contains tannin, as well as scordein and an oil. Formerly employed as a sudorific, scordein (scordium) was once believed to be an antidote for poisons, a tradition that appears in Pliny[87] and Dioscorides.[88]

Two kinds of *strychnoi* follow the *panakē*. One type induces sleep (*hypnōdēs*), while the second variety is called *manikos*. For the sleep

82. Cf. Pliny, *Natural History*, XXIII, 63, with *HP*, IX, 9.4.

83. Cf. Dioscorides, II, 164, and Pliny, *Natural History*, XXV, 133, and XXVI, 149.

84. By Hort, *Theophrastus*, II, 476, and Gow and Scholfield, *Nicander*, p. 235. Cf. Dioscorides, IV, 150, and Pliny, *Natural History*, XX, 3.

85. See also *HP*, IX, 14.1 and 2.

86. *HP*, IX, 9.5. Cf. *HP*, VII, 6.2, and Dioscorides, III, 98.

87. Pliny, XXIV, 130-131 (*Chamaedys herba*), XXV, 63, 100, and 127 (*scordion = scordotis*).

88. Dioscorides, III, 97, and 98. Pliny (note 87, above) may reflect the confusion of names in his Greek sources. In *HP*, IX, 9.5, and Dioscorides, III, 98, one meets χαμαίδρυς; in Dioscorides, III, 97, χαμαίδρυς = τεύκριον, and in Dioscorides, III, 111, χαμαίδρυς = σκόρδιον. The confusion is also mirrored in Bernhard Langkavel, *Botanik der spaeteren Griechen* (Berlin, 1866; reprinted Amsterdam: Hakkert, 1964), p. 59. Modern nomenclature makes the "wall germander" and the "water germander" into one species, going back, so it seems, to Theophrastus, who has only χαμαίδρυς. Theophrastus's σκόροδον (σκόρδον) is always garlic.

inducer, one soaks the root in wine, after the bark of the root has been bruised, and then drinks the wine thus treated to bring on drowsiness. The plant here in IX, 11.5, also appears in VII, 15.4, and is the famous deadly nightshade (*Atropa belladonna* L.),[89] or the belladonna leaf. Quite familiar to modern pharmacologists, the extract contains atropine, hyoscyamine, scopolamine, asparagine, choline, chrysatropic acid, atroscine, leucatropic acid, and phytosterol. Modern physicians will sometimes use belladonna as an anticholinergic, and veterinarians employ it to suppress the symptoms of heaves; its former broad veterinary use as an antispasmodic in colic, tetanus, cough, bronchitis, and dyspnea has been supplanted by more uniformly acting drugs. Theophrastus's (and Nicander's) "sleep inducer" would indeed promote relaxation, if the dose were as diluted as *Historia Plantarum* IX, 11.5, suggests. Unfortunately, there are numerous side effects – some quite serious – if the dose is anything other than minute. Such effects would be quite similar to those observed with atropine sulfate, which include xerostomia, brachycardia, mydiasis, blurred vision, and urinary retention.[90]

Stryknos manikos causes insanity (IX, 11.6). This is the thorn apple (*Datura stramonium* L.), again quite familiar in modern pharmacology.[91] The leaves contain 0.25-0.45 percent alkaloids (atropine, hyoscyamine, and scopalamine), plus some proteins and albumin; the seeds have the same constituents, but in lesser quantity. In modern medicine, the extract is called stramonium, and is used as an anticholinergic and antiasthmatic agent, as well as in the treatment of Parkinson's disease. Since 1967, however, the drug of choice has been levodopa. Theophrastus's *manikos* has four basic uses: one drachma improves one's mood; two drachmae cause temporary insanity and delusions; three drachmae cause permanent insanity (here mixed with *opon kentauriou* [*Centaurea salonitana* L. ?]); and four drachmae kill a man.[92] In many

89. Nicander, *Theriaca*, 74 and 878: simply *στρύχνον*, which is probably *στρύχνον ὑπνωτικοὐ*.

90. Dioscorides, IV, 72.1-2: *στρύχνον ὑπνωτικόν*. In IV, 72.2, one reads *ταύτης ὁ φλοὶος τῆς ῥίζης οἲνω ποθεὶς δραχμῆς μιᾶς ὁλκὴ ὑπνωτικήν*. Dioscorides notes that the effect (*δύναμιν*) of the juice is less than that of the poppy (*τῆς μήκωνος*). Galen, XII, 145-146 (*περὶ τρύχνουὴ στρύχνου*), also picks up the traditional description, except that the account seems a conflation of *HP*, IX, 11.5 and 6; Galen's *στρύχνον* includes both *στρύχνον ὑπνωτικόν* and *στρύχνον μανικόν*, given separate entries by Theophrastus and Dioscorides.

91. A. F. Blakeslee's *The Genus "Datura"* (New York: Ronald Press, 1959) is a standard reference.

92. The *drachmē* = 52.8 grains = 3.41 grams; the *oxybaphon* = 1/8 pint = 0.06 liters. Scarborough, "Nicander's Toxicology," pp. 6 and 11 with nn. 56 and 115a.

respects, IX, 11.6, is a forecast of the "herbals affecting the mind" found in IX, 18.3-11, followed by reemphasis on the fact that *manikos* causes madness in IX, 19.1. Dioscorides, IV, 73.2, has roughly the same measures for the effects of *manikos*: one drachma gives pleasant visions (or fantasies); two drachmae make one "out of his head" for three days;[93] and four drachmae kill. Dioscorides, unlike Theophrastus, includes an antidote (*antipharmakon*), which is *melikraton*, the honey-water drink seen in *Historia Plantarum*, IX, 11.2.[94]

Three types of spurge (*tithymalloi*) are in *Historia Plantarum*, IX, 11.7-9. These are from the numerous species in the genus *Euphorbia*, which have milky juice and flowers with no petals or sepals. *E. hirta* L. and *E. pilulifera* L. are both very common in India, and possibly some information on these two species came to Theophrastus as a result of Alexander's campaigns there. *E. peplus* L. and *E. paralias* L. are two other candidates for the list. Dioscorides, IV, 164.1-9, has seven varieties. Hort and his sources offer the following nomenclature: *tithymallos* (IX, 11.7) = *E. peplus; tithymallos ho arrēn* (IX, 11.8) = *E. Sibthorpii* (Wimmer offers *E. Characias* [p. 546]); *tithymallos ho myrtitēs* (IX, 11.9) = *E. Mysinites* (same as Wimmer, p. 546). Comparative readings from Dioscorides, IV, 164, and Pliny, *Natural History*, XXVI, 62-66, lead to similar, imprecise conclusions. Whatever the exact species, all the *Euphorbia* contain several resins and an unstable glucoside, widely used in medicine until quite recently in the treatment of asthma and bronchitis. Theophrastus's account says that the dried fruit is given in an unspecified drink (presumably wine), the juice from the whole plant functions as a bowel purge, and the fruit is called a "nut" (*kaletai kauron*).[95] There are two methods of administration: dry the *kauron*, clean it, wash it in water again, then give it to drink mixed with two parts of "black poppy," which all together equal one *oxybaphos*.[96] This concoction is particularly good as a "phlegm-purger from the bowels." The second method involves grinding up the *kauron* in sweet wine, or giving the nut with dried sesame (*Sesamum indicum* L.) to be chewed

93. *δύο δὲ δραχμαὶ ποθεῖσαι ἐξιστάνουσιν ἄρχι τριῶν ἡμερῶν.* In IV, 73.1, Dioscorides gives the other names for *μανικός*: *πέρσειον, περισσόν, ἄνυδρον, πεντόδρυον, θρύον,* and *ὀρθόγυιον* (ἐκαλεσαν). In Pliny, XXI, 177-179, the name seems to be derived from *ἐρυθρόν.*

94. This is probably the honey-water drink, as in Oribasius (quoting Antyllus), V, 29.7, and V, 14.1 (quoting Galen), contrasted with the honey-milk drink, offered in libation to the powers of the underworld (*Odyssey*, X, 519).

95. Cf. *De Causis Plantarum*, IV, 6.9.

96. See note 92, above.

up. No result is specified, but probably the bowels are purged again.

In IX, 11.10 and 11, occur two varieties of *libanōtis* (with fruit: *Karpimos*; and lacking fruit: *akarpos*). These two types are related to the well-known rosemary (*Rosmarinus officinalis* L.), long employed in the manufacture of perfumes, Eau de Cologne, and toilet soap.[97] By comparing IX, 11.10, with Dioscorides, III, 74.1, and Galen, XII, 60 (and the odd *libanōtis kachryphoros* of Nicander, *Theriaca*, 850), one is reasonably assured that Theophrastus's *libanōtis karpimos* is the rosemary frankincense, *Lecokia cretica* L.; *Libanōtis hē akarpos* is probably the sterile rosemary, *R. sterile*, or *Lactuca graeca*, as in Dioscorides, III, 74.4. According to Theophrastus, the root of the *karpimos* is beneficial for wounds and for "women's matters,"[98] given in dry black wine, and for difficulty in urination (strangury), for ophthalmia and conjunctivitis,[99] and to promote milk in women. *Akarpos* (IX, 11.11) has a root that purges "both ways: up and down," with the upper part of the root for vomiting, the lower part for the bowels. Also *akarpos* functioned as the ancient equivalent of paradichlorobenzene crystals: it kept moths from eating one's clothes. *R. officinalis* contains about 1 percent oil, resin, and the bitter principle (flowers), and oil and tannin (leaves). The leaves were used in medical practice as an emmenagogue, and the tannin would have beneficial effect, especially on open wounds.

Two kinds of *chamaileōn* follow (*cf.* VI, 4.3). *Chamaileōn ho leukos* (IX, 12.1) is the white pine thistle (*Atractylis gummifera* L.). Theophrastus says that the root is to be cooked, chopped up, and eaten like radishes for treatment of diarrhea. For treatment of flatworms,[100] the

97. A good, short summary is in Albert F. Hill, *Economic Botany* (New York: McGraw-Hill, 1952), pp. 185-186.

98. *καὶ πρὸς τὰ γυναικεῖα.* Soranus (ed. Ilberg), II, 24.51, suggests *ὁ λιβανωτός* (the real frankincense) in the treatment *περὶ ἄφθης* (thrush).

99. *πρὸς τὰς στραγγουρίας καὶ πρὸς τὰ ὦτα καὶ ἄργεμα καὶ πρὸς ὀφαλμίας.* "For the ears" may be similar to the following "for the eyes." *ἄργεμα* are rather curious. Pollux, *Onomasticon* (ed. E. Bethe [Stuttgart: Teubner, 1966; reprint of 1900-1937 ed.]), II, 65: *ἄργεμος[ον]* = *λεύκωμα.* In Dioscorides, III, 84, and Galen, XIV, 775, and Aetius, VII, 39, this means a "spot" in the eye, a thickening of the cornea, an anterior synechia causing a dense white cicatrix of the cornea. Unless Theophrastus or his source is prescribing a kind of pleasant-smelling eye wash (or salve) made from the rosemary frankincense, the text makes little sense.

100. This may be an echo of Aristotle's observations in *Historia Animalium*, V, 19 esp. 551a8-14 and 551b27-30. The flatworm probably is one of the cyclophyllidean tapeworms, common as parasites in man.

victim was to eat some raisins first, then to drink an *oxybaphon*[101] of the scraped root in wine. *Leukos* is fatal to dogs: one mixes it in a meal paste with oil and water to kill them. Likewise, *Leukos* is used to kill pigs: one mixes it with a spurge, *rhaphanos hē oreia* (probably *Euphorbia Apios* L.).[102] *Leukos* is useful in sweet wine for unspecified complaints of women.[103] Last, a little folk tradition peeps through in the account of *leukos*: if a sick man is washed with *leukos* (in wine) for three days – and lives – he will recover.[104]

Atractylis gummifera L. yields, by hydrolysis, the poisonous glucoside atractylic acid, in the form of its potassium salt. A highly toxic substance, atractylic acid (or atractyligenin) produces convulsions of a hypoglycemic nature, like strychnine. Atractylic acid would be quite poisonous, but could function as a circulatory stimulant in the manner of a bitter tonic. The plant might be effective against tapeworms, but the side effects would not warrent its use in heavy doses. It appears that the folk traditions have a clearer notion of *A. gummifera.*[105]

Chamaileōn ho melas is *Cardopatium corymbosum* L., the dark pine thistle. Theophrastus (*Historia Plantarum*, IX, 12.2) says that this is beneficial against leprosy, if mixed with vinegar; likewise, a plaster can be made, also useful against leprosy. *Melas* is also fatal to dogs – or ticks on a dog.[106] Dioscorides, III, 9.2, more or less repeats the notion that vinegar and *melas* cure leprosy, and adds that "passed through a hollow quill, [they] will break up a bad tooth." The substance may have had some use as a mild analgesic for toothache, but it is ineffective against leprosy. Until recently, the ethyl asters of some acids in chaulmoogra oil (from the Burmese tree, *Hydnocarpus Kurzii* [the seeds within the velvety fruit]) provided an effective, if painful, chemotherapy for leprosy. Modern drugs of choice are among the sulfones, especially dapsone (4,4'-sulfonyldianiline).

Three kinds of *mēkōnes* constitute the listings in *Historia Plantarum*, IX, 12.3-5. All appear to be wild poppies, none of which is the famous

101. See note 92, above.

102. Cf. Dioscorides, IV, 175 (which Wellmann [ed., *Materia Medica*, II, 324] asserts comes from Diocles, owing to the similarity to Theophrastus, *HP*, IX, 9.6).

103. Pliny, XXII, 21.45-47, picks up this tradition among others; XXII, 45: "Hac mastiche utuntur mulieres." There is no trace in Soranus.

104. One is reminded of Cato, *On Agriculture*, 157.10 (where Cato is extolling the medical virtues of cabbage): "Item pueros pusillos si laves eo lotio, numquam debiles fient." Scarborough, *Roman Medicine*, pp. 17-21 (on Cato).

105. Cf. Nicander, *Theriaca*, 656, and Dawkins, "Greek Names for Plants," p. 5.

106. Hort, Theophrastus, II, 279, n. 7: κύνας may be κυνορραϊστας, dogticks, as conjectured by Reinesius from Pliny's *ricinos canum.*

opium poppy (*Papaver somniferum* L., or *P. album* Mill.). *Mēkōn hē keratitis* (IX, 12.3) is the horned poppy (*Glaucium flavum* L. [Hort gives var. Serpierii]), the fruit of which "has the power to clean out the bowels," and the leaf removes *argema* from sheep.[107] *Mēkōn hē rhoias* (IX, 12.4) is called the corn poppy in North America (*Papaver rhoeas* L.; Hort offers *P. hybridum*), and is a bowel purge. *Mēkōn hē Hrakleia*, "frothy poppy" (IX, 12.5; *Silene venosa*, so Hort thinks), cleans as an emetic, and is employed in mead as a treatment for epileptics.[108]

There is a curious absence in this section: the opium poppy, which appears only once in the entire *Historia Plantarum*, and that reference is a very brief notice in I, 12.2, in a section on saps. The fig and the poppy have milky saps. And that is all. Even this one citation may be in doubt, because the Greek text is quite corrupted.[109] Given the fame and widespread employment of *Papaver somniferum* L. in classical antiquity (references begin with Homer, *Iliad*, VIII, 306), there may be good reason why Theophrastus declined to include it in his herbs and herbals. Almost all other sources in Greek and Roman pharmacy and medicine include the opium poppy, and the list is impressive: Nicander,[110] Theocritus,[111] Dioscorides,[112]

107. See note 99, above.

108. Cf. Dioscorides, IV, 64, and Pliny, XX, 205-206; Dioscorides, IV, 64, and Pliny, XIX, 167-169; and Dioscorides, IV, 66, and Pliny, XX, 207.

109. Hort, *Theophrastus*, I, 86, n. 4.

110. *Theriaca*, 946; *Alexipharmaca*, 433-440 (in list of poisons); Athenaeus, XV, 683f-684a (from Nicander, *Geo* ˙˙*a*; frag. 74 in Gow and Scholfield). Nicander has *P. rhoeas* in *Theriaca*, 851, and *Glaucium flavum* in *Theriaca*, 852.

111. Theocritus, *Idylls*, VII, 157; XI, 57-58. *Scholia on Theocritus: Idylls* (ed. F. Dübner), III, 29: τηλέφιον δὲ ἐστι τὸ φύλλον τῆς μήκωνος. A. S. F. Gow, *Theocritus*, 2 vols. (Cambridge: Cambridge University Press, 1952), II, 70, notes that the scholiast seems uncertain, because a second reading appears.

112. Dioscorides, IV, 64.1-7, is an extended account, beginning with the definite distinction of cultivation: μήκων · ἡ μὲν τίς ἐστιν ἥμερος καὶ κηπευτή. Dioscorides' authorities have warnings: Erasistratus (quoted by Diagoras) thought the use of the opium poppy was inadvisable for eye or ear problems, because it dulled vision and caused sleep (IV, 64.6); Andreas is quoted (ibid.) as saying that it causes blindness; Mnesidemus (ibid.) thought the opium poppy had two uses: for the odor and as a sleep inducer. The odor and bright color of the opium poppy figure in numerous similes in Greek and Roman poetry, as indicated by the references in Saara Lilja, *The Treatment of Odours in the Poetry of Antiquity* (Helsinki: Societas Scientiarum Fennica [*Commentationes Humanarum Litterarum*, 49], 1972), pp. 193-195. Dioscorides, IV, 64.5, also remarks that there are some "fake" opium products, suggesting (1) great demand for the genuine article and (2) willing customers for the adulterated juice. Earlier (IV, 64.3), he has written πλείων δὲ ποθεὶς βαπτίζει ⟨ὕπνῳ⟩ ληθαργωδῶς καὶ ἀναιρεῖ.

Celsus,[113] Pliny,[114] and Galen,[115] among many. Theophrastus's silence, however, may have a simple explanation, because the juice of *P. rhoeas* does have a small amount of opium, and would be a mild narcotic and anodyne. In IX, 16.8, *mēkōn* is coupled with *kōneion*, suggesting a hemlock poppy, another plant altogether. It may be that the "cultivated" poppy was not common in Theophrastus's time, and that he would not have recognized the substance as either more useful or more dangerous than other "saps." Some support for this conclusion lies in the treatment that Celsus gives to the poppy: in *De medicina*, V, 27.12B-C, Celsus does not include the poppy in his list of poisons, which suggests he knew only of a mild variety; he does, however, recommend the juice of *papaver* (probably *P. rhoeas*) as an internal medicine to induce sleep and relieve pain, and he advises its external application to alleviate pains in the parts.[116] Theophrastus's notice of

113. See note 116, below.

114. Pliny has a great number of vague references to *papaver*. The following passages are quite definitely about the opium poppy: XVIII, 229 ("visque somnifera etiam sativo"); XIX, 168-169 (beginning with "papaveris sativi tria genera"); XX, 61-64 (where Pliny has ignored the warnings in Dioscorides, IV, 64.6, "as sanat omnia oculorum vitia cum lacte mulierum, argema" [see note 99, above] nubiculas, cicatrices adustionesque omnes, praecipue caligines" [61]; the listing continues, with the *sucus* curing bowels, snakebites, the stings of spiders and scorpions, etc. Pliny quotes Crateuas [63] as recommending this poppy juice for dropsy); XX, 198-203 (authorities quoted: Diagoras, Iollas, Erasistratus, Andreas; this time, Pliny also quotes the warning of Diagoras and Erasistratus [200] in contradiction to XX, 61); XXI, 70 (probable); XXVI, 44 (probable); XXVI, 74 (probable); XXIX, 43 (doubtful); XXX, 60 (probable). The rest of Pliny's references to *papaver* are either to another kind, or are to the use of the poppy as a comparison. Index listings appear in L. Ian and C. Mayhoff, eds., *C. Plinius Secundus: Naturalis Historia*, 6 vols. (Leipzig: Teubner, 1865-1898; reprinted 1970), VI, 289-290, and vol. VII of the Loeb *Pliny: Natural History*, ed. and trans. W. H. S. Jones (Cambridge, Mass.: Harvard University Press, 1956), p. 527.

115. Galen, VI, 548 (= G. Helmreich, ed., *Galeni De Alimentorum Facultatibus*, 31 [*Corpus Medicorum Graecorum*, V, 4, 2 (1923)], p. 258); XII, 72-74; XIII, 37-47 (some collected recipes and authorities). There is enough evidence to suggest that Galen may have encouraged Marcus Aurelius in the use of the drug for its well-known effects; see Thomas W. Africa, "The Opium Addiction of Marcus Aurelius," *J. Hist. Ideas, 22* (1961), 97-102. But maybe mandrake was involved; see E. C. Witke, "Marcus Aurelius and Mandragora," *Class. Phil., 60* (1965), 23-24.

116. Celsus, II, 32 (sleep); V, 23B (part of an antidote), 25.4 (*silvestris papaveris* in the making of *catapotia*, used for sleeping pills, etc.); III, 10.2 (bread soaked *papavere* applied to the head for headache); 18.2 (a drink of *papaver* mixture for sleep); IV, 17.1 (*album papaver* added to the diet for treating kidney disease); 27.1E (from a fragmented text on *coeuntia*, including *nigrum papaver*); 31.6-7 (*papaveris cortices* and *sucus papaveris* in a remedy for joint pains).

Silene venosa in the treatment of epilepsy would refer to the "mild" variety, and the reference in *Historia Plantarum*, IX, 12.5, has parallels in Dioscorides (IV, 66) and Pliny (XIX, 21, and XX, 207).

In *Historia Plantarum*, IX, 13, there appear six plants in rapid order: *nymphaia* (13.1), *hē Skythikē* (13.2), *hē aristolochia* (13.3 = [more or less] IX, 20.4), *to ereuthedanon* (13.6), *skorpios* (13.6), and *polypodion* (13.6). Book IX, 13.4-5, gives a short digression on the color and taste of some plants, suggesting the classification observed in *Causis Plantarum*, VI, 4.5. *Nymphaia* is most probably a yellow water lily (*Nuphar luteum* [L.] Sibth. & Sm.), from which is extracted nupharidine. Theophrastus says that it functions as a wound-clotter (*ischaimon*) and is useful in a drink (wine? water?) for *dysenteria*. *Hē Skythikē* is the "Scythian root" or licorice (*Glycyrrhiza glabra* L.), still useful as a demulcent and expectorant. In Theophrastus, the plant is employed for asthma, dry cough, and as a thirst quencher (he says that with mare's cheese, the Scythians use this root to go without water for twelve or thirteen days); and mixed with honey, the root is good for wounds.[117] *Aristolochia* is a birthwort (probably *Aristolochia rotunda* L.), which Theophrastus recommends for wounds of the head, other wounds, and for what appears to be snakebite.[118] The substance is a sleep inducer, and is useful "for the womb" (*pros hysteran*). There are three methods of preparation and use: as a plaster, steeped in water, and given shredded in honey or olive oil. From the *Aristolochia* spp. comes aristolochic acid, which is employed as an aromatic bitter, and which produces toxic effects in laboratory animals (cardiac and respiratory arrest). *To ereuthedanon* is madder (*Rubia tinctorium* L.), which Theophrastus says is used as a diuretic and for pains in the loins.[119] Extracted from *R. tinctorium* are ruberythric acid and rubiadin. *Skorpios* is a plant sometimes called leopard's bane, one of the composite herbs in the genus *Doronicum*, usually having alternate, clasping leaves and yellow flowers (another plant called leopard's bane is *Arnica montana* L., from northern Europe, which yields tannin, resin, arnicin, arnidiol, and anthoxantine, used as a topical counterirritant). The plant described in Book IX, 13.6, has what appears to be the well-known notion of "signatures," because the root looks like a scorpion. It will, therefore, be effective against scorpion stings. The root would have some small

117. Cf. Scribonius Largus, *Conpositiones* (ed. G. Helmreich [Leipzig: Teubner, 1887]), LXXV. Scarborough, "Asclepiades," pp. 48-49. Dioscorides, III, 5.

118. Cf. Nicander, *Theriaca*, 509-519; Pliny, XXV, 95; Dioscorides, IV, 4.

119. Cf. Pliny, XIX, 47, and Dioscorides, III, 143.

benefit as a counterirritant against scorpion stings,[120] and Theophrastus and his sources have recorded a useful remedy.[121] Ending this section is the curious notice of *polypodion*, which is a fern in the genus *Polypodium* (probably *P. vulgare* L.) with creeping rootstalks, deeply pinnatifid evergreen fronds, and round, bare sori. Again the "doctrine" of signatures appears: not only is *polypodion* useful as a bowel purge, it is a potent charm against *polypoun* ("polyp") because the root looks like an octopus (*polypous*).[122]

After an important description of what drugs will keep – and what that will not[123] – as well as further definition by way of geographical and topographical location,[124] one comes to a short section on the *pharmakōdeis* native to the island of Crete (IX, 16.1-3). Here are *to diktamnon* (16.1), *to pseudodiktamnon* (16.2), and *Heteron diktamnon* (16.3). All three are dittanies, labiate plants. *Diktamnon* is probably the Cretan dittany (*Origanum Dictamnus* L.), said by Theophrastus to be used in difficult childbirth,[125] given in water. *Pseudodiktamnon* and

120. Experimental evidence shows that thiamine deficiency elevates the toxic action of scorpion venom. See Max W. McIntosh and Dean D. Watt, "Molecular Aspects of Neurotoxic Principle in Venom of the Scorpion *Centruroides sculpturatus*," in Findlay E. Russell and Paul R. Saunders, eds., *Animal Toxins* (Oxford: Pergamon Press, 1967), pp. 41-46 (esp. pp. 43, 45-46), and "Biochemical-Immunochemical Aspects of the Venom from the Scorpion *Centruroides sculpturatus*," ibid., pp. 47-58.

121. Cf. Dioscorides, II, 11-12, 33, and 78; IV, 51.

122. Cf. Dioscorides, II, 35 (ζῷα); II, 49; IV, 186.

123. *HP*, IX, 14.1-4. Some examples: ὁ μὲν γὰρ ἐλλέβορος καὶ τριάκοντα ἔτη χρήσιμος, ἡ δὲ ἀριστολοχία πέντε ἢ ἕξ, χαμαιλέων δὲ ὁ μέλας τετταράκοντα, κενταυρὶς δὲ δέκα ἢ δώδεκα (14.1). A pest of these stored roots is σφονδύλη (14.3), some kind of beetle. Section 14.4 is omitted in the MS called U*. Einarson, "The Manuscripts of Theophrastus's *Historia Plantarum*," *Class. Phil.*, *71* (1976), 68-70, and Hort, *Theophrastus*, II, 288, n. 4.

124. *HP*, IX, 15.1-8. E.g., φαρμακώδεις ... δοκοῦσιν εἶναι τόποι μάλιστα τῶν μὲν ἔξω τῆς Ἑλλάδος: Etruria, Latium, and Egypt (15.1); Ethiopia, Scythia, India (15.2 [this last looks like pure legend]); Thrace (15. 3). τῶν δὲ περὶ τὴν Ἑλλάδα τόπων φαρμακωδέστατον: Pelion in Thessaly, Telethrion in Euboea, Arcadia, and Laconia (15.4). Arcadia has cows (and thus the Arcadians drink cows' milk), two kinds of hellebore, carrot (?), a saffron-bay, spurge, marsh mallow, birthwort, hartwort, two kinds of στρύχνος (15.1), the "squirting" cucumber (making ἐλατήριον), and τιθύμαλλος (15.6), and πανάκεια. Most of these plants are in Laconia, too. Achaea has tragacanth (15.8).

125. Soranus (ed. (Ilberg), III, 38.5 (δίκταμνον is part of hot concoctions for the treatment of μύλη [lit. "millstone"] of the uterus); IV, 13(65).2 (rejection of δίκταμνον, among other herbals, recommended by Hippocrates [*Women's Diseases*, I, 77 (ed. Littré. VIII, 170-172)] for rapid childbirth); IV, 14(I 71).2 (Euryphon of Cnidos makes a diuretic to pull out afterbirth [χόριον] from

heteron diktamnon are, as Theophrastus says, much the same as *diktamnon*, except that *pseudodiktamnon* and *heteron* are weaker. *Pseudodiktamnon* appears, however,[126] to be *Dictamnus albus* L., sometimes called fraxinella or gas plant, because it emits a "burning" vapor. *D. albus* is a perennial, rutaceous plant, yielding dictamine (4-methoxyfuro [2, 3-b] quinoline). Even more confused is the account of *heteron*, and Theophrastus's notice does not allow definite identification (Hort offers *Ballota acetabulosa* for *pseudodiktamnon*, and *B. Pseudodictamnus* for *heteron diktamnon*).[127]

To akoniton is Theophrastus's beginning subject in his consideration of harmful plants, and the passages on *akoniton* appear jumbled and occasionally corrupt (IX, 16.5-6). The confusion of the Greek text is illustrated in the development and almost immediate contradiction in the account: *akoniton* can be mixed to give death calculated in advance (two, three, six months, one or two years); it causes a very painful, lingering death, with the body wasting away, and there is no known *lutikon pharmakon* ("counteracting medicinal").[128] The next sentence in 16.5 is contradictory: "Countryfolk occasionally can save someone with honey and wine and similar things."[129] It appears that the two types of traditions – folk and learned – have been set side by side for comparison. Then follow some extremely corrupted passages (16.6) that seem to be about *ephēmeron* (rendered by Hort as "meadow-

---

δίκταμνον καὶ ἐλελίσφακος; rejected in IV, 15 [I 72] with *πάντα δὲ μοχθηρὰ τὰ προειρημένα. δίκταμνον* appears in a gynecological context in the Hippocratic *corpus*, as prescribed by Euryphon, in *Women's Diseases*, I, 78 (ed. Littré, VIII, 176-179), and in *Nature of Women*, 32 (ed. Littré, VII, 346-350).

126. *HP*, IX, 16.2: *διαθερμαίνει γὰρ ἀπὸ μικροῦ σφόδρα. τιθέασι δὲ τὰς δεσμίδας ἐν νάρθηκι ἢ καλάμῳ πρὸς τὸ μὴ ἀποπνεῖν.* See Ronald Good, *The Geography of the Flowering Plants*, 3rd ed. (London: Longman, 1971), pp. 192 and 344.

127. See Hort, *Theophrastus*, II, 484 and 445.

128. *HP*, IX, 16.5: *λυτικὸν δὲ φάρμακον οὐχ εὑρῆσθαι, καθάπερ ἀκούομεν ἑτέρων τι φύεσθαι.* Wimmer, ed., p. 157, conjectures *ἕτερον τι φυόμενον* for the end of the sentence. Hort, *Theophrastus*, II, 300. accepts Schneider's conjecture *ἑτέρων*, together with an emended reading from the Codex Urbinas (U), and the early printed editions (Editio Aldina, Venice, 1495-1498 [Ald.] and Editio Heinsii [Heinsius], Leiden, 1613 [H]). See the fuller account in Einarson, "Manuscripts of Theophrastus's *Historia Plantarum*," pp. 67-76.

129. *HP*, IX, 16.5: *ἀλλὲ τοὺς ἐγχωρίους ἀνασώζειν τινὰς μέλιτι καὶ οἴνῳ.* Hort, *Theophrastus*, II, p. 300, attempts reasonable readings from U and the Codex Medici (M: two, but in very close agreement), while a gloss *εὕρηνται* appears in Ald. and H. Hort's text is the same as Wimmer's p. 157.

saffron") and countermeasures.[130] In 16.7 (after a confused passage about *ephēmeron* being taken by slaves to fake death to outwit masters, then fooling themselves by dying), the text returns to *akoniton*, "which is useless to those who do not understand it." In fact, "one is not supposed to possess it, under the penalty of death."[131] And – seemingly in the carefree manner of a folk tradition – this presumed "legal" statement is followed with the notion that the time that *akoniton* takes to kill is equal to the time since it was gathered.

Even with the confusion in the Greek text of IX, 16.4-7, one perceives a murky theory of toxic action, especially in the choice of *lutikon* to describe what moderns would call an "antidote." As an adjective in the ordinary Greek of Theophrastus's time, *lutikon* is "able to loosen,"

130. U, M, and Ald. all have different versions, largely irreconcilable. Wimmer's readings (pp. 157-158) are as uncertain as those of Hort (II, 300). Hort (ibid., n. 4) states that the passage "is confused, and the text is probably defective." Hort accepts an emendation proposed by Guilandinus (16.6: ἢ τῷ λειρίῳ; Wimmer: ἢ τῷ αἰρίῳ, from Ald. and H) on the basis of Dioscorides, IV, 84.

131. This may refer to the Athenian officials who administered poison to those condemned to death (e.g., the famous passages in Plato, *Phaedo*, esp. 63d5-e5 and 117b6-9). Κώνειον was the preferred poison, as Theophrastus indicates below (*HP*, IX, 16.9). In Attic law, the *archon basileus* had charge of cases involving poison in homicide (Aristotle, *Athenian Constitution*, 57.2-3), so it may be that he had appointed assistants to aid in carrying out sentences that employed poison. If one extrapolates that no "expert" testimony really mattered in Attic trials (e.g., the "evidence" given by a surgeon, on wounds, in Demosthenes, *Against Conon*, 11-14, is no more weighty than other witnesses; also see Demosthenes, *Against Evergus*, 67, and Lysias, *On the Refusal of a Pension to an Invalid*, 13-14, where *no* medical "evidence" appears; a modern court would demand it), then no "expert" in poisons was involved. Antiphon, *Orations*, I (rendered as "Against a Step-Mother on a Charge of Poisoning" by K. Freeman, *The Murder of Herodes* [New York: Norton, 1963], pp. 86-94), esp. 7, proves that poisons were readily available to citizens in Athens in the late fith and early fourth centuries B.C. General background (procedure, etc.) is given in A. R. W. Harrison, *The Law of Athens*, 2 vols. (Oxford: Clarendon Press, 1968-1971), esp. II, 9 and 134. See also Christopher Gill, "The Death of Socrates," *Class. Quart.*, *67*, n.s. *23* (1973), 25-28. Darrel W. Amundsen and Gary B. Ferngren, "The Physician as an Expert in Athenian Law," *Bull. Hist. Med.*, *51* (1977), 202-213, deftly analyze the basic question of "expert medical testimony." Amundsen and Ferngren note that two problems cause difficulty in the investigation of this question: (1) the lack of detailed evidence and (2) "the predominant tendency of modern scholars to base their conclusions on comparisons of Athenian private procedure with the much more rigidly defined modern usages" (p. 213). The authors, however, make the important point that Athenian law and its private procedure *could* allow such expert testimony "when [it was] deemed desirable by the individual" (ibid.).

which then is extended into the more specific "laxative."[132] In a medical or pharmacological context, it then can mean "able to loosen [that which tightens]," particularly a harmful substance ingested.[133] The account in Nicander (on hemlock) supports this conclusion,[134] and Gill has shown that Plato left the "choking" out of the *Phaedo* for his own illustrative purposes when discussing philosophic points.[135]

To akoniton is wolf's bane (or monk's hood, friar's cowl, or mousebane), *Aconitum napellus* L., one species in the large genus *Aconitum.*[136] A well-known toxic substance, aconite, was employed as a febrifuge and gastric anesthetic in medical and veterinary practice. No longer used in the pharmacopeia of modern medicine, aconite is sometimes used by veterinarians to treat laminitis in horses. The most powerful of the aconites is *Aconitum Ferox* Wall., the Indian aconite (also called bikhroot, bish, visha, and bishma), used until quite recently by Indians as an arrow poison to kill large animals. Given the confused state of the text in IX, 15.2, it is quite possible that Theophrastus had indeed "heard" stories about Indian arrow poison, as they were filtered through travelers' accounts, along with the tales that came from Somalia and Ethiopia.[137]

132. Athenaeus, III, 92c (quoting Mnesithius = frag. 36, in Janine Bertier, *Mnésithée et Dieuchès* [Leiden: Brill, 1972], p. 194), and Pseudo-Aristotle, *Problems*, 949a5.

133. Later theories of toxic action (those of Galen, etc.) did not employ the laxative notion, but modified it to mean a "drawing out" of the poisons, as well as a way of correcting the imbalance in the innate heat caused by the poison. Galen, IV, 584; X, 896; XI, 761 and 823. Scarborough, "Nicander's Toxicology," p. 10 and n. 114. Walter Pagel, "Peripheral Venous Flow 'Ascending' to the Heart (Ficinus 1489) and the Spread of Poison," *Episteme, 6* (1972), 128-134 (esp. 129).

134. Nicander, *Alexipharmaca*, 186-194.

135. Gill, "Death of Socrates," pp. 25-28 (esp. pp. 25 and 28).

136. Good, *Flowering Plants*, p. 85: there are over 200 species in *Aconitum.*

137. *HP*, IX, 15.2, indicates the muddled and questionable nature of Theophrastus's sources with εἴπερ ἀληθῆ λέγουσιν. The only arrow poison identified by Hort (*Theophrastus*, II, 290-291, and 485) is the ῥίζα θανατήφορος, "Somali arrow-poison, *Acokanthera Schimperi.*" Called Abyssinin or carissin, the glycoside in the root, bark, and seeds of *A. schimperi* (A. DC.) Beth & Hook. is the active principle of carissin, or African arrow poison. The state of the text in *HP*, IX, 15.2, suggests conflation, since Ethiopia and Scythia have the poison, followed by ἐν Ἰνδοῖς, where the text becomes extremely corrupt. E.g., ἥ τε δυναμένη τὸ αἷμα διαχεῖν καὶ οἷον ὑποφεύγειν makes little sense, unless one assumes a "flight" of arrows, rather than blood. These passages in *HP*, IX, are illustrative of the need for a critical edition. ἃ δή φασιν εὑρῆσθαι πρός τε τῶν ὀφιδίων τῶν θανατηφόρων suggests a filtered story about Indian cobras and the like, compacted with other tales of arrow poisons, antidotes, and drugs. Even after Alexander's expedition, "India" simply meant Ethiopia and the

Thus, in addition to Diocles of Carystos,[138] and the *rhizotomoi-pharmacopōlae,*[139] Theophrastus employed some garbled tales that had trickled in from the "East" to Greece over several centuries. There are, of course, some instances in the *Historia Plantarum* that indicate clear contact and awareness of Alexander's discoveries in Media and India,[140] but even in these passages there is an uncertainty that mitigates against any systematic collecting of data on plant lore from the expedition of Alexander into India.[141]

More important to Theophrastus than odd stories from India, Ethiopia, and points east are the local authorities he cites for some of his account on hemlock. In IX, 16.8, we are told that Thrasyas of Mantinea discovered – so it was said – the painless death from the juices of hemlock (*kōneion*) and poppy (*mēkōnos*) and other such plants. No more information follows on the poppy, so that confusion appears between the two (earlier in IX, 12.3-5, no opium poppy appears), as the Greek *kōneiou . . . mēkōnos* (perhaps rendered "hemlock poppy" or "poppy hemlock") would suggest (IX, 16.8). Thrasyas made small doses of the poison (a drachma or so), which worked very well, and kept indefinitely. Thrasyas's student Alexias was also skilled in these matters. Neither Thrasyas nor Alexias is known from other sources, unless the "Thrasea the surgeon" of Scribonius Largus (208 Helmreich) and Galen (XIII, 741) is the same as Theophrastus's Thrasyas (Galen gives a recipe of Thrasea [*Tharseos* in the Kühn text] called the Indian"). It is probable that Thrasyas and Alexias were either informants (like the Satyrus in *Historia Plantarum*, III, 12.4) or deceased predecessors, given

---

Somali coast (Strabo, I, 61, and XV, 86-87) and the *Indica* of Ctesias "showed [that the Greeks] could not tell true stories of distant lands from false ones" (M. Cary and E. H. Warmington, *The Ancient Explorers* [Harmondsworth: Penguin Books, 1963], p. 80). See also Truesdell S. Brown, *The Greek Historians* (Lexington, Mass.: D.C. Heath, 1973), pp. 77-86 (esp. pp. 81-83); Ctesias knew of Scylax, probably through Herodotus. In addition to Brown's notes for the sources on Ctesias, see H. H. Wilson, *Notes on the Indica of Ctesias* (Oxford: Ashmolean Society, 1836), a pioneering work employing Sanskrit and Persian comparisons.

138. See notes 9, 10, and 17, above.

139. See note 17, above.

140. Theophrastus's notices on "India" show a fuzziness, even in the context of Alexander's expedition; see e.g., *HP*, IV, 1 (εἶναι μυθολογοῦσι and λέγεται [Wimmer] on Indian ivy and Alexander). Hort, *Theophrastus*, I, 310-311, thinks the text is defective. See Wimmer, ed., under Ἰνδοί.

141. The exception may be the description of some flora by the admiral Androsthenes on a voyage from the Indus to the Persian Gulf: *HP*, IV, 7.7, and V, 4.7-8; see *De Causis Plantarum*, II, 5.5 (on the island of Tylos [Bahrein]: teak wood, calamader wood, and peculiar qualities of rain on the island).

Theophrastus's habit of not naming contemporary authorities.[142] The clipped description in *Historia Plantarum*, IX, 16.8-9, on the dosage fairly well agrees with the methods described in Plato's *Phaedo*, 63d5-e5 and 117b6-9, and Thrasyas and Alexias probably lived at least a generation before Theophrastus. Likewise, the description of the better "preparation of *kōneion*" (IX, 16.9) seems enough like the picture (however mauled) in the *Phaedo* to indicate that Theophrastus's information emerged around 400 B.C. He says that previously (*proteron*) the Cheans (Ceos) used *kōneion* like everyone else, simply shredding it up. Somebody from Ceos was the source of this small bit of recent history. Now – Theophrastus continues – the method is much better: one strips off the outer shell, removing the husk because this part is not easily assimilated;[143] then one bruises it in a mortar, runs it through a fine sieve, and finally sprinkles it on water to drink.[144]

Kōneion is the famous hemlock quaffed by Socrates in 399 B.C.[145] The plant is *Conium maculatum* L., and bears various popular names, including poison parsley and spotted cowbane, as well as the usual hemlock. *C. maculatum* yields coniine (conicine; cicutine; 2-propylpiperidine) that causes the classic symptoms: weakness, sleepiness, nausea, vomiting, difficult respiration, paralysis, asphyxia, and death. Two modern derivatives are part of the pharmacopeia: coniine hydrobromide and coniine hydrochloride. Both are occasionally employed as antispasmodics, and both derivatives are highly toxic.

Theophrastus develops further his ideas on toxic action, first mentioned in *Historia Plantarum*, IX, 16.4-7. In IX, 17.1, he returns to hellebore to illustrate how one could build resistance to toxic drugs, as did Thrasyas by eating hellebore. In IX, 17.2, Theophrastus proposes that *asynetheia* ("unfamiliarity") may be the reason that some *pharmaka* give toxic, rather than beneficial, effects. Thrasyas had proved that once the *physis* of man's body had accepted (*prosdexamenēs*) *pharmaka*, the

142. See Benedict Einarson and George K. K. Link, eds., *Theophrastus: De Causis Plantarum* (Cambridge, Mass.: Harvard University Press, 1976), I (bks. I and II), xix-xx: "Other writers on agriculture are occasionally mentioned, but only when (like the philosophers) they were no longer living . . . It was good form not to mention a contemporary by name."

143. *HP*, IX, 16.9. Cf. *De Causis Plantarum*, I, 14.4.

144. Cf. Plato, *Phaedo*, 117a. Hans Gossen, "Schierling," *RE*, suppl. vol. VIII (Stuttgart, 1956), cols. 706-710.

145. Although Plato uses only φάρμακον in the *Phaedo*, the traditional view that Plato's φάρμακον = κώνειον is well argued by John Burnet, ed., *Phaedo* (Oxford: Clarendon Press, 1911), Appendix I, and accepted by R. Hackforth, trans., *Plato's Phaedo* (Cambridge: Cambridge University Press, 1955), p. 194.

physis overcame (*katakratousēs*) them, and they were no longer *pharmaka*. Like Plato before him in the *Phaedo*, Theophrastus generally uses *pharmakon* to mean "drug," while rarely one reads *thanatēphoros* when he means "deadly drug" or "poison" (for example, *Historia Plantarum*, IX, 16.7).[146] Later medical and toxicological authorities employ a more specific vocabulary,[147] but this notion of "overcoming" the poison became quite popular among rulers who feared assassination by poisoning.[148] Mithridates VI of Pontus became quite famous for his antidote concoctions, which he presumed gave him immunity from the insidious assassin armed with poisons.[149]

With the exception of IX, 18.3-11, the remainder of the passages about herbs and herbals in *Historia Plantarum* discusses a curious mixture of plants, ingredients, and folk traditions. Book IX, 18.3-11, is an extended section on substances that "have effect on both the body and the powers of the mind" (18.3).[150] These passages deserve detailed analysis, because they include a number of *pharmaka* that have *dynameis* for both men's and women's sexual problems. Consequently IX, 18.3-11, is a rich source of aphrodisiac lore, beginning with the observation that most of the ingredients that follow act "like squill" (18.3-4).[151] The major authority cited by Theophrastus in these passages is Aristophilus of Plataea (18.4), who seems to have been a drug-vendor a specializing in love potions. Many of the traditions have complex histories, and many of the plants named are puzzling.

Odds and ends remain. *Akantha* appears in IX, 18.1. This is used for fractures, coughs (mixed in sweet wine), and various wounds (mixed in olive oil).[152] *Akantha* is gum arabic, or acacia, the dried gummy exuda-

146. Other references in *HP* for θανατήφορος are: IX, 13.4; 15.2; 16.4. In *De Causis Plantarum*, θαναθήφορος occurs in VI, 4.5 and 5.5.

147. E.g., Nicander, Galen, and Philumenus.

148. E.g., Attalus III of Pergamon. See Galen, XII, 252, and XIII, 416.

149. Galen, XIV, 2 (Mithridates and Attalus), XIII, 23, 52-54, 329-331, XIV, 2-3, 152-154, 283-284; Pliny, XXV, 6-7; Aulus Gellius, *Attic Nights*, XVII, 17. See Gilbert Watson, *Theriac and Mithridatium* (London: Wellcome Historical Medical Library, 1966), pp. 33-44.

150. Without warning, Hort in *Theophrastus* omits both text and translation of *HP*, IX, 18.3-11. The text with a Latin translation is in Wimmer, ed., pp. 159-161.

151. Squill is *Urginea maritima* (L.) Baker. A basic reference is Jerry Stannard, "Squill in Ancient and Medieval Materia Medica, with Special Reference to Its Employment in Dropsy," *Bull. N.Y. Acad. Med.*, *50* (1974), 684-713 (esp. 686-696).

152. Cf. Dioscorides, III, 146, and Pliny, XX, 84.

tion from the stems and branches of *Acacia senegal* (L.) Willd. and other species of African acacia.[153] The gum contains tannin. Medically, acacia is used as a demulcent, and once was employed as a colloidal solution (intravenous) for shock and edema. Veterinarians use acacia as a demulcent for mild diarrhea in small animals, foals, and calves. *To thleyphonon* (18.2) is another name for *skorpion* (wolf's bane, in the genus *Aconitum*), useful against scorpion's sting (see IX, 16.5-6, above). *Strychnos ho manikos* (IX, 19.1) is the same as the thorn apple, which caused madness in IX, 11.6, above. Also in IX, 19.1 is the root of the *onothēras* (= *daphnē hē agria*),[154] which when mixed with wine elevates the mood. *Onothēras* is oleander (*Nerium oleander* L.), from which one gains oleandrin (folinerin), used in modern medical practice for cardiac insufficiency; oleandrin is a powerful diuretic. In IX, 19.2, Theophrastus scorns the use of charms and amulets (*alexipharmaka*), which seem to have been quite popular in his time. The term *alexipharmakon* soon took on the specific meaning in Greek of "antidote," best illustrated in Nicander's poem bearing the name.

Heleiochrysos (19.3), *peperi* (20.1), the Cnidian *kokkos, peukedanon, daukon* (20.2), *ampelos hē agria* (= *mēlōthron*), *drakontion, thapsia* (20.3), *to tēs ebenou xylon, aristolochia* (20.4), *skammōnia*, and *pteris* (20.5) are the plants and substances listed in the last section of *Historia Plantarum*. One medicinal appears in *On Odors* by Theophrastus: *to megaleion* (35). *Heleiochrysos* is useful for burns (mixed with honey) and for *ta daketa* ("stings" or "bites" of venomous animals).[155] This is probably the gold flower (*Helichrysum siculum* L.), also recorded in Nicander, *Theriaca*, 625, as a remedy for poisonous bites. It has had little use in the pharmacopeia since the eighteenth century. *Peperi* is used, says Theophrastus, as an "aid" against hemlock, like frankincense (*ho libanōtos*: in the *Boswellia* spp., yielding olibanum as a gum resin).[156] *Peperi* is pepper (*Piper nigrum* L.), which gives piperine (1-piperoylpiperidine), toxic to houseflies, but harmless to humans. Ingestion of large amounts of black pepper might cause vomiting. *Knidios kokkos* (= *kneōron*) appears also in *Historia Plantarum*, VI, 1.4, as a spinless low-growing shrub. In IX, 20.2, the "Cnidian berry" has many

153. Kordofan gum (from the Sudan; *Acacia verek* Guill. & Perr.) is considered better than the old "gum arabic," or gum Senegal. See C. L. Mantell, *The Water-Soluble Gums* (New York, 1947).

154. Cf. Dioscorides, IV, 117, and Pliny, XXVI, 111.

155. Galen, XIV, 231, is much clearer: τῶν δακετῶν θηρίων. Cf. Dioscorides, IV, 57; Pliny, XXI, 168 and 169; and Vettius Valens (ed. Kroll), 127.29.

156. Cf. Dioscorides, II, 159, and Athenaeus, II, 73.

uses: its heating quality (*thermotēti*), along with its power to open up the bowels, and its use in pills to prevent throat burns make the *kokkos* quite beneficial.[157] *Kokkos* is from *Daphne gnidium* L., sometimes called the olive spurge, dwarf bay, mazereon, magell, and a number of other names, which yields (from the seed) a fixed oil and acrid resin, and (from the bark) mezerein and daphnin. A combined extract called mezereum was formerly used in medicine as a vesicant and epispastic. *Peukedanon* is also "heating" (*thermatikon*), and is used to make a sweating ointment, and the root is for the spleen.[158] *Peukadanon* is the sulfur wort (*Peucedanum officinale* L.), which gives (from the root) peucedanin (4-methoxy-5-isopropylfuro [1,3:6,7] coumarin), used in experimental animals in the investigation of antineoplastic agents. *Daukon* is some kind of wild carrot,[159] recommended as *thermatikon.*

Ampelos hē agria is also *thermatikon* and *drimu* ("pungent"), and is used as a hair remover, freckle remover, skin and leather smoother.[160] The plant is bryony (*Bryonia alba* L. or *B. dioica* Jacq.), which contains many "pungent" and toxic substances, including bryoamarid glycoside, bryonin, bryonidin, bryonicine, an oil, and resin. Once employed by physicians and veterinarians as a purgative, bryony has been replaced by more uniform drugs. *Drakontion* is a root that stops coughs when mixed with honey, and is probably the edderwort (*Dracunuculus vulgaris* L.).[161] *Thapsia* is again (as in IX, 8.3) *Thapsia garganica* L. ("the deadly carrot"), which purges "up and down" and which removes bruises.[162] Again Theophrastus lists *aristolochia*, as he did in IX, 13.3, with basically the same suggestions for its use. *Skammōnia* is the scammony (*Convolvulus scammonia* L.), as in IX, 9.1; here, in IX, 20.5, Theophrastus says that only the juice is useful, while in IX, 9.1, both the root and juice are included. No benefit comes in either listing, nor is there any more medicinal information in IV, 5.1. It appears that something has been omitted in the MSS,[163] as comparison with other Greek

157. Cf. Pliny, XXVII, 70; Dioscorides, I, 36; and Pliny, XV, 25; XXIII, 89.

158. Cf. Pliny, XXV, 117.

159. Probably *Malabaila aurea* L. here in IX, 20.2 (and IX, 15.8), as contrasted with δαῦκον in *HP*, IX, 15.5. Galen, VI, 654, and XI, 862, seems to be writing about another species. Cf. Dioscorides, III, 72, Nicander, *Theriaca*, 94, 858, 939; *Alexipharmaca*, 199; and *Scholia on Theriaca*, 94.

160. Cf. Dioscorides, IV, 181-183; Pliny, XXIII, 19 and 21; Galen, XI, 826.

161. Cf. Dioscorides, II, 167; Pliny, XXIV, 89.

162. Cf. Dioscorides, IV, 153; Pliny, XIII, 125 and 126.

163. Einarson, "Manuscripts of Theophrastus's *Historia Plantarum*," p. 70: "even in U* the concluding passage (9.19.4 through γίνεσθαι in Wimmer's text) is evidently incomplete."

and Roman medical sources would indicate.[164] Greek and Roman physicians valued scammony as a purgative, and it continued to be used until quite recently, because of its constituents, which include starch, ipuranol, a reducing sugar, a methylesculetin, dihydroxycinnamic acid, and resin (8-13 percent). *Pteris* is the male fern (*Dryopteris filix-mas* [L.] Schott.), which "expels the flat worm."[165] Modern medicine still values this very reliable antihelmintic, used as the oleoresin of aspidium (an ether extract of the male fern), which has at least 24 percent crude filicin. In humans, the drug is a stable antihelmintic, with various side effects (headache, yellow vision, colic, dizziness, and so on), that are easily controlled. Veterinary medicine uses the oleoresin of aspidium in the treatment of taeniasis, and against liver flukes in ruminants. This is one of the few pharmaceuticals from antiquity that has retained its value, in an era of ever more sophisticated laboratory synthesis.[166]

In *On Odors*, 35, *megaleion* is recommended as being a great help for all sorts of wounds. In *Historia Plantarum*, IV, 2.1 and 2.6, one finds a *balanos*, from which is made (*Odors*, 29) *megaleion* out of burnt resin,[167] and oil. Pliny (XIII, 13) says that the medicinal was named after Megallos, who invented it. *On Odors*, 35, notes that it is most effective when mixed with cassia cinnamon and myrrh. *Balanos* is probably *Balanites aegyptica* L., an Egyptian plant that bears a fruit like an acorn (hence the name).[168] The benefit for wounds came from the myrrh, *Commiphora myrrha* (Nees) Engl.[169] The last "herbal" would not fit Theophrastus's original definition, given in the beginning sections of this essay, but it would fit his notions of beneficial or harmful plants and their derivatives. In *Historia Plantarum*, IX, 20.4, one reads of the interesting *to tēs ebenou xylon*, ebony wood from *Diospyros ebenum* Koenig, the Macassar ebony, most common in India and Sri Lanka. This reference might be derived from some reports from India that appear in IX, 20.4, and the context of IV, 4.6, confirms this suspicion. In IV, 4.5, Alexander has ordered his men not to eat mango,

164. E.g., Pseudo-Aristotle, *Problems*, 864a4 and b13; Dioscorides, IV, 170, and V 73; Nicander, *Alexipharmaca*, 565; Pliny, XIV, 110 (as in Dioscorides, V, 73).

165. See also note 100, above. Cf. Pliny, XXVII, 145.

166. Hill, *Economic Botany*, p. 264, with a short summary. Harry F. Dowling, *Medicines for Man* (New York: Knopf, 1973), pp. 14-17, is very negative about the use and usefulness of ancient drugs: "Less than two dozen effective drugs were known before 1700" (p. 14). Aspidium appears on his short list.

167. Cf. Pliny, XIII, 7; Dioscorides, I, 58.3, and IV, 157.

168. *HP*, III, 8.3 (acorn), and IV, 2.6 (tree which has βάλανοι).

169. Cf. Celsus, V, 27 (myrrh for burns); Majno, *Healing Hand*, pp. 216-219.

and IV, 4.6, mentions the two kinds of ebony that occur in India. The second species is most likely *D. melanoxylon* L., which also occurs in northeastern Africa. It is probable that Theophrastus had some direct account of Alexander's expedition in India, but it seems that he combined this report of ebony wood with other, more local information.[170] In IX, 20.4, one reads that the wood, when rubbed on a whetstone, is useful for the eyes.[171] A section on ebony in Dioscorides (I, 98.1-2) solves the puzzle, because he picks up the same treatment, vaguely noted in Theophrastus; Dioscorides specifies the ebony and the manner of preparation of the eye salve. He says that the wood becomes yellow when rubbed on a whetstone, and that of the two kinds (Ethiopian and Indian), the Ethiopian is the better, because the Indian variety is streaked and spotted; furthermore, some try to sell other kinds of wood (like the acanthus) as if they were ebony (*Materia Medica*, I, 98.1). The eye salve (*kollyrion*) is prepared as follows (I, 98.2): the scrapings or dust of the ebony wood is steeped in Chian wine for a day and a night, then beaten into the consistency of eye salves (*kollyria*). Another method is to beat the scrapings and dust first, then sift then, and then soak them in the wine; some will use water instead of wine. A third method is to burn the dust and scrapings in a bowl, and then to wash the coals as one did white lead (*molybdos*).[172] Theophrastus has recorded a fragment of an apparently well-known remedy, and the state of the text may explain the strange omission of many details.[173]

There are forty-three major herbs and herbals (omitting IX, 18.3-11) in *Historia Plantarum* IX and *On Odors*. Five are toxic: mandrake (IX, 9.1), hellebore (IX, 9.2 and 10.1-4), the *strychnoi* (IX, 11.5-6), wolf's bane (IX, 16.4-7), and hemlock (IX, 16.9). There is one wood (Ethiopian or Indian ebony: IX, 20.4), and the male fern (IX, 20.5). Additionally, there is one animal product: the curd of the monk seal (IX, 11.3). There are no minerals, but *On Stones*, 23-24, notes that *smaragdos* is "good for the eyes."[174] The vehicles are wine, vinegar, honey, and water. If

170. "Local" in this case means Egypt, where the name originated. Herodotus, III, 97; Theocritus, XV, 123. Other references in *HP* suggest a kind of combination: I, 5.4 and 5; V, 3.1 and 2.

171. Cf. Pliny, XXIV, 89.

172. Cf. Galen, XI, 867-868.

173. Ebony dust (appearing in Dioscorides, I, 98) is omitted in Harald Nielsen, *Ancient Ophthalmological Agents*, trans. from the Danish by L. McBride (Odense: Odense University Press, 1974).

174. *On Stones* (ed. Eichholz, p. 64): *ἡ δὲ σμάραγδος . . . καὶ πρὸς τὰ ὄμματα ἀγαθή*. *σμάραγδος* may be green basalt, or green Aswan granite

Wellmann is correct,[175] Theophrastus derived many of his remedies from the works of Diocles, but it is clear that Theophrastus was a shrewd, independent collector of data in his own right,[176] including information on medicinals. The list of herbals assembled in *Historia Plantarum* IX became the direct ancestor of all later drug treatises in antiquity, and many traces of Theophrastus's (and Diocles's) original observations survive in the *Materia Medica* of Dioscorides. The analysis of the various plants and plant derivatives shows that the Greek *rhizotomoi* and drug-vendors had collected much valuable information on the medical employment of plants, and Theophrastus invented a format for this type of information that would be followed after his own time. Dioscorides adds many other names for the plants, so that the modern scholar can, in the majority of cases, key the genera and species, and thereby determine medical utility. Theophrastus's herbs and herbals show that, in the fourth century B.C., *pharmaka* were well known, and those that were especially beneficial and harmful had been carefully studied. It is to Theophrastus's credit that he used information supplied by the root-cutters and drug-vendors, who could either verify or refute many notions that might have become "common knowledge."[177]

(Eichholz, p. 103). Sometimes, according to Galen (XI, 867-868), ebony was confused with "stones."

175. See notes 13-17, above.

176. Sources and references are collected in Einarson and Link, eds., *Theophrastus: De Causis Plantarum*, xix-xxiii.

177. Lynn Thorndike, "Disputed Dates, Civilization and Climate, and Traces of Magic in the Scientific Treatises ascribed to Theophrastus," in Charles Singer and Henry E. Sigerist, eds., *Essays on the History of Medicine Presented to Karl Sudhoff on the Occasion of his Seventieth Birthday* (London: Oxford University Press, 1924), says Theophrastus "assures us that many remedies and antidotes have been brought to human notice by the example of animals who employ them" (p. 79).

V

Nicander's Toxicology I: Snakes

"IT SEEMS," wrote Galen, "that there is nothing more dangerous in life than poisons, and [the bites] of noxious animals."[1] He continues to say that one may avoid most dangers by fleeing from them, but poisons and venomous animals are treacherous enemies, since, if one is careless, he can take poison by mistake, or he falls victim to a quick bite without warning.[2] The great Roman physician thus sums the normal gloom and frustration expressed by many Greek and Roman writers about wounds from snakes, spiders, scorpions, and the cases of poisoning that occurred both accidentally and with intention. Rulers lived in fear of crafty poisoners, and a few—Attalus III of Pergamon, and Mithridates VI of Pontus are famous for this—went as far as to experiment on themselves and others in hopes of developing immunity over the long range against the assassin bearing insidious potions.[3] More common, however, were the occasionally fatal bites suffered by farmers in their fields dealt by hidden snakes, or troublesome wounds that developed from spiders, scorpions, and other inconspicuous creatures. Poisoning could result from a numerous array of plants as well, and tradition had compiled many antidotes that were assumed effective against poisons. Some were put down by Galen in his "theriac" books,[4] and there was constant hope that a panacea would emerge from the welter of remedies.[5] Sometimes the seasonal variation was cited as the only real cure, much as Vettius Valens writes that Sagittarius signals the end of the time in which "four-footed beasts fall from the bites of venomous animals."[6]

Greek sources in toxicology are a well developed and specialized portion of medical literature. Collections of antidotes against known poisons, both organic and inorganic, most likely were part of the ancient literatures of the Near East,[7] but it is not until the *Peri thēriōn* ("On Poisonous Animals") by Apollodorus that a Greek treatise took up the special study of poisons. Apollodorus lived sometime in the third century B.C.,[8] and may have owed much in medical theory to both Aristotle and Diocles of Carystos.[9] The *Peri thēriōn* is lost except for quoted extracts in a number of later authors including Athenaeus,[10]

Aelian,[11] Pliny,[12] and Galen,[13] who knows of Apollodorus through Sostratus.[14] It is probable that Dioscorides and Pliny derive much more material from Apollodorus than they cite in specific,[15] while it is certain that Nicander took his poison-lore directly from Apollodorus.[16] One of the scholiasts on Nicander mentions a second work by Apollodorus, a *Peri thanasimōn* or *dēlētēriōn pharmakōn* ("Poisons"),[17] which may be embedded in later writers without citation. Several of these later writers, including Nicander, borrowed Apollodorus directly: Numenius, Heracleides of Tarentum, Sostratus, Sextius Niger, and Archigenes.[18] Aelian purloined Sostratus' excerpations, Pliny and Dioscorides borrowed Niger's quotations, and the mysterious Aemilius Macer made a summary of poison-lore from Apollodorus and Nicander.[19] This complex textual history indicates the fundamental nature of the original *Peri thēriōn* by Apollodorus, which forms the base for most later Greek and Roman toxicology. Since Apollodorus' work has been lost, one must depend on the difficult poems by Nicander, whose extant *Theriaca* and *Alexipharmaca* provide the best cohesive sources for classical toxicology. Some additional materials and explanations are given by Philumenus,[20] and Galen, but the great majority of poison-lore emerges in Nicander.

Nicander made his home at Clarus, a small temple-precinct a few miles west of Colophon on the coast of Lydia in western Asia Minor.[21] Interpretation of evidence concerning the century of Nicander's life leads to contradictory conclusions, but modern scholars lean to a date in the late second century, since the biographical entry in the Byzantine *Suda* mentions an Attalus,[22] and context suggests this is Attalus III of Pergamon (*c.* 170–133 B.C.; ruler of Pergamon, 138–133 B.C.). Located about seventy miles north of Colophon,[23] Pergamon was the dominant Hellenistic power in western Asia Minor, until Attalus III willed the kingdom to Rome.[24] Attalus III was also famous for his study of poisonous plants, animals, insects,[25] and the discovery of some useful plasters.[26] He also composed works on agriculture, cited by later Roman au-
* thorities.[27] Nicander, the poet of Colophon-Clarus, probably wrote his *Theriaca* and *Alexipharmaca* in the intellectual atmosphere created by Attalus.

Nicander shows no competence in the subjects or specifics of poisons and toxicology in either the *Theriaca* or the *Alexipharmaca*. Likewise, he borrowed a number of other works as the base of his poetic expositions, in which he had no expertise: his *Prognostics* were a mere paraphrase of a Hippocratic treatise;[28] a *Georgica* revealed ignorance of its subject;[29] the *Ophiaca* may be another poison-poem, but the two fragments extant may not accurately represent the whole;[30] an *Oetaica* probably took up fish,[31] the *Heteroeumena* was about mythological changes,[32] but so little remains of Nicander's *Thebaica*, *Sicelia*, and *Europia* that themes and contents cannot be assumed.[33] Perhaps they were "geographical" exercises, ancestors of the works of Strabo and Stephen of Byzantium. There is a *Hymn to Attalus* extant in the scholia on the *Theriaca*,[34] and three epigrams in the *Greek Anthology* are attributed to Nicander.[35] Only the *Theriaca* and *Alexipharmaca* have survived intact, and they exhibit an ignorance of the summarized toxicology,[36] apparently well delineated by Apollodorus. Nicander was far more interested in the forms of his poems than he was in their content, and his syntax and vocabulary in the two poems are artificial, strained, obtuse, and intentionally obscure.[37] He invented endings when it suited his purposes,[38] and classical scholars have had great difficulties with the structure and individual lines from the two extant poems. The *Theriaca* and *Alexipharmaca* are valuable to medical historians because they plagiarize the solid materials of Apollodorus, whose *Peri thēriōn* exists only in fragments.

Nicander's toxicology is based upon his descriptions of venomous animals and plants followed by their antidotes. Contained in the *Theriaca* and *Alexipharmaca* are snakes, lizards, tortoises and turtles, frogs and toads, scorpions, spiders, various insects (moths, flies, bees, wasps, hornets and beetles), and botanical lore connected with poisons. In many cases, identity of the plants is more assured than nomenclature for snakes and spiders, and other better known poisonous denizens.[39] Nicander himself notes that one species may have more than one name.[40] Even with cross-identification with Modern Greek for some of the plants, one must exercise due caution, although plants are less likely than animals to be commonly called by more than one name in the same region. This may be the case since there was a specialized literature on plant classification, beginning with Theophrastus' *Enquiry into Plants.* By contrast, with the exception of Nicander, Philumenus, and Pseudo-Dioscorides, there is little to suggest a comparable genre on poisonous animals.[41] The medical writers do have much information about poisons and their antidotes,[42] but they form secondary matter, even in the pages of Dioscorides.[43]

Like Vettius Valens marks the end of the snake-season,[44] Nicander speaks of its beginning: "But especially during the summer you must be constantly guarding against venomous beasts, seeing the Pleiades rise, those smaller stars brushing the tail of Taurus."[45] However, before giving the snakes their names and characteristics, he lists numerous preventive measures, prophylactic notions that apparently had wide credence in the Hellenistic east. To ward off snakes and their "hot and harmful doom,"[46] one charred tined stag horn, fired dried lignite, put fern into the fire, along with frankincense root, garden cress, roe-horn, black cumin, sulfur, bitumen, galbanum, nettle, and powdered cedar wood.[47] The object was to produce "a smoky and repellant stench," which would "clear hollow caves and depressions and you can sink to the ground and gain your fill of sleep."[48] Essentially the same method is followed in the modern Middle East to clear caves, but smoking and burning straw or hay perform the function, with few added chemicals, excepting gasoline.[49] The various ingredients in Nicander's smoking concoction might make it smell rather nice (the cedar and frankincense,[49a] especially), but the effective agent is smoke. Likewise the majority of the numerous components that Nicander says to "spread around" one's sleeping place,[50] have little impact on snakes or scorpions, although thyme has a sweetish odor, which would smell pleasant in the mixture. Nicander also lists prophylactic ointments, which would have an unknown effect, since one of the major ingredients in the salves was silphium, an extinct species possibly of the onion or garlic family.[51] The last prevention, prescribed by Nicander, is pure folk medicine. One was to catch two of the poisonous snakes while they were mating at a crossroads, dump them into a mixture of stag marrow (thirty drachmas' worth), rose oil, ordinary olive oil, and wax, and heat it all in a pot. After a good softening of the snake tissues has taken place, one had to pull out the vertebrae (the poet says that the poison comes from the snake's backbone), and pound everything together with mortar and pestle. Spread over the arms and legs, the resultant ointment fended off snakes and other poisonous animals.[52] If, however, one could not prepare himself, he should at least know the types of snakes he would encounter, "especially when you are fasting, a time when disaster strikes a man."[53]

FIRST on Nicander's list of deadly snakes is the *dipsas*.[54] This is the "Male Viper," which does not help modern identification very much. Philumenus gives a description of the *dipsas*,[55] noting that it was about a "cubit long" (*c*. 1½ feet),[56] tapering, spotted black and yellow, and with a very narrow head. Sostratus, as quoted by Aelian,[57] says that the *dipsas* is white with two black stripes on the tail. According to Aelian, the snake has many names: *presteres* ("inflaters"), *kausones* ("burners"), *melanurus* ("black-tail"), *ammobates* ("sand crawler"), and *kentris* ("stinger"). Somewhat muddled at best, these descriptions of appearance, habits, habitat, or results of their bites, disguised in the names, can only suggest several species. Other ancient authors add further details. In a short essay, *Peri tōn dipsadōn* ("The Dipsads"), Lucian characterizes the snake as being typical of the awful animal life of Libya, which includes a nasty winged scorpion. The worst, however, is the *dipsas*, which is not particularly large, looks like a viper, and has a strong bite that excretes a thick poison that causes immediate pain that burns and corrodes, setting victims "on fire as if they were lying on a funeral pyre."[58] The wound from the *dipsas* causes extreme thirst, which Lucian writes (now quoting "the doctors") results because "the thick poison flows easier if it receives moisture from drinking, becoming more liquid naturally, and thus spreads over a greater area."[59] Lucian merely mentions Nicander's work without specifying any passages,[60] but the symptomatology is similar enough to *Theriaca*, 334–342, to suggest direct borrowing. Lucan, *De bello civili*, contains a section on the miserable conditions and terrible animal life in Libya, including *torrida dipsas*.[61] Symptomatology from the bite of the *dipsas* receives its most gruesome description from Lucan, and again the common source seems to be Apollodorus or Nicander. The wound was not particularly significant, but soon "there was a feeling of fire inside... the poison dried up the moisture around the vital organs... there was not sweating... no tears from the eyes... the victim lapped up salt water happily... finally opening up his veins with his sword and drank his own blood" before he died unaware that he had been poisoned.[62] Lucan may know the prophylactic measures described in *Theriaca*, 57–79, since he sneers at any prevention from piling up twigs and plants.[63] The scholiast on *Theriaca* has a section entitled *Peri dipsados*, which gives a slightly different description from that of Nicander, Lucian, Sostratus, and Philumenus.[64] Now the snake has a "flat head."

A second example from Nicander's *Theriaca* also shows the difficulty in assigning modern nomenclature to the snake described. The *sēps* is the second variety on Nicander's list of twenty types of dangerous snakes.[65] Like the *dipsas*, the *sēps* has various descriptions. Colors vary for the *sēps*, "constantly taking the color of the place in which it makes its hole."[66] Lucan says the snake is small,[67] and Philumenus' *sēps* is the same as the snake called *sēpedōn* by Nicander, *Theriaca,* 320.[68] The context of Nicander, Lucan, and Philumenus shows that the snake lives in Libya and Egypt, but Pausanias describes a *sēps* he has seen in Arcadia in Greece.[69] The snake, however, is rare in Arcadia.[70] In the Frazer translation of Pausanias, the description of the *sēps* runs: "It is like a very small adder, is ash-colored, and spotted irregularly; its head is flat, neck thin, belly large, tail short. Like the crested snake, it moves with a sidelong motion, crab-fashion."[71] In his commentary on Pausanias, Frazer notes that French surveyors thought Pausanias' picture of the *sēps* was excellent: "a better description could not have been given by a naturalist who had made a special study of reptiles."[72] Aelian repeats Nicander's line that the *sēps* changes color with the ground over which it moves.[73] If Philumenus' *sēps* is the same as the *sēpedōn* in Nicander, then the snake was about "two cubits" (*c.* 3 feet) long, tapering in shape, and it moved slowly in a forward, straight manner;[74] it had a flat head and was spotted white all over.[75] The total description from all sources results—again—in a muddled picture that could apply to several species.

Sēps, *sēpedōn*, and *dipsas* are names that indicate what happens when the venom of these snakes enters a victim ("decay," "putrifaction," and "thirst-provoking" respectively).[76] Local necrosis does develop from the bites of the *Viperidae*, and extremely advanced cases show lymphatic spread, but analysis of this aspect leads only to vague notions that can be appropriate for numerous species. The descriptions of physical characteristics may allow some tentative identification, especially if one limits the scope to North Africa, and—to account for Pausanias' *sēps*—Greece. Thus the South American Dipsas (*Dipsas bucephala* Boulenger) is ruled out immediately.[77] Recalling also Nicander's warning that there may be several names for the same snake,[78] one can suppose that the "several names" are, indeed, separate species.

Nicander's *sēps* is distinguished by its chameleon-like ability to blend into the surroundings, a quality that would describe several species in the genus *Cerastes*. A probable identification here would be *Cerastes cornutus* Boulenger,[79] or *C. cerastes* Andersson.[80] Pausanias' *sēps* is most likely *Vipera ammodytes* Sonnini/Latrielle,[81] the same as the *Coluber ammodytes* L. chosen by Frazer.[82] A modern description of the Egyptian Sand Viper (*Cerastes cornutus* Boul.) keys Nicander's picture rather well. The snake is "... a desert type of pallid hue which varies according to the hues of the sandy surface in different areas... [and] runs as fast as a crab over the sand dunes at the edge of the desert, then seems to sink from sight."[83] Lucan echoes this portrayal of the small snake (about 2 feet long), moving very rapidly.[84] The *dipsas* comes closest to *Cerastes vipera* Boul.,[85] in Nicander, Philumenus, and Lucian. All of the species identified are members of the family *Viperidae* in north Africa, southeastern Europe and western Asia Minor.

Two of the snakes in Nicander are easily identified. The *aspis* (*Theriaca,* 158, 190, 201, and 359) is the asp, or Egyptian Cobra, *Naja Haje* Merrem [=*Coluber haje* L].[86] The *kerastēs* (*Theriaca,* 258, 261, 276, 294, and 318) is the Horned Viper, *Cerastes cornutus* Boul., in this case with the definite erect and ribbed horn-like scale above the eye.[87] By contrast, all but one of the remaining varieties of snakes in the *Theriaca* cannot be identified: *kenkrinēs* (463), *skytalē* (384 and 386), *typhlōps* (492), *dryinas* (411),, *hydros* (414), *chersydros* (359), *akontias* (491), *amphisbaina* (372 and 384), *myagros* (490), *elops* (490), *libys* (490), *molouros* (491), *echis* (9, 129, 130, 209, 223, 259, 517, 545, 642, 653, and 826), and the *echidna* (129, 209, 232, 334, 517, and 673); the *echis* and *echidna* are probably of the *Viperidae*. A textual insertion by Nicander may key the last species: the *haimorrois* (282, 305, 315, 318, and 321). Gow and Scholfield gained expert opinion on the identity of this snake, and the question turned on whether or not Nicander "added" horns to his description. The species would be *Echis carinatus* without the horns,[88] and ". . . . a hypothesis that Nicander was embellishing his authority, or that his authority was mistaken, would cause us no great discomfort."[89] *Haimorrois* is *Echis carinata* Wagler,[90] also in the *Viperidae*. Nicander's snakes, in so far as they can be identified, are members of *Elapidae* (the Egyptian Cobra) and *Viperidae*.

"The clinical picture following snake bite often may serve indirectly to identify the responsible snake and determine treatment accordingly,"[91] runs a modern summary of symptomatology. Nicander and his source recognized this principle, and there is a distinction among the sequelae from the various snakes. *Dipsas* produces an oozing, oily wound, and the skin around the wound puckers up into a lump that can be green, pink, or bright red; or small pimple-like blisters spread around the wound, which appeared in the center of a scorched area.[92] Sometimes open sores appear which give off a dark blue ooze, and *dipsas* bites may also produce the following symptoms: vomiting, sometimes of "bile from the stomach"; general weakness; thirst; shivering; a moist sweating; and various color changes of the body, including a jaundiced yellow, a lead grey, and a blue-green like the "flowers of copper."[93] The *kerastēs* bite gives a wound that looks like a wart surrounded by watery blisters. Pain is no more intense than for other snake bites, but there is pain in the groin and a weakness in the joints, accompanied by a flushed appearance over the whole body. If the victim survives nine days, he survives.[94] The *haimorrois* produces far nastier results: a swelling that is dark; pain that "freezes the heart"; and vomiting of water from the stomach. A day later, blood escapes from the nose, throat and ears, and from under the fingernails, and the urine becomes bloody; the gums swell and become clammy, and the teeth become loose.[95] The *sēpedōn* causes a black poison to invade the whole body, and the victim loses his hair, including his eyelashes. A chalky rash, like leprosy, rapidly spreads over the body, along with small eruptions that have appeared on the limbs.[96] The *chersydros* is coupled with the *aspis*, and the symptoms are vivid: the skin becomes dry and bloated with putrid sores that break open from the bottom, exposing a clammy wound, and the victim experiences sudden swellings on the limbs which come and go erratically.[97] Other symptoms are described for other varieties of snakes, but are extremely vague. Nicander includes the dragon and the gecko in this section.[98] The first is a mythical animal (it is harmless to man, says the poet), and the second is not poisonous.

Nicander gives symptomatology for *dipsas, kerastēs, haimorrois, sēpedōn,* and *aspis/chersydros*. Modern nomenclature classes the first four among the *Viperidae*, and the fifth as a member of the *Elapidae*. A twentieth century symptomatology for these two families reveals interesting parallels with Nicander's descriptions. Careful studies of *Viperidae* bites and their clinical manifestations have been undertaken in the Middle East, especially in Israel.[99] Most bites occur on the hands and feet, much like Nicander indicates snakes bite farmers, herdsmen, and woodcutters in his time.[100] Immediately after the bite from one of the *Viperidae*, there appears a tender local swelling that spreads proximally during the first hours. Swelling can involve the whole body over a period of days. Shortly, hemmorrhagic or serous blisters appear around the wound, while subcutaneous hemorrhages accompany edema, and large hematomata and ecchymoses may also appear. Often lymphangitis and lymphadenitis go hand in hand with nausea, vomiting, abdominal pain, diarrhea, and peripheral shock, all within the first hour. Angioneurotic edema, uticaria, and severe swelling of the lips and face soon occur, and dehydration becomes a complication from the severe gastrointestinal disturbances. Internal organs experience hemorrhage, and melena, hematemesis, and epistaxis may accompany jaundice and hematuria. The victim may recover in a few days, with the swelling and bleeding receding. In severe cases, death may occur from shock during the first 24 to 48 hours. Sometimes, delayed shock will cause tachycardia, rapid respiration, profuse sweating, and a rise in temperature with a fall in blood pressure. Renewed edema accompanies new subcutaneous hemorrhages and occasionally hematuria and bloody diarrhea. Some victims die within 48 hours after the onset of delayed shock, while others recover over a long period. Other observable symptoms include engorged fingernail beds, due to the dilation of the capillary network throughout the body. Experimental evidence shows that death from *Viperidae* venom results from respiratory failure,[101] and the variation in patient response is interlocked with individual sensitivity.

Nicander's symptomatology for the *Viperidae* include small blisters around the site of the bite, swelling over the whole of the body, thirst, vomiting, epistaxis, bleeding from the ears and throat, blood escaping from under the fingernails, hives like one expects in general uticaria, hair loss, swollen gums, loose teeth, and a "freezing pain" around the heart. With the exception of the "thistle-down" loss of hair,[102] Nicander's symptoms match rather well the clinical picture presented in modern practice. Symptoms for the *Viperidae*, as a whole, show careful observation of particular sequelae, even through the strainer of Nicander's overweening and difficult poetic lines. Apollodorus, indeed, must have been a splendid clinician.

NICANDER'S portrait of *Elapidae* poisoning seems brief, given the fame of the *Naje Haje* Mer. Again, however, there is accuracy in Nicander's "... no deadly swelling with inflammation, but the man dies without pain, and a slumberous lethargy brings life's end."[103] The clinical features of elapid envenomation result from the presence of neurotoxins in the venom, which will, in turn, present different symptomatology from viperid poisoning. Swallowing and respiration paralysis are among the classic symptoms of elapid poisoning, and other signs are drowsiness, vertigo, and increasingly shallow breathing. There is no swelling or edema at the site of the wound, and no myalgia.[104] Many victims cannot sit up or lift their heads, and the drowsiness often leads into unconsciousness. Apollodorus has given Nicander a fairly precise distinction between the elapids and viperids, in terms of clinical signs. Our poet, however, cannot resist the urge to embellish his *aspis*, even after he has given the essential symptomatology in *Theriaca*, 187–189. *Theriaca*, 360–365, has the *aspis* (if Nicander truly links the *chersydros* with the *aspis*, and context says he does) produce putrid sores, and dry, ugly skin. Rare cases do display these sequelae, but the normal course of symptoms have already been given in *Theriaca*, 187–189. In this matter, Nicander has again revealed his ignorance of real snakes and their bites, while preserving the markedly good description from Apollodorus in the previous section on *Naja Haje* Mer.

Nicander does not give a theory of toxic action. Lucian, however, gives a summary of commonly held medical theory on toxic mechanisms in his own time (*c.* A.D. 120–180[?]), but he simply states that the thick poison of the *dipsas* is more destructive when it becomes more watery as the victim gulps moisture from any source.[105] It is to Galen (*c.* A.D. 129–200) that one turns for an explanation of how poisons work. In the massive writings of the polymath philosopher-physician are a number of works that deal specifically with this question, and all are cast in the mold of the Hippocratic humors. The Hippocratic, *On the Nature of Man*, for example, sets the tone that would be followed by many commentators in later centuries. The treatise asserts that the substances of the body are composed of the four humors: blood, bile, black bile, and phlegm.[106] Furthermore, the unknown author "proves" his theory with drugs: "if you give a man a drug which draws out phlegm, he will vomit phlegm,"[107] and the humors will vary according to the seasons since "if you will give the same man the same drug four times in the year, his vomit will be most phlegmatic in the winter, most liquid in the spring, most bilious in the summer, and blackest in autumn."[108] Thus, for the Hippocratic writer, the nature of the humors—and their seasonal variations—determined drug action. Galen employs almost identical logic when he writes of poisons and their actions in humans. In his *On Humors*,[109] Galen repeats many of the notions in the Hippocratic *On the Nature of Man*, including how changes occur according to the season.[110] Basic is the Qualitative Theory of Matter,[111] which had antecedents in the pre-Socratic philosophers. Galen expresses some of his drug theory in *On the Natural Faculties*,[112] where he writes: "Some drugs purge away the yellow bile, others purge away the black bile, some others will rid the body of phlegm, while others will eliminate the excess water."[113] Elsewhere, he likens the action of poisons to the action of a magnet on iron. Since the magnet has "changed" the nature of the iron with an alteration of the "peculiar quality" of the iron through the special quality of the magnet, the action of poisons—and their special qualities—alter the humors of the body.[114] The concept in Lucian's *Dipsads* is explained: the *dipsas*-poison, being thick like phlegm, will have greater effect with the addition of more water. Treatment, by implication, would be to "dry" out the victim, to get the phlegm back to its natural state.

At the conclusion of his antidote and remedy section, Nicander writes, "You will find that these medicaments will protect you against snakes."[115] The previous drug lore receives little organization as the poet arranges his material in a manner that has little to do with the subject matter. Within the class of "simple remedies," there are "compound" ones that bear no relation to one another, except as remedies. Nicander begins by listing the All-Heal (*Theriaca*, 508), but is confused when he equates this plant with Chiron's Medicinal

Root (500–502), which is there because it "bears the name of Centaur, son of Cronos" (501). Then in rapid order, the poet lists the "root of the Birth-Wort" (509–519: *aristolocheia*), the "root of Treacle-Clover" (520–527: *trisphyllon* or *minyanthes*), followed by a fustic (529: *thapsos*), agnus castus (530), savin (531, if *nēris* is correct), rue (531: *pēganion=pēganon* of *Alexipharmaca*, 413), savory (*Theriaca*, 531: *thymbrē*), asphodel (534: *asphodelos*), and something called *helxinē* (537). Now one is supposed to "crumble it all into a *cotyle* of vinegar or wine or even water" (539–540).[115a]

AN investigation of the medicinals in this short section of the *Theriaca* (500–540) reveals the problems and incredible confusion that Nicander has infused into his poem, unlike his source, Apollodorus, who has kept precision as his mark.[116] The "Medicinal Root of Chiron" (*Cheirōnos riza*) could be either *Centaurium umbellatium* Gilib. (*Erythraea centaurium* Pers.), or *C. spicatum* (L.) Fern. (*Erythraea spicata* (L.) Pers.), which was used as a bitter tonic, mild sedative, and analgesic. Even though *Centaurium* spp. do contain varying amounts of gentiopicrin, amarogentin, and gentisin, they cannot be the *panakeion* purported in *Theriaca*, 508. The birth-wort would be among the *Aristolochia* spp., which has aristolochic acid, which is mildly toxic, causing respiratory and cardiac arrest in experimental animals. At one time, the chemical was used as part of an aromatic bitter, a tradition that may go back to Nicander's line to "mix a drachma's worth in a drink of tawny wine" since it resembled the "boxwood of Oricus" (515–519), which has a distinctive odor. Treacle-Clover or Brief-Flower may be doubtfully identified as *Psoralea bituminosa* L., an extract from which was used in pleuritic pain. Gow and Scholfield write that the text in this section is very corrupt,[117] and that the prescription directions may not make any sense.

If indeed Nicander means *thapsos* in *Theriaca*, 530, the victim might feel cheated, since this is *Rhus cotinus* L., the source of a yellow dye called Zante fustic. In *Alexipharmaca*, 570, "fustic" is correct, but here in *Theriaca*, 530, it makes no sense to give the victim of snakebite an extract which produced a yellow-brown dye. A small textual emendation solves the puzzle. Gow and Scholfield note that it would be easy for the poet to alter "...the metrically intractable *thapsia*" to *thapsos*,[118] although Gow and Scholfield do not state that Nicander did this. *Thapsia* as an emendation for *thapsos* does make sense, and this would make the plant *Thapsia garganica* L., whose root has a sharp, milky sap, and was used as a remedy for many complaints. Support for the emendation is in parallel passages found in Theophrastus, Dioscorides, and Pliny.[119] There is no doubt about *agnos*, which is *Vitex agnus-castus* L., the "Monk's Pepper Tree," used as an anti-spasmodic drug.[120]

Nēris (*Theriaca*, 531) causes some difficulty, since this would be savin, derived from *Juniperus sabina* L. Nowhere else is this oil prescribed as an antidote for poisons, but Dioscorides (IV, 181) proclaims the great value of *nērion* for the bites of poisonous creatures. *Nēris* is most likely Nicander's poetic adaptation of *nērion*, which is oleander, *Nerium oleander* L. Oleander has been used as a diuretic and in cases of cardiac insufficiency due to its varying amount of oleandrin or folinerin. *Pēganion* (*Theriaca*, 531: rue, *Ruta graveolens* L.=the *rutē* in all but two citations by Nicander[121]) is given high marks by the poet, and ancients and moderns agree.[122] Rue has rutin (rutoside; quercetin-3-rutinoside) employed as a carminative and rubefaciant, and in modern times to decrease capillary fragility.[123] The savory is from the *Satureia* spp., the asphodel is probably *Asphodelus ramosus* L.,[124] but the *helxinē* is an insoluble quandry. Dioscorides twice names the plant (IV, 39, and IV, 85), and the plant can be rendered "convolvulus" and "pellitory" respectively, but Nicander's plant lives in moisture, which makes cross-identification with Dioscorides' *helxinē* impossible. In Nicander, the *helxinē* of *Theriaca*, 537, is the same as the *klybatis* of the same passage, which means the plant could be the *koulybateia* of *Theriaca*, 589 and 851. Tentative identification of *helxinē* as *Helxine soleirolii*, and *klybatis*=*koulybateia* as *Poterium officinale* by Gow and Scholfield and their references,[125] leaves the same quandry. The poet has muddled the description so badly that an actual species or genus cannot be identified.

Of the ten substances in forty lines (500–540) of the *Theriaca*, presumably useful against snakebite, two can be identified through textural emendation, four are in the 'probable' class, three are readily keyed, and one remains insoluble. Of the nine that can be identified with reasonable assurance, five substances would be of some benefit (esp. oleander and rue), while one is toxic in its own right.

Continuing, Nicander lists the *echis* of Alcibius (*Theriaca*, 541), followed by horehound (550: *prasion*). Not even the scholiasts know who Alcibius might be, and *echis* is the same word used to name the "male viper" in several places in the *Theriaca*.[126] Dioscorides (IV, 24 and 27) has two plants called *Alkibiadeion* that are helpful against snakebite, but an antidote named for the famous Alcibiades of Athens (*c.* 450–404 B.C.) is even more bizarre than the unknown Alcibius, especially in light of the scholiasts' silence. Later, however, Nicander says that this plant (rendered by Gow/Scholfield as "viper's bugloss;" *Theriaca*, 637–640) looks like an alkanet, which would make one of the three varieties (three have emerged from 541 and 637–640) *Alkanna tinctoria* (L.) Tausch. The root of *A. tinctoria*, which contains a red-brown dye, was formerly used in medicine as an astringent, and contains tannin, one of the best natural antidotes. Horehound is *Marrubium vulgare* L., containing marubiin as a bitter principle, and volatile oil that have been employed as a bitter tonic, expectorant, and diaphoretic. *Prasion* is also the term Nicander uses for horehound in *Alexipharmaca*, 47, but in *Theriaca*, 555, the equivalent is *meliktaina*, while in *Theriaca*, 554 and *Alexipharmaca*, 47, its equivalent is *meliphyllon*. Nicander adds (*Theriaca*, 677) that *melissophylon* is another alternate name. In this case, what appears to be a good example of Nicander's muddling, is explicable thanks to another reference in Dioscorides, and one in Theophrastus. Theophrastus, *Enquiry into Plants*, VI, 1.4, mentions the *melissophylon* next to the *prasion* and *konyza* in a listing of spineless plants, and Dioscorides, III, 104, says it was occasionally called *melittainon*, *melettaina*, and *meliphyllon*. Thus Nicander's *prasion* is simply a chosen alternative name, although *melissophylon* has been identified as *Melissa officinalis* L., which is called "balm" along with many other fragrant plants.[127] *Prasion* and the bugloss were to be taken as "shoots with wine" (*Theriaca*, 550–551).

Now Nicander gives a compound recipe, beginning with peeled brain-membranes from a "domestic fowl."[128] added to *polyknēmon*, *origanon*, and the tip of a boar's liver, cut so that one got the "tip of the lobe which grows from the 'table' and inclines toward the gall-bladder and the portal fissure." One was to drink these ingredients either mixed or separately in wine or vinegar. *Polyknēmon* (559) may be the same as the *euknēmon* of *Theriaca,* 648 and *Alexipharmaca,* 372. The plant is rendered "field basil" by Gow/Scholfield, but basically remains an unknown species. *Origanon* is marjoram among the *Origanum* spp., used as a stimulant rubefacient. After this compound remedy, the poet continues with a multi-ingredient listing. *Kyparissos* leaves (564), *panakes* (565), *kastoros ouloon orchin* (565), and likewise the testicle of the "Nile-horse" (566: *hippou ton Neilos*) all were to be taken by drachma's weight, soaked in water, and shredded together in a vessel. *Kyparissos* is probably the cedrolrich evergreen cypress, *Cupressus sempervirens* L., *panakes* has been discussed above (lines 500–508 of the *Theriaca*), and beaver testicle (accompanied here by hippopotamus testicle) was the presumed source of "castoria," famed in antiquity for its stench. *Castor fiber* L. indeed did produce the substance, but it came from the preputial follicles, not the testicles. Dioscorides, II, 23, specifically recommends hippopotamus testicle (*orchis hippopotamou*) taken in wine as a good remedy against snakebite (*pros herpetōn dēgmata*), and in *Materia Medica,* II, 24, is a longer section giving the virtues of beaver testicle as a remedy. Nicander does not give instruction for the administration of the concoction after one has soaked and shredded it.

More ingredients follow. *Habrotonon* (574), *daphnē* (574), *amarakos* (575), and *tamisos* (577) were to be mixed well (two drachmas' weight) in four *cyathi* of old wine. *Habrotonon* is wormwood, also appearing in *Theriaca,* 66 and 92, and *Alexipharmaca,* 46, which is the same as *apsinthion* in *Alexipharmaca,* 298. The plant is *Artemisia absinthium* L., the dried leaves and flowering tops containing absthin, anabsinthin, and dark green or brown volatile oil (mainly thujone). *A. absinthium* has been used as a bitter tonic and anthelmintic, and thujone is slightly toxic, causing convulsions in heavy doses. *Daphnē* is bay, or bay berries, sometimes known as sweet bay, *Laurus nobilis* L. This ingredient appears again in *Theriaca,* 943, and *Alexipharmaca,* 198. *Amarakos* is sweet marjoram, *Maiorana hortensis* Moench., and appears as *sampsychon* in *Theriaca,* 617. *Tamisos* is a bit more complicated than the previous vegetable ingredients, and is puzzling until the matter is explained by the scholiast on *Theriaca,* 577. Nicander has amalgamated a good deal of agrarian and zoological lore into these few lines, when he speaks of *tamisos* (rendered here as "curd") from a young hare, or from a deer called *prox,* or "the seminal purse which is cut from a stag."[130] *Tamisos* appears as *puetia* in *Alexipharmaca,* 68, and is curdled milk taken from the stomach. The scholiast on Nicander, *Theriaca,* 577,[131] notes that Greeks used curdled milk from the stomachs of various animals in the making of cheese. The enzyme (rennin) would still be active, and an expert could tell his cheese by the particular odor of the "curd" used in its preparation.[132] By contrast, modern dairies set their cheeses by coagulating milk proteins with rennet at 30°C, and the special texture and taste of the finished cheese will depend on the particular bacteria and molds used in the ripening process. Sap of the fig tree was a well known vegetable coagulant of milk,[133] but preference for quality in cheeses gave Greeks and Romans their choice of "curds" from various animals in making their cheeses.[134] Thus Nicander is recommending slightly curdled milk as part of his antidote, a seemingly odd notion that has recently received some confirmation in laboratory experiments with calcium and snake venom.[135] Comparison, however, of Nicander's mangled account of the internal anatomy of the ruminants, with that of Aristotle, *Historia Animalium*, 507b2–12, shows the poet's lack of knowledge. Aristotle clearly describes the four-chambered arrangement of the digestive system in animals that chew their cuds, and such information was generally available in Nicander's time, even if he had not seen for himself. The untrained eye easily detects the gross divisions between the rumen and reticulum, and between the omasum and abomasum, and it may be that Nicander is attempting to disguise complete ignorance of local sacrificial animals; few, indeed, would take the trouble to look for a *prox* or stag, and then to examine carefuly the divisions of his stomach. The complete antidote (the wormwood, bay berries, sweet marjoram, and the curd, if the previous beaver- and hippopotamus-testicles are not included) was to be taken as weights of two drachmas in four *cyathi* of old wine.

ANOTHER antidote follows. *Polion (Theriaca*, 583), *kedros* (583), *arkeythis* (584), *boupleuros* (585), *cyparissos* (585), and the puzzling *helxinē=koulybateia* (589), were to be ground in a round mortar, and then a *cotyle* of barley gruel, two *cyathi* of old wine, and two *cyathi* of olive oil were to be mixed with it. One presumes the mixture was drunk, although the poet does not say. *Polion* may be a hulwort, *Teucrium polium* L., and it appears again in the *Alexipharmaca*, 305. *Kedros* is the cedar, *Juniperus excelsa* L., rich in cedrol. *Arkeythis* is the berry of *Juniperus communis* L., but can also be the extracts from the wood and tops. Juniper berry was well known in earlier pharmacy since it contains volatile oil (various amounts of juniperin, resin, proteins, formic, acetic and malic acids) once used as a diuretic; the basic substance in the juniper oil, however, is cadinene (sesquiterpenes) which is a topical keratolytic and antipruritic agent. *Kyparissos* is the cypress, as in *Theriaca*, 564. *Helxinē* remains unknown as in *Theriaca*, 539. This recipe would be soothing for dry skin.

Next Nicander suggests 1/6 *cotyle* of pitch (*pissa:* 594), mixed with the central pith of the *narthex* (595) and the grated root of *hippeion marathon* (596). *Narthex* is the Giant Fennel, and the *hippeion marathan* (*=hippomarathon*) is most likely the Horse Fennel. Narthex thus is probably *Ferula communis* L., and *hippomarathon* may be identified as *Prangos ferulacea* Lindl. Fennels contain up to 4% volatile oil. One takes the pitch and grated fennels, adds them to the juniper berries (as in *Theriaca*, 584) and celery seeds (*selinon:* 597), mixing (if we understand the context) it all in the "full depth of an *oxybaphon*."[136] Celery seeds (*Apium graveolens* L.) also have volatile and fixed oils, a bitter extractive, and resin. The mixture might work rather well as a purgative.

Nicander continues to cast substances into recipes, all presumed antidotes for poisonous snakebite. Now we meet *hippeion selinon* (599), *smyrna* (600), and *kyminon hēmeron* (601) to be taken [?] in three *cyathi* of wine. Only the *smyrna* is given measure: two drachmas. *Hippeion selinon* (*=hipposelinon*) may be the seeds of Alexanders (*Smyrnium olustratum* L.). The *smyrna* is myrrh, the famous gum-resin from the Arabian tree, *Commiphora myrrha* (Nees) Engl. Pleasant smelling, myrrh is an antibacterial substance with not less than 30% alcohol soluble extract. Myrrh's constituents are well known to pharmacologists: 2 to 8% volatile oil and bitter principles, 25 to 40% resin (myrrhin), and 57 to 61% gum. Medically, myrrh makes a good carminative and topical stimulant in the oral cavity. Cumin is an aromatic stomachic, employed in the relief of nausea and flatulence. Perhaps this antidote did just that: calmed the stomach.

The next recipe is a marvellous jumble. *Nardos* (604), one drachma of milk, a crumbled freshwater crab, *iris* (607), *ereikē* (610), *myrikē* (612), *konyza* (615), *aktē* (615), *sampsychon* (617), *kytisos* (617), and *tithymallos* (617) all are pounded [?] in a mortar, and then taken in $^{1}/_{10}$ *chous* of wine. *Nardos* is spikenard (*Nardostachys jatamansi* DC.) which contains starch, pectin, sugar, and resin. The active agent is a volatile oil of unknown composition. Once used in the treatment of rheumatic fever, various dermatoses, and even syphilis, nard is no longer part of the pharmacopeia.[137] The "freshwater crab" (*Theriaca*, 605) is the common *Thelphusa fluviatilis* L., which also appears in recipes of Dioscorides (II, 10) and Pliny (*Natural History*, XXXII, 53). *Iris* is *Iris florentina* L., with constituents of iridin, isophthalic acid, a camphor-like substance, gum, tannin, sugar, and oil. Isophthalic acid is a mild irritant, while tannin is again a natural antidote for poisons. The iris extract can be used as an astringent in gastric bleeding and in the treatment of diarrhea. Nicander lists *iris* again in *Alexipharmaca*, 406. *Ereikē* is heath, *Erica arborea* L., listed again in *Alexipharmaca*, 451. *Myrikē* is tamarisk frond, *Tamarix tetranda* L., or *T. gallica* L. *Konyza* is fleabane (*Inula* spp. in Nicander; US spp. *Conyza*), containing tannin and gallic acid. *Aktē* is elder, *Sambucus nigra* L. *Sampsychon* is marjoram again. *Kytisos* is "tree medick" ([?] *Medicago arborea* L.), and *tithymallon* is probably spurge (either *Euphorbia peplus* L., or *E. hirta* L.), having resins and an unstable glucoside. Spurge extract has been used in treatment of asthma and bronchitis. The iris and fleabane, with their tannin, would be useful against internally consumed poisons, but would have little effect against the systemic distribution of snake venom. The milk is given in so small an amount that it too would have little effect.

Theriaca 620–624 has three antidotes, derived from animals: frogs boiled in vinegar, the liver of the biting snake taken in wine, and the head of the snake taken in water or in wine. The poet does not say if one were to drink the boiled frog in the vinegar, but Dioscorides (II, 26) writes that frogs "are an antidote (*antipharmakon*) against all [poisonous] snakes." Furthermore, Dioscorides continues, if frogs are "made into a light soup with salt and olive oil, the mixture is beneficial for chronic inflammations of the tendons [or sinews];" and vinegar, water, and frog's blood are also of help for toothache. It appears that Nicander has picked up only a hazy notion of the ingredients in the recipe that is given by Dioscorides. Nicander records the frogs and the vinegar, but bungles their use and combination. Galen (XII, 262) also mentions frogs' blood as generally beneficial.

The remainder of the snake-antidote section of Nicander's *Theriaca* (625–713) repeats many of the substances in the previous recipes, and with the exception of preparation instructions for turtle blood (700–713) and skinning a weasel (689–694), there are few definite directions for administration of the substances. New materials in this last section, not including the turtle blood and skinned weasel, are: *helichrysos* (625), the gold-flower ([?] *Helichrysum siculum* L. or *Achillea santolina* L.), which appears as well in a fragment of Nicander's *Georgica;*[138] *korkoros* (626), the blue pimpernel (*Anagallis arvensis* L.); *rhamnos* (630), which may be of the *Rhamnus* spp., but cannot be identified further; *ēryngos* (645), of the *Eryngium* spp.; *akanthos* (645), either *Acanthus mollis* L., or *A. spinosis* L., the same as *paidos erōs*, appearing in a fragment of Nicander's *Georgica;*[139] *erinos* (647), a campanula (*C. ramosissima* [?]); *annēson* (650), the anise seed (*Pimpinella anisum* L.), containing volatile oil, starch, protein, and a fixed oil, and used as a carminative; *chamaileos* (656), one of two varieties of pine thistles (*Cardopatium corymbosum* L., and *Atractylis gummifera* L.), keyed through Modern Greek;[140] *kotylēdōn* (681), probably the navelwort (*Umbilicus pendulinus* L.); *pyritis* (683), perhaps a bindweed (*Convolvulus arvensis* L.) or, since *pyritis=pyrethron* in other sources (*e.g.* Dioscorides, III, 73, and Galen, XII, 110), perhaps one of the following spp.: *Anacyclus pyrethrum* DC, used to increase salivary flow, or *Chrysanthemum cinerariaefolium* Vis., or *C. coccineum* Wild., most famous as the "Dalmatian insect powder" (the volatile oil, pyrethrin, pyretol, etc., useful as a scabicide, and in veterinary practice against external parasites); and *skolopendreion* (684), "Hart's Tongue" (*Phyllitis scolopendrium* (L.) Newm. Except for the *pyritis*, these substances are either harmless or pleasant.

NICANDER ends his snakebite remedy section with two suggestions that may appear bizarre to modern observers. The skinning of a weasel (*galeē:* 689), at first reading, does not seem related to snakebite, but the ingredients are clear: a weasel skin, stripped of fur over a "blazing fire" and treated with salt.[141] Then the poet says to rub the dried weasel skin with a "rasp as though it were a frail silphium or a round cake of dried milk, grating it into the wine."[142] Silphium, as noted above,[143] is possibly an extinct plant of the onion or garlic family, dried milk might have some small benefit against poisons, but the weasel-skinning may simply be a poetic device to illustrate the "grating" method for either silphium or cheese. Slivers of cheese in wine? Dioscorides, II, 25, helps us understand at least the essential notion. In discussing the weasel (*galē* in Dioscorides), he notes that one takes out the bowels, salts the rest, keeps this remnant a long time—being sure to dry the weasel in the shade—and then "it is a very good remedy for every kind of snakebite when two drachmas of it are taken in wine." This is the "domestic weasel" (*galē katoikidios*) kept as a house pet, presumably for rat control. Galen knows of this antidote,[144] but says he has never tried it.

Nicander's last recommendation is not as botched as is the weasel-skinning. He writes (700–713) that the blood of a sea turtle should be drawn off, especially the livid thin part (the serum), which in turn, should be allowed to dry, and then the clotted blood should be broken up into measures of four drachmas. To the turtle blood, one added two drachmas of cumin, and the curd (*tamisos*) from the stomach of a hare. Gow and Scholfield suggest this last section is very corrupt,[145] but that the ingredients are very clear. Cross-checking the recipe in

Dioscorides (II, 79. 2), we find almost the same suggestions: "... blood of a sea turtle taken with wine and the curd from a hare and cumin, is beneficial against the bites of poisonous animals (*pros thēriodēgmata*)."[146] Dioscorides does not, however, list simply turtle blood (both a land and sea turtle) as an antidote; *Materia Medica*, II, 79, has a listing of the numerous animals whose blood could be used against poisons and other complaints. Included are geese, ducks, pigeons, partridges, male and female goats, deer, hares, dogs (against rabies), the two kinds of turtles, bulls, horses, chameleons, green frogs, and a woman's menstrual blood. The blood of deer, goats, and turtles are particularly good antidotes against poisons, and Nicander—probably using Apollodorus—has given turtle blood first priority. The sea turtle is most likely *Thalassochelys caretta* L., an identification confirmed when Nicander, *Alexipharmaca*, 558, describes his *chelynē* with "weak flippers."

In Nicander's snake antidotes, there are fifty-one different plants or plant derivatives. Ten animal products are recommended, but only one mineral product (salt) is included. Of the fifty-one plants, most are listed only once, with the exception of marjoram (five citations), bugloss (four), All-Heal (three), and two each for savory, cumin, *helxinē*, cypresses, basil, juniper berries, and celery. Among the animal products, only one of the ten is given more than once (*tamisos*, twice), and the salt appears only in relation with the preparation of the weasel skin. Nicander's basic medium is wine, followed by vinegar, water, and olive oil. His prophylactic measures show twenty-seven plants, four animals products, and two minerals (if bitumen is correct for *asphaltos* in *Theriaca*, 44 and 525). Eleven of the plants that appear in the prevention suggestions (cedar, cumin, All-Heal, hulwort, bugloss, marjoram, wormwood, fleabane, agnus castus, juniper berries, and asphodel) reappear in the antidotes. None of the animal products among the prophylactics (stag marrow, a green caterpillar, wax, and mating poisonous snakes) reappears in the antidotes, unless one considers the snake head of *Theriaca*, 624, a duplication.

By modern standards, most of the ingredients in Nicander's antidotes for snakebite had little effect, unless their generally soothing properties are considered. The curd, rue, and tannin in several of the plants, plus those that promote rapid evacuation of the bowels would have salutory results from poison ingestion, but minimal effect on the various venoms. Even though the essential concept of using blood (for the manufacture of antivenin in modern treatment) in snakebite is the same in ancient and modern practice, Greek and Roman toxicology did not include formal notions of immunology, although the famous experiments of Mithridates VI of Pontus show practical knowledge of gradual buildup of immunity from ingested poisons. Snake venom, and its neurotoxic or vascular action, was treated as if the victim had "eaten" the poison, and any positive action by the calcium in curd, the components of rue, or any "immune" factor in the type of animal blood suggested, would generally be neutralized by the digestive process.

Fatality statistics, however, provide a needed perspective about Greek toxicology related to snakebite. A modern authority states that "Venomous snakebites are not always fatal. Even in India where snakes are found in large numbers, only 30–40% of snakebites result in death."[147] Another writer on the *Naja naja* goes even further: "The fangs are small and will not penetrate the leather of ordinary hunting shoes... First aid with cobra bite may be primarily of a psychological nature... The mortality due to snake bite recorded in 1953 in India was 15,000 per year; considering the population... this is about 0.-0041%... more people are killed by the bite of the cobra than by any other snake."[148] One study, quoted in a number of modern accounts on venom toxicity, suggests that folk tales about the utter lethality of *all* bites from poisonous snakes are quite a distance from reality. "As for snake bite in general, elapid bite is not synonymous with envenomation. Indeed, out of Reid's 47 cobra-bitten patients, 25 or 53% had no or negligible symptoms."[149] Reid suggests another factor in the assumption of fatalities from poisonous snakes: newspaper copy. "Even in India and Southeast Asia, where snakebite is comparatively common, cases frequently receive unwarranted prominence in the local press,"[150] and he writes in another essay, "... when poisonous snakes bite man, over one half will escape without poisoning."[151] There is no doubt of the potential toxicity of the various species under consideration—and they include the snakes of Egypt, the Middle East, and Greece, that figure in the works of Apollodorus/Nicander—but statistical analysis of snakebite incidence and sequelae indicates that most bites cause little more than annoyance. Reid and others offer optimistic prognosis for those victims who do develop symptoms from snake venom,[152] but few records have been kept on patients recovering on their own when antivenin is readily available.

One other aspect of snakebite calls for comment. Higginbotham and Clark have shown that normal tissue has an instant defensive response to venom, and that tissue mast cells rapidly release their heparin under the stress of local envenomation. They believe experimental evidence proves that the heparin-containing granules "... are readily ingested by local fibroblasts [and] may serve as a means for sequestration of venom constituents and transportation of this noxious material to appropriate cells for detoxification... [this] is an important factor in both natural and acquired resistance to this type of injury."[153] Greek and Roman toxicologists would not, of course, view snakebite in these terms, but they would recognize that some persons had greater "immunity" to snake bites than others, and they would recognize sequelae in cases of severe envenomation. Importantly, Apollodorus and all later commentators on snakebite noted the beneficial nature of the animal and plant preparations, even with their minimal physical results in cases of serious poisoning. It seems that Greeks and Romans were also prone to exaggerate the terrors of poisonous snakes (witness Lucan among others), while even Nicander's bumbling summary of Apollodorus recognizes the essential benefit of applied remedies. These would, in Reid's phrase, fight the psychological symptoms and aid recovery.

NOTES

1. Galen (ed. C. G. Kühn), XIV, 230–231.
2. *Ibid.*, 231.
3. Attalus III: Galen, XII, 252, and XIII, 416. Mithridates of Pontus: Galen, XIV, 2 [both Mithridates and Attalus]; XIII, 23, 52–54, 329–331; XIV, 2–3, 152–154, 283–284. Pliny, *Natural History*, XXV, 6–7. Aulus Gellius, *Attic Nights*, XVII, 17. Gilbert Watson, *Theriac and Mithridatium* (London: The Wellcome Historical Medical Library, 1966), 33–44.
4. Galen, XIV, 1–209 (*De antidotis*), and 210–310 (*De theriaca*). Galen's compilation talents included pharmacy and pharmacology. The great polymath recorded an enormous variety of material on pharmacology from

earlier authors, and the mass of matter—as well as its variety and occasionally disfigured form (Galen did *not* always quote accurately)—has defied scholarly assessment. A solid beginning, however, is Cajus Fabricius, *Galens Exzerpte aus älteren Pharmakologen* (Berlin/New York: Walter de Gruyter, 1972); Jutta Kollesch offers good criticism of the book in a review of Fabricius that appeared in *Deutsche Literaturzeitung für der internationalen Wissenschaft*, Jhrg. 94, Heft 3 (März, 1973), 202–206.

5. Watson, *Theriac and Mithridatium*, passim.
6. Vettius Valens (ed. G. Kroll [Berlin: Weidmann, 1908]), *Anthologiarum*, II, 40 (p. 127, lines 27–30).
7. *e.g.* E. A. Wallis Budge, ed., *Syrian Anatomy Pathology and Therapeutics or "The Book of Medicines"* (London: Oxford University Press, 1913; 2 vols.), I, 596 [Syriac text], and II, 709 [translation]. Many of these recipes probably go back into Assyrian times.
8. A. S. F. Gow and A. F. Scholfield, eds., and trans., *Nicander: The Poems and Poetical Fragments* (Cambridge: University Press, 1953), 18. Franz Susemihl, *Geschichte der griechischen Litteratur in der Alexandrinerzeit* (Leipzig: Teubner, 1891–1892; 2 vols.), I, 784–785. M. Wellman, "Apollodorus," in *Paulys Real-Encyclopädie der classischen Altertumswissenschaft* (Stuttgart, 1894), Vol. I, pt. 2, Nr. 69, col. 2895. This multi-volume encyclopedia will be abbreviated as *RE* in further citations.
9. Gow/Scholfield, *Nicander*, 23 n. 2, citing M. Wellman, "Das älteste Kräuterbuch der Griechen," in *Festgabe für Franz Susemihl* (Leipzig, 1898), and another essay by Wellmann in *RE*, V, col. 802.
10. The latest edition of the scholia on Nicander's *Theriaca* is Annunciata Crugnola, ed., *Scholia in Nicandri Theriaka* (Milan: Istituto Editoriale Cisalpino, 1971). *Scholia on Theriaca*, 715 [p. 262 Crugnola] shows that Apollodorus lived after Aristotle and shortly before Erasistratus. Athenaeus, *Deipnosophistae*, XV, 681d, and *Scholia on Theriaca*, 715 and 858, give the title as Περὶ Θηρίων.
11. Aelian, *On the Characteristics of Animals*, VIII, 7.
12. Pliny, *Natural History*, XXI, 116; XXII, 19, 31, and 59; XX, 25 and 86.
13. Galen, XIV, 181 and 184.
14. Galen, XIV, 184.
15. Susemihl, *Geschichte*, I, 784.
16. Gow/Scholfield, *Nicander*, 18.
17. *Scholia on Alexipharmaca*, 594.
18. Numenius of Heraclea (*fl. c.* 250 B.C.): wrote a Θηριακά in verse based on Apollodorus like the work of Nicander (*Scholia on Theriaca*, 637).

    Heracleides of Tarentum (*fl. c.* 75 B.C.): wrote a Θηριακά (Galen, XIV, 7, and Susemihl, *Geschichte*, I, 784 n. 49).

    Sostratus (*fl. c.* 150 B.C. [?] in Alexandria): made a paraphrase of Nicander, borrowed by Aelian (Galen, XIV, 184). M. Wellmann, "Sostratus, ein Beitrag zur Quellenanalyse des Aelian," *Hermes*, XXVI (1891), 321–350, and Susemihl, *Geschichte*, II, 444–445 and nn. 168–175.

    Sextius Niger (fl. in reign of Augustus ? [27 B.C.–A.D. 14]): medical and pharmacological authority for Dioscorides and Pliny. Wilhelm Schmid, ed., *Wilhelm von Christs Geschichte der griechischen Litteratur*, 6th ed. (München: Beck, 1912–1924; 3 vols.), II, 453 and n. 5. Martin Schanz and Carl Hosius, *Geschichte der römischen Litteratur*, 4th ed. (München: Beck, 1927–1935; 3 vols.), II, 359. M. Wellmann, "Sextius Niger, eine Quellenuntersuchung zu Dioscorides," *Hermes*, XXIV (1889), 530–569. Jerry Stannard, "Pliny and Roman Botany," *Isis*, LVI (1965), 420–425 [421 and n. 12].

    Archigenes (*fl.* in Rome under Trajan [A.D. 98–117]): works lost except for fragments, especially in Galen, who quotes him rather frequently. Galen, XX, 56–57 (index of most reffs.). E. Rohde, "Aelius Promotus," in *Kleine Schriften* (Tübingen, 1901), I, 380–410.
19. Aelian and Sostratus: M. Wellmann, "Sostratus," *Hermes*, XXVI (1891), 321–350. Pliny and Dioscorides: Jerry Stannard, "Pliny and Roman Botany," *Isis*, LVI (1965), 420–425. Aemilius Macer: Susemihl, *Geschichte*, I, 785, and n. 53. W. Morel, "Iologica," *Philologus*, n.s. XXVIII (1928), 345–389.
20. M. Wellmann, ed., *Philumeni de venenatis animalibus eorumque remediis* (Leipzig: Teubner, 1908; *Corpus Medicorum Graecorum*, X 1, 1). Hans Diller, "Philumenos," *RE*, Vol. XX, part 1 (Stuttgart, 1941), Nr. 7, cols. 209–211. Philumenus was a contemporary of Galen (*c.* A.D. 129–200).
21. Gow/Scholfield, *Nicander*, 4–5. Esther V. Hansen, *The Attalids of Pergamon*, 2nd ed. (Ithaca, New York: Cornell University Press, 1971), 423–31 [424]. Hansen calls Nicander the author of "...the only complete works extant of any Pergamene..." [427].
22. *Suda, s.v.* Νίκανδρος Ξενφάνους, Κολοφώνιος [A. Adler, ed., *Suidae Lexicon*].
23. This may be why the *Suda* has an Attalus.
24. Hansen, *Attalids of Pergamon*, 130–65.
25. Justin, *Epitoma historiarum Philippicarum Pompei Trogi* [ed. O. Seel (Teubner, 1972)], XXXVI, 4. 3. Plutarch, *Demetrius*, 20. Galen, XII, 252; XIII, 416; XIV, 2.
26. Galen, XIII, 409–16. Pliny, XXXII, 87. Celsus, V, 19. 11.
27. Varro, *Rerum rusticarum*, I, 1. 18. Columella, *De re rustica*. I, 8.
28. *Suda, s.v.* Νίκανδρος. *μεταπέφρασται δὲ ἐκ τῶν* Ἱπποκράτους Προ *γ νωστικῶν*.
29. Cicero, *De oratore*, I, 69.
30. Gow/Scholfield, *Nicander*, 143, has two fragments, numbered 31 and 32, with commentary, 204–5.
31. Gow/Scholfield, *Nicander*, 139, has two fragments, numbered 16 and 18, with brief commentary, 202–3.
32. Gow/Scholfield, *Nicander*, 143–45, has four fragments, numbered 43, 50, 59 and 62, with commentary, 205–8.

33. Gow/Scholfield, *Nicander,* 139, has one fragment of the *Thebaica,* numbered 19; 139–41, two fragments of the *Sicelia,* numbered 21 and 22; 141, two fragments of *Europia,* numbered 26 and 27; commentary, 203–4.
34. *Scholia on Theriaca* (ed. Crugnola), p. 33.
35. *Greek Anthology,* VII, 435 and 526; XI, 7. Numbered as 105, 106, and 107 in Gow/Scholfield, *Nicander,* 163–5.
36. Gow/Scholfield, *Nicander,* 18.
37. generally, Hermann Klauser, "De dicendi genere in Nicandri Theriacis et Alexipharmacis quaestiones selectae," *Dissertationes philologae Vindobonenses,* VI (1898), 1–92, and W. Kroll, "Nikandros," *RE,* Vol. XVII, part 1 (Stuttgart, 1936), Nr. 11, cols. 250–65. One essay illustrates: I. Cazzaniga, "Nicandro Theriaca *v.* 60," *Rivista di Filologia e d'Istruzione Classica,* XLI (1963), 461–9.
38. Aldo Bartalucci, "Gli aggettivi in -ΕΙΣ in Nicandro," *Studi classici e orientale,* XII (1963), 118–44.
39. R. H. Dawkins, "The Semantics of Greek Names for Plants," *Journal of Hellenic Studies,* LVI (1936), 1–11. Very important are illuminated manuscripts on botany, where they have survived. Identification of plants in Dioscorides was aided immeasureably by the Codex of Dioscorides of Byzantine origin. E. Emmanuel, "Étude comparative sur les plantes dessinées dans le Codex Constantinopolitanus de Dioscoride," *Schweizerische Apotheker-Zeitung,* L (1912), 45–50, and 64–72.
40. *Theriaca,* 522, 537, and 554; *Alexipharmaca,* 36–41, and 47.
41. Dioscorides, *Materia Medica* (ed. M. Wellmann), II, has a good deal of poison-lore embedded, but vague descriptions (similar to those in Nicander) characterize these sections.
42. *e.g.* Celsus, V, 27, and VII, 5. 5, and Galen (note 4 above).
43. Unless, of course, one includes Pseudo-Dioscorides, Περὶ δηλητηρίων φαρμακῶν and Περὶ ἰοβόλων, as does C. Sprengel in his edition of Dioscorides (in C. G. Kühn, ed., *Medicorum Graecorum Opera quae exstant* [Vols. XXV and XXVI] Leipzig, 1829 and 1830). Max Wellman in his edition of Dioscorides, *Pedanii Dioscurides Anazarbei De materia medica* (Berlin, 1906–14; 3 vols,; rptd. Berlin: Weidmann, 1958) does not include these two treatises in the "genuine" Dioscorides *corpus.* John M. Riddle, "Dioscorides," in *Dictionary of Scientific Biography,* IV (New York, 1971), 119–23 [122].
44. Vettius Valens, II, 40 (also note 6 above).
45. *Theriaca,* 121–23.
46. *Theriaca,* 35–6. trans. Gow/Scholfield, *Nicander,* p. 31.
47. *Theriaca,* 39–56.
48. *Theriaca,* 53–56.
49. In participating in an archaeological expedition at Machaerus, Jordan (east rim of the Dead Sea) in the summer of 1968, I was informed by our Jordanian hosts that this was the "standard" method. Those scorpions that did not scuttle out of the cave were killed by the smoke. No dead snakes were ever found.
49a. Nicander seems to have confused the "root" of the frankincense with its bark. It is not recorded whether there would be a fragrance from burning the root, since the incense is derived from the gummy exudation gained from wounding the bark of the tree above the ground. H. J. Carter, "Frankincense in Arabia," *Journal of the Bombay Branch of the Royal Asiatic Society,* II (1848), 380–90, gives a description of collection methods, followed to the present time: "The gum is procured by making longitudinal incisions through the bark in the months of May and December, when the cuticle glistens with intumescence from the distended states of the parts beneath; the operation is simple, and requires no skill on the part of the operator. On its first appearance, the gum comes forth white as milk, and according to its degree of fluidity, finds is way to the ground, or concentrates on a branch near the place from which it first issued, from whence it is collected by men and boys employed to look after the trees by the different families who possess the land in which they grow." Quoted in Guido Majno, *The Healing Hand: Man and Wound in the Ancient World* (Cambridge, Mass.: Harvard University Press, 1975), 212. Majno also provides a microscopic diagram showing the "small canals and larger cavities" under the bark that fill with the oleo-gum-resin.
50. *Theriaca,* 57–99.
51. John Scarborough, "The Drug Lore of Asclepiades of Bithynia," *Pharmacy in History,* XVII (1975), 43–57 [53 with n. 101]. It is also possible that silphium was derived from an umbelliferous plant closely related to *Ferula assa-foetida* L. A. C.Oersted, "Beitrag zur Deutung der Silphium-Pflanze," *Zeitschrift für Ethnologie,* III (1871), 197–203.
52. *Theriaca,* 98–114. The idea that poisonous snakes can be used for protection against their own bites, is a very old and universal one. Immunity to snakebite has been claimed by every snake-charming tribe and snake-worshipping sect. Amulets, talismen, divine protection, and—like in Nicander—ointments, salves, plasters, herbal concoctions, and matter from poisonous snakes all have been employed. Little scholarship exists in anthropology on this aspect of tribal life, but isolated reports exist on practices in Africa and India. M. Oldfield Howey, *The Encircled Serpent* (London: Rider and Co., 1928), 250, has the account of how Zulus "inoculate" themselves against snakebite. Every October, those undergoing the ceremony have a piece of skin cut from the back of the left hand, and snake venom mixed with saliva is rubbed into the wound. T. R. Fraser, "Address on Immunisation against Serpent's Venom and the Treatment of Snake Bites with Antivenene," *British Medical Journal,* I (1896), 957–60 [959], notes that swallowing dried venom glands and poison gave Bushmen immunity against "... yellow cobras [and] horn and night adders." Arthur Loveridge, "Notes on Snakes and Snake Bites in East Africa," *Bulletin of the Antinvenin Institute of America,* I (1927), 106–9, records how one "snake man" claimed immunity since he let the young of poisonous snakes bite him every now and then. The basic concept is, of course, preserved in the production

of antivenins (either monovalent or polyvalent) by using horses, gradually given immunity to snake venom over a minimum period of 3 months. The horse produces antibodies (proteins of the immune globulin type) which neutralize specifically the injected venom. The horse is bled, and the serum (containing the antibodies) is separated off. Fractionation (*e.g.* addition of ammonium sulfate followed by filtration or centrifugation) often is employed to separate the antibody-containing globulin from the crude serum. Good shelf life comes from lyophilization. On the process of preparation of one polyvalent antivenin: Sherman A. Minton, Jr., "Paraspecific Protection by Elapid and Sea Snake Antivenins," *Toxicon,* V (1967), 47–55. A good summary of immunity-stories and modern techniques is in Sherman A. Minton, Jr., and Madge Rutherford Minton, *Venomous Reptiles* (New York: Charles Scribners' Sons, 1969), 83–99.

53. *Theriaca,* 115–17. The same notion is repeated in Celsus, V, 27. 10: Illud ignorari non oportet, omnis serpentis ictum et ieiuni et ieiuno magis nocere; ideoque perniciosissimae sunt cum incubant, utilissimumque est, ubi ex anguibus metus est, non ante procedi quam quis aliquid adsumpsit.
54. *Theriaca,* 125; also 334–42 (symptoms).
55. Philumenus, 20.
56. In Latin, this is the *cubitus,* while in Greek, the more-or-less equivalent measure was the πῆχυς. Originally, the measure was the length of the human arm from the elbow to the wrist, or to the tip of the forefinger. The Greeks generally used the measure from the elbow to the tip of the forefinger, which meant that a Greek πῆχυς was about 1½ feet, and the Roman *cubitus* was a little less. The πῆχυς was divided by the Greeks into 2 spans (σπιθαμαί), 6 hand-spans (παλαισταί), and 24 finger-breadths (δάκτυλοι); the Romans also had 6 hand-spans (*palmi*) and 24 thumb-breadths (*pollices*) in their *cubitus.*
57. M. Wellmann, "Sostratus," *Hermes,* XXVI (1891), 321–50.
58. Lucian, *Dipsads,* 4.
59. Lucian, *Dipsads,* 5.
60. Lucian, *Dipsads,* 9.
61. Lucan, IX, 718.
62. Lucan, IX, 737–60.
63. Lucan, IX, 841.
64. *Scholia on Theriaca,* 334.
65. *Theriaca,* 115–487. The Dragon and the Gecko are among the "snakes."
66. *Theriaca,* 148–49.
67. Lucan, IX, 764 and 766.
68. Philumenus, 23.
69. Pausanias, *Description of Greece,* VIII, 4. 7.
70. Pausanias, *Description of Greece,* VIII, 16. 2.
71. Pausanias, *Description of Greece,* VIII, 4. 7.
72. J. G. Frazer, trans., and commentary, *Pausanias's Description of Greece* (Cambridge: University Press, 1898; 6 vols.; rptd., New York: Biblo and Tannen, 1965), IV, 193. Frazer thinks it is *Coluber ammodytes* L.
73. Aelian, XVI, 40.
74. Philumenus, 23.
75. *Ibid.*
76. *cf.* Lucan, IX, 609–10.
77. George Albert Boulenger, *Catalogue of the Snakes in the British Museum* (London: Trustees of the British Museum [Natural History], 1893–96; 3 vols.), III, 460–2.
78. note 39 above.
79. *Catalogue Snakes British Museum,* III, 502–3; "horns" do *not* always occur.
80. Konrad Klemmer, "Classification and Distribution of European, North African, and North and West Asiastic Venomous Snakes," in Wolfgang Bücherl, Eleanor E. Buckley, and Venancio Deulofeu, eds., *Venomous Animals and their Venoms* (New York/London: Academic Press, 1968), Vol. I, 309–25 [315].
81. *Ibid.,* 316.
82. note 72 above.
83. Raymond Ditmars, *Snakes of the World* (New York: Macmillan, 1952), 184 and plate 48.
84. Lucan, IX, 764.
85. *Catalogue Snakes British Museum,* III, 503–4. Klemmer, "Classification," in *Venomous Animals,* I, 315.
86. Klemmer, "Classification," in *Venomous Animals,* I, 313.
87. *Catalogue Snakes British Museum,* III, 502–3. Also note 79 above.
88. Gow/Scholfield, *Nicander,* 175 n. 282.
89. Gow/Scholfield, *Nicander,* 176 n. 282.
90. Klemmer, "Classification," in *Venomous Animals,* I, 315.
91. André de Vries and Eleanor Condrea, "Clinical Aspects of Elapid Bite," in Lance L. Simpson, ed., *Neuropoisons: their Pathophysiological Actions* (New York/London: Plenum Press, 1971), Vol. I, 1–20 [1].
92. *Theriaca,* 235–41. The snake also gives thirst in *Theriaca,* 338–42. *cf.* Lucian and Lucan, notes 58–62 above.
93. *Theriaca,* 242–57.
94. *Theriaca,* 271–81.
95. *Theriaca,* 298–308.
96. *Theriaca,* 326–33.
97. *Theriaca,* 359–365.

98. *Theriaca*, 438–57 (dragon). *Theriaca*, 483–87 (gecko). Another mythical "king of snakes" is in *Theriaca*, 396–410.
99. S. Gitter and A. de Vries, "Symptomatology, Pathology, and Treatment of Bites by Near Eastern, European, and North African Snakes," in *Venomous Animals*, I, 359–401 [esp. 363–64].
100. *Theriaca*, 1–7.
101. J. A. Vick, "Effect of Actual Snakebite and Venom Injection on Vital Physiological Function," in A. de Vries and E. Kochva, eds., *Toxins of Animal and Plant Origin* (New York/London/Paris: Gordon and Breach, 1973), Vol. III, 1001–11 [1007].
102. *Theriaca*, 329.
103. *Theriaca*, 187–89. trans. Gow/Scholfield, *Nicander*, p. 41.
104. John H. Brown, *Toxicology and Pharmacology of Venoms from Poisonous Snakes* (Springfield, Illinois: C. C Thomas, 1973), 150.
105. Lucian, *Dipsads*, 5.
106. *On the Nature of Man*, V, 3–4: *φημὶ δὴ εἶναι αἷμα καὶ φλέγμα καὶ χολὴν ζανθὴν καὶ μέλαιναν.*
107. *On the Nature of Man*, VI, 20: *τὰ α'υτὰ δὲ πάσχουσι καὶ 'υπὸ τῶν φαρμάκων τῶν τὸ φλέγμα 'αγόντων.* Previously, the author of the treatise has made the same point for drugs that draw out bile, which give vomiting of bile, then blood.
108. *On the Nature of Man*, VII, 67–71, as trans. by G. E. R. Lloyd, *Polarity and Analogy* (Cambridge: University Press, 1966), 75.
109. Galen, XIX, 485–96.
110. Galen, XIX, 487–96 [esp. 491].
111. S. Sambursky, *The Physical World of Late Antiquity* (London: Routledge and Kegan Paul, 1962), 40–43. John Scarborough, *Roman Medicine* (London: Thames and Hudson, 1969), 117.
112. Galen, II, 40.
113. *On the Natural Faculties*, I, 13. Scarborough, "Asclepiades," *Pharmacy in History*, XVII (1975), 46 and nn. 47 and 48.
114. Galen, VIII, 422–23 [esp. 423]: *'οταν γὰρ ε'υχύμω τινὶ φύσει, δεδιῃτημένῳ τε κατὰ πάντα τρόπον 'υγιεινῶς 'εζαιφνίδιος γένηται θάνατος, οἷος 'επὶ τινι τῶν δηλητηρίων θαρμάκων, εἶτα πελιδνὸν, ἢ μέλαν, ἢ ποίκιλον, κτλ.* Elsewhere, Galen notes that venom "penetrates" into the body, disturbing the "innate heat" (Galen, IV, 584 [*De semine*, I, 16: here on "plague" venom]); treatment for poisoning would take the form of "drawing out" by devices (*e.g.* cautery, cupping, caustic substances) the poison gaining entrance into the "interior," and any remedies that do work seem to be found only by trial-and-error, and they act "in sympathy" (Galen, X, 896; XI, 761 and 823). Some of these notions of toxic action were believed well into the Renaissance. W. Pagel, "Peripheral Venous Flow 'Ascending' to the Heart (*Ficinus*, 1489) and the Spread of Poison," *Episteme*, IV (1972), 128–34.
115. *Theriaca*, 714: Καὶ τάδε μέν τ' 'οφίεσσιν 'αλεζητήρια δήεις. A. S. F. Gow, "Nicandrea," *Classical Quarterly*, XLV (1951), 95–118 [97: 'αλεζιάρη]. The article is a series of corrections and additions to the listings (esp. for Nicander) in the Liddel and Scott, *Greek-English Lexicon*, 9th ed. He remarks that sometimes even "... the scholiasts are visibly guessing, and their guesses are visibly ridiculous" [95].

115a. Greek weights and measures are, to a certain degree, uncertain (see note 56 above). Gow/Scholfield, *Nicander*, 224, provide some equivalents, which have been adapted from H. Nissen, *Griechische und römische Metrologie*, and the measures provided in Liddell and Scott. The weights and measures that occur in the present essay are:

(1) Liquid and Dry Measures
kyathos = 1/12 pint = 0.04 liters
oxybaphon = ⅛ pint = 0.06 liters
kotylē = ½ pint = 0.27 liters
(2) Liquid Measure
chous = 6 pints = 3.2 liters
(3) Dry Measure
choinix = 2 pints = 1.22 liters
(4) Measure of Length
pēchys = 1 foot, 5¼ inches = 44 mm.
(5) Weights
obolos h 8.8 grains = 0.57 grams
drachmē = 52.8 grains = 3.41 grams

116. M. Wellmann, "Apollodorus," *RE* (Stuttgart, 1894), Vol. I, part 1, Nr. 69, col. 2895. Celsus, V, 27. 8: *panaces* for bite of *chelydrus*. Nicander does *not* specify which snake, but perhaps Apollodorus did.
117. Gow/Scholfield, *Nicander*, 180 n. 526.
118. Gow/Scholfield, *Nicander*, 24.
119. Theophrastus, *Enquiry into Plants*, IX, 9. 1 and 5–6. Dioscorides, IV, 153. Pliny, XIII, 124.
120. Scarborough, "Asclepiades," *Pharmacy in History*, XVII (1975), 50.
121. *'ρυτή*: *Theriaca*, 523; *Alexipharmaca*, 306, 528, and 607.
122. Rue references in Greek and Roman medical sources are very common. *E. g.* Celsus, V, 4 [rue seeds for "opening pores"]; II, 31 [increases urine]; III, 20. 4 [in treatment of "lethargy"]: IV, 27 B [in treatment of female hysteria]; IV, 28.2 [in treatment of *profusio seminis*, probably gonorrhea]. There are many references to rue in Galen, including XIV, 140 [for mushroom poisoning].

123. A basic reference is J. Q. Griffith, Jr., *Rutin and Related Flavonoids* (Easton, Pennsylvania: Mack, 1955).
124. 'ασφόδελος is probably *Asphodelus ramosus* L.; the plant appears in *Theriaca*, 73, as μολόθουρος, and may be the same as 'ολόσχοινος in *Alexipharmaca*, 147; if so, the plant is the club rush, *Scirpus holoschoenus* L., as in Theophrastus, *Enquiry into Plants*, IV, 12. 1, and IX, 12. 1, and Dioscorides, IV, 52.
125. Gow/Scholfield, *Nicander*, 24 and 181 n. 537.
126. *Theriaca*, 9, 129, 130, 223, 259, 517, 545, 642, 653, and 826.
127. A. S. F. Gow, *Theocritus* (Cambridge: University Press, 1965; 2 vols.), II, 82–83.
128. trans. Gow/Scholfield in *Theriaca*, 557–58.
129. *Ibid.*, 559–61.
130. As translated by Gow/Scholfield, *Theriaca*, 579. The editors of Nicander here have rearranged an apparently corrupt text, and this had been line 586 in earlier editions of the *Theriaca*. This notion seems to be reflected in Dioscorides, II, 41, where αἰδοῖον 'ελάφου, taken in wine, is recommended for the bite of a viper. Pliny, XXVIII, 150, also has a notice of this kind: (cervi) *testes vel genitale* and *venter*.
131. *Scholia on Theriaca*, 577.
132. Oribasius (ed. J. Raeder, *Collectionum medicarum reliquiae; Corpus Medicorum Graecorum*, VI, 1,1 [Leipzig: Teubner, 1928–33; 4 vols.]), I, 99: τυρὸς δὲ πᾶς χείρων μέν 'εστι τῶν εἰρημένων ἥκιστα δ' 'ὰν λυπήσειεν αἴγειος ταμισίνης ἐὐώδης μὴ παλαιὸς 'ολίγος, καὶ μᾶλλον 'οπός, quoting from Diocles of Carystos.
133. Homer, *Illiad*, V, 902, and Aristotle, *Historia Animalium*, 522b2 [vegetable coagulant: fig "juice"]. Modern experiment verifies that the latex from a fig tree does clot milk. Guido Majno, *The Healing Hand: Man and Wound in the Ancient World* (Cambridge, Mass.: Harvard University Press, 1975), 151–52.
134. Columella, VII, 8. 1, recommends lamb or kid; the Byzantine *Geoponica*, 18. 9, recommends kid. Nicander likes rabbits.
135. G. L. McGrew and B. D. Johnson, "*In vivo* Effects of Selected *Crotalus* Venoms on Serum Magnesium and Calcium," in *Toxins of Animal and Plant Origin*, Vol. III, 1039–54. E. R. Trethewie, "The Pharmacology and Toxicology of the Venoms of the Snakes of Australia and Oceania," in *Venomous Animals*, Vol. II (1971), 79–101 [88: "Tazieff and Trethewie... have reduced the effect of cardiotoxin from *N. nigricollis* with calcium"].
136. *Theriaca*, 598.
137. Scarborough, "Asclepiades," *Pharmacy in History*, XVII (1975), 47 and n. 68.
138. Athenaeus, XV, 684D. Frg. 74. 69 (Gow/Scholfield, *Nicander*, 154).
139. Athenaeus, XV, 684B. Frg. 74. 55 (Gow/Scholfield, *Nicander*, 154).
140. R. M. Dawkins, "The Semantics of Greek Names for Plants," *Journal of Hellenic Studies*, LVI (1936), 1–11 [5].
141. *Theriaca*, 690–3.
142. *Theriaca*, 696–7, as rendered by Gow/Scholfield, *Nicander*, p. 75.
143. note 51 above.
144. Galen, XII, 362; Aetius, II, 166; and Paul of Aegina, VII, 3. Philumenus, 33, records that the domestic weasel is useful against snakes. Plutarch, *Moralia: On Moral Virtue*, 446E, notes pet weasels were regarded like cats, which the Greeks also kept as pets. Otto Keller, *Die antike Tierwelt* (Leipzig, 1909; rptd. Hildesheim: Olms, 1963; 2 vols.), I, 164–71 [weasels], and 67–81 [cats].
145. Gow/Scholfield, *Nicander*, 183–4 n. 709.
146. Galen, XIV, 184, quotes the recipe as that of Apollodorus through Sostratus. Nicander, *Alexipharmaca*, 585, follows Apollodorus (as does Dioscorides, II, 79. 2) on how toads are also good antidotes.
147. D. K. Chaudhuri, S. R. Maitra, and B. N. Ghosh, "Pharmacology and Toxicology of the Venoms of Asiatic Snakes," in *Venomous Animals*, II, 3–18 [4].
148. P. J. Deoras, "The Story of Some Indian Poisonous Snakes," *Ibid.*, 19–34 [25–6].
149. André de Vries and Eleanor Condrea, "Clinical Aspects of Elapid Bite," in *Neuropoisons*, I, 1–20 [6]. H. A. Reid published an article on his observations in Malayan snakebite in the *British Medical Journal*, II (1964), 540, as listed by de Vries and Condrea, 20. H. Alistair Reid, "Symptomatology, Pathology, and Treatment of Land Snake Bite in India and Southeast Asia," in *Venomous Animals*, I, 611–42, gives many statistics and much data to support this point.
150. H. Alistair Reid, "Symptomatology," in *Venomous Animals*, I, 614. The idea is repeated by Reid in "Clinical Aspects of Animal Toxins," in *Toxins of Animal and Plant Origin*, III, 957–83 [esp. 958–60].
151. Reid, "Clinical Aspects," *Toxins*, III, 960.
152. Reid, "Symptomatology," *Venomous Animals*, I, 611–42, with sources and authorities, 641–2.
153. R. D. Higginbotham and J. H. Clark, "Significance of the Local Tissue Responses to Venoms in Normal and in Sensitized Mice," in Findlay E. Russell and Paul R. Saunders. eds., *Animal Toxins* (Oxford: Pergamon Press, 1967), 337–49 [349]. Materials used were Na heparinate (117 U per mg. Upjohn Co.), egg white lysozyme (3 x crystallized, Nutritional Biochemicals Corp.), and venoms of Russell's viper (*Vipera russelli*), eastern cottonmouth moccasin (*Agkistrodon p. piscivorus*) and western diamondback rattlesnake (*Crotalus Atrox*), on male mice of the Fairfield-Webster strain weighing 19–21 g [337].

VI

Nicander's *Toxicology*

II: Spiders, Scorpions, Insects and Myriapods

Part I

Nicander of Colophon, who probably lived in the time of King Attalus III of Pergamon (reigned 138–133 B. C.), is the author of two poems, the Theriaca *and* Alexipharmaca. *Both works are fundamental for the understanding of Greek pharmacology and toxicology, because the poet based his difficult lines on data and treatises that have not survived. Earlier authors that include Diocles of Carystos and Apollodorus provided Nicander with his subject-matter: snakes, poisonous arthropods, venomous fish and amphibians, poisonous plants and concoctions, and other presumably dangerous creatures. The generally obtuse* Theriaca *and* Alexipharmaca *provided a summary of Greek and Hellenistic ideas of toxicology, and later Roman authors — Philumenus, Pliny, and Galen are but three — employed Nicander for much of their data on toxicology. The various species of venomous snakes, sequelae of their bites, and their antidotes as given by Nicander, are summarized in* Nicander's Toxicology, I: Snakes, PHARMACY IN HISTORY, *19 (1977, 3–23).*

Introductory Remarks: Greek and Roman Sources on Medical Entomology

Nicander seems fairly confident as he describes snakes and their characteristics, and the *Theriaca* has specific remedies for various types of venomous snakes and their bites as they were known in Hellenistic times.[1] By contrast, the consideration of arachnids, insects, and myriapods contained in the *Theriaca* and *Alexipharmaca* is often brief, obscured, truncated, and so clipped as to be unintelligible without recourse to other sources; on the other hand, the section in the *Theriaca* on scorpions is overly verbose, giving presumed varieties in some detail, but the account fails to distinguish remedies for the specific "types." As with his data on snakes, Nicander drew materials from the lost works of Apollodorus,[2] and probably also from earlier treatises that date from the time of Aristotle and Theophrastus.

Théodoridès has noted how many of the Greek assumptions about medical zoology were transmitted in Byzantine manuscripts throughout the long history of the Byzantine Empire, and moreover that these re-copied works were accompanied by illustrations.[3]

Illustrated manuscripts of Nicander's *Theriaca* also demonstrate how long-lived were the details that Nicander summarized from earlier works on poisonous arthropods; one quite late Greek manuscript (Bologna, Bibl. Univ. Codex 3632, esp. fol. 417^v: late fifteenth or early sixteenth century) pictures Nicander's poisonous creatures, including seven distinct varieties of scorpions.[4] Thus, much as there is a long history of illustration in medical botany, that goes back at least to Crateuas,[5] there is a lengthy history of artistic representation accompanying copies of Nicander's works, confirming the popularity of these summaries of toxicology by a Hellenistic poet. Alongside Philumenus,[6] Pseudo-Dioscorides,[7] and certain parts of Aristotle, Theophrastus, Pliny, and Galen, Nicander's *Theriaca* and *Alexipharmaca* became a major source of information on poisons and poisonous creatures until well into the Renaissance. One has only to cite the yet unedited and unpublished lengthy commentary on the Pseudo-Dioscorides *Poisons* by Prosper Alpinus, written between 1599 and 1610,[8] to perceive how important were these kinds of tracts at the beginnings of modern toxicology.

Even though spiders and scorpions were known to be occasionally harmful from earliest times,[9] such animals were apparently considered simply nuisances except in famous cases where large numbers appeared and caused widespread havoc.[10] Spiders are quite shy—even the Black Widow[11]—retreating rapidly at the approach of larger animals, and scorpions, stinging insects, and myriapods would cause concern particularly in rural societies. This basic context may explain why the ancient literature on these creatures is so limited: folk traditions often were snubbed (although Theophrastus gives them full treatment in the medical sections of *Historia Plantarum*, IX),[12] and farmers or agricultural workers rarely put their experiences into writing. There are, however, notable examples in Nicander, Theophrastus, and other sources that show how accurate were the observations by rural inhabitants, and later agricultural manuals—for example the *Geoponica*, the *Mulomedicina Chironis*, and Vegetius' *Mulomedicina*—record the blunt, precise views of farmers on poisonous animals, especially relating to their horses, cows, and oxen.[13] Nicander, of course, is not interested in such matters, but wishes to adapt earlier medical and toxicological works for his *Theriaca* and *Alexipharmaca*, poems that baffle while preserving a solid substratum of information derived usually from Apollodorus.

Spider superstitions have been, and remain, world-wide.[14] As Bristowe points out,[15] a prominent belief in classical antiquity drew attention to the color of the spider's web: if white, good fortune would follow; if black, disaster was imminent.[16] In addition to venerated beliefs that spiders could forecast the weather, exemplified wisdom and cunning, and could generally foretell the future, there are numerous examples of presumed medical uses and powers associated with spiders. Recording of these superstitions in the nineteenth century revealed a wide range of employment: spiders eaten by the handful with bread and butter cure constipation; a live spider, hung in a bag over someone with whooping cough guarantees recovery; anointing victims of smallpox and plague with an "oil of spiders and earthworms" is beneficial; and an ointment and drink made from the large Mygale spiders of Mexico helps in the treatment of leprosy. Bristowe expresses amazement at how powerful these notions remain in the twentieth century: " ... more remarkable is the long list for which tinctures prepared from the bodies of spiders are still recommended in homeopathic medicine!"[16a] Thus it is not surprising that the scientific study, classification, and analysis of spiders is in its early development,[17] compared to the sophisticated fields of myrmicology,[18] the taxonomy of insects,[19] or the habits of the honeybee,[20] to choose three related areas at random. Comstock's *Spider Book* (1912) remains standard for North America, while Kobert's *Giftspinnen* (1901) indicates vividly how little investigation of spiders and scorpions had gone before this pioneering summary.[21] There is, of course, a large literature on the Black Widow (*Latrodectus* spp.), some poisonous scorpions, and increasingly on the Brown Recluse spider (*Loxosceles* spp.),[22] but one must still refer to articles of the 1890's in *Nature* for a full description of the fascinating solifuge,[23] a creature that figures in Nicander's *Theriaca*, 729–733. Cloudsley-Thompson provides a modern synopsis in his *Spiders Scorpions Centipedes and Mites*, but there are obvious gaps in our knowledge of this elusive animal. Medical entomology is a well-developed modern specialty,[25] but again modern research has concentrated on those spiders, scorpions, insects, and myriapods that pose danger to man, according to the modern assumptions of biochemistry, coupled with the increasing availability of anti-venin.[26] Thus, in contrast to the relatively abundant modern sources on spiders and related animals, ancient documents like Nicander's *Theriaca* and *Alexipharmaca* not only tell us what Greek antiquity thought important about such creatures, and their effects on man,[27] but they also inform us about the assumptions that characterized medical entomology in the west until the late nineteenth century.[28]

Until Linnaeus' *Systema Naturae* (1st ed., 1735; 10th ed., 1758), Aristotle's system of classification of *entoma* ("animals that are incised," or "cut into segments") in the *Historia Animalium* remained the most useful, and subsequent accounts in classical antiquity are generally derivative.[29] In the various sections of the *Historia Animalium*, one meets scorpions,[30] spiders (of two kinds),[31] numerous insects,[32] centipedes,[33] millipedes,[34] and several other kinds of "segmented" animals,[35] but not the solifuge. In the same era,[36] Diocles of Carystos practiced medicine and wrote many medical treatises including one that considered medically important *entoma*,[36a] and the lost Aristotelian *Medical Practice* most likely was the base for Diocles' tract, *Wild Herbs*, which is extant only in clipped fragments.[37] In turn, as shown by Wellman, Diocles' writing formed a major part of the foundation for Apollodorus, who became the base for Nicander's obtuse poems.[38] Apollodorus' observations on poisons and poisonous creatures provided Nicander with usually accurate data, and Nicander was not the only author to purloin Apollodorus' materials: Aelius Promotus, Sostratus, Pseudo-Dioscorides, Pliny, Philumenus, and Galen are but a few of the authorities who borrowed heavily, either directly or indirectly, from Apollodorus.[39] Unfortunately, Nicander became the "preferred authority" rather than Apollodorus or Sostratus, in an age that seemed to chose learned argument as distinguished from direct observation, as a passage from Philumenus shows.[40] It is clear that Apollodorus also wrote on poisonous creatures other than snakes:. quotations in Pseudo-Dioscorides, *(Poisonous) Animals*,[41] Pliny,[42] Nicander, and Galen,[42a] show indirect and direct usurpation from Apollodorus. One can place the initial study of medical entomology in the Peripatetic school of Aristotle, to be augmented by Theophrastus and Diocles,[43] and brought to fruition by Apollodorus and Sostratus.

The Galenic *Antidotes* summarized Greek and Roman knowledge of poisonous creatures, especially snakes, spiders, and scorpions, but later authors continued to borrow from the earlier Hellenistic and early Roman imperial sources: Aelian (c. A.D. 170–235) wrote *On Animals*, which lifted matter from numerous sources in zoology and toxicology, including Apollodorus, Sostratus, and Nicander; Oribasius (c. A.D. 320-c. 400), whose massive *Collectiones medicae* was the first to excerpt Galen, and also includes Nicander among the
* huge number of carefully cited authorities; Aetius of Amida (late 5th century A. D.), compiled *Libri medicinales* and a work now mistitled *Tetrabibloi*, which continued the handbook style, quoting hundreds of earlier authorities, especially Galen (spiders appear in *Libri medicinales*, XIII, 16, and *Tetrabibloi*, IV, 1. 18); Alexander of Tralles (probably *fl.* in the reign of Justinian (A. D. 527–565) whose wide-ranging interests included poison lore and worm-infestation as seen in the *Letter on Helminths*, and who quoted Galen among his sources; Paul of Aegina (late 6th century A. D.), who composed a medical handbook in seven books, and scorpions, spiders, centipedes, and insects figure in V, 5–9, derived from Pseudo-Dioscorides, Nicander, Aelius Prom-
* otus, Aelian, Galen, and probably Dioscorides; Nonnus Theophanes (reign of Constantine VIII Porphyrogenitus (A.D. 913–959), whose *Epitome de curatione morborum* again borrowed early classical sources, and the consideration of spiders (270) appears to rest on Nicander and Dioscorides; and one may also mention the curious versification of Aelian's materials, written by Manuel Philes in the 14th century.[44] Nicander's own *Theriaca* and *Alexipharmaca* maintained their own textual tradition, and, as the illustrated manuscripts of late Byzantine times demonstrate, the two poems retained a long-lasting popularity, in spite of their opaque phrases, which gave rise to much speculation on the part of numerous scholiasts.

NICANDER (*Theriaca*, 714) separates his snakes and snakebite account from the following sections on spiders and scorpions: "You will find that these *(previous)* remedies will protect you against snakes." This is evidence that Nicander's major source (Apollodorus; Nicander had *no* competence whatever in toxicology)[45] had delineated snakes from other poisonous creatures, giving a separate class of remedies for spider bites and the stings of scorpions and insects. Even Nicander's manner of organization mirrors that of his source,[46] and one may feel confident in assuming that Apollodorus had also provided a clear, generally accurate account of spiders, scorpions, insects, and the two myriapods. It appears, however, that these creatures were less flashy than snakes, so that Nicander has mauled the data even more than he did in the snakes and snakebite sections of the *Theriaca*. Sometimes poetic allusion and license take open precedence over facts, and recovery of species among the spiders, scorpions, and insects is fraught with complicated difficulty.

Phalangia

The bite of a venomous spider is serious, as Celsus notes,[47] and treatment becomes more complex than even the *chlydrus*-snake: "added to the treatment by surgery, the person bitten (by a *phalangium*) should be plunged often into a hot bath." Celsus *phalangium* is the *phalangion* of Nicander's *Theriaca*, 715–724, and ultimately derives from Aristole's two-part distinction: *phalangia* and *arachnai*.[48] The question of what the Greeks meant by *phalangia* as opposed to *arachnai* is partially answered by Philumenus, the scholiasts commenting on the *Theriaca*, and by lexicon-compilers of late antiquity. Philumenus has two separate sections for the *phalangia* (six poisonous kinds)[49] and the *arachnai* (along with the *tetragnatha*, "four-jawed"), not believed to be as harmful.[50] The *Scholia on Theriaca* tells us that "the first of the *phalangia*" (in Nicander's passage) "is called *rhōx*, because it (looks like) a shiny grape being carried along."[51] Hesychius' *Lexicon* lists *kokkos* ("berry" or "grape") as the same as a type of *phalangion*.[52] Thus it may be that originally the "grape-" or "berry-like" spiders were meant by *phalangia*, and Nicander/Apollodorus have taken this original name and subsumed varieties under it. Therefore the first of the *phalangia* (in both Nicander, *Theriaca*, 716, and Philumenus, *Poisonous Animals*, 15. 1–2) is the *rhōx*, another word for "grape" or "berry" as found in Aristotle[53] and Dioscorides.[54] This grape-*rhōx* is colored like "black/pitchy smoke,"[55] which in the Greek displays what Nicander probably thought was his poetic skill. *Rhōx* in the plural can mean "fingertips," according to Pollux,[56] Soranus,[57] and Rufus,[58] and Nicander follows this allusion to the manner in which the spider walks with "(having legs that crawl successively."[59] *Theriaca*, 718, shows careful observation (by Apollodorus), since the line contains *esklēken*, which captures the modern notion of "chitinous," that is "hard" more than "dry."[60] The summary-description of the creature called *rhōx* in *Theriaca*, 716–719, gives a sooty-black, shiny grape that walks on its 'fingertips' with legs that move in synchronous succession.

Symptoms of the *rhōx* bite follow in *Theriaca*, 719–724; the spider is now called "the *rhōx* sooty like pitch" (*rhōx pissēen:* 719). The skin does not appear to be wounded; there is shivering of the arms and legs; the skin and penis become rigid, and priapism occurs with oozing; there is a numbness below the groin, accompanied by weakness in the knees.

Nicander's description of the *rhōx* (with help from Philumenus and other sources), coupled with the symptomatology, suggests one or more of the species in the genus *Latrodectus*. The essential description gathered from all sources is of a creature whose external appearance is like a grape, usually shiny black to mottled gray. *Latrodectus* is indeed noted for its bulbous, shiny black appearance, and one live specimen observed in California in 1972 was about the size of a very large grape.[61] Modern nomenclature for spiders is in disarray,[62] but Bucherl's recent listing gives six species of *Latrodectus* of world wide distribution.[63] Two (perhaps three) species would fit Nicander's *rhōx*, given the geographical limitations of Greece, Asia Minor and the Middle East, and Egypt: *Latrodectus mactans* (Fabricius), which is cosmopolitan, and the most probable subspecies is *L. mactans tredecimguttatus* (Rossi);[64] *L. pallidus* Cambridge, which has been observed in southern Russia, Syria, Palestine, and from Iran west through Libya; and *L. dahli* Levi, observed in Iran.[65] This is, of course, the infamous Black Widow, one of the two poisonous spiders that occur in the United States.[66] The Black Widow has received great attention from medical entomologists, and uniquely, scientific investigation of this genus was well under way by the seventeenth century.[67] All modern texts of medical entomology and clinical parasitology devote extended sections to the Black Widow,[68] and the literature describing research into the physiology and biochemistry of *Latrodectus* has been enormous.[69]

Symptoms of the bite of the various species of *Latrodectus* are well known and fairly specific. First occurs a sharp pain at the site of the wound, which disappears rapidly and usually is gone within four hours. Soon begins the abdominal muscular rigidity, becoming boardlike (thus the often mistaken diagnosis of appendicitis), to be followed by abdominal cramps. Other signs are profuse sweating, congestion of the eyes and face, and excessive sensitivity of the skin. Children may suffer convulsions. Priapism and ejaculation are also clinical manifestations,[70] and Maretić notes that untreated *Latrodectus* victims have an " ... illness up to eight days" and that " ... the prognosis is in general favorable, but fatalities do occur."[71] It is established that the venoms of *Latrodectus* are highly labile proteins with neurotoxic action,[72] and Frontali and Grasso gave gained five protein fractions from the venom of the Italian *L. mactans tredecimguttatus;* only one of these fractions is fatal to mammals, while two others kill only insects.[73] Of course, Greek toxicology did not view poison action in terms of protein fractions, but the comparison of symptoms and causes can lead to species identification in the texts of Greek and Roman authors. The description of the spider, as well as the essential similarity of clinical symptoms of Latrodectism, rather well keys Nicander's *rhōx* as *Latrodectus mactans* (Fabricius).

The second spider on Nicander's list is called *asterion* (*Theriaca*, 725–728). Gow and Scholfield translate this as "the starlet,"[74] but something akin to "the glitterer" might be closer. Curiously, *asterion* does not appear in Philumenus, and the Scholiasts add nothing, nor does the prose-summary by Eutecnius.[75] Gow and Scholfield propose that this variety is simply a variant of *Latrodectus mactans tredecimguttatus*,[76] implicitly dismissing identifications given by Kobert and others. This is probably correct, but spider nomenclature is in such confusion that it is quite understandable why so many variants have been offered for Nicander's *asterion* over the past fifty years.[77] Symptoms of the bite of the *asterion* (*Theriaca*, 727–728) are shivering, sleepiness, and weak knees.

The third kind of *phalangion* in Nicander's catalogue is called the *kyaneon*,[78] rendered by Gow and Scholfield as "blue spider."[79] This seems a good guess, given the normal meaning of the word in Greek, but something appears to have been omitted from Nicander's account. *Kyaneon* is distinguished by its rapid movement (*pedēoron: Theriaca*, 729), and its hairiness (*lachnēen: Theriaca*, 730). There is no description. Symptoms are a terrible wound from the bite, and the vomiting of spider web threads (*arachnēenta: Theriaca,* 733).[80] The *kyaneon* might prove a complete mystery, were it not for a series of textual borrowings by a number of ancient sources. As expected, Pliny picks up this account,[81] and we read about something called *caeruleus* ("the blue one"), "covered with black hair."[82] Moreover, the bite of the *caeruleus* causes the vomit of spider web, along with the dimming of the vision.[83] This last is probably a rendition of the very odd phrase in *Theriaca,* 732,[84] also re-done by Eutecnius in the *Paraphrase.*[85] Pliny then (*Natural History,* XXIX, 86–87) proceeds to list two other kinds of spiders, the wingless hornet and the *myrmecion* (summarizing *Theriaca,* 738–751) with some description. Next Pliny (*Natural History,* XXIX, 87) rather abruptly remarks, "there are two kinds of *tetragnathii.*" For these creatures, there is a short description by Pliny, seemingly picking up from the source that had just offered the *caeruleus,* "covered with black hair." It appears that Nicander and Pliny have followed the same source in *Theriaca,* 715–758 and *Natural History,* XXIX, 86–87, but Nicander has truncated the account of the *kyaneon* (presumably to fit his sense of poetic diction), and Pliny has given *caeruleus* (= *kyaneon*) covered with black hair (Nicander has only "hairy") but no further description. Shortly come the *tetragnathii,* which never appear in any of the extant texts of Nicander, but which appear in Philumenus, *Poisonous Animals,* 35, and in a number of other Greek and Latin sources. The scholiasts on *Theriaca* merely add that *kyaneon* runs very rapidly and is black,[86] and Eutecnius simply says that *kyaneon* is "large and not slow."[87] It is probable that Pliny's *caeruleus* (= Nicander's *kyaneon*) is the original source's *tetragnatha,* which both Nicander and Pliny have butchered. It can be assumed that Apollodorus had *tetragnatha,* which Nicander found poetically intractable; Pliny probably was using a Latin translation/summary (Aemilius Macer?[88]) of Nicander, plus a text of * Apollodorus,[89] which he found to include *tetragnatha,* so he added it at the end of this section of *Natural History,* XXIX, on spiders.

Tetragnathii are "the four-jawed ones," a striking description. Greek and Latin authors do mention this creature from time to time, and Pliny has apparently forgotten that he had considered it in an earlier book of the *Natural History* (VIII, 104)[90] calling it *solipuga.* A further point of confusion is Philumenus' listing of the *tetragnathon* in the same passages with *arachnai,* since one assumes that Nicander's *phalangia* ultimately derived from Aristotle's two-part distinction between *arachnai* and *phalangia.* Steier, however, admits that this distinction is quite uncertain,[91] and Aristotle's *Historia Animalium,* IX, 39 (622–623) adds to that uncertainty.[91] Given the frequent equivalence and use of *phalangion* for *arachnē,*[93] and *vice versa,* it appears that Aristotle may have suggested such a distinction, and that some later authors—including Apollodorus and Philumenus—chose to ignore it. Even Kobert expresses his quandary about the "two kinds" in antiquity.[94]

The first extant source on *tetragnatha* is in a fragment of Agatharcides' * *Erythrean Sea,*[95] where "scorpions, *phalangia* and *tetragnatha* live in great abundance" in the land to the south (context is for Ethiopia). Strabo, *Geography,* XVI, 4. 12 (C 772), picks up this tale, saying that there is an area south of upper Egypt which is empty of people, who fled because of the large numbers of scorpions, *phalangia,* and *tetragnatha.*[96] Aelian, *On Animals,* XVII, 40 more-or-less repeats the story, even though Aelian says "India," which could also be Ethiopia, given the notions of continental geography in those times.[97] Pliny, *Natural History*, VIII, 104, also has borrowed a version of the account in Agatharcides/Strabo, calling the creatures *solpugae;* the wording in Pliny is almost identical with the Agatharcides/Strabo/Aelian version of *tetragnatha*. Thus *tetragnatha* = *solpugae*. Other sources confirm this. Solinus, *Polyhistor*, IV, 3, says that the *solifuga* is a poisonous spider, and that it is so called because it " ... flees the day."[98] In his catalogue of horrid Libyan animals, Lucan, *Civil War*, IX, 837, includes a *salpuga*.[99] Festus likewise speaks of a *solipugna* which is an " ... evil sort of animal ... hiding from the sun."[100]

Solpuga = *tetragnathon* without much doubt, which leads one back to Nicander's *kyaneon*. Pliny may have rearranged materials from his multiple sources, when he saw that Nicander's account did not give the detail he found in Apollodorus, but one may ask why — other than the lengthy poetic intractibility of *tetragnathon*—Nicander chose *kyaneon as his "term" to replace tetragnathon*. The Greek lexica provide some clues. Normally, the word would mean "blue" or "the color of the heavens," as Hesychius suggests. He also notes that the word can be "blue-black" or "black," and has association with snakes and "Ethiopians."[101] Pollux in his *Onomasticon* has the word among color-terms that describe the various types of men, which means his *kyaneon* stands for "black," and the following *melan* would mean "jet black."[102] One cannot assume "blue" here. The final clue emerges from the Byzantine *Suda*,[103] where *kyaneoi* first means "black ones," but then follows another definition that reads "dark-gleaming, spread out *(petasmata)*." *Petasmata* is the term used by Aristotle, *Historia Animalium*, 541b7, to describe the tentacles of an octopus as they are "spread out." Returning to the *Suda* entry, next one reads that *kyanochaitēs* means "black-haired" (*melanothrix* = *kyanothrix*), a term applied to describe the god, Poseidon. If Nicander saw *tetragnathon* in his text of Apollodorus, he may have thought he could display both his pedantic knowledge of synonyms as well as his command of the verses of Homer with the use of *kyaneon*. It may seem somewhat strained—this is quite typical of Nicander's poetry—but it may be that he intended the reader to recall Homer, *Iliad*, XI, 629, as well as understand that *kyaneon* would mean "hairy, spread-out [legs] that were black," an exceedingly obscure substitute for the absolutely clear *tetragnathon*. The Homer passage (*Iliad*, XI, 628–629) is in the context of Nestor's cup, and the mixing of a potion by Hecamede. The table (*trapezan:* 628) on which the potion is set has "feet of black (or "blue-black:" *kyanopezan:* 629). Nicander's substitute word presumably means a creature that is black, has legs that are spread out, and is very hairy. What is lost in this series of muffled literary allusions is the chief characteristic of the creature: its four jaws.

Those four jaws key the animal as one of the elusive solipugida, or solifugae, often called Wind Scorpions or False Scorpions. They form a separate order (*Solifugae)* among the arachnids, and " ... the hairy body is divided into two parts ... the chelicerae are extremely well developed, forming two powerful pincers with which the prey is destroyed. Sometimes these are as long as the entire prosoma and they are possibly for their size the most formidable jaws in the animal world."[104] Most common in North Africa is *Galeodes arabs* C. L. Koch, which will attain a width (legs included) of five inches (13

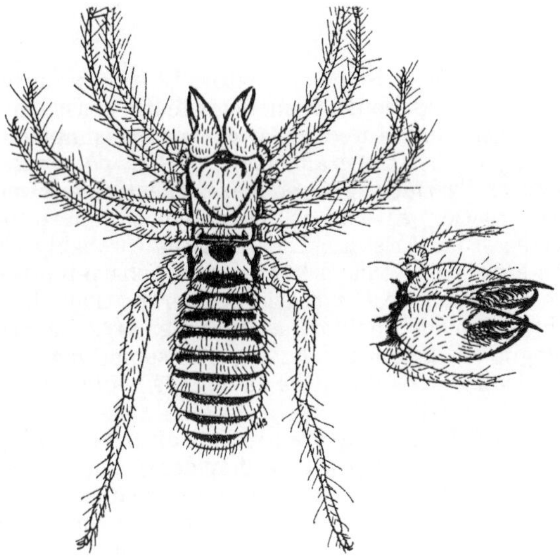

***Galeodes arabs*, dorsal aspect. African & Near Eastern Solifuge. after Savory 17 cm (7"). (*drawing by Lysa Scarborough*).**

cm).[105] No other arachnid is so "hairy" in appearance, and to the "... casual glance, it looks like a ball of fluff."[106] The bite of the solifuge is painful, but not poisonous,[107] and the " ... long-legged forms can run at great speed so that they resemble balls of yellow thistledown blown over the desert."[108] Some examples of the Egyptian varieties range in color from light yellow-brown to brownish-black,[109] but the Indian species (*Galeodes fatalis* Pocock) will generally be black.[110] Steier's rather wild guess of "cantharid" for Nicander's *kyaneon* can be dismissed,[111] but given the muffled nature of the poet's substitution for an apparently accurate description by Apollodorus, one can easily understand Steier's baffled reaction to the passage. Gow and Scholfield simply list authorities, with a reference to Pliny, *Natural History*, XXIX, 86.[112] Whatever medical treatment might later be prescribed by Nicander would be unnecessary, because no poison is involved. A danger might be from infection in the wound, which could be serious, since the solifuge will occasionally consume small birds, lizards, and the largest of insects; the large pincers can inflict a deep and jagged injury.

A fourth *phalangion* appears in *Theriaca*, 734: the *agrōstēs*, rendered by Gow and Scholfield as "huntsman."[113] The creature is described as being like the "wolf spider" in form,[114] and its bite is harmless to man.[115] The "wolf spider" (*lykos*) of Aristotle, *Historia Animalium*, 632a1, and Philumenus, 15. 2, is indeed one of the trap door spiders, but only one species spins a web, while Aristotle believes all kinds are web-spinners. Again, Nicander has taken a simple term, *lykos*, and made a poetic substitution with *agrōstēs*, which may be understood if the normal meaning ("crafty," as in *Alexipharmaca*, 473, or "rustic," as in Theocritus, *Idylls*, XXV, 48) is set side-by-side with other meanings. For Nicander, the basic meaning would most likely be derived from Homer, and *Odyssey*, XVI, 218, has *agrōstēs*, "hunter." If one adds the curious use of the term by Aristotle, *Historia Animalium*, 552a15, and Theophrastus, *Historia Plantarum*, I, 6. 10, to describe grass "with dog's teeth," to Theophrastus' context describing how the roots of some plants "choose to turn downward by choice" so that those roots are naturally strong, as well as to Aristotle's statement that ticks come from dog's-tooth grass, one may discern faintly why Nicander substituted *agrōstēs* for the simple, clearly descriptive *lykos*. The *ho agrōstōr* ("the crafty one") of *Alexipharmaca*, 473, coupled with the *agrōstēs* of *Theriaca*, 734, squeezes the Homeric meaning ("hunter") together with "rustic," as well as the notion of "sharp-toothed-strong-at-the-base" derived from Aristotle/Theophrastus (probably through Apollodorus); Nicander's creature is thus a hunter/crafty/sharp-toothed/with strong legs, much more satisfying to the poetic desiderata than the bland, clipped *lykos*. The bite of the spider would be, as Nicander says, harmless, so its inclusion in the catalogue of dangerous *phalangia* is something of a mystery. Philumenus, 15. 2, also includes the *lykos* among his *phalangia*, but his authority is Nicander.

Generally speaking, superficial wounds are common after venom injection from the various species in the genus *Lycosa* (wolf spiders), but temperature changes can alter the behavior of the normally harmless creatures. In Brazil, *Lycosa erythrognatha* " ... is handsome and harmless during warm weather, but irritable and aggressive when there is no sun for several days."[116] Even when *Lycosa* spp. bite, there is local necrotic action only, with no general symptoms, and the local pain never is prominent. *Lycosa* venoms are cytotoxic,[117] and there is an anti-venin from the Butantan Institute called *Anti-licōsico* for individuals particularly sensitive to cytotoxic venom.[118] Perhaps Apollodorus had observed that *lykoi* were quite unpredictable, becoming aggressive on cloudy days, and thus placed them among the dangerous *phalangia*, to be followed in that classification by Nicander and Philumenus.

The fifth spider in Nicander's list is the *sphēkion* (*Theriaca*, 738), probably best translated as "wasp spider" or "spider wasp." The creature is reddish, and "like the horse in high spirit,"[119] which is not very helplful in keying the genus or species. Following Nicander alongside Apollodorus, Pliny says that this spider differs from the wasp only in having no wings, and that its bite makes the victim emaciated.[120] There are no parallel passages in Oppian, Theocritus, or elsewhere in Nicander, and the scholiasts and Eutecnius add nothing to the understanding of *Theriaca*, 738. The ancient lexica provide no zoological definitions, and Bussemaker's identification of the creature as a "solipuge" is merely a guess without verification.[121] The total description (Nicander and Pliny) is of an animal that is reddish, one of the "spider" group, and looks like a wasp without wings. The "high-spirited horse" causes one to think of spiders that "leap" or "jump," and perhaps Apollodorus had observed some species in the large number of genera in the Family *Salticidae* (jumping spiders), especially *Sarinda* spp. There are a number of species in *Sarinda* that have perfected a protective mimicry,[122] and the full range of distastful (to birds and other spider enemies) imitations is represented: ants, wasps, "bugs" (*Hemiptera*), beetles, and even scorpions.[123] Corollary to various European species, the eastern United States has *Sarinda hentzi*, which is indeed "reddish" (reddish-orange), and looks *exactly* like a "wasp without wings." *S. hentzi* is quite small (0.2": 6mm), but some of the European species in *Sarinda* are somewhat larger. It seems reasonable to presume that Apollodorus (followed by Pliny) had seen some of these "jumping spiders," and Nicander has preserved a shadow of his source with the "spirited horse" phrase. Jumping spiders can inflict a painful bite, but there are no significant symptoms. Nicander records none, and Pliny's line noting the bite of the spider "makes the victim thin" may have come directly from Apollodorus. There is no explanation for this notion, if it did come to Pliny from Apollodorus. As Gow and Scholfield write,[124] *Theriaca*, 738–746, is a mass of confusion.

Nicander's sixth *phalangion* is called *myrmēkion* (*Theriaca*, 747), and may be rendered "ant-spider."[125] This creature, as the name suggests, resembles an ant, has a red neck, a body colored like dust, a broad speckled back, and a head that is dark and quite small.[126] The scholiasts record that this sixth kind of *phalangion* in *Theriaca* is called *myrmēkion* "because it looks like an ant," and "Sostratus calls it *myrmēkeion*, Heracleoticon calls it *myrmēka*, and all the others call it *myrmēkoeidēs*."[127] Philumenus has *to myrmēkion* as one of his six *phalangia*, and says it is thus called because it looks like a big ant;[128] then he quotes Nicander, *Theriaca*, 748–749, as his description. In this case, Philumenus is quite right in his choice, because the description in *Theriaca*, 747–751, with Philumenus' added word "big" to "ant," keys the creature. A modern description of the Family *Mutillidae* ("velvet ants" in the United States), especially of *M. europea* (like the American *Dasymutilla occidentalis* L.), rather well keys Nicander's *myrmēkeion:* "The female is apterous with the thorax and propodeum usually fused into a single plate ... Both sexes are black to reddish in colour, often with spots or bands of silvery pubescence and generally velvety appearance."[129] The *Mutillidae* are wasps, and the wingless female is the creature in Nicander and Philumenus. American species are somewhat larger, and the females appear like large, wingless, red wasps,[130] although a quick glance would make them very large, velvety ants.[131] In Europe, *M. europea* is parasitic on bumblebees, and the "ant" can inflict a nasty sting. The venom would thus be that of a wasp, and there are individuals who are extremely sensitive to wasp venom.[132] That sensitivity is classed as "allergic" and the symptoms as anaphylactic. Treatment would be local, and Habermann notes that a topical antihistamine has proven useful against wasp stings.[133]

Theriaca, 752–758, is a very confused section, describing when harvests are done "without sickles," swarms of *phalangia* emerge to cause havoc. Although Gow and Scholfield are tempted by similar accounts of the Black Widow appearing in large numbers during harvests in southern France,[134] Nicander says that the creatures are "like cantharids."[135] This is, indeed, a blister beetle, and most probably the infamous "Spanish-Fly" (*Cantharis vesicatoria* L.),[136] rejected by Gow and Scholfield.[137] Nicander's symptoms are decisive: babbling, delirium, and watery eyes.[138] Pliny describes "swarms" of cantharid beetles,[139] and a Galenic listing says that *phalangia* can also mean *kantharides*.[140] Much clearer and more to the point is Nicander's account of the *kantharis* in *Alexipharmaca*, 115–127. Here the creature eats wheat,[141] and the substance made from the beetle smells like pitch and tastes much like juniper berries. For someone who has taken the concoction made from *kantharides*, there is a biting sensation to the lips followed by similar feelings in the stomach; shortly come sharp pains in the belly and the bladder, and grave discomfort in the chest, especially at the point of the xiphisternum. Last occur fainting spells and delusions.[142]

Learned argument in antiquity debated which part of the cantharid beetle's body produced the powerful drug (known in modern pharmacy as cantharidin), and Pliny quite rightly guessed the elytra.[143] The present drug is prepared from the dried specimens of *C. vesicatoria*, using the elytra alone, since they contain more of the active principle (cantharidin) than all of the other parts combined, even though the third accessory glands of the male *C. vesicatoria* are quite rich in cantharidin.[144] Symptomatology for cantharid poisoning includes severe gastroenteritis, nephritis, fainting, and possible death, even from small amounts.[145]

The *Phalaina-Kranokolaptēs*

Before Nicander considers scorpions, he inserts an incredibly garbled section on something that has characteristics of both a moth (or butterfly) and a large wasp (*Theriaca*, 759–768). Gow and Scholfield lean toward the notion that this is the fabled "winged scorpion,"[146] reported in a number of other ancient sources.[147] There may be, however, more to it than this. First, *Theriaca*, 760, calls the creature *phalaina*, a "moth," and then comes the description of a creature with "dense and downy wings," quite recognizable as a moth or butterfly. Next (as translated by Gow and Scholfield): "Its terrible head nods ever in grim fashion and is hard, and its belly is heavy; its sting it plants in the top of a man's neck or his head ..."[148] One can, as do Gow and Scholfield, assume that the creature is in the same class as the griffin or the unicorn, but it is quite possible that Nicander has sandwiched an account of a moth together with a description of a large wasp. In light of the fact that "... lepidopterism was first observed only at the end of the last century (1891),"[149] Nicander's "poison moth" warrants close examination. The zootoxic genus of moths, *Zygaena*, inhabits northern Italy,[150] and it has wide distribution (esp. *Z. laeta*) in southern Europe. Entomologists remain uncertain concerning the taxonomy of the genus,[151] and *Z. laeta* certainly could not be classed as having a "terrible head," nor frightening with its length of 16 mm. The fact remains, however, of the poisonous flechettes borne by species in *Zygaena*. "Rossi treated the golden zootoxic secretion of *Zygaena* with hydrolizing products, obtaining a fixed atoxic fraction and a toxic volatile fraction whose nature is ketonic or aldehydic. Inoculation in mice and frogs produces paralysis and death."[152] In humans, severe dermatitis, accompanied by dizziness, nausea, dyspnea, and related symptoms can occur, especially in individuals who are particularly sensitive to the ketone-like venom.[153] It seems reasonable to suggest that Nicander's source knew some data about *Zygaena*, perhaps through the medium of folk-tales, which even Theophrastus respected.[154] If true, then Apollodorus would have been quite willing to incorporate such facts in his lost works, but one can only wonder what form the information took, given the state of the text in Nicander.

The scholiasts tell us that the creature was also known as *kranokolaptēs*,[155] and Philumenus, 15. 1 and 5, has *kranokolaptēs* as his sixth type of *phalangion*. The scholiasts further add that another name is *kephalokroustēs* ("head-that-strikes"), and it has four wings, as well as a sting hidden by its neck, beneath the head.[156] In a fragment of the lost treatise on dangerous animals by Sostratus,[157] one learns that the *kranokolaptēs* frequents the Persea-tree,[158] and when drowned in oil, it becomes an antidote—presumably against others of its kind. Another description in Philumenus (15.5) of the *kranokolaptēs* as "long and green" brings to mind the praying mantis, but Philumenus' description is almost unique among the sources, and the mantis has no resemblance whatever to the gemstone figure of the winged scorpion.[159] That figure has four wings, greatly resembling the wings of the *Zygaena*, but no moth has a sting, clearly stated as a nasty characteristic of *kranokolaptēs* by both the scholiasts and Philumenus. If Nicander (or his source) has compacted a poisonous moth with a large wasp, a suitable suggestion for the latter would be one of the cosmopolian genera of Cicada Killers (the most common North American species is *Sphecius speciosus* [Drury]. These large wasps generally have a gold and black coloration, and most stings received come on the neck and head. *Theriaca*, 762, would seem to be about a wasp, but Nicander apparently says that the creature is related to scorpions, noting that the "wings are joined by a membrane."[160] This tempts one in the direction of bats, but nothing else in the texts supports this hunch. If two creatures—a moth and a wasp—are reflected (and an equally strong case can be made for the mythical winged scorpion), then the venoms involved would be from the poisonous flechettes of the female moth, and the usual wasp venom. One can conclude that Nicander's *phalaina* = *kranokolaptēs* = *kephalokroustēs*, but identification of the genus (or genera) remains quite uncertain.

Scorpions comprise *Theriaca*, 769–804. There are nine kinds: *leukos* (*Theriaca*, 771: "the white kind") is harmless; *pyrsos* (772: "the red kind") moves very rapidly, causes a burning fever in the mouth, convulsions as if the victim is on fire, and a great thirst; *ho zophoeis* (775; "the dark gray [?] kind"[161] causes a fearful agitation and *typsis* (perhaps "beating" [of the heart?]); *chloaōn* (777: "the green kind") causes shivering and an awful wound; *empelios* (782: "the pale yellow kind"[162]) causes swollen testicles;[163] two other kinds (786–796) merely are described as being like a crab on the seashore, and like a crab; *melichlōron* (797: "the honey-colored kind") has a sting that is tipped in black, and the scholiasts say that this type looks like a "spinning whorl;"[164] and the last variety is again the winged scorpion (799–804), "the one with bent 'hands',[165] colored flame red."[166] This last scorpion kills children instantly.

Aristotle had recognized that some scorpions were harmless, while others living in different places were dangerous: at Pharos, the sting of a scorpion was harmless, but the scorpion of Caria (Asia Minor) was fatal to man and pig.[167] One can ascertain two "kinds" of scorpions from this terse description in *Historia Animalium*, but Nicander's *Theriaca* is the first extant source that lists the known "kinds" in classical antiquity. Again, Apollodorus' observations were the foundation for Nicander's lines.[168] In the case of scorpions, it is certain that Nicander borrowed directly, because Pliny, *Natural History*, XI, 86–91, quotes Apollodorus by name as his authority on scorpions. Pliny writes that Appollodorus had distinguished nine kinds, mainly by their colors, "an utterly useless way," since one could not tell which of the nine was least harmful.[169] Pliny also quotes Apollodorus on the winged scorpion,[170] which suggests that Apollodorus had compacted two creatures into one, seen in Nicander's *phalaina/kranokolaptēs*.[171] Having rejected Apollodorus' "color scheme," Pliny gives an even vaguer description of symptomalogy than had Nicander.

Aristotle's basic idea of locale combined with Apollodorus' observations of varying color-types proves to be essentially correct. Modern identification rests not only on the shape of the sternum, and spurs between the last two leg-segments, but also on coloration and locale. Balozet carefully describes the "geography of scorpionism (in northwestern Africa) which corresponds to the habitat of this species [*Androctonus australis* (L.)],"[172] and then follows a detailed listing of limited areas like "south and west of the Atlas." Wilson carefully notes the colors of the various scorpions in Egypt, and describes *Buthus Quinque-striatus* [= *Leiurus quinquestriatus* (H. and E.)] as being "... sandy yellow in color tending to brown."[173] Curiously, Wilson also describes a species he calls *Prionurus Citrinus*, which is greenish yellow,[173a] thus verifying the almost unique report of a "greenish" scorpion found in Philumenus.[174] Apparently Wilson's "greenish yellow" Egyptian scorpion has been subsumed within a newer nomenclature, since Balozet recognizes only the following in North Africa and the Middle East as being truly dangerous: *Androctonus australis* L.; *Buthus occitanus*, Am.;[175] *Buthacus arenicola* E. Sim.; *Androctonus amoreuxi* Aud & Sav.; *A. aeneas* C. L. Koch; *A. hoggarensis* Pallary; *Leiurus quinquestriatus* H. & E.; *Androctonus crassicauda* Olivier; and *Buthus judiacus*.[176] The very large—and most famous African black scorpions—from the *Pandinus* spp., as well as comparable giants from southern Asia (*Heterometrus* and *Palamneus* spp.) are only "slightly venomous" in spite of their large size (up to 7 inches/17 cm).[177]

The common yellow *Buthus occitanus*, which ranges on both the northern and southern shores of the Mediterranean, is probably Nicander's *empelios* (*Theriaca*, 782), and *Leiurus quinquestriatus* is the *melichlōron* of *Theriaca*, 797. Perhaps the large *Pandinus* spp. are intended when Nicander writes of those scorpions "like crabs" and "like crabs on the seashore" (*Theriaca*, 786–796), and Nicander's *zophoeis* (*Theriaca*, 775) is to be identified as one of the very common and harmless *Euscorpius* spp., which rarely exceed 2 inches (5 cm) in length. Nicander's *leukos* (*Theriaca*, 771) is not a separate kind of scorpion, but the appearance of newly born scorpions, which have mounted their mother's back. The young are born alive, and depending on the species and the season, will remain on the mother's back from ten days to three weeks, until the first moult. *Leukos* quite certainly is harmless. The rest (excluding the winged scorpion of *Theriaca*, 799–804) probably are *Androctonus* spp., which can according to their surroundings, appear "reddish-gold," "greenish," and so on. If Nicander's *phalaina/kranokolaptēs* is *not* a moth/wasp, then another of the poisonous *Androctonus* spp. can be assumed. If *Pandinus* is correct for the two "crab-like" scorpions, and *Euscorpius* is Nicander's *zophoeis*, then at least three types of scorpions in *Theriaca* are harmless. Even if *phalaina* is not a scorpion, there would be some danger from the poisonous flechettes of a female moth. Of the nine varieties listed by Apollodorus/Nicander, five are definitely dangerous, with a sixth being either a myth, or a "scorpion story" founded on rare observations of desert winds "blowing" scorpions off the ground,[178] or a compaction of two venomous insects into one.

Wilson established that the active principle of *L. quiquestriatus* consisted of at least two "proteids,"[179] and recent research has demonstrated some variation in the number of protein fractions in the active principle among various species of scorpions. Two remains the correct number for *Androctonus*, according to Balozet,[180] while research on the nature and biochemistry of scorpion neurotoxins has identified important components within the polypeptide chains. Niu and Frankel-Conrat have pinpointed the C-terminal residue in Toxin I, of *Androctonus australis* by hydrazinolysis, and shown it to be threonine,[181] and Rochat and colleagues have taken this method among others to isolate eleven neurotoxins from scorpion venoms.[182] Thus all symptoms in mammals from scorpion stings will be in direct proportion to the amount of neurotoxin injected, which is related to the mass/size of the victim. Wilson, however, had demonstrated that several mammals were immune to scorpion venom (the jerboa, desert fox [fennec], and a desert rat [*Gerbilus pyramidum*], while the venom was very toxic to ordinary white rats, guinea pigs, and humans.[183] In modern terms, this specific immunity is related to the particular reactions among species to the various fractions,[184] much as seen among victims of spider bites.[185]

"Scorpion stings always occur under accidental circumstances, more often at night than during the day, and more often when the weather is stormy, the temperature is elevated, and the wind hot."[186] So reads a modern description of the setting of scorpion envenomation in north Africa, which is not too dissimilar in context from Nicander's farm workers and fishermen. One scorpion (*Theriaca*, 800) brings death instantly to children, who remain the majority of fatalities from scorpion stings. Balozet gives figures of deaths among infants and children (apparently up to age 10) that suggest why Nicander would have written his blunt line: infants received 411 stings, with 32 deaths; children received 5211 stings, with 191 deaths. By comparison, adults received 13,130 stings, with 145 deaths, while elderly victims numbered 1412 with 18 deaths. Respectively, 7.78%, 3.66%, 1.10% and 1.27% were fatalities from the sting of *Androctonus australis*.[187] These numbers and percentages represent sixteen years of records kept in Algeria, and one may ask how many thousand scorpion stings—and infant deaths—went unreported. Unlike the frequently overblown reports of snakebite fatalities,[188] scorpion envenomation is a serious problem in north Africa, Egypt, and the Middle East, as well as Mexico, and the American southwest. It is ironic that the sensationalist press has made so little of this, especially when infants and children are most frequently stung, and most frequently die.

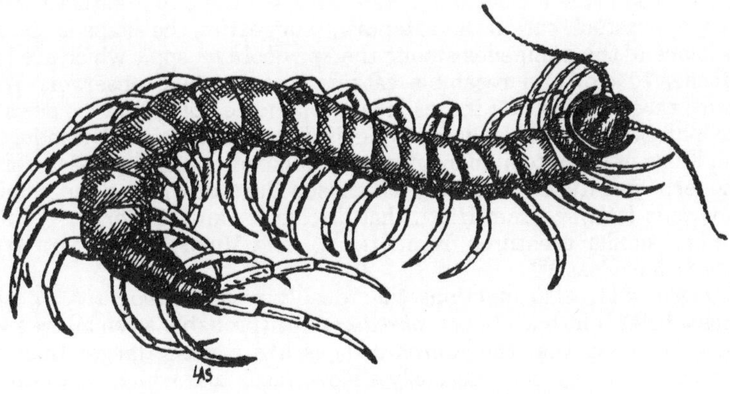

Scolopendra heros. **Arizona Scolopendromorph. after Strekalovsky 15 cm (6″).**
(drawing by Lysa Scarborough).

Nicander's symptomatology for scorpion envenomation shows rather precise observation by his source (Apollodorus): thirst, a "burning fever" in the mouth, swollen testicles, *typsis* (a beating of some kind), shivering convulsions, and death to children. Modern symptomatology does include some of these: first comes an extremely sharp pain at the site of the sting, shortly replaced by a prickling and spreading of that latter sensation, to be followed by a numbness; after a time (within two to three hours), the victim becomes agitated, cramps occur in the muscles of the abdomen, limbs, and pharynx; children have convulsions; in males, priapism is a common clinical manifestation; the blood pressure falls, usually causing the patient to faint; salivation is markedly increased, and there is heavy lacrimation and profuse sweating; pulse rates increases, commonly becoming arrhythmic, and the respiration becomes very irregular, sometimes being of the Cheyne-Stokes variety. When death occurs, it is always a result of respiratory paralysis.

Other Creatures: Insects, Myriapods, and "Miscellaneous"

Nicander now considers what he apparently thought were miscellaneous poisonous animals. *Bembix* next appears in *Theriaca*, 806, as does *melissa*. *Bembix* is one of the numerous types of bumblebees ("humblebees" in Europe), and *melissa* is the common honeybee. The scholiasts add nothing, except to note that *bembix* is black and like a wasp,[189] while Pliny (*Natural History*, XI, 75) writes that *bombyx* is a large "Assyrian" type of bee or wasp. Any venom would be that of an ordinary beesting, which is rarely fatal to patients highly allergic to the venom of bees and wasps.[190] Nicander has no symptoms, except "death" (*Theriaca*, 807).

* *Theriaca*, 811, contains the *ioulos*, which Gow and Scholfield identify as a "woodlouse,"[191] following the Liddell/Scott/Jones who say "a creature like a centipede, probably the woodlouse."[192] Other sources, however, prove both Gow and Scholfield, and Liddell/Scott/Jones incorrect. In Theophrastus,[193] *ioulos* means "catkin," or "tendril," but the key text that clearly identifies the *ioulos* is Galen, *Use of Parts*, III, 2.[194] We read that " ... the whole bodies ... of the *ioulos* and the centipede have been greatly lengthened ... ,"[195] showing that Galen has made a clear distinction between the two creatures. Together with Theophrastus' "catkin" and "tendril," suggesting the shape of the animal, *ioulos* is one of the millipedes among the *Spirobolidae* spp., which are long (up to 4 inches/10 cm) and resemble catkins to the casual observer. Woodlice (*Isopoda*) rarely exceed 1.1 inches in length, and do not match the descriptions in Theophrastus, Galen, and Aristotle[196] for the *ioulos*. If Nicander, or his source, knew of harm to humans from any millipede, it has not been verified in the modern literature. Cloudsley-Thompson does describe a large millipede (*Rhinocricus lethifer*) from Haiti, that discharges an acid spray,[197] and there seem to be similar creatures from Greece, Asia Minor, and Egypt. Woodlice are utterly harmless.[198]

Theriaca, 811, also mentions the "deadly wasp" (*oloos sphēx*), and 812 contains a brief reference to *pemphrēdōn oligē* (probably a "small tree wasp"). The scholiasts say that the *pemphrēdōn* is like a wasp, larger than an ant, smaller than a honey bee, variously striped black and white, and that it uses hollow oaks for nesting.[199] Nicander gives no symptoms, and one can assume only that these two creatures are wasps.

Theriaca, 812, has *amphikarēs skolopendra*, "the two-headed centipede ... which can bring death to a man from both ends" (812–813). Even the scholiasts dismiss this notion as absurd,[200] stating that this idea is refuted by Aristotle. Aristotle does discuss the centipede,[201] and one reference from the *Historia Animalium* explains why Nicander says "two-headed:" Aristotle writes that "long insects [*entoma*] with many feet can live a long time after they have been cut in two; the severed part can move either backwards or frontwards, as happens with the *skolopendra*, as it is named."[202] Nicander has mauled this clear account to make a "two-headed" *skolopendra*, and a preceding passage in *Historia Animalium*,[203] saying how *entoma* generally live after being cut in two, and how the cut part must retain the head to remain alive, may also be in Nicander's mind as he put down this line about the "two-headed *skolopendra*." One could reason, perhaps, that since Aristotle has just written that the head of the *entomon* must be retained for it to remain alive after it is cut in two, and since he also follows this passage with an account of the two halves of the cut *skolopendra* living and moving, it must follow that each half has to have a head.

Cloudsley-Thompson regards even the large centipedes as not particularly dangerous to man: "... centipedes are for the most part comparatively innocuous members of the community of animals. Even the large scolopendras do not bite unless molested and will always try to escape rather than fight."[204] Bucherl (quoted by Cloudsley-Thompson)[205] has established that the venom of several species of scolopendra are indeed venomous, and that "... human mortality cases after Scolopendra bites have been reported, but it seems that they may not stand up against exact analysis."[206] Turk has given a vivid case history of the results of a bite from a small centipede (85mm) in southern France (Cassis, near Marseilles, in 1949): the victim was bitten on the second finger of the right hand, and in about 15 minutes the finger was swollen greatly, the pain being like that from a sting of a large wasp; after 60 minutes, the right hand was swollen to twice its normal size, but was not painful to the touch; three days later, all effects had disappeared.[207] In his experiments (on white mice) with scolopendra venom, Bucherl has observed other symptoms: sweating, vomiting, respiratory failure, convulsions, and "... death, followed by immediate tetanus. Undoubtedly, this is a neurotoxic venom, actng chiefly on the bulbar centers."[208] Probably the uncertainty concerning centipede venom rests on the small amount of research that has been conducted on the subject.[209] Typical is the report in Cloudsley-Thompson about the large, green California *Scolopendra heros* (which can be 6 inches/15cm long), "... greatly feared not only on account of its poisonous bite but because it also produces a reddish streak where it has crawled upon the body."[210]

Several species are possible as Nicander's *skolopendra: Scolopendra morsitans* L., which can be 120mm in length, having varying coloration, from lemon yellow to reddish yellow, to olive or dark green; *S. subspinipes* Leach, to 230 mm, with brown head and first tergite, and dark green body; *S. valida* Lucas, to 160 mm, with olive green, olive brown, or chestnut brown coloration. These three are most likely to have been noticed in classical antiquity, because of their large size and geographical distribution (esp. *S. valida*). Two other species are remotely possible: *S. claviceps* C. L. Koch (80 mm) and *S. dalmatica* C. L. Koch (80 mm).[211] Viewing the gross aspects of the larger centipedes (*Scolopendromorpha*) may also help explain why Nicander (or his source) might believe that the animal had two heads, and that both could bite. A ventral view of the postcephalic segment reveals a very prominent pair of venom jaws, while the last pair of legs are modified into lengthened prehensile limbs, which can deliver a firm pinch.

Theriaca, 815–834, introduces six other creatures, almost at random: a "shrewmouse,"[212] the "seps" (which is a snake or lizard),[213] a salamander, two poisonous fish, and a "sea snake." The salamander and fish will be considered in a later article in this series; the "seps" is a probable duplication of *Theriaca*, 147 (although it is *sepa* in 817, which could mean "lizard"),[214] and the "sea snake" (*drakonta*: 828) is most likely a fish. No symptoms are contained in this incredibly confusing section of the *Theriaca*, except for some muddled allusions to problems from one of the fish.

Two beetles remain in Nicander's catalogue of dangerous insects. The blister beetle of *Alexipharmaca*, 115–127, and *Theriaca*, 752–758, has been considered previously.[215] The second creature is called *bouprēstis*, and Nicander considers it in a distinct section of the *Alexipharmaca* (335–346). Like some of the other substances in the *Alexipharmaca*, the *bouprēstis* is a "concoction" that is poisonous, made from an insect called *bouprēstis*. Nicander says it tastes like *litron* (*Alexipharmaca*, 337),[216] and smells awful. It causes pains at the "mouths of the stomach" that come and go (338–339), stops the urine, causes a throbbing in the lower bladder, and the belly feels inflated as when there is dropsy around the navel (341–342). In addition, the skin on the victim's limbs becomes taut. Nicander adds that the creature is aptly named, because cows will eat it and thence become bloated: thus "cow-inflater" (344–346).

The scholiasts also make comment on the combination of medical and agricultural lore in this passage,[217] and they note that Aristotle had already written about the harm that could come to farm animals from eating this insect. In *Historia Animalium*, 604b18, Aristotle tells us that there is little hope for a horse that has swallowed a *staphylinos*, which is about the size of a *sphondylē* ("knucklebone").[218] Curiously, *Historia Animalium*, 604b15–18, says that horses with *kardian algēsē* ("heart pain") display a tightness of the flanks, some kind of bladder problem, urine retention, and a tautness of the haunches, causing the horses to draw up their hooves; these symptoms of "heart pain" are almost identical with Nicander's symptoms from ingestion of *bouprēstis*, perhaps suggesting that the poet has taken his source and compressed *bouprēstis* with some previous drug or affliction.

Other sources help identify *bouprēstis*. In both the Hippocratic *corpus*[219] and Galen,[220] this creature is employed as a medicine for various ailments. Pliny writes that the *buprestis* is rare in Italy, and that it looks a scarab beetle with long legs.[221] He adds that when cattle eat the *buprestis* by mistake, they swell up and burst. Aelian follows the same source used by Pliny.[222] The later agricultural writers pick up the tradition, first recorded in Aristotle. Vegetius says that the *buprestis* looks like a spider, and when farm animals eat them in their hay, they swell up.[223] According to Vegetius, the first signs of *buprestis* in stock are small and frequent stools.[224] The *Mulomedicina Chironis* also states that the *buprestis* looks like a spider, and problems arise for animals when they eat it in their hay.[225] The *Geoponica* (like Vegetius) says that wine will help ease the problem of *bouprēstis* infestation in farm stock.[226] The key reference, however, comes in Galen, where "the *bouprēstis* is an animal that looks like the *kantharis*,"[227] which means that the *bouprēstis* is one of the blister beetles. Hesychius, by contrast, following Theophrastus, makes *bouprēstis* into a type of wild herb,[228] while Pliny (following Aristotle[229]) says that the drink of a woman's milk is effective against the poison of the *buprestis*.[230] Pliny thus reflects the medical/veterinary tradition, and Hesychius/ Theophrastus represent a separate botanical/veterinary tradition in classical sources.

The summary of descriptions in our authorities is of a creature that looks like a spider, cockroach, leech, a scarab beetle with long legs, and which lives on plants, probably a wild herb called *lachanon*. Its close association with *kantharis* in Galen and Hippocrates (and the specific directions to use the elytra in making *bouprēstis*-medicine) makes it fairly certain that the creature is one of the blister beetles, most likely the common *Meloe variegatus* Donov. The appearance of this beetle, with its short elytra and bronzed-black body could, indeed, be something like a cockroach or leech. From the descriptions, the beetle could not be the very common *Cantharis vesicatoria* L., which is an attractive metallic green, with full-length elytra. Although Leitner will not commit himself on the identity of *buprestis* in Pliny,[231] it appears that Gossen's guess of M. variegatus,[232] using Tauschenberg,[233] is quite correct. *M. variegatus* is not as rich in cantharidin as *C. vesicatoria*,[234] but all species of Meloidae have an abundance of cantharidin in their elytra. Thus *bouprēstis* is something like a "weak" cantharid concoction, rightly described by Galen as a "uterine contractor."[235]

Summary of Creatures

In *Theriaca*, 715–836, and *Alexipharmaca*, 115–127, 335–346, the following animals can be identified with fair assurance: *rhōx* (Black Widow spider), *asterion* (a variation of the Black Widow), *kyaneon* (a solifuge), *agrōstēs* (a wolf spider), *sphēkion* (a jumping spider), *myrmēkeion* (the velvet ant, a wasp), *katharis* (a blister beetle), *leukos* (the harmless young of scorpions), *zophoeis* (a harmless scorpion), *empelios* (a poisonous scorpion), *melichlōron* (a poisonous scorpion), two kinds of large harmless scorpions, two variations ("red, and "green") of poisonous scorpions, *bembix* (bumblebee), *melissa* (honeybee),[236] *sphēx* (a wasp), *pemphredōn oligē* (a small wasp), *bouprēstis* (a blister beetle), *ioulos* (a large millipede), and *skolopendra* (a large centipede). Of the twenty-two creatures in Nicander's listing, which can be keyed, seven are dangerous to man in their natural state (the Black Widows, four of the scorpions, and perhaps the centipede), two are poisonous when made into drugs (the two blister beetles), two are utterly harmless (the *leukos* and the millipede), and the remainder (including the "winged scorpion," if it is a moth/ wasp) inflict bites and stings generally annoying but usually far from fatal.

(See footnotes, beginning on page 22)

References

Abbreviations employed:

HA: Aristotle, *Historia Animalium*
HP: Theophrastus, *Historia Plantarum*
LSJ: Henry George Liddell, Robert Scott, and Henry Stuart Jones, *Greek-English Lexicon*, 9th ed. with supplement (Oxford: Clarendon Press, 1968)
RE: Paulys Realencyclopädie der classischen Altertumswissenschaft

1. John Scarborough, "Nicander's Toxicology, I: Snakes," PHARMACY IN HISTORY, 19 (1977), 3-23. H. Gossen u. E. Steier, "Schlange," *RE*, II A I (Stuttgart, 1921), cols. 494-508 (esp. 500-504). W. Morel, "Iologica," *Philologus*, 83 (1928), 345-389. Sometimes, later writers, who borrowed Nicander's snake-names, became confused by similarities in place-names: Morel, 356-357 [Aelian]. Plant-names occasionally displayed the same manner of local associations in classical antiquity: Françoise Skoda, "Associations d'idées et métaphores dans quelques dénominations de plantes en Grec ancien," *Annales de la Faculté des Lettres et Sciences humaines de Nice*, No. 21 (1974), 131-139.
2. Apollodorus lived sometime in the third century B.C. Scarborough, "Nicander's Snakes," PHARMACY IN HISTORY, 19 (1977), 3-4, with nn. 8-20. M. Wellmann, "Apollodoros," *RE*, I, part 2 (Stuttgart, 1894), Nr. 69, col. 2895.
3. J. Théodoridès, "Remarques sur l'iconographie zoologique dans certains manuscrits médicaux byzantins et études des miniatures zoologiques du Codex Vaticanus Graecus 284," *Jahrbuch der Österreichischen Byzantinischen Gesellschaft*, 10 (1961), 21-29, with plates Nos. 1-4.
4. Zoltán Kádár, "Anfänge der zoologischen Buchillustration," *Das Altertum*, 19 (1973), 88-95 [93-95, with plate No. 5]. The scribe/artist seems unsure how many legs should be on a scorpion: three kinds have six pairs of legs, while four have seven pairs. Scorpions have five pairs, including the "claws." A "portrait" of Nicander appears in the famous Vienna Codex of Dioscorides, fol. 3^v (reproduced in full color in Kurt Weitzmann, *Late Antique and Early Christian Book Illumination* [New York: George Braziller, 1977], p. 62 [plate 16]). Nicander is one of seven famous pharmacologists and physicians pictured, and his account of snakes and snake bites forms part of this beautiful codex (*vid.* esp. fol. 441^r, with its six snakes and a lizard). *Vid.* also n. 362 below. Kádár has recently published *Survival of Greek Zoological Illuminations in Byzantine Manuscripts* (Budapest: Akadémiai Kiadó, 1978). The Vienna Codex has recently been published in facsimile, with an accompanying volume of listings and commentary: Hans Gerstinger, *Dioscurides: Codex Vindobonensis med. gr. 1 der Österreichischen Nationalbibliothek* (Graz: Akademische Druck-u. Verlagsanstalt, 1970). Fols. 393-437 contain part of the curious *Paraphrase of Nicander's Theriaca* by Eutecnius, and fols. 438-459 are the *Paraphrase of the Alexipharmaca* by Eutecnius; both have numerous illustrations of snakes, spiders, scorpions, a few insects, and the mysterious *ioulos* [nn. 191-196 below] and what presumably is a centipede. (fol. 422^r). The scribe/illustrator has reversed the *ioulos* and the centipede; the "centipede" is flat and cylindrical, while the *ioulos* is flat and not cylindrical, with a pair of pincers at its posterior. In fol. 416^r appears the equally puzzling *kyaneon* [nn. 94-110 below], painted light grey and mottled black, and which has the correct number of appendages for a solifuge. Among the scorpions (6 varieties, fols. 419^v-421^v), only one (fol. 421^v) has the correct number of limbs (four pairs of legs + two claws).
5. Crateuas was physician to Mithridates VI of Pontus (120-63 B. C.), and like his king, was known as an eminent herbalist. Pliny, *Natural History*, XXV, 8, tells us that Crateuas prepared an illustrated herbal (pinxere namque effigies herbarum atque ita subscripsere effectus. verum et pictura fallax est coloribus tam numerosis ...), and those paintings may be the direct ancestors of the plants pictured in the Vienna Dioscorides. M. Wellmann, *Krateuas* (Berlin: Weidmann, 1897 [*Abhandlungen der königlichen Gesellschaft der Wissenschaften zu Göttingen*, philologisch-historische Klasse, N. F. Bd. 2, Nr. 1]), 3-6. Charles Singer, "The Herbal in Antiquity and its Transmission to Later Ages," *Journal of Hellenic Studies*, 47 (1927), 1-52 [5-18]. Quite often, Byzantine scribes made compilations of the pharmacology found in Crateuas, Dioscorides, and Galen. M. Wellmann, "Zu Galens Schrift *περὶ κράσεως καὶ δυνάμεως τῶν ἁπλῶω φαρμάκων Hermes*, 38 (1903), 292-304. Not only did Pliny take great interest in the works of Crateuas and his royal patron, but many Roman sources record numerous substances and remedies for poisons, derived from the court of Pontus. Georg Harig, "Die antike Auffassung vom Gift und der Tod des Mithridates," *Schriftenreihe für Geschichte der Naturwissenschaften. Technik und Medizin* [= *NTM*], 14 (1977), 104-112. W. Morel, "Gifte," *RE*, Supplementband V (Stuttgart, 1931), cols. 223-228.
6. Philumenus *fl. c.* A. D. 180, and is the author of an extant *On Poisonous Animals and Cures*, which seems to have been part of a larger encyclopedic work on medicine. The standard text is M. Wellmann, ed., *Philumeni De venenatis animalibus eorumque remediis* (Leipzig: Teubner, 1908 [*Corpus Medicorum Graecorum*, X 1, 1]). There are numerous parallel passages in the text of Philumenus that markedly resemble sections in the Pseudo-Dioscorides *On Poisons* and *Booklet on* [*Poisonous*] *Animals* (*vid.* n. 7 below). Hans Diller, "Philumenos," Nr. 7, *RE*, XX, part 1 (Stuttgart, 1941), cols. 209-211. Texts (with German translation) of a Latin rendition of several treatises by

Philumenus—orinally in Greek—are in T. Puschmann, herausg. u. ubers., *Nachträge zu Alexander Trallianus: Fragmente aus Philumenus und Philagrius* (Berlin, 1887; rptd. Amsterdam: Hakkert, 1963), 16–73. These short excerpts are rich in pharmacology, applied to ailments suggested by the titles: *De reumate ventris, De dysenteria reumatica, De coeliacis*, and *De tenesmo*.

7. Renaissance scholars accepted the two works *On Poisons* and *Booklet on [Poisonous] Animals* as part of the genuine Dioscoridean *corpus*, but since about 1800, most scholars have accepted the unsupported judgment of J. A. Fabricius (ed. Harles), *Bibliotheca Graeca* (Hamburg, 1794), IV, 679–680, who rejected both works as spurious. C. Sprengel included the two treaties in his edition of Dioscorides (in C. G. Kühn, ed., *Medicorum Graecorum Opera*, Vols. XXV and XXVI; *On Poisons* and *Booklet on [Poisonous] Animals* in Vol. XXVI [Leipzig: C. Cnobloch, 1830], with the Latin titles *De Venenis eorumque praecautione et medicatione* [pp. 1–41], and *De iis, quae virus eiaculantur, animalibus libellus, in quo et de rabioso cane* [pp. 42–91].), but M. Wellmann omitted them from his edition of Dioscorides (*Pedanii Dioscuridis Anazarbei De materia medica* [3 vols., 1906–1914; rptd. Berlin: Weidmann, 1958]), although he did include the *On Simple Drugs* [Vol. III, pp. 151–317], believed to be spurious by many scholars. Sprengel's text of *On Poisons* and *On [Poisonous] Animals* remains the most recent, and depends upon the MSS listed by Hermann Diels, *Die Handschriften der antiken Ärzte* (Leipzig: Zentralantiquariat der Deutschen Demokratischen Republik, 1970; rpt. of essays that appeared in the *Abhandlungen der Preussischen Akademie der Wissenschaften*, philosophisch-historische Klasse, 1905–1907), pt. II, pp. 31–32. The text of Philumenus seems to expand upon materials in Pseudo-Dioscorides (*e.g.* Philumenus, 32 [Wellmann, pp. 35–36] compared with Pseudo-Dioscorides, *[Poisonous] Animals*, 5 [Sprengel, p. 67], "On Centipedes"), but the major sources for Philumenus' details about spiders, scorpions, insects, and myriapods appear to be Apollodorus and Sostratus (n. 2 above: Apollodorus; n. 127 below: Sostratus), although Apollodorus is "filtered" through Nicander. Pseudo-Dioscorides *Poisonous Animals* may represent an independent tradition in Greek and Roman lore on these creatures, and the numerous parallels to the tract in Philumenus suggests a compaction in *On Poisonous Animals and Cures* of Apollodorus, Nicander, Sostratus, and Pseudo-Dioscorides. *Vid.* John Riddle, "Dioscorides," *Dictionary of Scientific Biography*, Vol. IV (New York: Scribners, 1971), 119–123, and M. Wellmann, "Dioskurides," Nr. 12, *RE*, V, part 1 (Stuttgart, 1903), cols. 1131–1142.
8. Venice, Biblioteca Communale Bertoliana, MS 7. 3. 34 (509, formerly 6. 9. 11). Alpinus was born in Marostica (near Venice) in November, 1553, and died in Padua in January, 1617.
9. *E.g.* E. Wallis Budge, ed. and trans., *Syrian Anatomy Pathology and Therapeutics or "The Book of Medicines,"* 2 vols. (London: Oxford Univ. Press, 1913), Vol. II (trans.), 24–25, 523–524, 543–545, 548, 577, 617, and 688 (mostly scorpions). Much of the "data" may go back to Assyrian times. Egyptian papyri provide other glimpses of real-life reaction. Marcus N. Tod, "The Scorpion in Graeco-Roman Egypt," *Journal of Egyptian Archaeology*, 25 (1939), 55–61. Ancient magical lore often mentions scorpions, either as charms, or in terms of spells and incantations to ward off being stung, or to inflict such stings on an enemy. *E.g.* K. Preisendanz, *Papyri Graecae magicae: Die griechischen Zauberpapyri*, Zw. verb. Aufl. (Stuttgart: Teubner, 1974), Vol. II, p. 8, lines 194–197 [VII, 194–197]. *Cf.* Campbell Bonner, *Studies in Magical Amulets chiefly Graeco-Roman* (Ann Arbor: Univ. Michigan Press, 1950 [Humanistic Series, Vol. 49]), 77–78, and S. Eitrem, "Der Skorpion in Mythologie und Religionsgeschichte," *Symbolae Osloensis*, 7 (1928), 53–82 [esp. 68–70].
10. *E.g.* the stories in Agatharcides, Strabo, and Aelian. *Vid.* n. 95 below.
11. John Henry Comstock, *The Spider Book*, rev. and ed. by W. J. Gertsch (Ithaca, New York: Cornell Univ. Press [Comstock Publishing Associates], 1940), 348. J. L. Cloudsley-Thompson, *Spiders, Scorpions, Centipedes, and Mites*, 2nd ed. (Oxford: Pergamon Press, 1968), 209–214.
12. Lynn Thorndike, "Disputed Dates, Civilization and Climate, and Traces of Magic in the Scientific Treatises ascribed to Theophrastus," in C. Singer and H. Sigerist, eds., *Essays on the History of Medicine Presented to Karl Sudhoff . . . on his Seventieth Birthday* (Oxford and Zürich: Oxford Univ. Press and Verlag Seldwyla, 1924), 73–86 [79–85]. *Cf.* Juliette de Baïracli Levy, *Herbal Handbook for Farm and Stable*, 2nd ed. (London: Faber, 1973), 17: " . . . especially to farmers who consider herbal veterinary treatment out-of-date and worthless: their own beasts will convince them that there is a great deal in natural medicine."
13. Nicander, *Theriaca*, 1-7, and 108–114, as two examples among many. Theophrastus, *HP*, IX, 8. 5–8. John Scarborough, "Theophrastus on Herbs and Herbal Remedies," *Journal of the History of Biology*, 11 (1978) [in press]. *Vid.* nn. 223-226 below [*Geoponica* and other agricultural manuals].
14. Raymond W. Thorp and Weldon D. Woodson, *The Black Widow Spider* (New York: Dover, 1976; rpt. of 1945 ed.), 3–20.
15. W. S. Bristowe, "Spider Superstitions and Folklore," *Transactions of the Connecticut Academy of Arts and Sciences*, 36 (1945), 53–90 [58].
16. Pausanias, *Description of Greece*, IX, 6. 5–6 (Bristowe does not give specific references). Pliny, *Natural History*, XI, 79–85, is a good representative short summary of Greek and Roman spider lore and superstitions. Not surprisingly, fact and fancy are meshed together: Democritus is cited along with an unnamed authority (Aristotle, *HA*, 623a30) to illustrate the conflicting theories explaining how spiders make their webs [XI, 80]; the spider web is an architectural marvel [XI, 81–82]; spiders capture young frogs and lizards [XI, 84], as well as *sunt ex eo* [the spider] *et auguria*, which include higher webs forecast the rising of rivers, and a large number of webs forecasts rain; and "father

spiders" aid in the incubation of the young, which always devour the mother and then sometimes the father after they have hatched [XI, 85].

16a. Bristowe, "Spider Superstitions," *Connecticut Academy*, 36 (1945), 63–66 [weather forecasting], 60 [wisdom and cunning], 58–60 [foretelling the future], and 68 (constipation, jaundice, whooping cough, smallpox, plague, and leprosy; homeopathic medicine). *Cf.* Charles J. Hempel, *New Homeopathic Pharmacopoeia and Posology* (New York: William Radde, 1850), 83. *Vid.* also W. S. Bristowe," Facts and Fallacies about Spiders," *Proceedings, South London Entomological and Natural History Society*, 5 (1928–1929), 12–13. Line one is well worth quotation: "I am used to be looked upon as an oddity by my friends for collecting spiders, though why an interest in spiders should be regarded as something rather degrading when no similar stigma attaches to Lepidopterists I cannot see."

17. Theodore Savory, *Arachnida*, 2nd ed. (London/New York: Academic Press, 1977), 3–14. Cloudsley-Thompson, *Spiders ... Mites*, vii–xv.

18. William Morton Wheeler, *Ants* (New York: Columbia Univ. Press, 1910), remains a standard reference.

19. The great majority of articles in entomology journals are concerned with taxonomy. To take coleoptera as an example, *vid. The Coleopterists Bulletin*, Vol. 30 (1976) which contains 70 articles in 368 pages, and 39 consider taxonomy. Edward T. Schenk and John H. McMasters, *Procedure in Taxonomy*, 3rd ed. (Stanford: Stanford Univ. Press, 1959), gives the basic methodology, but far more readable is George Gaylord Simpson, *Principles of Animal Taxonomy* (New York: Columbia Univ. Press, 1969).

20. Two standard monographs will illustrate: R. E. Snodgrass, *Anatomy of the Honey Bee* (Ithaca, New York: Cornell Univ. Press [Comstock Publishing Associates], 1956), and Karl von Frisch, *The Dance language and Orientation of Bees*, trans. by Leigh E. Chadwick (Cambridge, Mass.: Harvard Univ. Press, 1967). *Vid.* also Florence Naile, *America's Master of Bee Culture: The Life of L. L. Langstroth* (Ithaca, New York: Cornell Univ. Press, 1942; rptd. 1976).

21. Comstock, *Spider Book*, remains a standard text. Rudolf Kobert, *Beiträge zur Kenntniss der Giftspinnen* (Stuttgart: Ferdinand Enke, 1901).

22. George Marx, "On the Effect of the Poison of *Latrodectus mactans* Walck. Upon Warm-Blooded Animals," *Proceedings of the Entomology Society, Washington* 2 (1891), 85–86, is a sturdy example of work in the late nineteenth century. *Vid.* Kobert, *Giftspinnen*, 37–70, and 100–129, for European investigation prior to 1900. *Vid.* nn. 26, 62–67, and 70–73 below. R. W. Thorpe and W. D. Woodson, *Black Widow* (Chapel Hill: Univ. North Carolina Press, 1945), provided the best summary before the 1950's. [rptd. as *Black Widow Spider*, 1976; vid. n. 14 above].

23. W. L. Distant, "Are the Solipugidae Poisonous?" *Nature* (London), 46, no. 1185 (July 14, 1892), 247 [a short paragraph on how the Cape Wagtail attacked the solpuga]. R. I. Pocock, "The Nature and Habits of Pliny's Solpuga," *Nature* (London), 57, no. 1487 (April 28, 1898), 618–620. Short summaries are in Keith R. Snow, *The Arachnids* (New York: Columbia Univ. Press, 1970), 62–63, and Savory, *Arachnida*, 233–244.

24. Cloudsley-Thompson, *Spiders ... Mites*, 107–123.

25. Two older, somewhat outdated medical entomology texts, set the standards for their modern successors: E. Martini, *Lehrbuch der medizinischen Entomologie* (Jena: Gustav Fisher, 1925), and William B. Herms, *Medical Entomology*, 3rd ed. (New York: Macmillan, 1939). *Vid.* also H. M. Parrish, "Deaths from Bites and Stings of Venomous Animals and Insects," *A. M. A. Archives of Internal Medicine*, 104 (1959), 198–207.

26. Scarborough, Nicander's Snakes," PHARMACY IN HISTORY, 19 (1977), 5–6, with n. 52. E. C. Faust and P. F. Russell, *Craig and Fausts Clinical Parasitology*, 7th ed. (Philadelphia: Lea & Febiger, 1968), 713–944, with bibliographies to 1967. George Cheever Shattuck, *Diseases of the Tropics* (New York: Appleton-Century-Crofts, 1951), 741–783 [essential bibliography on the Black Widow to 1950, pp. 782–783].

27. J. L. Cloudsley-Thompson, *Insects and History* (London: Weidenfeld and Nicolson, 1976), 1–75. Günter Morge, "Entomology in the Western World in Antiquity and in Medieval Times," in Ray F. Smith, Thomas E. Mittler, and Carroll N. Smith, eds., *History of Entomology* (Palo Alto: Annual Reviews, 1973), 37–80. F.S. Bodenheimer, *Materialen zur Geschichte der Entomologie bis Linné*, 2 vols. (Berlin: W. Junk, 1928–1929); nicely summarized by F. A. Dixey in *Nature*, 123 (June 22, 1929), 935–937, and *Nature*, 125 (March 29, 1930), 483–485. L. O. Howard, *A History of Applied Entomology* (Washington, D. C.: Smithsonian Institution, 1930 [Smithsonian Miscellaneous Collections, Vol. 84]), 207–212: "Early European Economic Entomology."

28. B. Jaeger, *The Life of North American Insects* (New York: Harper, 1859), passim. The standard survey of American (and some European) entomology from the beginnings to 1930 is H. O. Essig. *A History of Entomology* (1931; rptd. New York: Hafner, 1965). *Vid.* also Howard, *History of Applied Entomology*, passim, and Herbert Osborn, *Fragments of Entomological History* (Columbus, Ohio: Pub. by author, 1937).

29. Wilhelm Capelle, "Zur Entomologie des Aristoteles und Theophrast," *Rheinisches Museum für Philologie*, n.f. 105 (1962), 56–66. *Vid.* Aristotle, *HA*, 487a32–35, and 523b13, alongside 531b20–532a4.

30. *HA*, 501a31; 532a16; 555a23–26; 557a27; 557b10; 602a28; 607a15–20 and 29.

31. *HA*, 622b27: τῶν δ' αραχνίων καὶ τῶν φαλαγγίων ἔστι μὲν πολλὰ γένη (text becomes confused). *HA*,

552b22–24: the ichneumon-wasp kills *φαλάγγια*, which cannot be anything other than the wolf spiders, excluding Black Widows, scorpions, etc.

32. *E.g.* the famous account (very correct in some ways, very incorrect in others) of bees: *HA*, 551a29; 553a17–554b21, which parallels the equally famous account in *Generation of Animals*, 759a8–760b33. G. E. R. Lloyd, *Aristotle* (Cambridge: Cambridge Univ. Press, 1968), remarks that "... although his discussion of this problem [the generation of the three types of bees] is in many ways an unfortunate one, he ... lays down an extremely important methodological principle ... theories must wait on evidence, and he reversed Plato's view that abstract argument is more trustworthy than observation" (pp. 78–79).

    Four distinct beetles appear: rose chafers (*HA*, 523b19 and 25), the dung beetle (*HA*, 490a15 and 17; 552a17; 601a4), the blister beetle (*HA*, 531b24; 542a9), the stag beetle (*HA*, 531b24; 532a27). There are wasps, hornets, ants, flies, moths, butterflies, etc.
33. *HA*, 489b22; 523b18; 532a5; 621a9.
34. *HA*, 523b18; *cf. Theriaca*, 811: *ἴουλος*. *Vid.* nn. 192–196 below.
35. Various worms, *e. g.* the "glow-worm" (*HA*, 523b20).
36. Werner Jaeger, *Diokles von Karystos*, Zw. Aufl. (Berlin: de Gruyter, 1963), esp. 186–236. Scarborough, "Nicander's Snakes," PHARMACY IN HISTORY, 19 (1977), 3, with n. 9. M. Wellmann, "Das älteste Kräuterbuch der Griechen," in *Festgabe für Franz Susemihl* (Leipzig: Teubner, 1898), 1–31 [esp. 23–25].

36a. M. Wellmann, *Die Fragmente der sikelischen Ärzte Akron, Philistion, und des Diokles von Karystos* (Berlin: Weidmann, 1901), Frgs. 135 (quoted in Athenaeus, *Deipnospohistae*, VII, 320d) and 145 (quoted in Pseudo-Dioscorides, *[Poisonous] Animals*, Prooemium [ed. Sprengel, p. 48]), from Diocles' *Healthy States, to Pleistarchus* (Wellmann, pp. 172 and 187).

37. Wellmann, "Kräuterbuch," *Festgabe Susemihl*, 23. This was the *περὶ λαχάνων* (*On Wild Herbs*), cited by Galen (ed. C. G. Kühn [Leipzig, 1821–1833; 20 vols. in 22; rptd. Hildesheim: George Olms, 1964–1965]), XVIII, part 1, 712 (= *Commentary IV on Hippocrates' On Joints*, 30. Galen, XIX, 89 (*Galen's Exegesis of Hippocratic Words*, Beta), curiously cites *On Wild Herbs* (to explain *βούπρηστις*, a type of blister beetle [*vid.* nn. 219–234 below]), but under the name of Dioscorides. Wellmann, *Die Fragmente ... des Diokles*, 192–195 (14 fragments from Diocles' *Wild Herbs*). What little is known of the Aristotelian *Medical Practice* is contained in eight fragments and testimonia in Plutarch, Pliny, Diogenes Laertius, Michael Psellus, and Caelius Aurelianus. A. Heitz, ed., *Fragmenta Aristotelis* (Paris: Didot, 1886), pp. 216–218.
38. Wellmann, "Kräuterbuch," *Festgabe Susemihl*, 28. M. Wellmann, "Apollodoros," *RE*, I, part 2 (Stuttgart, 1894), Nr. 69, col. 2895. Franz Susemihl, *Geschichte der griechischen Litteratur in der Alexandrinerzeit* (Leipzig: Teubner, 1891–1892; 2 vols.), I, 784–785. Scarborough, "Nicander's Snakes," PHARMACY IN HISTORY, 19 (1977), 3 with n. 8.
39. Scarborough, "Nicander's Snakes," PHARMACY IN HISTORY, 19, (1977), 3–4, with nn. 9–19.
40. Philumenus, 15.3 (ed. Wellmann, p. 19): Nicander, *Theriaca*, 749, is the cited authority for one of the spiders, and is quoted verbatim.
41. Pseudo-Dioscorides, *[Poisonous] Animals*, 19 (ed. Sprengel, p. 77): "Some Commonly-Held Treatments for [the Injuries] from Poisonous Animals." *Cf.* Galen, XIX, 194 (*Proper Diet in Acute Diseases from Hippocrates*, 2). Otto Schneider, *Nicandrea* (Leipzig: Teubner, 1856), 182.
42. Direct quotations from Apollodorus occur in Pliny, *Natural History*, XX, 86; XXI, 116; XXII, 19, 31, and 59; and XXIV, 167. Apollodorus' *Poisonous Animals* (on scorpions) is quoted in XI, 87–88, and his tract *Advice to King Ptolemy on What Wines to Drink* appears in XIV, 76. A section of a work by Apollodorus on medical plants (some kind of gladiolus [*cypiros*]) is in XXI, 116.

42a. Galen, XIV, 181 (*Antidotes*, II, 13: one of the "Various Remedies against Phalangia"), and XIV, 184 (*Antidotes*, II, 14: a "Remedy against Snakebite, Invented by Apolodorus and Praised by Sostratus").

43. Theophrastus, *HP*, IX, passim. Wellmann, *Die Fragmente ... des Diokles*, 117–207. Jaeger, *Diokles*, 186–223.
44. Aelian: text ed. and trans. by A. F. Scholfield, *Aelian: On the Characteristics of Animals*, 3 vols. (Cambridge, Mass.: Harvard Univ. Press, 1958–1959 [Loeb]). Aelian's *Varia Historia* has been recently re-edited by M. R. Dilts (Leipzig: Teubner, 1974). W. Schmid u. Otto Stählin, *Wilhelm von Christs Geschichte der griechischen Litteratur*, Sechs. Aufl. (Munich: Beck, 1912–1924; 2 vols. in 3 parts), II, part 2, 789, with n. 5 [Nicander, Apollodorus, and Sostratus as sources for Aelian, and listing of a series of articles on the subject by M. Wellmann in *Hermes*].

    Orbasius: text. ed. by J. Raeder, *Oribasii Collectionum medicarum reliquiae* (Leipzig: Teubner, 1928–1933; rptd. Amsterdam: Hakkert, 1964; 4 vols. [*Corpus Medicorum Graecorum*, VI 1, 1–VI 2, 2]). Raeder also edited Oribasius' *Synopsis ad Eustathium* and *Libri ad Eunapium* (Leipzig: Teubner, 1926; rptd. Amsterdam: Hakkert, 1964 [*Corpus Medicorum Graecorum*, VI3]). Oribasius was chief physician and close friend of the emperor Julian (A. D. 361–363). *Vid.* H. O. Schröder, "Oreibasios," *RE*, supplementband VII (Stuttgart, 1940), cols. 797–812.

    Aetius of Amida: text of *Libri medicinales*, I–VIII, ed. A. Olivieri (Leipzig: Teubner, 1935 [*Corpus Medicorum Graecorum*, VIII, 1], and Berlin: Academiae Litterarum, 1950 [*Corpus Medicorum Graecorum*, VIII 2]) in two volumes. Books IX–XVI are in preparation for the *CMG*, ed. V. De Falco and F. Sbordone. Book XIII has been edited by S. Zervos, *Aetios aus Amida: Unveröf-*

fentliche Werke altgriechischer Ärzte, 2 (Athens, 1908). *Tetrabibloi* awaits editing. *Vid.* W. A. Greenhill, "Aetius," in W. Smith, ed., *Dictionary of Greek and Roman Biography and Mythology* (London: John Murray, 1870; 3 vols.), I, 53-54; Heinrich Haeser, *Lehrbuch der Geschichte der Medicin*, Drit. Bearb., Vol. I (Jena: Hermann Dufft, 1875; rptd. Hildesheim: Olms, 1971), 457-458; A. Corlieu, *Les médecins grecs depuis la mort de Galien jusqu'a la chute de l'Empire d'Orient* (Paris: J. B. Baillière, 1885), 118-122; and Schmid/Stählin, *Christs Geschichte*, II, part 2, 1098, with n. 4.

Alexander of Tralles: text. ed. Theodor Puschmann, *Alexander von Tralles* (Vienna, 1878-1879; rptd. Amsterdam: Hakkert, 1963; 2 vols.). *Letter on Helminths* is in J. L. Ideler, ed., *Physici et Medici Graeci* (Berlin, 1841-1842; 2 vols.; rptd. as 1 vol., Amsterdam: Hakkert, 1963), I, 305-311 = Pushmann, ed., II, 586-593. Haeser, *Lehrbuch*, I, 458-459; Corlieu, *Les médecins grecs*, 130-137; Owsei Temkin, "Byzantine Medicine: Tradition and Empiricism," *Dumbarton Oaks Papers*, 16 (1962), 97-115 [100, with nn. 24 and 25] = Owsei Temkin, *The Double Face of Janus and Other Essays in the History of Medicine* (Baltimore: Johns Hopkins Press, 1977), 202-222 [206, with nn. 24 and 25]; Schmid/Stählin, *Christs Geschichte*, II, part 2, 1098-1099, with nn. 5, 10-14.

Paul of Aegina: text ed. I. L. Heiberg as *Epitomae medicae* (Leipzig: Teubner, 1921-1924 [*Corpus Medicorum Graecorum*, IX 1 and 2]; 2 vols). Still useful is the rich commentary and translation by Francis Adams, *The Seven Books of Paulus Aegineta* (London: Sydenham Society, 1844-1847; 3 vols.). Schmid/Stählin, *Christs Geschichte*, II, part 2, 1099, with nn. 4-5; Corlieu, *Les médecins grecs*, 140-146.

Nonnus Theophanes: text ed. J. S. Bernard (Gotha, 1794-1795; 2 vols.). Schmid/Stählin, *Christs Geschichte*, II, part 2, 1099, with n. 7. H. Schoene, "Zwei Listen chirurgischer Instrumente," *Hermes*, 38 (1903), 280-284 [by Nonnus Theophanes]. Corlieu, *Les médecins grecs*, 151-152.

Manuel Philes: Karl Krumbacher, *Geschichte der byzantinischen Litteratur*, Zw. Aufl. (Munich, 1897; rptd. New York: Burt Franklin, 1958; 2 vols.), 775. Schmidt/Stählin, *Christs Geschichte*, II, part 2, 788. K. Vogel, "Byzantine Science: Zoology," in J. M. Hussey, ed., *Cambridge Medieval History*, Vol. IV: *The Byzantine Empire*, part 2: *Government, Church and Civilization* (Cambridge: University Press, 1967), 284-286 [285].

45. Scarborough, "Nicander's Snakes," PHARMACY IN HISTORY, 19 (1977), 4-5, with nn. 28-38.
46. Wellmann, "Kräuterbuch," *Festgabe Susemihl*, 27-31.
47. Celsus, V, 27. 9.
48. Aristotle, *HA*, 662b27
49. Philumenus, 15 (ed. Wellmann, pp. 18-21).
50. Philumenus, 35 (ed. Wellmann, p. 38).
51. *Scholia on Theriaca*, 715a (ed. Annunciata Crugnola, *Scholia in Nicandri Theriaka* [Milan: Cisalpino, 1971], p. 262), followed by Eutecnius, *Paraphrase*, 715 (ed. Isbella Gualandri, *Eutecnii Paraphrasis in Nicandri Theriaca* [Milan: Cisalpino, 1969], p. 59).
52. Hesychius, *Lexicon* ed. minor (ed. M. Schmidt [Jena: Duftius, 1867]), col. 1329. *Suda, s.v.* *φάλαγγες καὶ ὁ ἀράχνης δὲ, ὅν ἔνιοι καλοῦσι φαλάγγιον.* also *s. v.* *φάλαγξ* and *φαλάγγια* which show the confusion: *φάλαγξ: ἀράχνιον τι* ("some [kind of] spiderweb"); *φαλάγγια:ζῶόν τι τῶν δακέτων ἐστὶ τὸ φαλάγγων* (ed. Ada Adler, *Suidae Lexicon*, Pars IV: *Pi-Psi* [Stuttgart: Teubner, 1971; rpt. of 1935 ed.], pp. 695-696).
53. Aristotle, *HA*, 550a28.
54. Dioscorides, IV, 51 (ed. M. Wellmann, *Dioscurides De Materia medica* [Berlin: Weidmann, 1958; 3 vols.; rpt. of 1907-1914 ed.], Vol. II, p. 207).
55. Nicander, *Theriaca*, 716: *ὁ μὲν αἰθαλόεις ῥώξ.* Pliny, *Natural History*, XIV, 74, makes *αἰθαλόεις* into a grape grown in Egypt.
56. Pollux, *Onomasticon*, II, 146 (ed. Eric Bethe, *Pollucis Onomasticon*, Fasc. Prior: Lib. I-V [Stuttgart: Teubner, 1967; rpt. of 1900 ed.], p. 128, esp. line 8).
57. Soranus, *Gynecology*, I, 3. 2, and IV, 8. 1 (ed. J. Ilberg, *Sorani Gynaeciorum libri* [Leipzig: Teubner, 1927; *Corpus Medicorum Graecorum* IV], pp. 4 and 138).
58. Rufus, *Names for the Parts of the Body*, 85-86: *τὰ δὲ ἔσωθεν πέρατα τῶν δακτύλων, ῥᾶγες, καὶ κορυφαί* (ed. Ch. Daremberg and Ch. Émile Ruelle, *Oeuvres de Rufus d'Éphèse* [Paris: 1879: rptd. Amsterdam: Hakkert, 1963], p. 144).
59. Nicander, *Theriaca*, 717: *ἐπάσσοτεροις ποσὶν ἕρπων.* My translation gives the sense only.
60. A. S. F. Gow, "Nicandrea," *Classical Quarterly*, 45 (1951), 95-118 [108: *s.v.* *σκέλλω*]. *Cf. Theriaca*, 766, 785, and 789; *Alexipharmaca*, 491.
61. I observed a female *Latrodectus mactans* (Fabricius) in Fresno, California, July, 1972. Her globulous abdomen was *c.* ¾ inches (20 mm) in diameter.
62. Savory, *Arachnida*, 103-112. Cloudsley-Thompson, *Spiders ... Mites*, 186-187. H. W. Levi, "The Number of Species of Black Widow Spiders (Theridiidae: Latrodectus)," *Science*, 127 (1958), 1055.
63. Wolfgang Bücherl, "Spiders," in Wolfgang Bücherl and Eleanor E. Buckley, eds., *Venomous Animals and their Venoms*, Vol. III: *Venomous Invertebrates* (London/New York: Academic Press, 1971), 197-277 [217-220].
64. *Ibid.*, 219, with synonyms in nomenclature.
65. *Ibid.*, 220.
66. *Vid.* n. 22 above. The other US species is normally called the Brown Recluse (*Loxosceles* spp.), and an equally venomous species (*L. laëta* Nicolet = *L. rufipes* Bücherl) occurs in South America. Unlike the

large bibliography available on the *Latrodectus*, the literature on the *Loxosceles* is widely scattered and sparse. Study of the *Loxosceles* spp. is in its beginnings, and " ... the classification of the loxoscelids continues in a confused state ... about 50 different species have been described ... [from most species] described by different authors we know only one male, one female, or one young." Bücherl, "Spiders," in *Venomous Invertebrates*, 216. *Vid.* H. Schenone, L. Semprevivo, and E. Schirmer, "Consideraciones a propósito de dos casos de loxoscelismo cutáneo-viseral," *Boletin Chileno de Parasitologia*, 14 (1959), and A. Vukuric, "Loxoscelismo cutáneo-visceral mortal," *Ibid.*, 17 (1961), 25-27. *Loxosceles* spp. occur in the Middle East, and since its medical symptomatology is so distinct from the *Latrodectus* spp., one may presume that the Greek toxicologists may have had similar distinct observations, perhaps meshed with snakebite symptoms in our present texts. P. Efrati, "Bites by *Loxosceles* Spiders in Israel," *Toxicon*, 6 (1969), 239. In *Loxosceles* poisoning, local necrosis is prominent, as distinguished from the neurotoxic action of *Latrodectus* envenomation. F. E. Russell, W. G. Waldron, and W. B. Madon, "Bites by the Brown Spiders *Loxosceles unicolor* and *Loxosceles arizonica* in Californa and Arizona," *Toxicon*, 7 (1969), 109, have observed similar contrasts in two North American species. H. Alistair Reid, "Clinical Aspects of Animal Toxins," in A. de Vries and E. Kochva, eds., *Toxins of Animal and Plant Origin*, Vol. III (London: Gordon & Breach, 1972), 957-983 [963], remarks that Russell *et. al.* " ... postulate an auto-pharmacological response to the venom as a mechanism in causing necrosis, rather than a direct cytolytic effect of the venom." In the gross aspects, the whole clinical picture resembles envenomation from bites of *Viperidae*. Scarborough, "Nicander's Snakes," PHARMACY IN HISTORY, 19 (1977), 7-9, with nn. 76, and 99-102. *Cf.* H. T. Kirby Smith, "Specific Treatment of Black Widow Spider Bite," *Southern Medical Journal*, 38 (1945), 696-698, and Y. Constant and P. Gouere, "Sur les phénoménes d' aranéisme provoqué par *Latrodectus menavody*," *Bulletin d. Société Pathologie exotique*, 41 (1948), 234-237. *Vid.* Reid, "Clinical Aspects of Animals Toxins," in *Toxins of Animal and Plant Origin*, Vol. III, 980-983, for listing up to 1972.

67. Kobert, *Giftspinnen*, Chs. IV. "Historisch-Litterarisches über Lathrodectes aus den letzten zwei Jahrhunderten," and VIII, "Eigene Berichte über Lathrodectsbisse bei Menschen." There is also evidence of interest in what was generally called the "tarantula," especially the "Italian tarantula." Kobert, 28-36. One finds scattered reports in the nineteenth century on the "tarantula" in North America. *E.g.* B. Dowler, "Remarks on the Natural History of the Tarantulidae and Other Arachnidans, and on the Alleged Poisonous Effects of their Bites," *New Orleans Medical and Surgical Journal*, 16 (1859), 786-796. A. Fatal [*sic!*], "Spider Bite," *Medical News, Philadelphia*, 43 (1883), 307. J. B. Crandall, "Tarantula Bite with Recovery," *Leavenworth Medical Herald*, 1 (1867-1868), 389-391. R. Menger, "Essay on Injurious Insects, Parasites, and Reptiles of Texas," *Texas Courier-Record of Medicine* [Fort Worth], 2 (1884-1885), 262-270.
68. W. R. Horsfall, *Medical Entomology* (New York: Ronald Press, 1962), 24-31.
69. *E.g.* David S. Smith and Findlay E. Russell, "Structure of the Venom Gland of the Black Widow Spider *Lactrodectus mactans*. A Preliminary Light and Electron Microscopic Study," in Findlay E. Russell and Paul R. Saunders, eds., *Animal Toxins* (Oxford: Pergamon Press, 1967), 1-15, and J. W. Abalos and E. C. Baéz, "The Spider Genus Latrodectus in Santiago del Estera, Argentina," *Ibid.*, 59-74, each with lengthy bibliographies. *Vid.* nn. 22, 26, and 66 above, and nn. 70, and 72-73 below.
70. Zvonimir Maretić, "Latrodectism in Mediterranean Countries, Including South Russia, Israel and North Africa," in Bücherl and Buckley, eds., *Venomous Invertebrates*, 299-310 [300].
71. *Ibid.*, 301. *Vid.* also the two "classic" essays in this field: V. L. Kellogg, "Spider Poison," *Journal of Parasitology*, 1 (1915), no. 3, 107-112, and W. J. Baerg, "The Effects of the Bite of *Latrodectus mactans* Fabr.," *Journal of Parasitology*, 9 (1923), no. 3, 161-169.
72. John D. McCrone and Robert J. Hatala, "Isolation and Characterization of a Lethal Component from the Venom of *Latrodectus mactans mactans*," in Russell/Saunders, eds., *Animal Toxins*, 29-34 [esp. 33]: "The venom of *L. mactans mactans* can be separated into 7 protein and 3 non-protein fractions by means of vertical acrylamide gel electrophoresis. The only fraction that is lethal to mammals is protein fraction B. This fraction ... is 20 times as lethal as the whole venom and is very labile."
73. N. Frontali and A. Grasso, "Separation of Three Toxicologically Different Protein Components from the Venom of the Spider *Latrodectus tredecimguttatus*," *Archives of Biochemical Biophysics*, 106 (1964), 213.
74. Gow/Scholfield, *Nicander*, 77.
75. Eutecnius, *Paraphrase*, 725-733 (ed. Gualandri, p. 59, lines 20-25).
76. Gow/Scholfield, *Nicander*, 184 n. 725, quoting from T. Thorell, *Synonyms of European Spiders* (no date or place given), 508.
77. *Vid.* nn. 63-64 above.
78. *Theriaca*, 729-733.
79. Gow/Scholfield, *Nicander*, 77.
80. *Cf.* Aristotle, *HA*, 622b12, and Paul of Aegina, V, 6.
81. Pliny, *Natural History*, XXIX, 86.
82. *Ibid.*: lanugine nigra.
83. *Ibid.*: caliginem concitans et vomitos araneosos.
84. *νύξ δὲ περὶ κροτάφοις.*
85. Eutecnius, *Paraphrase*, 725-733 (ed. Gualandri, p. 59, line 30): *καὶ ὡς νύκτα ὁρᾶν.*

86. *Scholia on Theriaca*, 729 (ed. Crugnola, p. 266).
87. Eutecnius, *Paraphrase*, 725–733 (ed. Gualandri, p. 59, lines 26–29).
88. Scarborough, "Nicander's Snakes," PHARMACY IN HISTORY, 19 (1977), 4, with n. 19. A.S. Hollis, "Aemilius Macer, *Alexipharmaca?*" *Classical Review*, 87 n.s. 23 (1973), 11: "Most scholars have seen [in Ovid, *Tristia*, IV, 10. 43–44] a reference to three works by Macer, (a) *Ornithogonia* (no doubt inspired by the Greek poem of Boeus or Boeo), (b) *Theriaca* (following Nicander), and (c) *de Herbis*, a poem on salutory medicines." W. Morel, "Iologica," *Philologus*, 83 (1928), 345–389: "Die für die folgenden Untersuchungen wichtigsten Schriften sind die Theriaka des Lehrdichters Nikander von Kolophon, ihre uns nicht erhaltene lateinische Übertragung von Aemilius Macer und die Schrift von eines Arztes Philumenos ... "[345]. Morel believes that Macer's *Theriaca* is the source for Lucan's snake-lore of Libya, and that Lucan had borrowed this data from Livy, who had, in turn, taken it from Macer [346]. Macer was a friend of Vergil and Ovid, and died in 16 B.C. M. Wellmann, "Aemilius Macer aus Verona," *RE*, I, part 1 (Stuttgart, 1892), Nr., 86, col. 567.
89. Pliny, *Natural History*, I, list of authorities (*ex auctoribus*) for Book XXIX, under medical writers (*medicis*). There may be other conflations involving the works of Xenocrates, Democrates, and Chrysippus, as well as Nicander (who appears under *medici*).
90. Pliny, *Natural History*, I, list of authorities for Book VIII: again Nicander and Apollodorus are included.
91. E. Steier, "Spinnentiere," *RE*, IIIA, 2 (Stuttgart, 1929), cols. 1786–1812 [cols. 1786–1787], esp. 1786: "Die Ableitung von *ἀράχνη* bezw. *aranea* und *φαλαγγίον* ist unsicher." But Steier presumes, in sum, the traditional view, citing no evidence.
92. *τῶν δ' ἀραχνίων καὶ τῶν φαλαγγίων ἔστι μὲν πολλὰ γένη, τῶν μὲν δηκιτῶν φαλαγγίων δύο, τὸ μὲν ἕτερον ὅμοιον τοῖς καλουμένοις λύκος, μικρὸν καὶ ποικίλον καί ὀξὺ καὶ πηδητικόν. κτλ.*
93. *Vid.* n. 52 above.
94. Kobert, *Giftspinnen*, 12–13.
95. Agatharcides, *De mari Erythraeo*, 44 [59]: C. Müller, ed., *Geographi Graeci minores*, Vol. I (Paris: Didot, 1882), pp. 150–151: *ὑπὸ πλήθους ἀπίστου σκορπίων καὶ φαλαγγίων, ἅς τετραγνάθους ὀνομάζουσιν ἔνιοι* Truesdell S. Brown, *The Greek Historians* (Lexington, Mass.: Heath, 1973), 183, with nn. 68–70: "[Agatharcides] was born about 202 B. C." [183]. *Erythraean Sea* was originally in five books.
96. *ὑπὸ πλήθους σκορπίων καὶ φαλαγγίων τῶν τετραγνάθων καλουμένων.*
97. M. Cary and E. H. Warmington, *The Ancient Explorers* (Baltimore: Penguin Books, 1963), 94–107.
98. Solinus, *Polyhistor* (ed. T. Mommsen, 2nd ed. [Berlin: Weidmann, 1895]), IV, 3: quod diem fugit.
99. Lucan, *Civil war*, IX, 837:Quis calcare tuas metuat, salpuga latebras?
100. Festus, *De verborum significatu*, 431 (ed. W. M. Lindsay [Leipzig: Teubner, 1913], p. 389).
101. Hesychius, *Lexicon* (ed. K. Latte [Copenhagen: Munksgaard, 1966], Vol. II), 4346–4348 (ed. Latte, Vol. II, p. 539): a) *κυάνεος · μέλας, σκοτεινός* b) ⟨*κυάνεος*⟩ *ἐλέλικτο δράκων · μέλας ἐν τῷ ἀναφορεῖν *κυανέων ·* Μαύρων L Αἰθιόπων **κύανον · εἶδος χρώματος οὐρανοειδές.*
102. Pollux, *Onomasticon*, VII, 129 (ed. Bethe, Vol. II [Leipzig: Teubner, 1931], p. 87).
103. *Suda*, *s.v.* *κυάνεοι* (A. Adler, ed., *Suidae Lexicon*, Vol. III [Leipzig: Teubner, 1933], p. 203): *κυαναυγῆ [= μελαναυγής] πετάσματα.*
104. Cloudsley-Thompson, *Spiders ... Mites*, 107.
105. *Ibid.*, 108.
106. Savory, *Arachinida*, 240.
107. W. L. Distant, "Are the Solpugidae Poisonous?" *Nature* [London], 46, no. 1185 (July 14, 1892), 247, followed by all subsequent authors. R. I. Pocock, "The Nature and Habits of Pliny's Solpuga," *Nature* [London], 57, no. 1487 (April 28, 1898), 618–620 [619]: Mr. Carter of Madras allowed "... the solpuga, in the presence of natives, to bite his arm until the blood ran, without suffering anything worse than a passing pain from the wound ... [the natives] did not alter their judgement one whit ... of the deadly nature of the Jerrymanglum," even though the solpuge was proved to be harmless.
108. Cloudsley-Thompson, *Spiders ... Mites*, 112.
109. *Ibid.*, 108–109.
110. Pocock, "Pliny's Solpuga," *Nature*, 57, (1898), 618.
111. E. Steier, "Spinnentiere," *RE*, IIIA, part 2 (Stuttgart, 1929), cols. 1786–1812 [1800–1801].
112. Gow/Scholfield, *Nicander*, 184 n. 729. Philumenus, 35. 1, also displays this "common source," but Wellmann (p. 38) identifies it as Xenocrates, who thus becomes the source for both Pliny and Galen through Juba. *Scholia on Theriaca*, 715a, lists Juba and Apollodorus as the other writers on spiders.
113. Gow/Scholfield, *Nicander*, 77.
114. Nicander, *Theriaca*, 734.
115. Nicander, *Theriaca*, 737.
116. Bücherl, "Spiders," *Venomous Invertebrates*, 198.
117. *Ibid.*, 267.
118. *Ibid.*, 273.
119. Nicander, *Theriaca*, 738–739.
120. Pliny, *Natural History*, XXIX, 86–87: Etianum deterior a crabrone pinna tantum differens. Hic et ad maciem perducit.
121. U. Cats Bussemaker, ed., *Scholia et Eutecnii Paraphrasis in Nicandrum* and *Scholia et Parap-*

hrasis in Oppianum (Paris: Didot, 1849; in vol. titled *Scholia in Theocriti Idyllia*, ed. F. Dübner), 661.

122. Cloudsley-Thompson, *Spiders ... Mites*, 212.
123. *Ibid.*, with W. S. Bristowe, *The Comity of Spiders*, 2 (London, 1941).
124. Gow/Scholfield, *Nicander*, 184–185.
125. Gow/Scholfield, *Nicander*, 79, translate "antlet," which would not fit the larger size of the *Mutillidae*. *Vid.* nn. 129–131 below.
126. Nicander, *Theriaca*, 747–751.
127. *Scholia on Theriaca*, 747 (Crugnola, p. 270). Sostratus (*fl.* *c.* 50 B. C.[?] in Alexandria) made a paraphrase of Nicander, knew and improved on the observations of Apollodorus, and wrote outstanding treaties on toxicology. His works are lost with the exceptions of quotations in Celsus, Pliny, Galen (who knows Apollodorus through Sostratus), Aelian, Athenaeus, and several other extant authors. M. Wellmann, "Sostratus, ein Beitrag zur Quellenanalyse des Aelian," *Hermes*, 26 (1891), 321–350, collects the know fragments. Scarborough, "Nicander's Snakes," PHARMACY IN HISTORY, 19 (1977), 4 with nn. 14 and 18. Heracleoticon seems otherwise unknown.
128. Philumenus, 15. 1–3 (Wellmann, p. 19).
129. A. D. Imms, *A General Textbook of Entomology*, 9th ed., rev. O. W. Richards and R. G. Davies (London: Methuen, 1970), 719–720.
130. I collected several dozen specimens of *Dasymutilla occidentalis* L. in eastern Kansas in July and August, 1959. The females are rather aggressive and inflict a sting like that of a mud dauber wasp. *D. occidentalis* favors the larvae of *Phyllophaga* (June beetles) in eastern Kansas, and will paralyze them before dragging them into a burrow; eggs are then laid on the hapless grub.
131. Other US species are parasitic on bees and fly larvae, as well as *Phyllophaga*. The standard monograph remains C. E. Mickel, *Biological and Taxonomic Investigations on the Mutillid Wasps;* Vol. 143 (1928) of the *Bulletin of the US Natural History Museum* (Washington, D.C.).
132. E. Habermann, "Chemistry, Pharmacology, and Toxicology of Bee, Wasp, and Hornet Venoms," in Bücherl, ed., *Venomous Invertebrates*, 61–93. "In European countries, fatal accidents caused by hymenopteran venoms are more frequent than such accidents following other animal poisoning. They cannot be ascribed to true toxicity of bee, wasp, or hornet venoms, but must be catalogued among anaphylactic reactions" [87]. "Wasp venom contains histamine and serotonin" [62]. Table I, p. 62, also lists "wasp kinin," Phospholipase A. Phospholipase B, and Hyaluronidase, as other components of wasp venom.
133. *Ibid.*, 85.
134. Gow/Scholfield, *Nicander*, 185 n. 752 ff., citing J. H. Fabre, *Life of the Spider* (1912).
135. *Theriaca*, 755: κανθαρίδεσσι.
136. John Scarborough, "Some Beetles in Pliny's *Natural History*," *Coleopterists Bulletin* [Smithsonian Institution], 31 (1977), 293–296. Three other species in *Lyttinae* are also possible: *Lytta dives* Brullé (*cf.* Pliny, XXIX, 76, 93 and 94), *Lytta segetum* Fabr. (*cf.* Pliny, XXVII, 78), and *Lytta nuticollis* Muls. (*cf.* Pliny, XXIX, 94). All species produce cantharidin, but less than *Cantharis vesicatoria*.
137. Gow/Scholfield, *Nicander*, 185 n. 755.
138. *Theriaca*, 757–758. *Cf.* C. F. Lehmann, J. L. Pipkin, and A. C. Ressmann, "Blister Beetle Dermatosis," *AMA Archives of Dermatology*, 71 (1955), 36–38
139. Pliny, *Natural History*, XVIII, 7–78.
140. Galen, XIX, 731: ἀντὶ κανθαρίδων, φαλάγγια (in the tract entitled περὶ ἀντεμβαλλομένων ["Substitutions" or "Synonyms"]).
141. Nicander, *Alexipharmaca*, 115: σιτηβόρου. *Scholia on Alexipharmaca*, 115b (ed. Marius Geymonat, *Scholia in Nicandri Alexipharmaca* [Milan: Cisalpino, 1974]), p. 67: κανθαρὶς ζωύφιον μέλαν καθάπαξ τοῖς φυτοῖς λυμαινόμενον; but the scholiasts apparently have confused the blister beetle with the common dung beetle (115a): ... εἰσὶ τὰ κοπρόφορα καί σιτοφθόρα Also 115c shows that σιτηβόρου means "grain-eating" (σιτηβόρου] σιτοφάγου).
142. *Cf.* Dioscorides, II, 61. "Xiphisternum" would describe the point of the thorax as one reads of it in *Alexipharmaca*, 122–123: περὶψανσυσι δ'ἀνῖαι/ θώρηκος τόθι χόνδρος ὑπὲρ κύτος ἕζετο γαστρός. *Vid.* also Gow, "Nicandrea," *Classical Quarterly*, 45 (1951), 107, *s.v.* πλαδάω.
143. Scarborough, "Pliny's Beetles," *Coleopterists Bulletin*, 31 (1977), 295.
144. Imms, *Entomology*, 182, and 806–807, also reporting on accessory glands observed by H. Beauregard, *Les insectes vésicants* (Paris, 1890).
145. R. G. Todd, *Extra Pharmacopoeia Martindale*, 25th ed. (London: Pharmaceutical Press, 1967), 277, quotes three cases of death from extremely minute amounts of cantharidin ingestion, esp. *Pharm. Journal*, 2 (1953), 467: "An angler mixed cantharidin in ground-bait, cut his thumb in the process, sucked the cut thumb, and soon after complained of stomach trouble. Two days later he died from cantharidin poisoning." The two other cases involve 1 grain of cantharidin.
146. Gow/Scholfield, *Nicander*, 185–186 n. 759, and 186 n. 801. *Cf. Theriaca*, 801. Otto Keller, *Die antike Tierwelt* (Leipzig, 1909–1913; rptd. Hildesheim: Olms, 1963; 2 vols.), II, 479, reproduces an ancient gem (otherwise unattributed) with this winged scorpion (Keller's reference says "Im Londoner Gemmenkabinett habe ich mir (a. 1880) zweigeflügelte Skorpionenotiert," with a notation to his own *Tier-und Pflanzenbilder auf Münzen und Gemmen das klassischen Altertums* [co-authored with Imhoff-Blumer; Leipzig: Teubner, 1889], XXIV, 9).

147. *E.g.* Strabo, XV, 703 (quoting Megasthenes' account of India); Pausanias, *Description of Greece*, IX, 21. 6 (the creature was brought to Ionia by a Phrygian); Aelian, *On Animals*, XVI, 42. Other sources for the "winged scorpion" listed by Crugnola, ed., *Scholia on Theriaca*, 285, and Steier, "Spinnentiere," *RE*, IIIA, part 2, col. 1806.

148. Gow/Scholfield, *Nicander*, 79.

149. Hugo Pesce and Alvaro Delgado, "Poisoning from Adult Moths and Caterpillars," in Bücherl/Buckley, eds., *Venomous Invertebrates*, 119–156 [120].

150. *Ibid.*, 121 and 125, quoting M. Phisalix in *Animaux venimeux et venins* (Paris: Masson, 1922), Vol. I, 343–356.

151. Imms, *Entomology*, 546–547.

152. Pesce/Delgado, "Poisoning from Moths," *Venomous Invertebrates*, 125.

153. *Ibid.*, 129–131.

154. Scarborough, "Theophrastus on Herbals," *Journal of the History of Biology*, 11 (1978), n. 177.

155. *Scholia on Theriaca*, 760a and b (Crugnola, pp. 273–274).

156. *Scholia on Theriaca*, 763a (Crugnola, p. 275). The *κρανοκολάπτης* as a name, suggests how the Greeks took a description and expanded upon its presumed effects. Hesychius, *s.v. κράνα* (ed. Latte, Vol. II, p. 524) says that this is a synonymn for *κεφαλή* ("head"), and *s.v. κράνος* (ed. Latte, Vol. II, p. 524) is *περικεφαλαία* ("head-covering," *i.e.* "helmet"); but *s.v. περικεφαλαία* (Hesychius, ed. minor Schmidt, col. 1224): *ἡ ἐκ τριχῶν γεγουνῖα περιθετή. καὶ μέρος τι τῆς νεώσ. ἡ κάσ(σ)ις* where the description means a "wig." *περικεφαλαία* means simply "covering of the head [in nature]" in Antyllus (quoted by Oribasius [ed. J. Raeder, *Oribasii Collectionum medicarum reliquiae*, Vol. I (Leipzig: Teubner, 1928), VI, 36. 3 [Raeder, I, p. 187]), while in Soranus it is the specific name of a bandage that "goes around the head" (Soranus, ed. Ilberg, *On Bandages*, 24 [Ilberg, p. 163], with plate VI 24); in botany, *περὶ κεφαλαία* meant some sort of disease in oak trees (Theophrastus, *HP*, III, 13. 4). Of course, *κρανίον* means "upper part of the skull" (Aristotle, *HA*, 491a31, and Galen, II, 739 = *On Bones for Beginners*, 1), but *κρανία* is "spear" or "branch [of a tree]" in Galen, XII, 41 (= *Blendings and Dynameis of Simple Drugs*, VII, 47) and Dioscorides, I, 119 (*cf. κρανέα* of *Geoponica* [ed. H. Beckh; Leipzig: Teubner, 1895], X, 87. 4 [ed. Beckh, p. 322]). Numerous other meanings in other authors (Arrian, Homer, etc.: LSJ, 989, *s.v. κρανεία* etc.) include a special cherry and wood from that particular cherry tree.

The 'other half' of the term, —*λάπτης*, also has a variety of nuances. Hesychius, *s.v. κολάπτει · κλώθει πρὸς τῷ γόνατι, ἢ γλύφει* (ed. Latte, Vol. II, p. 500), a curious composite which can be rendered "it pecks [like a bird]: it spins on the knee, or it chisels [or carves]" or "it pecks [like a bird]: it spins in the crotch, or it chisels." "In the crotch" may be more correct, taking *Scholia on Theriaca*, 541a (Crugnola, p. 210) as a guide: *ὑπὸ ἔχεως πληγέντα τινὰ κατὰ βουβῶνα, τουτέστι τὸ γονάτιον Vid.* n. 163 below for *βουβῶνα · ὁ κολαπτήρ* ("chisel") is the basic noun, and *κολάπτω* is the basic verb which means "peck" like a hen (or any bird) as in Aristotle, *HA*, 609a35 and b6.

Why Nicander chose the common "moth" may be explained through a fragment of Sostratus (Frg. No. 2 Wellmann: "Sostratus," *Hermes*, 26 [1891], 346) contained in *Scholia on Theriaca*, 760b (Crugnola, p. 274): *καὶ γὰρ ἡ φάλαινα ζῷον, ἥτις νῦν ψώρα* ("moth"). *φάλαινα λέγεται ἡ παρ᾽ ἡμῖν λεγομένη ψυχή · ἔστι δὲ αὕτη ζωύφιον ᾗφασιν ἐμφερῆ τὸν κρανοκολάπτην. Cf.* Plutarch, *Moralia*, 636C (= *Table Talk*, 2. 2), derived from Aristotle, *HA*, 551a15–25 (*ψύχη* = moth or butterfly, which emerges from a caterpillar made dry, which then produces another creature, the *ψύχη*). Nicander's source (Apollodorus?) presumably also employed by Sostratus, would, in turn again reflect the Peripatetic notions of chrysalis-making, and the scholiasts would record the apparently odd "fact" that the *ψυχή* might carry within itself the life-giving properties for the *κρανοκολάπτης*. In sum, Nicander's *φάλαινα* is something that "spins" (like a spider; hence its position in the *Theriaca* between spiders and scorpions), "pecks" like a bird (presumably readers then would recall the myth of Prometheus, whose liver was "pecked" by an eagle), and perhaps looked like a "wooden chisel." That the creature "attacked the head" is self-evident from the name given to it, because one could presume multiple meanings from *κρανο-*, as the various references above might suggest. The simplest translation, however, of *κρανοκολάπτης* would be "creature with a head that pecks," but given Nicander's usual habit of poetic allusions (almost always very strained) the simple *φάλαινα* = *κρανοκολάπτης* probably contains *at least* all of the allusions adduced above. One is left with a "poisonous moth" that attacks like a large wasp.

157. *περὶ τῶν βλητῶν καὶ δακέτων (On Striking and Biting Animals)*. *βλητόν* here probably mirrors the manner in which snakes will sometimes strike. *Vid.* n. 127 above. *Scholia on Theriaca*, 763a and 764a (Crugnola, pp. 275–276) = Wellmann, "Sostratus," *Hermes*, 26 (1891), Frgs. Nos. 2 and 3 (pp. 346–347).

158. *Mimusops Schimperi*. Gow/Scholfield, Nicander, 192 n. 99, with sources.

159. n. 146 above.

160. Gow, "Nicandrea," *Classical Quarterly*, 45 (1951), 108, *s.v. στεγνός Vid.* also n. 170 below.

161. Nicander, *Alexipharmaca*, 501, has *νύξ* as an equivalent for *ζοφόεις Cf. Alexipharmaca*, 474, and Aretaeus (ed. C. Hude [Berlin: Academiae Scientiarum, 1958; 2nd ed.; *Corpus Medicorum Graecorum* II]), II, 9. 4; IV, 13. 3; and VII, 3. 7 (ed. Hude, pp. 50, 85, and 150), where *ζοφοειδής* or *ζοφώδης* means "color of an elephant."

162. Gow/Scholfield, *Nicander*, 81, translate *ἐμπέλιος* as "livid," but *Scholia on Theriaca*, 782a (Crug-

nola, p. 280): ἤτοι πελιδνός, ὁ ὠχρὸς λεγόμενος. ὠχρός is the "color of yellow bile" in Galen, XV, 554 (*Commentary II on Hippocrates' Diet for Acute Diseases*, 22) and the "color of egg yolks" in Aristotle, *HA*, 560a21.

163. Gow/Scholfield, *Nicander*, 81, translate, "it deals a stroke incurable upon the groin," but βουβῶσι (*Theriaca*, 784) probably is "testicles," given the βουβώνων of *Scholia on Theriaca*, 782a (Crugnola, p. 280). The scorpion would thus attack/cause swollen testicles, perhaps a veiled — or not so veiled — pun, like those seen in Aristophanes. *Vid.* Jefferey Henderson, *the Maculate Muse: Obscene Language in Attic Comedy* (New Haven: Yale Univ. Press, 1975), 125 (sect. 75, with nn. 96 and 97).
164. *Scholia on Theriaca*, 797a (Crugnola, p. 284): μελιτόχρουν and τὸ δὲ σπόνδυλος θηλυκῶς νῦν. A "womanly" σπόνδυλος is the circular whorl which would balance and twirl a spindle, as in Theophrastus, *HP*, III, 16. 4; Soranus, II, 41. 2 (ed. Ilberg, p. 84); and Pollux, *Onomasticon*, VII, 31 (ed. Bethe, Vol. II, p. 60).
165. Nicander, *Theriaca*, 799: ὁ τε ῥαιβὰ φέρει φλογὶ εἴκελα γυῖα. One would presume "legs" for γυῖα but Theocritus, XXII, 81, uses γυῖα to mean "hands."
166. *Vid.* nn. 146 and 156 above. With this added description, we have a creature with red legs, a biting head, and a green body (if Philumenus, 15. 5, is accepted), four wings, a sting underneath its neck, and shaped something like a sculptor's chisel.
167. Aristotle, *HA*, 607a13–20.
168. E. Steier, "Spinnentiere (Skorpione)," *RE*, IIIA, part 2 (Stuttgart, 1929), col. 1804: "Der einzige Autor, der verschiedene Arten des Skorpions unterscheidet, ist Nikander, dessen Quelle Apollodor war."
169. Pliny, *Natural History, XI*, 87: Apollodorus auctor est in novem genera descriptis per colores maxime, opere supervacuo, quoniam non est scire quos minime exitiales praedixerit.
170. Pliny, *Natural History*, XI, 88: Apollodorus idem plane quibisdam inesse pinnas tradit. It may be, however, that Pliny "solves" the mystery of the winged scorpion by his comment (heard or borrowed?): hoc malum Africae volucre etiam austri faciunt pandentibus bracchia ut remigia sublevantes. The image is striking: scorpions given the power of flight by the South Wind, which supports the creatures when they spread out their legs as if they were oars. Perhaps both Pliny and Nicander may reflect a source (Apollodorus?) which had observed the desert winds "blowing" scorpions along, perhaps — to the onlooker — looking like a "bat" with 'membranous' wings. *Vid.* n. 160 above.
171. nn. 146–160 above.
172. Lucien Balozet, "Scorpionism in the Old World," in Bücherl/Buckley, eds., *Venomous Invertebrates*, 349–371 [351–352]. *Vid.* also A.J. Alexander and D. W. Ewer, "Temperature Adaptive Behavior in the Scorpion, *Opisthophthalmus latimanus* Koch," *Journal of Experimental Biology*, 35 (1958), 349–359 [a south African scorpion that shows marked variations in habit, according to the temperature]. Cloudsley-Thompson, *Spiders ... Mites*, 88: "Most species have a very limited range."
173. William H. Wilson, "On the Venom of Scorpions," *Egyptian Government School of Medicine* [Cairo] *Records*, 2 (1904), 11–44, with plates I–III [11].
173a. *Ibid.* The US *Hadrurus hirsutus* [Arizona] is also usually green.
174. Philumenus, 15. 5.
175. Balozet, "Scorpionism," *Venemous Invertebrates*, 351, notes that *Buthus occitanus* occurs very commonly on the northern coasts of the Mediterranean (Spain, France, Italy, Greece, the Balkans, and the Greek Islands) and " ... are not really dangerous." Pliny., *Natural History*, XI, 88–89, says that Italian scorpions are harmless, while the nasty kind cannot live north of Sicily.
176. Balozet, "Scorpionism," *Venomous Invertebrates*, 351–352.
177. *Ibid.*, 352. An example of *Pandinus* in my collection measures 6½ inches in length.
178. n. 170 above.
179. Wilson, "Venom of Scorpions," *Egyptian School of Medicine Records*, 2 (1904), 22.
180. Balozet, "Scorpionism," *Venomous Invertebrates*, 354–355.
181. C. I. Niu and H. Frankel-Conrat, "Determination of C-Terminal Amino Acids and Peptides by Hydrazinolysis," *Journal of the American Chemical Society*, 77 (1955), 5882–5885.
182. H. Rochat, C. Rochat, C. Kupeyan, S. Lissitzky, F. Miranda, and P. Edman, "Structure of Scorpion Neurotoxins," in de Vries/Kochva, ed., *Toxins of Animal and Plant Origin*, Vol. II, 525–528.
183. Wilson, "Venom of Scorpions," *Egyptian School of Medicine Records*, 2 (1904), 36–38. The varanus lizard also proved immune. C. Todd in *Journal of Hygiene*, 9 (1909), 69–85, cited in Balozet, "Scorpionism," *Venomous Invertebrates*, 359, observed variations even among different breeds of dogs. Other authorities listed by Balozet (p. 359) have shown that cats, porcupines, hedgehogs, chickens, turkeys, toads and frogs "lack sensitivity" or are "almost completely resistant."
184. Balozet, "Scorpinism," *Venomous Invertebrates*, 354–360. E. Zlotkin, G. Fraenkel, F. Miranda, and S. Lissitzky, "The Effect of Scorpion Venom on Blowfly Larvae — A New Method for the Evaluation of Scorpion Venom Potency," *Toxicon*, 9 (1971), 1–8. I. Israeli-Zindel, E. Zlotkin, and A. Shulov, "The Resistance of Insects to the Venom of the Yellow Scorpion *Leiurus quinquestriatus*," in de Vries/Kochva, eds., *Toxins of Animal and Plant Origin*, Vol. III (1973), 933–939.
185. n. 73 above.
186. Balozet, "Scorpionism," *Venomous Invertebrates*, 360–361.
187. *Ibid.*, 362; compiled from data kept by the Service de Santé des Territoires du Sud (Algeria) from 1942 to 1958.

188. Scarborough, Nicander's Snakes," PHARMACY IN HISTORY, 19 (1977), 17–18.
189. *Scholia on Theriaca*, 805–812 (Crugnola, p. 286, lines 9–11).
190. E. Habermann, "Chemistry, Pharmacology, and Toxicology of Bee, Wasp, and Hornet Venoms," in Bücherl/Buckley, eds., *Venomous Invertebrates*, 61–93 [85–86]: "If man were in the same range of susceptibility as is the mouse and we assume 0.1 mg of dry substance per sting, then some thousands of bees would have to sting man (intravenously!) to reach a lethal dose." Modern medicine has seen a fascinating attempt to reverse assumptions concerning bee stings. Bodog F. Beck, *Bee Venom Therapy* (New York: Appleton-Century, 1935). Beck hoped that bee venom might provide a panacea for arthritis; unfortunately, empirical experience over a number of years has disproved this panacea, like all others.
191. Gow/Scholfield, *Nicander*, 83.
192. LSJ, 833.
193. Theophrastus, *HP*, III, 5. 5 and 7. 3 ("catkin"); III, 18. 11 ("tendril").
194. G. Helmreich, ed., *Galenus De usu partium* (Leipzig: Teubner, 1907–1909 [2 vols.]; rptd. Amsterdam: Hakkert, 1968), Vol. I, p. 129 (*Use of Parts*, III, 2).
195. *Ibid.*, lines 22–25.
196. Aristotle, *HA*, 523b18, and *Parts of Animals*, 682b3. The ἰουλος also figures in Aratus, *Phaenomena*, 957, where large numbers of ἴουλοι, climbing walls, are forecast of coming rain. The scholiasts, commenting on the *Phaenomena*, 957 (ed. J. Martin, *Scholia in Aratum vetera* [Stuttgart: Teubner, 1974], pp. 463–464), says that οἱ ἴουλοι are many-footed σκώληκες ("worms"), that live underground and do not appear during winter; and shortly (p. 464 Martin) the scholiasts note that some ἴουλοι are like σκολοπένδραι but others are like worms with countless feet (ἄλλοι δὲ τὸν σκώληκα τὸν μυρίοις ποσὶ). The scholiasts derive their millipedes-on-the-wall from Theophrastus, *Weather Signs*, 19.
197. Cloudsley-Thompson, *Spiders ... Mites*, 36. Recent research has confirmed that millipedes do produce a number of potent substances as natural defensive agents against their enemies, especially ants. Hydrogen cynanide: Hans E. Eisner, William F. Wood, and Thomas Eisner, "Hydrogen Cyandide Production in North American and African Polydesmoid Millipeds," *Psyche*, 82 (1975), 20–23, and C. Guldensteeden-Egeling, "Über Bildung von Cyanwasserstoffsäure bei einem Myriapoden," *Pflügers Archiv für Physiologie*, 28 (1882), 576–579; polyzonimine: J. Smolanoff, A. F. Kluge, J. Meinwald, A. McPhail, R. W. Miller, Karen Hicks, and T. Eisner, "Polyzonimine: A Novel Terpenoid Insect Repellent Produced by a Milliped," *Science*, 188 (1975), 734–736; and benzoquinone: J. Smolanoff, J. M. Demange, J. Meinwald, and T. Eisner, "1, 4-Benzoquinones in African Millipeds," *Psyche*, 82 (1975), 78–80.
198. One species (*Armadillium klugii* of Yugoslavia) does mimic *Latrodectus mactans* quite successfully, presumably to deter being eaten by lizards. H. W. Levi, "An Unusual Case of Mimicry," *Evolution*, 19 (1965), 261–262.
199. *Scholia on Alexipharmaca*, 183a (Geymonat, p. 88).
200. *Scholia on Theriaca*, 812b (Crugnola, p. 287).
201. Aristotle, *HA*, 523a31–532b26 and 523b17–18; *Parts of Animals*, 682a35.
202. Aristotle, *HA*, 532a1–5.
203. Aristotle, *HA*, 531b31–35.
204. Cloudsley-Thompson, *Spiders ... Mites*, 66.
205. *Ibid.*, 64–65.
206. Wolfgang Bücherl, "Venomous Chilopods or Centipedes," in Bücherl/Buckley, eds., *Venomous Invertebrates*, 169–196 (195).
207. F. A. Turk, "Myriapodological Notes, III. The Iatro-Zoology, Biology and Systematics of Some Tropical 'Myriapods,'" *Annual Magazine of Natural History*, 4[12] (1951), 35–48.
208. Bücherl, "Venomous Centipedes," *Venomous Invertebrates*, 194.
209. *Ibid.*, 193: "There is very little literature on venomous scolopendromorphs and the effect of their venoms on mammals and man. Some documents are often contradictory." Then follow reports of death in humans from centipede bites by Wood (1866), Chalmers (1915), Venzmer (1932), and Faust (1928).
210. Cloudsley-Thompson, *Spiders ... Mites*, 66–67.
211. *Ibid.*, 51, mentions a "North African *Orya barbarica* (Geophilomorpha)" which can measure 6 or 7 inches in length, and (p. 52) *S. cingulata* of the Mediterranean.
212. *Theriaca*, 816: μυγαλέη. Superstitions about harmful shrews appear in numerous sources, *e.g.* Aelian, *On Animals*, II, 37; Pliny, VIII, 227 and XXIX, 88. Aristotle, *HA*, 604b19, notes that the shrew causes blisters in farm animals, Gow, "Nicandrea," *Classical Quarterly*, 45 (1951), 96 with n. 2. Aristotle may indeed record the base for the superstition: "The shrew has toxic saliva which kills small prey; it causes a burning sensation if injected into humans." Anonymous, "Shew and Vole," *Wildlife*, 19 (1977), 137.
213. Scarborough, "Nicander's Snakes," PHARMACY IN HISTORY, 19 (1977), 6–7, with nn. 65–74, and 79–83.
214. Dioscorides, II, 65 (and Pliny, *Natural History*, XXIX, 102) say that σῆπα is but another name for χαλκιδικὴ σαύρα (*Chalcis*), "Chalcidean lizard." Philumenus, 35, puts X. σαμίρα with the salamander, and quotes Soranus in saying that the bite makes a blister that blackens and produces pus. *Scholia on Theriaca*, 817a (Crugnola, pp. 288–289) say that σῆπα = σαύρα, and the creature is

rather large ("four palms in length"), and has bronze lines on its back. Aristotle, *HA*, 604b23 has a χαλκίς = ζιγνίς, a small lizard, dangerous to farm animals, especially oxen. Gow/Scholfield, *Nicander*, 187 n. 817 for the overabundance of modern identifications.

215. nn. 134–145 above.
216. λίτρον = νίτρον. λίτρον is the "older" form, found in the Hippocratic *Epidemics*, II, 6. 9 and 29 (ed. E. Littré, Vol. V, pp. 134 and 138). Herodotus, II, 86 and 87, and Plato, *Timaeus*, 60d and 65d. Nicander's major source, Apollodorus, probably used the term because it was found in Theophrastus, *e.g. HP*, III, 7. 6. λίτρον = νίτρον = 'natron,' or "soda," sodium carbonate. Since Soranus, II, 13. 2 (ed. Ilberg, p. 60, line 11) has νίτρασμα meaning "soapy," one may suggest Nicander's λίτρον may be translated "soap." *Vid.* also n. 329 below.
217. *Scholia on Alexipharmaca*, 335–337 (Geymonat, 127–129).
218. Aristotle, *HA*, 604b18: καὶ ἐὰν σταφυλῖνον περιχάνῃ · τοῦτο δ'ἐστὶν ἡλίκον σφονδύλη. *Cf.* n. 164 above (σπόνδυλος).
219. *Nature of Woman*, 3 and 32 (ed. Littré, Vol. VII, pp. 316 and 360): βούπρηστις as part of a female pessary. *Diseases of Women*, I, 71 and 74 (ed. Littre, Vol. VIII, pp. 150 and 158): again βούπρηστις part of pessaries. *Infertile Women*, 221 (ed. Littré, Vol. VIII, p. 426): βούπρηστις honey, and myrrh, specifically recommending the wing-covers (elytra). Apparently, Soranus rejected βούπρηστις since it does not appear in the *Gynecology*.
220. Galen, VII, 139 (*Causes of Symptoms*, I, 7): "uterine contractor." XII, 364 (*Blendings and Dynameis of Simple Drugs*, XI, 45): the βούπρηστις is among the kind of animals that includes the κανθάριδος (considered in *Simple Drugs*, XI, 44), and acts in medications in the same manner. XIV, 141 (*Antidotes*, II, 7): βούπρηστις causes vomiting. XIV, 264 (*Theriac to Piso*, 13): βούπρηστις and κανθάριδος subsist on plants (p. 265 contains a quotation from Nicander, *Theriaca*, 231–232, on the number of teeth in the "male" and "female" viper, to illustrate the variations in danger between male and female of various poisonous animals). There are traces of Nicander's *Georgica* in Galen, XIV, 100–102 (*Antidotes*, II, 15: "On the Preparation of Theriac"), esp. line 16, p. 101, and line 40, p. 102. Otto Schneider, *Nicandrea* (Leipzig: Teubner, 1856), 101 n. 1. But quotations of Nicander, or information about Nicander in the Galenic *corpus*, must be treated with caution. *e.g.* Galen, XVII, part 2, 400 (*Commentaries on the Hippocratic Aphorisms*, 12), where one reads that Praxagoras was the son of Nicander. Schneider, *Nicandrea*, 19, n. 1, points out that this is a scribal gloss for Nicarchus, stated correctly in Galen, II, 141 (*Natural Faculties*, II, 9), and VII, 584 (*On Tremor, Rigor, Palpitation and Spasm*, 1). Other quotations from Nicander in the Galenic *corpus* come from *Theriaca* and *Alexipharmaca*. *E.g.* Galen, XII, 289 (*Blendings and Dynameis of Simple Drugs*, X, 16: "On Saliva") paraphrases *Theriaca*, 86; V, 275 (*Opinions of Hippocrates and Plato*, II, 8 = I. Mueller, ed., *De Placitis Hippocratis et Platonis* [Leipzig: Teubner, 1874; rptd. Amsterdam: Hakkert, 1975], p. 238) is a quotation of *Alexipharmaca*, 21–22 (*vid.* Gow/Scholfield, *Nicander*, 191 n. 19, on the difficulty of this passage about the "heart of the stomach"). Galen, XX, 429 (index entries for Nicander), has five more passages listed. Surprisingly, the Brasavolus index (Venice: Junta, 1609) to Galen has no entries for Nicander. Galen, XIX, 726 ("Substitutions" or "Synonyms," B: ἀντὶ βουπρήστεως, σίλφαι βδέουσαι ἢ βδελλα) the βούπρηστις is likened to a cockroach or a leech.
221. Pliny, *Natural History*, XXX, 30: Buprestis animal set rarum in Italia, simillimum scarabaeo longipedi.
222. Aelian, *On Animals*, VI, 35.
223. Vegetius, *Mulomedicina*, II, 79. 10 (ed. E. Lommatzch [Leipzig: Teubner, 1903], p. 167): Bestiolus etiam, qui appellatur buprestis, araneae similis, sicum faeno devoratis, fuerit animal praefocabit.
224. Vegetius, *Mulomedicina*, II, 142 (ed. Lommatzch, p. 238): stercora minutatim et frequenter reddit.
225. E. Oder, ed., *Mulomedicina Chironis* (Leipzig: Teubner, 1901), 453 (ed. Oder, p. 144) and 506 (ed. Oder, p. 165).
226. *Geoponica*, XVIII, 18 (ed. H. Beckh [Leipzig: Teubner, 1895], p. 479.
227. Galen, XIX, 89 (*Exegesis on Hippocratic Words*, B): βούπρηστις · τὸ δὲ ζῷον τὸ τῇ κανθαραίδι παραπλήσιον. Then the text tells us that the word also means "some kind of wild herb" mentioned by "Dioscorides" in the first book of his *Hygiene*, and also in his *On Wild Herbs*. Wellmann, *Die Fragmente ... des Diokles von Karystos*, p. 168, correctly recognizes that περὶ λαχάνων was authored by Diocles, not Dioscorides, and thus the Kühn text contains some kind of scribal error. Wellmann, p. 168, makes Galen, XIX, 89, into Frg. 124 of Diocles' lost work, περὶ λαχάνων Galen, XIX, 726 (*vid.* n. 220 above) compares the βούπρηστις to the cockroach or the leech, which means that the creature is always dark brown or black. The Hippocratic *corpus (vid.* n. 219 above) always has κάνθαρις and βούπρηστις together in remedies.
228. Theophrastus, *HP*, VII, 7. 3, and Hescychius, *Lexicon*, 955 (ed. Latte, Vol. I, p. 341): *s.v.* βούπρηστις · λαχάνου εἶδος.
229. Pliny, *Natural History*, XXVIII, 74, apparently following Aristotle's lost 'ιατρικά (ed. A. Heitz, *Aristotelis Fragmenta* [Paris: Didot, 1886; 2nd part of Vol. IV of *Aristotle: Opera Omnia*], p. 217 [Frg. 5]).
230. Pliny, *Natural History*, XXVIII, 74.
231. Helmut Leitner, *Zoologische Terminologie beim älteren Plinius* (Hildesheim: Gerstenberg, 1972), 63–64: "Unter dem Namen buprestis" verschiedene Arten der Familie Meloidae, Ölkäfer, Blasenkäfer, zu verstehen sind" [64].
232. H. Gossen, "Käfer," *RE*, X (Stuttgart, 1919), cols. 1478–1489 [col. 1480].

233. E. Tauschenberg, *Die Insekten*, Neu. bearb. C. W. Neumann (Leipzig, 1942), 270–272.
234. nn. 134–145 above. Scarborough, "Pliny's Beetles," *Coleopterists Bulletin*, 31 (1977), 293–296.
235. Galen, VII, 139 (*Causes of Symptoms*, I. 7).
236. The τενθρήνη of *Alexipharmaca*, 547 is Nicander's synonym for μέλισσα. Aristotle, *HA*, 629a31 has τενθρηδών as a kind of wasp, but Hesychius (ed. Schmidt), col. 1444, *s. v.* τενθρηδών, gives two meanings: the first is derived from Aristotle (ζῶον τῶν ἐντόμων καὶ κεντροφόρων παραπλήσιον σφηκί); the second says a "wild bee" (ἔνιοι ἀγρίαν μέλισσαν).

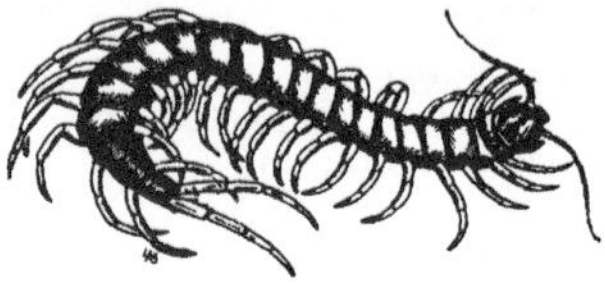

Nicander's *Toxicology*

II: Spiders, Scorpions, Insects and Myriapods

(Illustrated by Lysa Scarborough)

Part II

Remedies: The Blister Beetles

Only the two blister beetles (*kantharis*: *Theriaca*, 755, and *Alexipharmaca*, 115; and *bouprēstis*: *Alexipharmaca*, 335) have specific remedies prescribed by Nicander. As Gow and Scholfield remark, "the portentious list of simples which [are in *Theriaca*, 838–914] does not fulfil the apparent promise of [*Theriaca*], 837, for Nicander only once (867) condescends to tell us in what complaints these will be useful."[237] One can, therefore, gain a clear insight into an aspect of Greek toxicology from Nicander's remedies for the *kantharis* and *bouprēstis*, but understanding the antidotes for the other twenty (or twenty-two) creatures would require detailed comparison with other Greek and Roman authorities, as well as modern pharmacology, in order to specify utility in particular injuries. Below, the antidotes for blister beetles receive a full analysis, and four of the 107 substances in *Theriaca*, 837–956, are examined to illustrate the complex problems attached to the consideration of specific pharmaceuticals in Greek and Roman medicine. An appendix lists the remaining drugs and suggestions, with tentative identifications for each. It is unfortunate that Nicander has compacted so much lore into *Theriaca*, 837–956, since Aristotle speaks of "poison-vendors" who supply themselves with various spiders.[238] One would like to have the "full text" from which Nicander has borrowed his information, but only fragments have survived of Apollodorus, Diocles, and others, which could have given far greater detail about the fascinating details of Greek understanding of spiders, scorpions, insects, and myriapods.

As always, Nicander's antidote recipes are a bizarre amalgam of numerous traditions, and the remedies for *kantharis* poisoning are no exception. First the poet recommends (*Alexipharmaca*, 128) *glēchōn*, as part of a concoction that includes *kykeōna* (129), mixed with "river water" (*potamēisi*). The scholiasts sniff at the fancy "river water," remarking that this simply means "mix with water."[239] Recipe number one against *kantharis* ingestion is *glēchōn*, *kykeōna*, and water. The puzzling *glēchōn* is the same as *blēchōn* in other sources, and Dioscorides (III, 31) notes that *blēchōn* bears small, hairy leaves, and is rather short, as does Theophrastus, *Historia Plantarum*, IX,
* 16. 1. This plant is the European pennyroyal (*Mentha pulegium* L.), and it appears in the Hippocratic *corpus* as (*glēchōn*),[240] Herodas,[241] and Aristophanes' *Lysistrata* (89) and *Peace* (712), among others. Aristophanes tells us what pennyroyal was used for—in most cases—in Greek antiquity: as an abortificant. The two references in Aristophanes, taken together with Soranus' comments on *glēchōn*,[242] suggest that Nicander has totally failed to understand the pharmacology of his source (or sources). In *Lysistrata*, 89, one chuckles at the obscene pun on *blēchō*,[243] and in *Peace*, 712, there is another allusion to a woman's sexual attractiveness, with the recommendation of *kykeōna blēchōnian* (something akin to "pennyroyal potion") for too "much fruit." The playwright could assume that everyone would know these terms and understand the allusions, which tells much about "common knowledge" of both aphrodisiacs and abortificants, but one remains uncertain concerning the distinction between contraception and abortion among the Greeks.[244] Aristophanes has picked up the association of *blēchōn*/*glēchōn* with something called *kykeōna*, just as Nicander associates the two in his obscure recipe in *Alexipharmaca*, 128–129. Nicander would assume that *kykeōna* was well known to any pedant, since *kykeōn* was a venerated "potion," first given in Homer's *Iliad*, XI, 624 and 641,[245] and the drink (in Homer) contained grated cheese, Pramnian wine, and barley-groats. Nicander would be proud of his allusion to Homer, but he probably did not know why his source associated *kantharis* with *blēchōn*/*glēchōn* and *kykeōn*. *Kantharis*, as mentioned above, is the presumed aphrodisiac "Spanish Fly," and would have intimate connection with the common profession of prostitution in antiquity.[246] Prostitutes, of course, would use any compound that might guarantee them freedom from pregnancies, which pennyroyal could have done. The complete recipe in *Alexipharmaca*, 128–129, presumably against *kantharis* poisoning, includes grated cheese, Pramnian wine,[247] barley-groats, pennyroyal, and water. One was supposed to mix all these ingredients *en kymbeï*, which the scholaists say is another term for *oxybaphon*,[248] about ⅛ pint or 0.06 liters.

There is little doubt that Nicander's *glēchōn* is *Mentha pulegium* L., the pennyroyal. Distribution of the plant is throughout most of Europe (except northern Europe), the Mediterranean seaboard, and generally in the Middle East.[249] One of its distinguishing characteristics is its "hairy" appearance, with the corolla hairy outside, and the calyx slightly two-lipped, lobes unequal and hairy, and the throat closed by hairs.[250] Not only is pennyroyal an excellent natural insecticide,[251] its aroma is also somewhere between peppermint and camphor, giving it the strong, sweetish smell so highly recommended by Soranus in the delivery chamber.[252] Most important, however, is the medical use that pennyroyal—and its extract, the ketone Pulegone—has had in Europe until quite recently. "Pennyroyal Oil" or "Pulegium Oil" was commonly employed as an emmenagogue, and as an abortificant. In excretion, "Pennyroyal Oil" mildly irritates the kidneys and bladder, and reflexly stimulates uterine contractions. Although Greek sources indicate that pennyroyal was a common female contraceptive/abortificant, and apparently was known to all who would laugh at the puns in Aristophanes' *Peace* and *Lysistrata*, the modern extract of "Pennyroyal Oil" has caused extreme toxic effects. Convulsions result from as little as 4 ml.[253] "Pennyroyal Oil" contains not less than 85% Pulegone, while the natural extract found in the dried leaves and flowering tops of *Mentha pulegium*, *M. longifolia* (L.) Hudson, and *Hedeoma pulegioides* (L.) Pers. (US sp.) contains about 1% of the volatile oil, along with tannin and bitter principles. The ancient preparation apparently did serve well in its intended use, and its urinary effects were observed in conjunction with the action of *kantharis*,[254] explaining why Nicander would couple the two seemingly unrelated substances. This "recipe" of *Alexipharmaca*, 128–129, however, would be of little use against *kantharis* ingestion. In fact, it would make the problem worse.

Nicander's second remedy for *kantharis* poisoning (*Alexipharmaca*, 134–138) is *linoio speradessin*, in a rich broth made from a head of a hog, lamb, goat, or goose, given to the victim until he becomes sick, when one tickles his throat to make him vomit. Nicander's *linoio speradessin* is the same as the *linou sperma* of Thucydides,[255] *to linospermon* of Dioscorides,[256] Galen,[257] Artemiodorus,[258] and other sources,[259] and *to linosperma* of the *Geoponica*,[260] Galen,[261] and Alexander of Tralles.[262] This is "flax-seed," the same as linseed (*Linum usitatissimum* L.) from which is made the famous oil. In modern veterinary practice, linseed oil is employed as a laxative in large animals, and formerly veterinarians used the crushed seeds in a poultice for small animals, a practice that may have had its origins in the "Hippocratic" sources of the *Geoponica*.[263] In modern medicine, linseed oil has limited uses as a topical demulcent and emollient. The oil contains glycerides of linoleic, linolenic, oleic, stearic, palmitic, and myristic acids, and linoleic acid is one of the essential

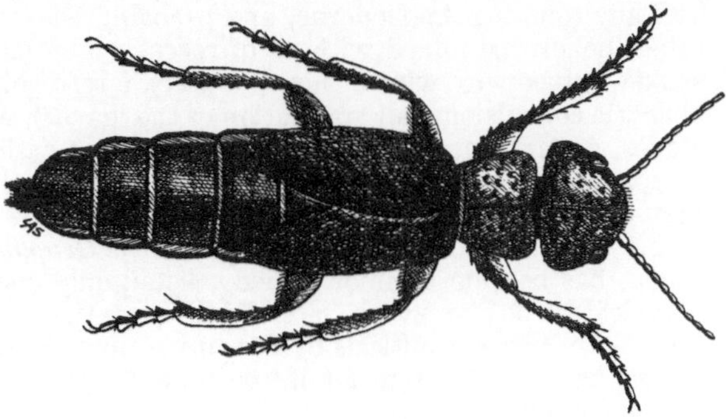

***Meloë variegatus*. Oil beetle. Central and southern Europe, Mediterranean littoral. Metallic gold-black to gold-green elytra, same for abdominal segments. after Boháč. up to 42 mm [1½"]**

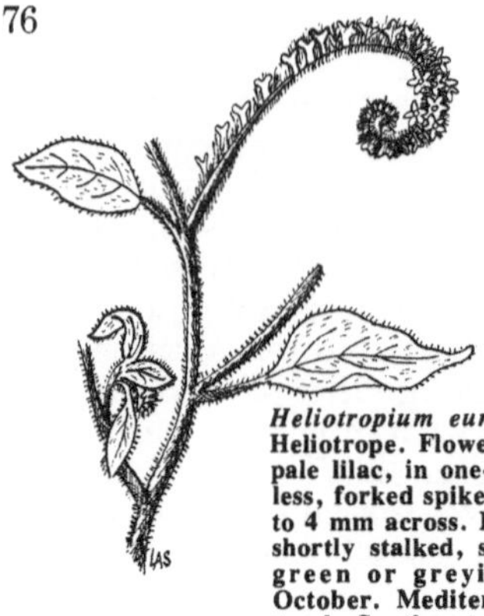

***Heliotropium europaeum* L. Heliotrope. Flowers white or pale lilac, in one-sided, leafless, forked spikes. Corolla 3 to 4 mm across. Leaves oval, shortly stalked, softly hairy, green or greyish. June–October. Mediterranean littoral, Southeastern Europe. After Polunin and Huxley (Everard).**

fatty acids (the Spartans were quite right to supply their troops with crushed linseeds).[264] Linoleic acid causes nausea and vomiting when administered in large doses.[265] If enough of the broth and linseed were given, as Nicander says "until the person is sick," and vomiting resulted, this would be an effective treatment for *kantharis* ingestion, if performed soon after the poisoning had taken place. It would not matter what kind of protein broth formed the medium, if it were coarse and perhaps repulsive enough.

Alexipharmaca, 139–140, gives the third "recipe" against *kantharis* poisoning: administer an enema using sheep's milk. This is worthless. A fourth (*Alexipharmaca*, 141) remedy is to drink some "creamy milk," which might help dilute the poison, if ingestion had occurred only a short while before. The fifth remedy (142–143) consists of drinking chopped, green vine tendrils and leaves *glykei*. Gow and Sholfield render the sense of *glykei* as "grape-syrup,"[266] but Hesychius suggests that this might be a form of "bitter" milk,"[267] which is "buttermilk." The scholiasts also remark that "buds" or "shoots" are meant in Nicander's *kaulea*,[268] so that the remedy has the victim drink sour milk with vine buds. Perhaps this too would make the patient vomit.

The sixth remedy given by Nicander for *kantharis* (*Alexipharmaca*, 144–146) is the root of *skorpiouros* administered "little by little" (*paura*) with honey. This recipe is rather puzzling, given the usual *skorpios* in Greek botany.[269] Fortunately, Dioscorides tells us that *skorpiouros* is another name given to *hēliotropion to mega*,[270] rather easily keyed as *Heliotropium europaeum* L.[271] Theophrastus and Galen give only one variety of *hēliotropion*,[272] but Dioscorides describes a second type called *hēliotropion to mikron*,[273] most likely the smaller *H. supinum* L.[274] Once again Apollodorus is the source of Nicander's crabbed reference, and again Pliny gives us the full range of uses to which this herb was put in antiquity:[275] with milk it acts as a gentle laxative, and taken "straight" it becomes a drastic purge; other uses recorded by Pliny (quoting Apollodorus, and probably Dioscorides) included headache relief (heliotrope mixed with oil of roses), an antidote against scorpions and snakes (mixed with wine or honey-water), a refreshing mouthwash, a cure for epileptic convulsions (an application of the leaves), a way to break up bladder stones, a wart remover, an aphrodisiac (mixed with honey), a charm against scorpions, and a number of other matters. Heliotrope appears in Soranus as part of a remedy for "the burning fever called *seiriasis*,"[276] the "dog-star fever" (*siriasis*) of Pliny.[277] By the time the *Geoponica* was compiled, *hēliotropion* has become a minor remedy, listed only once as one of a long list of botanicals to be given with water.[278] It seems that the plant had dropped out of the class of pharmaceuticals by Byzantine times, and its use in modern days is limited to its cultivation for its perfume.[279] Honey and heliotrope would at least be harmless.

Nicander's seventh remedy against *kantharis* is "four drachmas [*c*. 13.64 grams/211.2 grains] of Parthenian Earth" (*Alexipharmaca*, 148–149). No medium is specified. As usual, the poet has chosen to disguise something rather common in the cloak of allusion, which the scholaists explain. They tell us that Parthenius is another name for Samos,[280] but they admit some quandary about "Samothracian Earth," and whether or not "Parthenian Earth" applies to the whole island or to just a particular kind of "earth" found at one particular spot on the island of Samos. Pausanias clears up the confusion about Samothrace,[281] but most important for understanding Nicander's "Parthenian Earth" (= Samian Earth) is Theophrastus, *On Stones*, IX, 62–64. Here is a clear and detailed description of the mining process of "Samian Earth," an important commercial item for the island's economy. Theophrastus describes the dimensions of the mines[282] (*c*. 2 feet in diameter, not much smaller than the shafts of the silver mines at Laurium).[283] One presumes that slaves were used in mining Samian Earth, because inhalation of its fine dust causes emphysema and nodular pneumoconiosis.[284] Samian Earth is a very white, dense kaolin,[285] essentially a hydrated aluminum silicate (approx. $H_2Al_2Si_2O_8H_2O$).

Although Nicander is very brief in his notice of Samian Earth as a remedy in Greek pharmacology, other sources give full details. Dioscorides,[286] followed by Pliny,[287] and Oribasius,[288] provide the context omitted by Nicander. Dioscorides writes that Samian Earth is very white, and when it touches the tongue, it holds it like glue.[289] This is why, he continues, the substance is sometimes called *kollourion*,[290] often used in eye-salves. There are two kinds of Samian Earth: "ordinary" and "star" (*astēr*), which is thick and crusty like a whetstone.[291] *Astēr* is most likely a "trade mark" to signify the high quality of the Earth,[292] similar to the Lemnian "goat" on shipments of Lemnian Earth, stating this was, in effect "the best" Lemnian Earth.[293] Samian Earth, to return to Dioscorides' account, is excellent for the suppression of the spitting of blood, and given in a concoction with pomegranate flower is a cure for women who menstruate too heavily.[294] Samian Earth helps against bladder stones, and a most important use is its effectiveness against poisonous animal bites and as an antidote for poisons that might have been quaffed.[295] Galen gives a full summary of the uses of Samian Earth,[296] and it appears that it was a highly valued substance in the treatment of numerous ailments, including acute poisoning. One usually takes it in wine.[297] Presumably Nicander's "four drachmas of Parthenian Earth" would be taken in some amount of wine, although suspension of kaolin would be temporary. Greeks apparently knew of its total insolubility in water, because no source recommends that medium for the administration of Samian Earth.

Modern Americans are most familiar with kaolin in its prepared form, Kaopectate (Upjohn), which is a flavored suspension of kaolin, bentonite, and pectin, sold over the counter for treatment of mild diarrhea. Similar is Pectocel (Lilly), another flavored suspension containing kaolin and zinc phenosulfonate, and European products with kaolin include Tridia (Crookes), the various Kaylenes (Kaylene Chemicals), and K. L. N. Suspension (Maws). Kaolin is very much part of the modern pharmacopea; it is an excellent adsorptive agent, and if given by mouth, it adsorbs many toxic substances from the digestive tract, increasing the bulk of solid waste. In its numerous modern forms, kaolin compounds are commonly used for symptoms of enteritis, colitis,

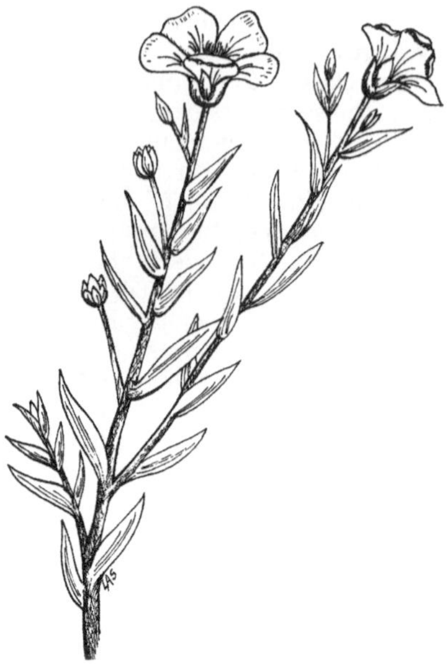

***Linum usitatissimum* L. Linseed; flax seed. Petals bright blue, 12–15 cm. Annual. Unknown in wild state. Cosmopolitan (England, Holland, Argentina, Egypt, Morocco, etc.). After Flück.**

cholera, and dysentery. Modern medicine also employs kaolin in the treatment of diarrhea associated with food poisoning and in cases of ingested poisoning with alkaloids. Nicander's "Parthenian Earth" would have had benefit for *kantharis* poisoning, but his suggested amount would have fallen far short if there had been more than minute quantities of *kantharis* ingested. Swift administration would have been essential, since cantharids are highly toxic.[298]

Pēganion is the basic substance in the eighth—and last—remedy Nicander prescribes for *kantharis* poisoning. One "crumbles" [*pēganion*] sprigs into the wine [?][299] kneading the herbs[300] with rose oil (*Alexipharmaca*, 154–155). Eight drachmas (27.3 grams/422.4 grains) is the recommended amount of wine, if that is the medium (Nicander does not say). Apparently if someone did not happen to have rose oil in his stock of handy medicinals, he could use the same combination of *pēganion* and wine [?], with oil of iris (*irineō: Alexipharmaca*, 155–156). *Pēganion* is rue (*Ruta graveolens* L.), which also figures in Nicander's snakebite remedies.[301] Greek and Roman sources have many references to rue,[302] and some of these help our understanding of Nicander's overly-abbreviated notice. Dioscorides tells us that the two kinds of *pēganon* (a "wild" and "garden-variety") are diuretic (*ourētika*) and produce menstrual blood; an *oxybaphon* (⅛ pint/0.06 liters) of rue seeds, taken in wine, is an antidote for poisonous drugs, and if one were to eat the leaves before taking the poison, they would prevent ill effects; and either eaten or quaffed, *pēganon* prevents conception.[303] In the Hippocratic *Regimen*, II, 54. 30, *pēganon* is recommended as a prophylactic against poisoning.[304] Plutarch's *Table Talk* notes that *pēganon* is very harmful to pregnant women,[305] and his source on the plant is "gardeners."[306] Even though Galen presents many recipes with rue (*e.g.* mixed with oil as a remedy for flatulence,[307] mixed with vinegar as an antidote against poison mushrooms,[308]) it is Soranus that gives uses and mixtures some clarity. In several passages, Soranus describes *pēganon* as part of a vaginal suppository, generally as a contraceptive or abortificant.[309] Once rue is suggested in the treatment of gonorrhea,[310] and once rue is the major ingredient of an emmenagogue.[311] The *Geoponica* picks up the tradition that made rue an emmenagogue,[312] and there are similar passages in Celsus,[312a] Rufus,[313] and Pliny.[314] Wellmann argues that Nicander had borrowed his data on *pēganon* directly from Apollodorus,[315] and that data, in turn, is most likely derived from the Peripatetic circle, especially Theophrastus.[316] The ancients believed that *pēganon* was not only a good antidote against poisons (Galen, quoting Asclepiades, specifies which poisons, *e.g.* mushrooms, aconite, cantharids),[317] but that it also was a reliable contraceptive/abortificant. Plutarch's coy allusions are filled out by Soranus, and it seems that Nicander has again merely excerpted only one aspect of a "famous" drug.

Rue has been used as a carminative, rubefacient, and is occasionally employed in the reduction of capillary fragility.[318] It contains rutin (rutoside; quercetin-3-rutinoside), and is part of the European pharmacopeia for the treatment of retinal hemorrhages in combination with ascorbic acid.[319] Rutin appears to have the ability to reduce capillary bleeding, but in its natural state, the amount of the rutin and volatile oil in *R. graveolens* would be so small as to have little effect. Yet the ancients were convinced of the great benefit of *pēganon*, and until the end of the nineteenth century, an infusion of rue oil was used as an emmenagogue, just as Soranus had prescribed.

Modern treatment of cantharid poisoning follows a standard course. The stomach of the victim is emptied by emetics or with a stomach tube. Sometimes, what is called medicinal charcoal will be administered, and demulcent drinks are recommended. Among Nicander's substances, only the Samian Earth (kaolin) would be of any benefit against cantharid poisoning, but the repeated urging to "get the victim to vomit" would have good results. Rue might have "smelled" like good medicine; pennyroyal would be harmful; while the remainder of the remedies in Nicander for cantharid poisoning would be harmless. One has the distinct impression, however, upon review of the ancient literature relating to cantharids and the solution made from their elytra that most "cases" were women, suggesting that our sources reflect problems among the ranks of prostitutes in particular. The association of pennyroyal with cantharids in the traditions recorded by Nicander, especially draws our attention to this aspect of ancient life, and reemphasizes the ordinary, everyday appearance of prostitution. Moreover, Celsus and Soranus record a fairly common incidence of gonorrhea.

Remedies for *bouprēstis* consist of figs in wine three years old (or fig-wine, three years old: *Alexipharmaca*, 347–348), milk and the "honey-sweet liquid" (351–352; presumably the same as the "wine" or "fig-wine" of 347–348), "crumbled fruit of the date palm" mixed with wine and dried wild pears, an ordinary pear, an olive, and some myrtle (353–355). Added to these Nicander suggests that one suckle milk (apparently human, if the scholiasts are right),[320] promote vomiting (356–363). The fig is the well known *Ficus carica* L., and the Hippocratic writers prescribe a decoction of figs in the treatment of sore tongue and inflamed throats.[321] Dioscorides and Plutarch speak of fig-wines,[322] and Galen suggests that figs with rue form a good antidote to poisons.[323] Moreover, Galen employs the same tradition used by Nicander, in which figs are part of the treatment for *bouprēstis* poisoning.[324] In Europe, figs are candied, made into a jam, brewed into an alcoholic drink called either fig wine or fig brandy, and are employed to make a laxative syrup and demulcent.[325] Figs contain 50–64% sugar, with small amounts of citric, acetic, and malic acids, as well as ficin, a proteolytic enzyme. Ficin has many modern industrial uses; a chillproofing agent in the brewing of beer; a shrinkproofing agent in the textile industry; a meat tenderizer; and an enzyme that is used for bating leather. Ficin can cause severe irritation to the eyes, skin, and mucous membranes. Nicander's figs would provide a mild laxative, not the best treatment for ingestion of a *cantharis*-type of solution.

Nicander prescribes twelve substances in either wine or water for blister beetle poisoning. Only the kaolin would be useful, while pennyroyal might be somewhat harmful. The rest of the ingredients would be either reasonably harmless or soothing.

***Theriaca*, 837–956**

There are 107 substances or treatments prescribed by Nicander for scorpion stings, spider bites, and wounds from insects and myriapods, in this extremely compacted and lengthy conclusion of the *Theriaca*. Other than plants and plant parts (roots, seeds, leaves), he suggests cautery (923–924), use of a cupping vessel to draw out the poison (921–922),[326] rabbit-curd (949),[327] an unknown moss or liverwort (945), a leech (930), a freshwater crab (949: *Telphusa fluviatilis*), sheep or goat dung (931–933), and three minerals: salt (948), a kind of iron ore called reddle (864–865),[328] and *nitron/litron*.[329] Below follows a commentary on three of the plants, and the goat/sheep dung, to illustrate the nature of Nicander's remedies, as well as to show the complicated state of his sources and the context of Greek and Roman pharmacology. The "Appendix" at the end of the text lists the remaining substances in *Theriaca*, 837–956, together with modern nomenclature and common names.

Theriaca, 839, prescribes *pentapetēlon*, a term found only in Andromachus (quoted by Galen) among other sources in Greek and Roman pharmacy.[330] Most authorities call the plant *pentaphyllon*, beginning with Theophrastus, *Historia Plantarum*, IX, 13. 5. From his description, as well as that of Dioscorides, IV, 42. 1–3, one can key this plant as one of the many species of *Potentilla*. Nicander's *pentapetēlon* = *pentaphyllon* is most likely *P. reptans* L., creeping cinquefoil, or possibly *P. recta* L., sulfer cinquefoil.[331] The plant found many uses in ancient drug prescriptions. The Hippocratic *Diseases*, II, 42 (Littré, VII, 58) suggests its use in tertian fever, and the Hippocratic *Wounds*, 20 (Littré, VI, 424), includes two varieties to be applied under bandages for the treatment of wounds and ulcers; the Hippocratic writer suggests *P. reptans*, as well as *P. argentea* L., hoary cinquefoil. Dioscorides, IV, 42. 1, lists seven alternate names for *pentaphyllon*, but Nicander's *pentapetēlon* is similar only to Dioscorides' *kallipetalon* or *xylopetalon*. In Dioscorides, the plant has many virtues: the root held in the mouth helps against toothache (IV, 42. 2 [Wellman, ed., II, p. 201]); it helps heal ulcers in the mouth (*Ibid.*); it soothes the windpipe if made into a gargle;[332] it is an aid against vomiting and diarrhea, and in a drink (of wine?) is good for arthritis and sciatic pains. The juice and the root are effective against poisons, as well as useful for liver and lung complaints.[333] In addition to Galen's description of *pentaphyllon* as one of the better "heating" and "drying" drugs,[334] there are numerous citations of the plant in Pliny,[335] and the *Geoponica*, II, 6. 29, includes it as effective in various complaints. Nicander's name for his cinquefoil may emerge from Apollodorus, but it seems Nicander "coined" the name (one could, after all, look up the other names) found in *Theriaca*, 839, borrowed only by Andromachus among later sources. It is significant that Galen's normal term for the plant is *pentaphyllon*, contrasted with his quotation of Andromachus' *Theriac*, which uses

Nicander's *pentapetēlon*. To Nicander, the incompetent botanist, one "five-petaled" or "five-leafed" plant was as good as any other, and it appears that the poet certainly did not comprehend his sources' careful descriptions and distinctions, especially the materials that had come to him from Theophrastus, Diocles, or Apollodorus.

Although Potentilla no longer is part of the pharmacopeia in the United States, *P. recta* remains an official drug in several European countries. Called Tormentil Rhizome, it is a red coloring principle containing not less than 15% tannin, and is employed as a tincture and internally and externally as an astringent. Preparations of Tormentil can be obtained in Austria, Portugal, Switzerland, and several other eastern European nations.[336] The tannin would be of some benefit, but the astringent qualities of the plant and its derivatives would not make it suitable in the treatment of poison ingestion, much as Galen suggests.[337]

Thridax appears in the long list (*Theriaca*, 838). Quite common in the drug recipes of antiquity, *thridax* is given careful consideration first by Theophrastus, who distinguished two varieties in *Historia Plantarum*, VII, 2. 4 and 9, and 5. 3.[338] This is lettuce, most likely "wild" lettuce, *Lactuca serriola* L., or *L. virosa* L. Even in modern times, the preparation has retained its ancient name, as the French call their Lactucarium "Thridace," which is the inspissated juice of *L. sativa*. The British Pharmaceutical Codex (1934) lists "Lactuca" as a mild sedative and hypnotic, useful in the treatment of irritable cough.[339] Martindale also informs us that the Portuguese have a Lactucarium called "Lettuce Opium," which is made into postilles and lozenges as a cough sedative. Another "Lettuce Opium" is the "German" Lactucarium, which is the dried milk-juice of *L. virosa* L., containing 0.2% lactucin, about 50% lactucerol, as well as smaller amounts of hyoscyamine, lactucic acid, caoutchouc, volatile oil, and mannite. Dioscorides, II, 136 (Wellmann, I, 207–208) tells how the ancients used the two varieties of lettuce (*L. sativa* and *L. serriola*: *thridax hēmeros* and *thridax agria*): *hēmeros* is generally beneficial for stomach complaints, inducing sleep in those persons who have frequent dreams and nightmares; *agria* is much like the poppy, and makes an excellent purge for the elimination of excess water, a good pain killer, emmenagogue, and antidote against scorpions and *phalangia* (II, 136. 3). The best drink is that mixed with poppy-juice (*mēkōn*), and the juice of *thridax agria* received careful preparation and storage, as Dioscorides says, "put up in newly-made pottery-jars" (II, 136. 3). Both Nicander and Dioscorides probably have extracted information from Apollodorus, or the preceding work by Diocles of Carystos.[340]

In the same line (*Theriaca*, 838), *anchousa* is prescribed. Not as common in the Greek and Roman writers on pharmacy, *anchousa* does have a respectable history as a valued remedy in classical antiquity.[341] Theophrastus, *Historia Plantarum*, VII, 8. 3, and 9. 3, mentions one general variety, while Dioscorides, IV, 23–25, lists three kinds. From these two major sources, one can key the plant, with some assurance, as an alkanet, especially the widely distributed *Alkanna tinctoria* (L.) Tausch, the famous "Dyer's Alkanet." Similar, but with more localized distribution are *A. orientalis* (L.) Boiss., *A. boetica* DC, *A. graeca* Boiss. & Sprun., and *Anchusa strigosa* Labill.[342] Alkannin and tannin are in the extract, and alkannin has been used as an astringent. Alkanna remains in the British Pharmaceutical Codex (1949), and is used for its red dye to color toilet preparations of either an oily or alcoholic nature, as a coloring in wine, and in microscopy for the detection of fats and oils.[343] The fullest account of its use in antiquity again is in Dioscorides (IV, 23–25 [Wellmann, II, 187–189]). His first kind of *anchousa*, which "some call *kalyx* and others *onokleia*" (IV, 23. 1) has roots that are useful for burns and old wounds, if the *anchousa* is mixed with wax and oil. Additionally, this type of *anchousa* is an abortive agent, given as a pessary (IV, 23. 2: *prostithemenē kai embrya kataspa*), as well as effective against leprosy (mixed with vinegar). Ointment makers also used the plant (the root with its dye) to thicken their various unguents. Dioscorides' "other kind" (IV, 24) is also called the [plant] "of Alcibiades,"[344] and is particularly effective against the bites of venomous animals, especially snakes, whether the plant is eaten, drunk, or hung about the neck. Furthermore, if one was chewing the plant (leaves?), and managed to spit into the mouth of a venomous snake, the spittle would kill the snake. The third variety (IV, 25) has the same potency in saliva as the previous *anchousa*, but the root of this third type, mixed in an *oxybaphon* (⅛ pint/0.06 liters) of wine with *hyssopos* (*Majorana hortensis* Moench) and *kardamon* (?*Lepidium* spp.), has the power to expell flatworms.[345]

Theriaca, 931–933, recommends a paste of sheep's dung mixed with wine or vinegar. This remedy for stings and bites has the long respect of Greek and Roman pharmacology, beginning with the Hippocratic writers.[346] Dioscorides, II, 80, is a long account of the various dungs used in medicine, and "pellets of goat/sheep dung" are useful in all sorts of ailments, including the bites of poisonous creatures (II, 80. 1 [Wellmann, I, 162]). A plaster of dung, mixed with vinegar or wine is particularly effective against the bites of snakes (II, 80. 2). Wellmann believes that the original notion of sheep/goat dung being effective against snakebite came from Apollodorus,[347] and recipes in Philumenus tend to support Wellmann's theory. Philumenus, 7. 6 (ed. Wellmann, p. 12) suggests goat dung, salt, rue, *kalaminthē* (*Mentha* spp., "mint"), and *skoroda* ("garlics:" *Allium sativum* L.) mixed in a plaster for poison snakebites, and 17. 10 (Wellmann, p. 24) recommends goat dung and wine in a plaster for snakebite. Pliny has many uses for dung in medicine,[348] and Galen also has a section on the tested virtues of goat manure in medicine.[349] Curiously, a paraphrase of Nicander (*Theriaca*, 86) has appeared only a few pages previous to Galen's account of goat dung,[350] much as Dioscorides, II, 79. 2 (Wellmann, I, 161) contains a paraphrase of *Theriaca*, 700–713. These passages are on the use of saliva,[351] and Schneider has shown that they are all derived from Apollodorus,[352] proved by the context of Galen's *Antidotes*.[353]

Cinquefoil, lettuce, alkanet, and sheep/goat manure represent well known and generally accepted pharmaceuticals in classical antiquity. Given the widespread cross-borrowing and repetition in our sources, Nicander's prescriptions (more correctly his clipped listings) mirror the numerous tracts on pharmacology that were available in his era, and *Theriaca*, 837–956, is a valuable catalogue that displays the detailed empirical knowledge in Greek toxicology and pharmacology in the second century B.C. Because we do not have a complete text of the works of Apollodorus,[354] nor do we possess more than fragments of Sostratus,[355] Krateuas,[356] Aelius Promotus,[357] or some of the earlier writers like Diocles of Carystos,[358] one must consult Nicander, Dioscorides, Pliny, Galen, Philumenus, and Oribasius to gain a full picture of the state of

Greek and Roman pharmacy and toxicology. In spite of his incompetence, Nicander provides a clear view of the pharmaceuticals in the second century B.C., and Dioscorides and Galen give better details and context, but Nicander is one of the important sources for the transmission of pharmaceutical information to the Roman world. This is especially true in toxicology, where numerous quotations in Pliny and Galen attest to the value placed on the *Theriaca* and *Alexipharmaca* by the Romans. A comparison of the plants and other substances in the following "Appendix" with Theophrastus, the Hippocratic *corpus*, Dioscorides, Galen, Philumenus, Celsus, Pliny, and Oribasius, would thus fill out many of the large gaps left in the summary of ancient drug lore by Schmidt.[359] Each has a rich history in classical antiquity, and one may be surprised at how many substances and ingredients in Nicander's compacted catalogue also function as contraceptives or abortificants. To take one example, the Hippocratic author of *Nature of Women*, 32 (Littré, VII, 350) suggests goat/sheep dung would make an excellent abortificant if prepared as a pessary. One can only reflect on the very common prescriptions that employ pennyroyal, cantharid beetles, and the like, and how so many seem to be directed at either the profession of prostitution or to "educated" women who wished to avoid pregnancies. These are reminiscent of the "folk" traditions in Theophrastus, *Historia Plantarum*, IX, 18. 3-11 (on aphrodisiacs), and Nicander's prescriptions of remedies for the bites and stings of spiders, scorpions, insects, and myriapods also have their important use in this little known aspect of Greek and Roman life.

Appendix

Ingredients and Substances in *Theriaca*, 839–956

Theriaca line no.	term	modern nomenclature	common name
839	*batos*	*Rubus ulmifolius* L.	bramble
840	*arkition*	*Inula* spp.; perhaps	
		I. conyza DC	ploughman's spikenard
		I. ensifolia	narrow-leaved inula
		I. viscosa (L.) Aiton	aromatic inula
840	*oxalis*	*Rumex acetosa* L.	sorrel; dock
840	*lykapsos*	*Echium* spp.; perhaps	
		E. italicum L.	pale bugloss
		E. vulgare L.	viper's bugloss
841	*kikama*	*Tordylium apulum* L.	hartwort
841	*tordelion*	*Tordylium maximum* L.	hartwort
841	*chamēlē pitos*	*Ajuga chamaepitys* (L.) Schreber	bugle; ground pine
842	*phēgos (phegou phloion)*	*Quercus macrolepis* Kotschy	Valonia oak (bark)
843	*kaukalis*	*Torilis japonica* (Houtt.) DC	upright hedge—parsley
843	*staphylinos* (seeds)	*Daucus carota* L.	carrot
844	*tremithos*	*Pistacia terebinthus* L. (= *terminthos*)	turpentine tree; terebinth
845	*phykos*	*Roccella tinctoria* C.	litmus; orchella-weed; lichen

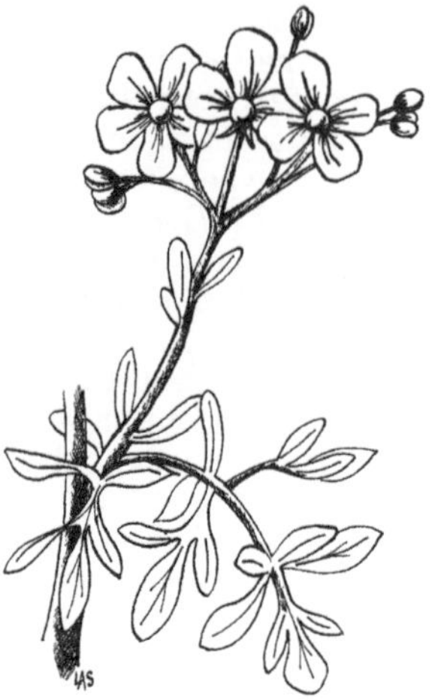

Ruta graveolens L. Rue. Flowers greenish-yellow, 12 mm in diameter. Petals four or five. Strongly-smelling, generally glaucous, woody-based shrub-like perennial to 80 cm. Leaves, two or three times cut into oval to spathulate segments 3 to 12 mm. Mediterranean littoral. May–July. After Flück.

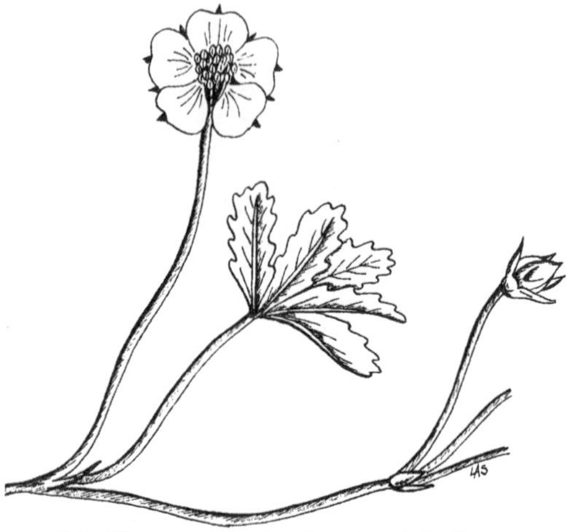

***Potentilla reptans* L. Creeping cinquefoil. Flowers light yellow to golden yellow. Flowering May–September (esp. June–July). Flowers 1½–2½ cm. across. All Europe, except Iceland. After Flück.**

Theriaca line no.	term	modern nomenclature	common name
846	*adianton*	*Adiantum capillis-veneris* L.	maidenhair fern
848	*smyrneion*	*Smyrnium perfoliatum* L.	perfoliate alexanders
849	*leukas*	*Lamium* spp.; perhaps	
		L. amplexicaule L.	henbit
		L. album L.	white dead-nettle
		or *Galeobdolon luteum* Hudson	yellow archangel
849	*ēnryngos*	*Eryngium creticum* Lam.	small-headed blue eryngo
850	*libanōtis*	*Lecokia cretica* L.	rosemary frankincense
850	*aparinē*	*Galium aparine* L.	goosegrass; cleavers
851	*koulybateia*	?*Parietaria officinalis* L.	erect pellitory-of-the-wall
		?*P. diffusa* Mert. & Koch	pellitory-of-the-wall
		?*Soleirolia soleirolii* (Req.) Dandy	mind-your-own business; mother of thousands
		(= *helxinē* and *klybatis*: *Theriaca*, 537)	
851	*mēkōn thylakis*	*Papaver rhoeas* L.	capsuled poppy; corn poppy
852	*mēkōn epitēlis*	*Glaucium flavum* Crantz[360]	yellow horned-poppy
853	*kradē*	*Ficus carica* L.	fig
854	*erinas*	*Ficus caprificus* L. (= *erineos*)	"wild" fig
856	*pyrakantha*	*Pyracantha coccinea* M. J. Roemer (= *oxykantha*)	fire thorn
856	*phlomos*	*Verbascum sinuatum* L.	mullein
857	*aigilōps*	*Aegilops ovata* L.	spikeweed
857	*chelidonion*	*Chelidonium majus* L.	greater celandine
858	*daukeion* = *daukos* = *staphylinos* (*Theriaca*, 843 above)		
858	*bryōnis*	*Tamus communis* L. (= *bryōnē* [*rhiza*])	black bryony

Theriaca line no.	term	modern nomenclature	common name
860	*peristerion*	*Verbena officinalis* L.	vervain
861	*rhamnos*	*Rhamnus catharticus* L.	buckthorn
863	*parthenion*	*Chrysanthemum parthenium* (L.) Bernh.	feverfew
864	*korkoros*	*Anagallis arvensis* L.	blue or scarlet pimpernel
864	*petalitis*	*Phyllitis vulgare* L. (= *phyllitis*)	hart's tongue fern
864–865	*miltos Lēmnis* ["Lemnian Earth"]	hematite	reddle
866–867	*sikuos agroteros*	*Ecballium elaterium* (L.) A. Richard	squirting cucumber
868	*paliouros*	*Paliurus spina-christi* Miller	Jerusalem thorn; Christ's thorn
870	*sidē*	*Punica granatum* L.[361]	pomegranate
872	*hyssōpos*	*Majorana hortensis* Moench[362]	sweet marjoram
872	*onōnis*	*Ononsis spinossa*, or *O. fruticosa* L.	restharrow
873	*tēlephilon*	? a poppy[363]	
874	*aglis*	*Allium sativum* L.	garlic
874	*korion*	*Coriandrum sativum* L.[364]	coriander
875	*konyza*	*Pulicaria dysenterica* L.) Bernh.	fleabane
876	*peperis*	*Piper nigrum* L.	black pepper
877	*Mēdōn kardamon*	*Lepidium sativum* L.	garden cress; pepperwort
877	*glēchōn = blēchōn*	*Mentha pulegium* L.[365]	pennyroyal
878	*strychnon*	various spp. possible	
		Solanum nigrum L.	black nightshade
		S. dulcamara L.	bittersweet; woody nightshade
		Datura stramonium L.	thorn apple
878	*sinēpi = napeion*	*Sinapis alba* L.	white mustard
879	*prason*	*Allium porrum* L.	leek
880	*knidē*	*Urtica pilulifera* L.	Roman nettle
881	*skilla*	*Urginea maritima* (L.) Baker[366]	squill
881	*bolbos*	*Muscari comosum* (L.) Miller	tassel hyacinth
882	*drakontion*	*Dracunculus vulgaris* Schott	dragon arum; edderwort
883	*rhamnos*	same as *Theriaca*, 861, above	
883	*peukē*	*Pinus nigra* Arnold	black, or Corsican pine
886	*skorpios*	*Heliotropium europaeum* L.	heliotrope; scorpionwort
887	*sidē*	*Nymphaea alba* L.	white water-lily
891	*pistakion*	*Pistacia vera* L.	Pistachio-nut tree
892	*kaukalis*	same as *Theriaca*, 843, above	
892	*myrton*	*Myrtus communis* L.	myrtle
893	*horminon*	*Salvia horminum* L.	red-topped sage
893	*marathon*	*Foeniculum vulgare* Miller	fennel
894	*eirysimon = erysimon*	*Sisymbrium officinale* (L.) Scop.	hedge mustard
894	*erebinthos agroteros*	*Cicer arietinum* L.	chickpea
896	*sisymbron*	*Nasturtium officinale* R. Br.	watercress
897	*melillōtus = lōtos*	*Melilotus officinalis* (L.) Pallas	common melilot
898	*oinanthē*	*Oenanthe fistulosa* L.	water dropwort
		O. crocata L. [Nicander says that the white blossoms are pounded in mortars by shepherds]	hemlock water dropwort; roots called "Dead Man's Fingers"
899	*lychnis* (seeds)	*Agrostemma githago* L.	corn cockle
899	*thryallis* (seeds)	*Plantago* spp.	
		P. indica L.	branched plantain
		P. major L.	great plantain
		P. ovata Forsk.	blond plantain
		P. psyllium L.	psyllium

Theriaca line no.	term	modern nomenclature	common name
900	*rhodon* (seeds)	*Rosa gallica* L. [Nicander has *rhodeon* at *Theriaca*, 103, and *rhodeon lipos at Alexipharmaca;* 155; the *rhodeon thyos* of *Alexipharmaca*, 452, probably obtained from *Rosa damascena* Mill.]	rose; Damask rose
900	*ias* (seeds)	*Matthiola incana* (L.) R. Br. [*ion* at *Theriaca*, 545, is *Viola odorata* L.]	stock; gilliflower; sweet violet
901	*poulygonon*	*Polygonum aviculare* L.	knotgrass
902	*psilōthron*	probably = *ampelos leukē*, or *a. agria*, since meaning is "depilatory." *Bryonia cretica* L.[367]	white bryony
902	*hyakinthos*	? *Hyacinthus orientalis* L.[368]	hyacinth
907	*tripetēlon*	*Psoralea bituminosa* L. [= *trisphyllon* = *triphyllon*]	pitch trefoil; treacleclover
907	*opos*	gum of silphium, an unknown extinct plant[369] [Nicander says to mix *opos* with *tripetēlon* in equal measure, making 3 obols/26.4 grains/ 1.71 grams]	
909	*herpyllos*	*Thymus serpyllum* L.	wild thyme; tufted thyme
909	*krēthmon*	*Crithmum maritimum* L.	rock samphire
910	*poiē kyapissos*	*Santolina chaemecyparissus* L. [= *chamikyparissos*]	lavender cotton
911	*annēson*	*Pimpinella anisum* L.	anise
911	*Libykē rhiza*	= *silphion* (*Theriaca*, 907, above)	
909–911:	mix the thyme, samphire, and lavender cotton + grated anise and *silphion* in a drink		
912–914:	shred the ingredients (*Theriaca*, 909–911) into a bowl, either together or separately, and drink in wine, or vinegar, or water, or milk		
915–920:	non specific; chew up leaves, roots, or seeds of handy plants; lay the half-masticated matter on the wound		
921–922	*sikūe chalkērea*	bronze cupping vessel	
923	*kradēs opon*	*Ficus carica* L.	fig juice[370]
925–929:	use a wineskin, made of goat's hide, and fill with wine; for a bite on the ankle or hand; tie cord at armpit or groin; put arm or leg inside full wineskin for a "wine bath"[371]		
930	*bdella*: let leeches feed on the wound		
931	*opon krommyon*	*Allium cepa* L. [drip on wound]	onion juice
931–933:	paste of sheep's dung with wine or vinegar		
934–956:	general panacea[372]		
937	*aristolochia*	*Aristolochia clematatis* L.	birthwort
937	*iris* (root)	*Iris florentina* L.	fleur-de-lis; white iris; orris root
937	*nardos* (root)	*Nardostachys jatamansi* DC	spikenard
938	*chalbanides rhizai*	*Ferula galbanifera* Boiss. & Buhs.	galbanum; kasnib; all-heal
938	*pyrethron*	*Anacyclus pyrethrum* (L.) Link	pellitory
939	*daukeion*	same as *Theriaca*, 858, above	
939	*bryōnē*	= *ampelos melaina* (*Theriaca*, 858, above	
940	*glykysidē*	*Paeonia officinalis* L.	peony
941	*helleboros melanochroos*	*Helleborus niger* L.	black hellebore; Christmas rose
941	*aphros litron*	= *nitron*: sodium carbonate	soda
942	*kyminon*	*Cuminum cyminum* L.	cumin

Theriaca line no.	term	modern nomenclature	common name
942	*konyza*	*Theriaca*, 875, above	
943	*staphis agrotera*	*Delphinium staphisagria* L.	stavesacre; licebane
943-944	*daphnē* (berries)	*Laurus nobilis* L.	laurel; sweet bay
944	*kytisos*	*Medicago arborea* L.	tree medick
945	*hippeios leichēn*	= *hippoleichēn*: a moss, or liverwort[373]	
945	*kyklaminos*	*Cyclamen graecum* Link	Greek cyclamen
946	*mēkōn* (juice)	*Papaver somniferum* L.	opium poppy
946-947	*agnos* (seeds)	*Vitex agnus-castus* L.	agnus castus; chaste tree
947	*balsamon* (resin or oil)	*Commiphora opobalsam* Engl.	balsam; Mecca myrrh tree
947	*kinamon*	*Cinnamomum cassia* Blume	cassia
948	*sphondyleion*	*Heracleum sphondylium* L.	hogweed; cow parsnip
948	*hals* (a bowlful)	sodium chloride	salt
949	*tamisos* (of *ptōx*)	= *puētiē*: rennet or curd from a rabbit[374]	
949	*karkinos*	*Telphusa fluviatalis* L.	river crab
951-952:	toss all ingredients into a mortar, and use a pestle to grind them up		
953-954	*aparinea chylon*	*Theriaca*, 850, above [pour *aparinea chylon* on dry ingredients]	juice of cleavers
954-956:	make round cakes of a drachma/52.8 grains/3.41 grams each, weighing each carefully with a balance; shake up in two *cotylai*/1 pint/0.54 liters of wine; drink		

References

Abbreviations employed:

HA: Aristotle, *Historia Animalium*
HP: Theophrastus, *Historia Plantarum*
LSJ: Henry George Liddell, Robert Scott; and Henry Stuart Jones, *Greek-English Lexicon*, 9th ed. with supplement (Oxford: Clarendon Press, 1968)
RE: *Paulys Realencyclopädie der classischen Altertumswissenschaft*

(Continued from PHARMACY IN HISTORY, Vol. 21, No. 1, p. 34)

237. Gow/Scholfield, *Nicander*, 188 n. 837.
238. Aristotle, *HA*, 622b33-623a2. *Cf.* Theophrastus, *HP*, IX, 16 passim.
239. *Scholia on Alexipharmaca*, 128 (Geymonat, p. 70).
240. *Diseases*, III, 17 (Littré, Vol. VII, p. 160): as a diuretic.
241. W. Headlam and A. D. Knox, eds., *Herodas: The Mimes and Fragments* (Cambridge: Cambridge Univ. Press, 1922), IX ("The Breakfast Party"), 13. Headlam/Knox, 405 n. 13, quote *Scholia on Aristophanes' Pax*, 712, for the definition of *βληχωνίαν* which becomes the meek "potion to allay overeating of fruit." It seems Headlam/Knox have chosen to ignore the blunt reference intended by Aristophanes (and the scholiasts). Herodas' *γλήχωνα κείνην* (*Mimes*, IX, 13) is in the same genre as Aristophanes' "potion of pennyroyal," prescribed for too much Opora, "fruit" or "sex." Henderson, *Maculate Muse*, 186, with n. 137. *Vid.* n. 243 below.
242. Soranus, *Gynecology*, II, 2. 2 (ed. Ilberg, p. 51): pennyroyal for sweet smell in the birth chamber immediately after partruition; III, 32. 5 (Ilberg, p. 115): pennyroyal in hot water bath to help loosen an "embedded clot" in the uterus (III, 32. 1: *τὸν ἐγκείμενον Θρόμβον* [Ilberg, p. 114]); III, 32. 6 (Ilberg, 115): a female suppository of pennyroyal for the same purpose; III, 38. 4 (Ilberg, p. 118): pennyroyal plaster for chronic affections of the uterus; III, 39. 2 (Ilberg, p. 118): rejection of steaming with pennyroyal for uterine problems; III, 39. 2 (Ilberg, p. 118): rejection of pennyroyal in drink of wine and honey for treatment; in the two previous citations, Soranus thinks pennyroyal is too harsh.
243. Henderson, *Maculate Muse*, 135: "Pubic hair is almost always conceived in agricultural terms as a flowering growth. *βλήχων* (or *βληχώ*) pennyroyal, is jokingly used by Lysistrata (89) to refer to the Boeotian girl's neatly depilitated *campus muliebris*, with a clever reference to the smooth, fertile plains of that region: *κομψότατα τήν βληχώ γε παρατετιλμένη* with neatly trimmed pennyroyal

plots. The pennyroyal posset (κυκεῶνα βληχωνίαν) recommended as a remedy for too much fruit (*Peace*, 712) contains an obscene allusion to Opora's sexual attractiveness." *Vid*. n. 241 above.

244. John Scarborough, *Roman Medicine* (London: Thames and Hudson, 1969), 101–102, with nn. 50–58.
245. *Vid*. nn. 78–104 above (the solifuge). ὁ κυκέων can also mean (in Homer) honey and magical drugs, *e.g. Odyssey*, X, 316 and 234 sq. *Vid*. nn. 241 and 243 above.
246. John Scarborough, *Facets of Hellenic Life* (Boston: Houghton Mifflin, 1976), 179–185.
247. "Pramnian" wine probably means simply the "best" wine. *I. e.* Hesychius (ed. Schmidt), col. 1270, *s.v.* πράμνιος οἶνος · ἔστι ἐγκώμιον οἴνου. Athenaeus, I, 28f., 30b–d, and 31d–e, gives the major conclusions from the arguments over the topic in antiquity. In ancient wine manufacture, the "best" wine was that which trickled out from the mass of untromped grapes. Scarborough, *Facets*, 67. *Geoponica*, VI, is one of the major sources for the process of ancient wine making.
248. *Scholia on Alexipharmaca*, 129f (Geymonat, p. 70).
249. George Usher, *Dictionary of Plants Used by Man* (London: Constable, 1974), 387.
250. Oleg Polunin, *Flowers of Europe* (London: Oxford Univ. Press, 1969), 367 (No. 1167).
251. Juliette de Baïracli Levy, *Herbal Handbook for Farm and Stable*, 2nd rev. ed. (London: Faber & Faber, 1975), 97–98.
252. Soranus, *Gynecology*, II, 2. 2 (ed. Ilberg, p. 51).
253. *Martindale*, 1544.
254. Galen, XI, 609 (*Blendings and Dynameis of Simple Drugs*, III, 23): as an extreme diuretic.
255. Thucydides, IV, 26. 8 (seige of Pylos, 425 B.C.), where poppy seeds, mixed with honey and crushed linseeds were the rations of the encircled Spartans.
256. Dioscorides, II, 103.
257. Galen, VI, 549 (*Dynameis of Foods*, I, 32 = G. Helmreich, ed., *De alimentorum Facultatibus* [Leipzig: Teubner, 1923; *Corpus Medicorum Graecorum* V 4, 2], pp. 258–259). Parallel sources listed by Helmreich, p. 258.
258. Artemidorus, *Onirocriticon*, I, 68 (ed. Roger A. Pack, *Artemidori Daldiani Onirocriticon* [Leipzig: Teubner, 1963], p. 75): "Sesame, linseed, and mustard predict good [luck in dreams] for doctors."
259. *E.g.* Alexander of Aphrodisias, *Problemata*, I, 67 (ed. J. L. Ideler, *Physici et Medici Graeci minores* [rpt. of ed. 1841–1842, 2 vols. in 1: Amsterdam: Hakkert, 1963], p. 22).
260. *Geoponica*, XVI, 20. 1 (ed. Beckh, pp. 465–466).
261. Galen, XII, 433 (*Compounding Drugs According to Parts of the Body*, I, 2), quoting from Cleopatra's book, *Cosmetic Preparations*.
262. Alexander of Tralles, III, 12 (ed. T. Puschmann [Vienna, 1878–1879; 2 vols.; rptd. Amsterdam: Hakkert, 1963], Vol. II, p. 87).
263. *Geoponica*, XVI, 20. 1 (ed. Beckh, pp. 465–466). The Hippocratic writers have numerous uses for linseed. Littré, X, 667 (index reffs. [Lin, graine de]).
264. Thucydides, IV, 26. 8 (n. 255 above).
265. T. P. Hilditch, *The Chemical Constitution of the Natural Fats*, 3rd ed. (London: Chapman and Hall, 1956), 175–180. E. W. Eckey, *Vegetable Fats and Oils* (New York, 1954), 535–547.
266. Gow/Sholfield, *Nicander*, 103.
267. Hesychius, 670 (ed. Latte, I, p. 381), *s.v.* γλυκεῖαν · τὸ γάλα, καὶ τὴν χολήν.
268. *Scholia on Alexipharmaca*, 142b (Geymonat, p. 70).
269. Theophrastus, *HP*, IX, 13. 6: σκορπίος is one of the *Doronicum* spp., probably "Leopard's Bane," possibly quite useful against scorpion stings. Vid. Scarborough, "Theophrastus on Herbals," *Journal of the History of Biology*, 11 (1978), n. 120. Theophrastus, *HP*, IX, 18. 2: σκορπίος is one of the numerous *Aconitum* spp. ("Wolf's Bane").
270. Dioscorides, IV, 190.
271. Oleg Polunin and Anthony Huxley, *Flowers of the Mediterranean* (London: Chatto and Windus, 1974), 149 (No. 385).
272. Theophrastus, *HP*, VII, 3. 1; 8. 1; 9. 2; 10. 5; 15. 1. Galen, XIX, 732 ("Substitutions" or "Synonyms," K: ἀντὶ κλινοποδίου).
273. Dioscorides, IV, 191.
274. Polunin, *Flowers of Europe*, 331–332 (No. 1045).
275. Pliny, *Natural History*, XXII, 59–61.
276. Soranus *Gynecology*, II, 55. 2 (ed. Ilberg, p. 92).
277. Pliny, *Natural History*, XXII, 59.
278. *Geoponica*, II, 5. 4 (ed. Beckh, p. 38).
279. Albert F. Hill, *Economic Botany*, 2nd ed. (New York: McGraw Hill, 1952), 187–188.
280. *Scholia on Alexipharmaca*, 149a–c (Geymonat, p. 78).
281. Pausanias, *Description of Greece*, VII, 4. 3: Thracian Samos colonized by Samians from *the* Samos, off the coast of southwestern Asia Minor.
282. Theophrastus, *On Stones*, 63–64 (ed. D. E. Eichholz, *Theophrastus: De lapidibus* [Oxford: Clarendon Press, 1965], p. 82, with commentary, pp. 130–131).
283. K. D. White, "The Birth of Mining," *Optima*, 5 (1955), 118.
284. *Martindale*, 709, quoting A. Granata in *Folia Medica*, 40 (1957), 329 = *Abstracts, World Medicine*, 22 (1957), 412.
285. Eichholz, 129.

286. Dioscorides, V, 153. 1-2.
287. Pliny, *Natural History*, XXXV, 191.
288. Oribasius, XIII, Γ. 3(ed. J. Raeder [Leipzig: Teubner, 1928-1933; rptd. Amsterdam: Hakkert, 1964; 4 vols.; *Corpus Medicorum Graecorum*, VI 1-2] Vol. II, pp. 162-163).
289. Dioscorides, V, 153. 1.
290. *Ibid.*: ἥν τινες κολλούριον καλοῦσιν *Vid.* also Harald Nielsen, *Ancient Ophthalmological Agents* (Odense [Denmark]: Odense Univ. Press, 1974), esp. p. 57. Still useful is the pioneering study by C. L. Grotefend, *Die Stempel der römischen Augenärzte* (Hannover: Hahn'sche, 1867).
291. Dioscorides, V, 153. 1: πλακώδης ὢν καὶ πυκνὸς ὡς ἀκόνη.
292. Eichholz, 130. Theophrastus, *On Stones*, 63.
293. Dioscorides, V, 97. Galen, XII, 170 (*Blendings and Dynameis of Simple Drugs*, I, 1. 2: "On Various Names given to Earths").
294. Dioscorides, V, 153. 2.
295. *Ibid.*
296. Galen, XII, 178-192 (*Blendings and Dynameis of Simple Drugs*, I, 1. 4: "On Samian Earth").
297. Dioscorides, V, 153. 2.
298. *Vid.* n. 145 above. W. Morel, "Gifte," *RE*, Supplementband V (1931), Cols. 223-228 [226].
299. Gow/Scholfield, *Nicander*, 105, guess "must" from context.
300. Nicander's word for 'herbs' is θρόνα. *Scholia on Alexipharmaca*, 155b (Geymonat, p. 80) simply says τὰς ἰατρείας, while in Theocritus, II, 59, the word means "those herbs used as drugs *and* charms." *Cf.* Nicander, *Theriaca*, 493 and 936.
301. Scarborough, "Nicander's Snakes," PHARMACY IN HISTORY, 19 (1977), 11-12, with nn. 121-123.
302. Curiously, the cognate ἡ ῥυτή is far less common in Greek than τὸ πήγανον = πηγάνιον. *Vid.* Nicander, *Theriaca*, 523, and *Alexipharmaca*, 306. Latin, however, chose *ruta* as the usual term for rue, perhaps because one of the earliest Greek physicians in Rome (Archagathus of Sparta, in Rome *c.* 220 B.C.) came from the Peloponnesus, where ἡ ῥυτή was the usual term, not πήγανον. LSJ, 1577. Scarborough, *Roman Medicine*, 38, 40, and 150. In Greek botany, Theophrastus, *HP*, I, 3. 4 and 10. 4, provides the first major reference to πήγανον, and Dioscorides, III, 45 and 46 has two kinds (πήγανον ὀρεινόν may be *Ruta halepensis* L., "mountain rue"). Both Galen and Pliny have numerous references and medical uses for rue, and the plant appears in almost all medical and pharmacological authors. Diocles, Frg. 138 (ed. Wellmann, pp. 174-175) shows that Nicander's "information" had once again filtered down to his own time from the traditions of the time of Aristotle and Theophrastus.
303. Dioscorides, III, 45. 1-5.
304. Littré, VI, 558.
305. Plutarch, *Moralia: Table Talk*, 647B: καὶ ὅλως πολέμιόν ἐστι ταῖς κυούσαις.
306. Plutarch, *Moralia: Table Talk*, 648D: οἱ κηπουροί.
307. Galen, X, 578 (*Method of Medicine*, VIII, 5).
308. Galen, XIV, 140 (*Antidotes*, II, 7: "From Asclepiades' *Antidotes for Lethal Drinks*"); XIV, 141 ("Against Cantharids") also suggests rue together with oil of iris.
309. Soranus, I, 35. 2 (ed. Ilberg, p. 24); I, 35. 5 (Ilberg 25); I, 63. 1 (Ilberg 47); I, 64. 2 (Ilberg, 48); III, 32. 6 (Ilberg, 115). I. 63. 1 gives a recipe for an abortificant/contraceptive (probably "contraceptive," if ἀτόκιον [Soranus, I, 60, ed. Ilberg, p. 45] is intended): 2 obols/17.6 grains/1.14 grams of rue seeds, 2 obols of opopanax gum, 2 obols of "Cyrenaic juice" (probably silphium), all ground up and coated with wax, and drunk in wine that has been watered down.'Οποπάναξ is *Opopanax Chironium* (L.) Koch, and is the same as the πάνακες τὸ Ἡράκλειον of Theophrastus, *HP*, IX, 11. 1 and 3. Scarborough, "Asclepiades," PHARMACY IN HISTORY, 17 (1975), 53, and "Theophrastus on Herbals," *Journal of the History of Biology*, 11 (1978), n. 69. Scarborough, *Roman Medicine*, 101-102, with nn. 50-55 (on contraceptives).
310. Soranus, III, 46. 3 (ed. Ilberg, p. 124).
311. Soranus, III, 16. 2 (Ilberg 104): rue + honey.
312. *Geoponica*, XII, 25. 2 (ed. Beckh, p. 373).
312a. *E.g.* Celsus, II, 22 and 31; V, 25. 5 and 27. 5.
313. Rufus, 431 (ed. Daremberg-Ruelle): in the "Remedies for Dessication of the Sexual Organ."
314. *E.g.* Pliny, *Natural History*, XIX, 156; XX, 131-142.
315. M. Wellmann, ed., *Dioscorides: Materia Medica*, Vol. II, p. 57; esp. Nicander, *Theriaca*, 531, and *Alexipharmaca*, 413.
316. Scarborough, "Theophrastus on Herbals," *Journal of the History of Biology*, 11 (1978), n. 69.
317. Galen, XIV, 135-144 (*Antidotes*, II, 6-7: "From the Fifth Book of Asclepiades' *Antidotes* as Recorded by Asonus," and "From Asclepiades' *Antidotes for Lethal Drinks*"). XIV, 139: aconite. XIV, 140: mushrooms. XIV, 141: cantharids.
318. Scarborough, "Nicander's Snakes," PHARMACY IN HISTORY, 19 (1977), 11-12, with nn. 121-123.
319. *Martindale*, 146.
320. *Scholia on Alexipharmaca*, 65a (Geymonat, pp. 52-53), citing Erasistratus' *On Poisons*. *Cf.* Pliny, XXVIII, 72 and 74, and Dioscorides, II, 70. 6.
321. *Diseases*, II, 28 and 31 (Littré, VII, pp. 46 and 48).
322. Dioscorides, V, 32 (συκῖτις). Plutarch, *Moralia: Dialogue on Love*, 752B (σύκινον πόμα).
323. Galen, VI, 793 (*Healthy and Unhealthy Nourishment*, 8) = G. Helmreich, ed., *De rebus boni*

malique suci (Berlin: Teubner, 1923; *Corpus Medicorum Graecorum* V 4, 2), 8. 5 (Helmreich, ed., p. 415).

324. Galen, XIV, 141 (*Antidotes*, II, 7: "From Asclepiades' *Antidotes for Lethal Drinks*"); Asclepiades/Galen say to promote vomiting, use warm milk, a decoction of figs, and a measure of nitron with water.
325. *Martindale*, 1272. Usher, *Dictionary of Plants*, 254.
326. *Cf.* John Stewart Milne, *Surgical Instruments in Greek and Roman Times* (Oxford: Clarendon Press, 1907), plates XXXIII–XXXV, with literary descriptions and sources, pp. 101–105. Scarborough, *Roman Medicine*, 46, with nn. 37–38 (p. 190); also plate 38. Nicander, *Theriaca*, 921, employs *σικύη* for "cupping vessel" or "bleeding cup," the most common term for the instrument in Greek sources.
327. *Cf. Theriaca*, 711 (*τάμισος*). Scarborough, "Nicander's Snakes," PHARMACY IN HISTORY, 19 (1977), 16–17, with nn. 145–146, and "Theophrastus on Herbals," *Journal of the History of Biology*, 11 (1978), nn. 70–71 and 72a (seal rennet). Erotian, T 32 (ed. Ernst Nachmanson, *Erotiani Vocum Hippocraticarum collectio cum fragmentis* [Gotoburg/Upsalla: Eranos' Förlag, 1918], p. 87). Hesychius, *Lexicon* (ed. Schmidt), col. 1434: *τάμισος · ἡ πυτία*. The Hippocratic *Diseases of Women*, II, 192 (Littré, VIII, 372):"Η *τάμισον ὄνειον καὶ σίδης γλυκείης ῥίζην καὶ κικίδα ἐξ ἴσου πάντα, κὰι ῥοιῆς. γλυκείης χυλὸν ξύν οἴνῳ*. Galen, XIX, 145 (*Exegesis of Hippocratic Words*, T).
328. *μίλτος Λήμνις*, which is red ocherous hematite, sometimes called "red chalk," and will be mixed with various types of clay; this "Lemnian earth" is thus a silicate of aluminum and iron. Edward Salisbury Dana, *Textbook of Mineralogy*, 4th ed., rev William E. Ford (New York: John Willey, 1949), 484.
329. *Vid.* Scarborough, "Asclepiades," PHARMACY IN HISTORY, 17 (1975), 49, and "Theophrastus on Herbals," *Journal of the History of Biology*, 11 (1978), n. 30. *λίτρον* = *νίτρον* which is sodium carbonate, $Na_2CO_3 \cdot HNaCO_3 \cdot 2H_2O$, sometimes called trona or urao. Dana, *Mineralogy*, 530–531.
330. Galen, XIV, 40 (*Antidotes*, I, 6: "The Elder Andromachus" *Theriac* Against Poisonous Snakes").
331. Polunin, *Flowers of Europe*, 166–167.
332. This seems to be the meaning: *καὶ τραχύτητας ἀρτηρίας ἀναγαργαριζόμενον παραιτεῖται.*
333. *ὁ δὲ χυλὸς τῆς ῥίζης ἁπαλῆς ποιεῖ πρὸς τὰ ἐν ἥπατι καὶ πνεύμονι πάθη καὶ τὰ θανάσιμα.*
334. Galen, XII, 96 (*Blendings and Dynameis of Simple Drugs*, VIII, 8).
335. Pliny, *Natural History*, XXV, 109, 128, 166, and 174; XXVI, 23–24, 26, 35, 90, 113, 116, 123, 126–127, and 131.
336. *Martindale*, 1420: Poland, Czechoslovakia, Hungary, Soviet Union, Yugoslavia.
337. n. 334 above.
338. *Cf.* Dioscorides, II, 136. Diphilus of Siphnos (as recorded in Athenaeus, II, 69e): John Scarborough, "Diphilus of Siphnos and Hellenistic Medical Dietetics," *Journal of the History of Medicine and Allied Sciences*, 25 (1970), 194–201. Rufus of Ephesus (ed. Daremberg-Ruelle), 430. Galen, XI, 887 (*Blendings and Dynameis of Simple Drugs*, VI, 6. 6: "On Lettuce"). Gargilius Martialis, XI: "De lactuca" (ed. V. Rose, *Plinii Secundi...Gargilii Martialis: Medicina* [Leipzig: Teubner, 1875], pp. 144–145). Pliny, *Natural History*, XX, 62, 64, and 68. *Geoponica*, XII, 13. 1–15 (ed. Beckh, pp. 357–359).
339. *Martindale*, 1531.
340. Wellmann, "Kräuterbuch," *Festgabe Susemihl*, 1–31.
341. *Cf.* Galen, XI, 811–813 (*Blendings and Dynameis of Simple Drugs*, VI, 1. 4: "The Four Ἀγχοῦσαι"). Pliny, *Natural History*, XXII, 48–49, 51–52; XXVII, 59. Hesychius, *Lexicon* Ed. Latte, Vol. I, p. 35), 924–925: *ἄγχουσα · ἡ κάλυξ* and *ῥίζια, ᾗ φυκοῦνται γύναια*. Oribasius, XI A, 5–6 (ed. Raeder, Vol. II, p. 81) = Dioscorides, IV, 23–24 Nicander, *Theriaca*, 541. Theophrastus, *Odors*, 31 and 33.
342. Polunin/Huxley, *Flowers of the Mediterranean*, 150–151. C. N. Goulimis, *Wild Flowers of Greece*, ed. W. T. Stearn, with paintings by N. A. Goulandris (Athens/Kifissia: Goulandris Botanical Museum, 1968), xxix: on Euboea appears "... the bright, yellow-flowered *Alkanna boeotica*."
343. *Martindale*, 556. Hill, *Economic Botany*, 131.
344. Scarborough, "Nicander's Snakes," PHARMACY IN HISTORY, 19 (1977), 12 with n. 126.
345. *Cf.* Theophrastus, *HP*, IX, 20. 5 (male fern as antihelmintic). Scarborough, "Theophrastus on Herbals," *Journal of the History of Biology*, 11 (1978), nn. 165–166.
346. *Nature of Woman*, 32 and 34 (Littré, VII, 350 and 372); *Diseases of Women*, II, 147 (Littré, VIII, 324); *Prognosis*, I, 41 (Littré, V, 520/522); *Coan Prognostics*, 471 and 591 (Littré, V, 688/690, and 722).
347. Wellmann, ed., *Philumenus*, p. 24: from Apollodorus'Ε*υποριστων*.
348. Parallel passages from Pliny listed by Wellmann, ed., *Dioscorides*, I, 161–163.
349. Galen, XII, 290–308 (*Blendings and Dynameis of Simple Drugs*, X, 18–29), esp. XII, 297–300 (*Ibid.*, X, 22: "Goat Dung").
350. Galen, XII, 289 (*Blendings and Dynameis of Simple Drugs*, X, 16: "Saliva").
351. *Cf.* Dioscorides, IV, 24 and 25.
352. Schneider, *Nicandrea*, 182.
353. Galen, XIV, 184 (*Antidotes*, II, 14).
354. Schneider, *Nicandrea*, 181–201, remains the best collection and commentary on Apollodorus.
355. M. Wellmann, "Sostratus," *Hermes*, 26 (1891), 321–350.
356. M. Wellmann, *Krateuas* (Berlin: Weidmann, 1897 [*Abhandlungen der königlichen Gessellschaft der*

Wissenschaften zu Göttingen, philosophisch-historische Klasse, Neue Folge, Band 2, Nr. 1]) = Fragments and Testimonia in Wellmann, ed., *Dioscorides*, Vol. III, pp. 139–146.

357. Erwin Rohde, "Aelius Promotus," *Rheinisches Museum*, n.f. 28 (1873), 264–290.
358. Wellmann, ed., *Die Fragmente der sikelischen Ärzte*.
359. Alfred Schmidt, *Drogen und Drogenhandel im Altertum* (Leipzig: J. A. Barth, 1924).

Notes to the Appendix

360. W. Thiselton-Dyer, "On Some Ancient Plant-Names," *Journal of Philology*, 33 (1914), 195–207 [204–205]:᾿Επιτηλίς = μήκων κερατîτις.
361. Nicander, *Alexipharmaca*, 489–491, lists perhaps four major kinds. Dioscorides, I, 110, has three kinds (γλυκεîα, ὀξεîα, οἰνώδης). Pliny, XIII, 112; XV, 39; and XXIII, 106, has nine or ten. Gow/Scholfield, *Nicander*, 198 n. 492: "Apart from Nicander and Pliny pomegranates do not seem to be prescribed in these cases [against poison fish]." *Vid.* also Theophrastus, *HP*, IV, 13. 2; Athenaeus, XIV, 650e; and Palladius, IV, 10 (ed. Robert H. Rodgers, *Paladii Rutilli Tauri Aemiliani: Opus agriculturae. De veterinaria. De insitione* [Leipzig: Teubner: 1975], pp. 122–127): "De pomis: Malum Punicum."
362. It is rather clear that *Hyssopus officinalis* L. is not the plant, although LSJ, 1905, translate "hyssop." The basic clue to the identity of the plant probably is the drawing of Dioscorides' *hyssopos* in the Vienna manuscript (*Codex Aniciae Julianae*: Vienna, Nationalbibliothek, cod. med. gr. 1; 491 fols. [fol. 359^{v}]). A. von Premerstein, K. Wessely, and J. Mantuani, *Dioscurides Codex Aniciae Julianae picturis illustratus, nunc Vindob. Med. gr. 1* (Leipzig, 1906). This plant appears to be one of the *Origanum* spp., and *Majorana hortensis* Moench (*Origanum majorana* L.) is the most likely candidate here in *Theriaca*, 872. John Scarborough, ed., Luis García Ballester, *Galen of Pergamon: Medical Practice and Philosophy*, trans. by Carl J. Post (Rome/Milan: Episteme Editrice [in press]), Ch. 5, "Pathology," editor's n. *111.
363. *Scholia on Theocritus*, III, 29 (ed. F. Dübner, *Scholia in Theocriti Idyllia* [Paris: Didot, 1848], p. 30), suggest some kind of poppy: τηλέφιλον δὲ ἐστι τὸ φύλλον τῆς μήκωνος; but the scholiasts are most unsure, also suggesting some kind or shrub with spiral seed pods. Literally rendered, the name means something akin to "loveless."
364. Dioscorides, III, 63, says that κόριαν is a vermifuge and aphrodisiac, but is a "mind-deranger" when taken in large doses. Galen, XIV, 139 (*Antidotes*, II, 7): τοîς δε χλωρὸν κορίανον πιοûσι βοηθεî οἶνος ἄκρατος ποθεὶς καὶ ζωμὸς ὄρνιθος λιπαρâς.
365. *Vid.* nn. 239–254 above.
366. Jerry Stannard, "Squill in Ancient and Medieval Materia Medica, with Special Reference to its Employment for Dropsy," *Bulletin of the New York Academy of Medicine*, 2nd series, 50 (1974), 684–713. *Vid.* Theophrastus, *HP*, IX, 18. 3–11 (ed. F. Wimmer, *Theophrasti Eresii Opera* [Paris: Didot, 1866; rptd. Frankfurt am Main: Minerva, 1964], pp. 159–161. Hort has omitted—without comment—both Greek text and translation of *HP*, IX, 18. 3–11, presumably due to its "offensive" contents, which caused George Sarton to remark, "... such prudishness in a scientific book is truly shocking (George Sarton, *A History of Science*, Vol. I: *Ancient Science Through the Golden Age of Greece* [Cambridge, Mass.: Harvard University Press, 1952; rptd. New York: Norton, 1970], 555, n. 96). The passages missing in Hort's Leob Theophrastus are translated (without comment) in Chalmers L. Gemmill, "The Missing Passage in Hort's Translation of Theophrastus," *Bulletin of the New York Academy of Medicine*, 49 (1973), 127–129.
367. Theophrastus, *HP*, IX, 20. 3: root used as a depilatory. Scarborough, "Theophrastus on Herbals," *Journal of the History of Biology*, 11 (1978), n. 160.
368. A very uncertain identification. A. S. F. Gow, *Theocritus*, 2nd ed. (Cambridge: Cambridge Univ. Press, 1952; 2 vols.), II, 200–201: "These flowers (for more than one seems to have borne the name [of ὑάκινθος]), after long discussion, have not been satisfactorily identified" [200]. Gow's collection of source references shows much confusion, although Theophrastus, *HP*, VI, 8. 2, has two kinds (ἡ αγρία and ἡ σπαρτή), and does class ὑάκινθος in his mountain plants.
369. Alfred C. Andrews, "The Silphium of the Ancients: A Lesson in Crop Control," *Isis*, 33 (1941), 232–236. *Vid.* also Scarborough, "Nicander's Snakes," PHARMACY IN HISTORY, 19 (1977), 5 with n. 51, and "Asclepiades," *Ibid.*, 17 (1975), 53 with n. 101, for further bibliography on silphium and suggested identifications. "An extinct species possibly of the onion or garlic family" seems about as close as we can come ("Nicander's Snakes," 5). *Cf. Alexipharmaca*, 202, 204, 309, 329, and 369 (juice); *Theriaca*, 85 and 697 (root); *Theriaca*, 911 below (root).
370. The notion that fig juice was useful in clotting blood goes back in Greek medicine to Homeric times. Since fig juice 'clotted' milk, analogy suggested it could also 'curdle' blood. "Disease causes bodily humors to clot, just as rennet causes milk to curdle." Guido Majno, *The Healing Hand: Man and Wound in the Ancient World* (Cambridge, Mass.: Harvard Univ. Press, 1975), 151–152, with nn. 61–63, p. 489. Majno proved that the Homeric poets were right, as far as the fig juice 'clotting' milk was concerned, but fig juice failed to clot blood—in fact it retarded the process.
371. A "wine bath" would indeed have much benefit for wounds resulting from spider bites, scorpion stings, and insect bites generally. "The antiseptic power of wine is no myth," and the antiseptic properties result from "... the anthocyanes, a subgroup in the large group of polyphenols present in

wine...[and also is] the principle pigment of red wines, malvoside or oenoside; there is a colorless equivalent for white wines...the bactericidal power of wine [increased] with age." Majno, *Healing Hand*, 186–188 [187], with nn. 248–265, p. 498. Majno tested Chianti, Beaujolais, Dôle du Valais, and a Spanish Rioja on *Staphylococcus aureus, Streptococcus pyogenes, E. coli, Proteus mirabilis*, and *Pseudomonas aeruginosa*: "After six hours, no live bacteria could be recovered, except a few stapylococci, but they too failed to grow after twelve hours" [187].

372. Various ingredients in Nicander's "panacea" continued to be valued in later theriacs, especially casia, various poppies and their juices, squill, iris, balsam, freshwater crab, rennets, "Lemnian Earth," salt, onion, wine, and black pepper. *Vid.* Gilbert Watson, *Theriac and Mithridatium* (London: Wellcome Historical Medical Library, 1966), 40–93.

373. *Scholia on Theriaca*, 945a (Grugnola, pp. 318–319) is a welter of information and pseudo-information on ἱππεῖον λειχῆνα. The scholiasts say that one should know that this is a growth on the knee of horses which is scraped off and given in a drink as a remedy for spider bites (τρίβοντας διδόναι πιεῖν τοῖς ὀφιοδήκτοις ἀλεξήτηριον). Another name for the "growth" is χελιδόνη, but Dioscorides, II, 43, says that λειχῆν is simply the normal callosity on the foreleg of a horse (the "chestnut"), which implies that the scholiasts have mauled the information they might have found in Dioscorides. The scholiasts add that ἱππεῖον λειχῆνα is also the name of an herb (βοτάνη θεραπευτική) also called ἱπποσέλινον (Alexanders: *Smyrnium olustratum* L.), used in the treatment of horses—an obvious guess that is founded only on the etymology of the word. *Smyrnium olustratum*, much like celery, appears in Theophrastus, *HP*, II, 2. 1, and Dioscorides, III, 67, but there is no trace in the *Geoponica*. One would be tempted to identify λειχῆνα as simply a lichen, but the context of Theophrastus, *Causis Plantarum*, V, 9. 10 (olives and olive trees with λειχήν) implies both a kind of lichen and a moss that grows on trees. Dioscorides, IV, 53, says that λειχήν is a kind of mossy plant (probably a liverwort) that grows on wet rocks. The Hippocratic *Aphorisms*, III, 20 (ed. W. H. S. Jones, *Hippocrates* [Loeb Classical Library; 4 vols.], Vol. IV, p. 128) has λειχῆνες side-by-side with λέπραι, making λειχήν a skin disease, and Aeschylus, *Libation-Bearers*, 281–282, speaks of λειχήν (probably leprosy here) have a "white down" (λευκὰς κόρσας; *cf. Leviticus*, XIII, 3) that could be likened to the appearance of the "downy" moss. Galen, XII, 342 (*Blendings and Dynameis of Simple Drugs*, XI, 21), simply records that λειχήν ἵππων with vinegar is a good remedy for poisonous animal bites. The sum of all sources leads one to conclude that some ancient writers are speaking of a lichen, some of a skin disease, while others (including probably Nicander) mean a moss or liverwort.

374. Scarborough, "Theophrastus on Herbals," *Journal of the History of Biology*, 11 (1978), nn. 70–80 (various animals and their curds in remedies).

VII

THE OPIUM POPPY IN HELLENISTIC AND ROMAN MEDICINE

WELL known from earliest Greek history,[1] the opium poppy (*Papaver somniferum* L.) occupied an important role in ancient pharmacy and medicine, and its use encompassed matters of dietetics as well as frequent employment as a soporific and general analgesic. Greco-Roman medicine and pharmacology incorporated a very succinct knowledge and command of the dangers and benefits in the use of the opium poppy, and actions of drugs were widely understood. Its harvesting, preparation, distribution, and application in general pharmacy and medical therapeutics all were sophisticated and as precise as was then possible. Our ancient sources attest repeatedly to this deep sophistication in the grasp and understanding of the opium poppy, and Hellenistic and Roman pharmacy had refined a lengthy and venerated tradition of multiple uses. Modern pharmacology and medicinal chemistry, of course, confirms much of this ancient expertise, even as we wrestle with the addictive effects of the major alkaloids commonly isolated and administered from the raw opium. One notes in the study of Hellenistic and Roman use of opium that the 'natural product' may have induced occasional addiction (and was certainly employed in suicides), but unlike the dangers explicit with the employment of morphine, codeine, thebaine, and other opium alkaloids in modern pharmacy and medicine, and ancients could presume their collected latex had benefits that far outweighed its dangers.

Homer's epics contain the first references in Greek literature to the opium poppy,[2] and one reads in the *Odyssey* that this drug is one which 'quiets all pains and quarrels'. One also hears that this beneficial substance is derived from a plant that grows in Egypt, a rather curious assertion since *Papaver somniferum* L. is native to Asia Minor, but a 'made in Egypt' label in Homer's day carried much medical weight. More curious is the lack of notice in our Greek sources of the opium poppy from Homer's time through the fifth century BC, and when Theophrastus considers *mēkōnes* in his masterful *Enquiry into Plants*,[3] there is but a brief notice of how one gathers the useful juice from the 'head' of the plant. In the Hippocratic corpus, there are thirteen references to the use of opium or the opium poppy,[4] and nine of these are nestled within the gynaecological tracts, suggesting employment among midwives but less frequent use by male physicians. In the Hellenistic Age, physicians were well acquainted with the dangers of opium poisoning, and added to the clipped references by Dioscorides[5] to the fears of the drug set down by Diagoras (*fl.* ?400 BC),[6] Andreas (d. 217 BC),[7] and Mnesidimus (*fl.* ?),[8] we have the rather accurate description of the results of fatal opium overdoses (and some antidotes) by Nicander of Colophon,[9] who lived in western Asia Minor about 130 BC. In the *De medicina* of Cornelius Celsus (*fl.* in the reign of Tiberius (AD 14–37)), one finds some possible references to the medical use of the latex of the opium poppy, but 'Celsus never alludes to the cultivated poppy from which opium is obtained', and since he '. . . does not include poppy juice in his list of poisons . . . he probably knew only a mild variety of the juice.'[10] Poppy tears (*lacrimae*) do figure in a number of Celsus' anodynes, but the source of these lozenges was probably the mildly narcotic *Papaver rhoeas*, not *P. somniferum*.

Dioscorides of Anazarbus (*fl. c.* AD 70) composed one of the most important works in all the history of medicine,[11] and his *Materia Medica*, IV, 64 (ed. Wellmann, II, pp. 218–21) contains the first and best summary of what the opium poppy 'did' in Hellenistic and Roman therapeutics. Dioscorides has used frequently various preparations of 'poppy-juice' in his own practice, extending over many years and several provinces in the eastern half of the Roman Empire. The traditions and practices recorded by Dioscorides throughout the *Materia Medica* often suggest clinical observations fused with folk medicine and a precise pharmacology, and it is what drugs 'do' when given to patients that occupies Dioscorides' major attention. Consequently, an organizing principle for the whole *Materia Medica* comes not through botanical morphology or an alphabetical listing of pharmaceuticals, but through what John Riddle has perceptively discerned as a 'drug affinity' system[12] – that is what happens when patients are given a particular drug or compound in the treatment of particular ailments. This is exactly the blueprint one meets in Dioscorides' account of the opium poppy: he begins with a general summary of where opium poppies grow (wild and cultivated), and proceeds with admirable clarity into general properties (in Greek *dynameis*) of the drug in its several forms, some special names applied to different kinds of poppies, preparation techniques, various applications in specific ailments, the detection of true opium from counterfeit lookalikes, and finally the most excellent description we have of the harvesting of the latex from the poppy capsules in Classical antiquity. In a departure, too, from his usual habits of not citing authorities from written works on pharmacology, Dioscorides suggests how earlier physicians had been quite in error in their fear of opium as an overly dangerous drug:[13] 'these very opinions are wrong, refuted through experience with the efficacy of the drug being observed in its results'. The names cited by Dioscorides – Erasistratus quoting Diagoras, Andreas, and Mnesidemus – indicate a debate and wide use of the opium poppy in medicinal pharmacy going back at least 400 years; it is little wonder that Theophrastus in his rightly renowned *Enquiry into Plants* does not emphasize the opium poppy among his limited listing of pharmaceuticals in Book IX,[14] since opinions among physicians and rootcutters varied so greatly. Comparison also with the accounts of opium in Pliny the Elder's *Natural History* to that in Dioscorides indicates some common sources of information (there is no evidence that Pliny knew the work of Dioscorides, or vice versa),[15] at least as such data were available on drugs from books; and to Dioscorides' list of written authorities on the opium poppy, Pliny adds Iollas, a name which appears in the *Preface* by Dioscorides to his *Materia Medica.*[16] Pliny designates 'the drug from the poppy capsule' in its Greek form, the *dia kōduōn*,[17] the term used continuously for this medicament from Pliny's day through the quotations in the works of Byzantine physicians.[18] In Galen's drug books, there is a list of embedded authorities on opium or the drug made from the opium poppy capsule,[19] and they range from Asclepiades and Themison,[20] to Damocrates' quoted poem *From the Poppy Capsule*,[21] a formula for the poppy capsule drug from the works of Soranus, mentions of similar formulas by Criton (physician to Trajan),[22] Heras,[23] and Galen's own version of the drug.[24] And with the exception of theriacs, as Galen relates the uses and properties of the opium capsule preparation, comparison with the text of Dioscorides reveals close parallels, showing that Dioscorides' explication incorporated the main lines of medical opinion on opium, accepted and followed by most learned physicians after *c.* AD 100. One can, therefore, take Dioscorides' *Materia Medica*, IV, 64, as representative of the best understanding in Hellenistic and Roman pharmacy of the properties, actions, and uses of the opium poppy. Dioscorides stands, moreover, in time on the bridge between Roman imperial medicine and the earlier heritages of Hellenistic practices, and his citations (for purposes of refutation) of Diagoras, Erasistratus, Andreas, and Mnesidemus give a glimpse of an earlier literature on pharmaceutical employment of the opium poppy and its latex.

Although Dioscorides was clearly a very skilled medical botanist, he spends few words on plant morphology, perhaps presuming that anyone interested in such matters would consult Theophrastus' very fine *Enquiry into Plants*. In beginning his section on the opium poppy, Dioscorides specifies that some varieties are 'cultivated and grown in gardens',[25] and that these garden poppies provide seeds made into a special bread recommended as particularly healthy by dieticians. The seeds of this garden variety poppy were also fit substitutes for sesame seeds, if the poppy seeds were mixed with honey, and this sesame seed replacement has the name 'common poppy' (Greek *thylaktis*),[26] with the plant bearing a white seed in a longish capsule. Dioscorides knew that poppy seeds had no narcotic properties, and his mention of white seeds from this cultivated type is strikingly verified by a modern description which notes that 'Seeds [are] used for preparation of emulsions (white-seeded varieties are preferred)',[27] even as poppy seeds 'contain no opium and are used extensively in baking and sprinkling on rolls and bread'.[28] Dioscorides' dietetic experts also knew how 'health-inducing' were these seeds, and modern food chemists have found goodly amounts of lecithin in poppy seed meal. It is significant that Dioscorides begins his section on the opium poppy with its dietetic uses, a signal not only of his organizational principles but also of the soon-accepted manner of compiling medical handbooks with initial chapters on healthy food-stuffs (usually plants) which also functioned as drugs.[29] And by commencing the account of the opium poppy with the garden variety, Dioscorides is suggesting two important aspects about Hellenistic and Roman understanding and use of the opium poppy: first, one can raise it in a garden for ordinary employment in the diet as bread and as a plant which yields a nourishing oil,[30] as well as some limited use as a narcotic; and, secondly, there is the assumption that uncultivated opium poppies provide the more potent latex, used almost exclusively as a drug. In speaking of the garden poppy, Dioscorides also includes two other kinds by way of introducing the more powerful varieties which will follow in the next section: there is a semi-wild poppy with a black seed called *pithitis* or *rhoias* – the corn poppy – so named 'from the latex (*opos*) flowing from it'; and a second kind is even less cultivated, which is smaller 'and more useful as a drug, having a longish capsule'.[31]

Turgidly Galen repeats[32] what Dioscorides had set down concisely 150 years previously regarding the properties of the opium poppy. In his usual terse and clipped manner, Dioscorides writes that 'a common property (*dynamis*) among [the kinds of poppies] is cooling',[33] and he proceeds immediately to say that the decocted leaves and capsules applied as fomentations bring on sleep. One may also drink this decoction for insomnia, but if the pharmacologist triturates finely the capsules and mixes this pounded poppy capsule in a poultice made from hulled barley and then formed into plasters, such a plaster could be used to treat inflamed boils (*phlegmonai*) and cases of St Anthony's fire (that is erysipelas). This is the weakest form of the drug, and its source is either a boiled down solution (here in water) or a combination of whole capsules and leaves with crushed barley, and Dioscorides' own experience with these preparations proved their usefulness in sometimes including slumber for insomniacs, and in successful treatment of skin problems, including reddened boils and the shiny and red lesions on the arms and legs or the face characterized by vesicles. Iranian folk medicine continues to employ for boils a paste made from compounded linseed (*Linum usitatissimum* L.), mallow (*Malva* spp.), and poppy,[34] and the modern pharmacopoeias record that the poppy capsule is mildly sedative.[35] And although opium does indeed have some bactericidal properties, one remains uncertain if Dioscorides' barley–poppy plaster would have been effective against the Group A beta-hemolytic streptococci causative of erysipelas, but it is probable that the mild analgesic itself alleviated the severe discomfort of patients afflicted by this superficial cellulitis.[36]

Immediately following his prescriptions for decocted poppy capsule and leaves, and the barley–poppy plaster, Dioscorides specifies another preparation technique for this mildly acting form of the drug: 'One ought to make it into lozenges – pounding them in a mortar while they are still green – and drying them to lay them up into storage, and thus employ it.'[37] Such lozenges, sometimes still called trochisks as borrowed directly from the Greek word, were easily stored and transported, and dried tablets retained their medicinal properties after they were remelted and used in plasters or in fomentations. It is in particulars like this that Dioscorides shows his practised experience with drugs, and parenthetically such specifics indicate that the best of the Greco-Roman physicians were also skilled pharmacists and compounders of drugs, as well as able medical botanists, quite capable of identifying plants in the field and gathering them for preparation as pharmaceuticals.

Next Dioscorides describes a slightly stronger form of the drug to be used as a 'pain-killing lozenge (*anōdynon ekleikton*) for coughs and tracheal discharges, as well as bowel conditions'.[38] The poppy capsules are to be boiled in water down to half the original volume, and then boiled again with honey until 'the moisture should condense out'. This process would give a syrup, which could be hardened into tablets, stored, and remelted for use as a Greco-Roman version of a cough medicine, or, sucked as would be modern cough drops, and gave the pain-killing remedy specified by Dioscorides. 'Poppy capsule . . . has been used as a liquid extract or syrup in cough mixtures',[39] showing that ancient applications of poppy for coughs have continued for two millennia. And as modern pharmacognosy texts repeatedly emphasize, 'Opium, while closely resembling morphine, exerts its action more slowly, and is therefore preferable in many cases, e.g. in the treatment of diarrhoea',[40] again a millennial-deep reflection of Dioscorides' recommendation that poppy capsules be used for 'conditions of the bowels'.

If one mixed *hyokistis* and *akakia* with the decocted honey–poppy capsule preparation, the compounded drug is 'more efficacious'[41] as a cough remedy and medicine for diarrhoea, and several other Roman writers agree with Dioscorides in recommending *hyokistis* and *akakia* for the control of both vomiting and diarrhoea.[42] The ever-cautious Soranus of Ephesus suggests the two in combination,[43] noting that these (among a number of substances) increase the effective properties of a 'styptic' or 'contracting action' (*stypsis*), that is what we would term adsorbent action in the digestive tract. The use of *akakia* in cough medicines is verified in modern practice: 'acacia is used as a demulcent in lozenges'.[44] *Akakia* is the famous 'gum arabic', the dried gum obtained from the stem and branches of *Acacia senegal* Willd., *A. arabica* Willd., and other species of *Acacia* in north and central Africa. Gum arabic's constituents explain – in modern terms – its well-known pharmaceutical properties, since it contains mostly arabin and the calcium salt of arabic acid along with traces of magnesium and potassium.[45] This natural combination makes gum arabic an excellent mucilage, tablet excipient, emulsifier, and thickener,[46] and adding *akakia* to the ancient version of the cough remedy made good sense in another way as well: Dioscorides has just mentioned putting the poppy capsule plus honey lozenges up for storage, and these trochisks would be employed later as needed; by adding and combining the opium poppy capsule and honey decoction with gum arabic, Greco-Roman pharmacologists were extending the effectiveness of the drug, or as the *Merck Index*, 11th edn, p. 11, notes, '[acacia is used] where flavor stability and long shelf life are important'.

Unlike the continued use of acacia in official medicine and pharmacy, the use of *hypokistis* had become 'obsolete' by 1830.[47] Well known to the Romans as an effective treatment for dysentery and milder forms of diarrhoea,[48] the juice of *Cytinus hypocistus* (L.) L., a member of the Rafflesiaceae (relatives of the mistletoe), has astringent properties and does retain a respected role in the folk medicine of southern Europe.[49] The modern pharmacopoeias do not include *Cytinus*, and there is little literature on its medicinal chemistry, but as a parasitic plant with bright yellow flowers growing from the roots of *Cistus* bushes (which produce balsams), it has been recorded clearly by Greco-Roman medical botanists in both its relation to the balsams and in its great usefulness in treatment of various diarrhoeas. As Dioscorides writes (perhaps quoting from Sextius Niger),[50] *hypokistis* has a property (*dynamis*) like that of *akakia*, but the *hypokistis* is 'more styptic and more drying'.[51] It appears that combining the *Cytinus* juice with gum arabic, and the decocted honey and poppy capsule preparation, would enhance the anti-diarrhoeal properties of this remedy, but as a therapy there might be some risk of constipation following milder cases of diarrhoea. Dysenteries are another matter altogether. Modern pharmacognosy does not detail why *Cytinus* has dropped out of use, even though folk medicine recognizes its value.

Perhaps the drying action of poppy seed oil engendered the belief that triturated poppy seeds quaffed in wine would alleviate diarrhoea and even hypermenorrhoea,[52] and the same assumptions appear to underlie the recommendation of applying a plaster of black poppy seeds with water to the forehead and temples to help insomniacs. Yet once Dioscorides has set down these ineffective suggestions, he tells us he is proceeding into data about the latex itself (*ho opos autos*), notably more cooling, thickening, and drying in its pharmaceutical properties than the poppy capsule preparations which have preceded: 'taken in as small a quantity as a bitter vetch seed, the latex is an anodyne and sleep-inducer, and it promotes digestion, being useful for coughs and intestinal conditions; but too much of the latex being drunk, it plunges one into lethargy in sleep, and it kills'.[53] Even as we read a reiteration of some uses of the opium poppy, met previously in the poppy capsule preparations, we also read that the latex by itself has fatal consequences if taken in too great a quantity. By citing the seed of the bitter vetch (*Vicia ervila* (L.) Willd. or *V. orobos* DC) as a 'unit of measure' or 'dosage', Dioscorides is making a very important point, well understood in Greco-Roman pharmacy: usually referred to in the plural in Greek, due to their small size, a seed of the bitter vetch by itself as a dosage unit would suggest the potency of such a measure of the opium poppy's latex, especially in an initial administration. Greco-Roman physicians were well aware that repeated use of raw opium (the latex) was – as we say – habit forming,[54] and that greater and greater dosages are required as time progresses to obtain the pleasurable effects, which include sleep accompanied by alluring dreams and visions.[55] Excessive and continued ingestion eventually leads to delirium and death, and as little as 300 mg of opium can be fatal to a human being[56] (it is on record, however, that some morphine addicts can tolerate 2,000 mg of morphine over a period of four hours). Approaching death is signalled by cold and clammy skin, a weak and rapid pulse, cyanosis, and (in modern diagnostics) pulmonary oedema, followed by a final pulmonary and circulatory failure.

Hellenistic and Roman medicine knew the dangers of the opium poppy's latex, and as early as the fifth century BC (if we have Diagoras' dates right) there was a firm opinion among physicians and pharmacologists that the opium poppy was in many instances too dangerous to employ as a drug. It is, however, in the hexameters of Nicander of Colophon (second century BC) that one initially gains a full view of Hellenistic recognition of opium poisoning, indicating lucidly enough how physicians and pharmacologists regarded the fatal potentials when someone quaffed too much of the 'tears of the poppy'.[57] Significantly, Nicander's verb is 'when they drink' (*pinōsin*),[58] showing that opium latex was well known as a drug in solution, and those who drink it 'fall completely asleep'. Also noteworthy is the similarity of Nicander's description of impending death to that given by modern physiological toxicologists:

> their extremities are chilled; their eyes do not open but are bound quite motionless by their eyelids. With the exhaustion an odorous sweat bathes all the body, turns cheeks pale, and causes the lips to swell; the bonds of the jaw are relaxed, and through the throat the laboured breath passes faint and chill. And often either the livid nail or wrinkled nostril is a harbinger of death; sometimes too the sunken eyes.[59]

Nicander's suggested antidotes include hot wine, and the syrup made from grapes, as well as the oil of roses, olive oil, the oil of the iris, and slapping the hapless victim on the cheeks, shaking him too, hoping that vomiting will follow, 'ridding him of the fatal affliction'.[60]

A precious moment of Roman pharmacy is the *Compositiones* by Scribonius Largus, a tract that records what a well-versed physician–pharmacologist would recommend in the reign of Claudius (AD 41–54).[61] Opium latex (almost certainly *Papaver somniferum* L. in the recipes of Scribonius Largus) is a frequent ingredient in eye-salves (here *collyria*), ranging from gentle ones (*collyria lenia*),[62] to harsher ointments (*collyria acria*).[63] Scribonius' grouping of recipes for itch-salve (*collyrium psoricum*) includes two formulas containing opium latex,[64] and a Roman pound of opium is part of a six-ingredient drug applied in the treatment of nasal polyps.[65] Dehydrated opium figures in a compound drug for difficult breathing,[66] and many *catapotia* ('pills' here to function like cough drops) for coughs feature opium as a prominent constituent.[67] Scribonius prescribes opium much less for internal afflictions,[68] and there appears to be some caution perhaps inherited in part from his Hellenistic Greek medical texts, a caution in recommending opium for internal consumption. In the section titled *Ad opium*,[69] Scribonius follows the main lines already observed in Nicander's *Alexipharmaca* regarding the signs of opium poisoning (head becomes heavy, cold sweat, laboured breathing, deep sleep), and getting the person to vomit – using a feather or leather strap in the back of the throat – after forcing down some water mixed with oil is the first recommendation. Wine, vinegar, more oil, rose oil, more vinegar, and mustard follow in succession: one wonders, indeed, if the feet and legs plastered with a solution of mustard pounded in vinegar[70] would prevent the patient from falling back into sleep. Keeping the victim awake was essential.

By Pliny the Elder's day (the *Natural History* was dedicated to Titus in AD 77), an overdose was a common manner of committing suicide, as in the case of the father of Publius Licinius Caecina,[71] a senator during the short reign of Galba (AD 68–9). Pliny adds weightily to his tale of P. Licinius Caecina's father, *item plerosque alios* ('and thus also several others'), indicating that opium poppy latex was ordinarily available and occasionally used to end one's life *cum valetudo inpetilibus odium vitae fecessit* ('when an unbearable disease had rendered life hateful'). There is no mention of physicians or other medical specialists who might have been involved in procuring the opium, so one assumes the drug was sold openly and anyone could purchase it at one of the numerous druggists' stalls, where one could buy any medicament desired.[72]

Pliny and his sources, one of whom was Sextius Niger, also known and used by Dioscorides,[73] were observing the effects of the 'crude' opium latex, a complex mixture of 'at least 50 alkaloids, with the major constituent being morphine'[74] (morphine averages about 16%),[75] and the 'natural' combination provides a far different physiological and biochemical action in the body compared to one of the alkaloids acting alone. In fact, until Friedrich Wilhelm Sertürner isolated morphine from raw opium (his classic paper on the topic was published in 1817),[76] the observed physiological and pharmaceutical properties of opium resulted only from the combination of effects from the raw opium's multiple alkaloids. And in contrast to the lay person's assumption that opium latex (used in whatever form) is as potent as morphine or its laboratory-produced product heroin (made from morphine by replacing both hydroxyls with acetyl $-COCH_3$), a toxic dose of opium must be ten times larger than an equivalence of morphine for fatal effects.[77] Crude opium contains morphine (up to 20%), noscapine (up to 8%), codeine (up to 2.5%), papaverine (up to 2.5%), thebaine (up to 2%), and smaller amounts of narceine, protopine, hydrocotarnine, and the other alkaloids, as well as meconic acid (the fifty alkaloids are largely combined with this organic acid) and some lactic and sulfuric acid among other constituents including up to 25% water.[78] Raw opium's analgesic action results generally from its morphine, which acts directly as a depressant on the thalamus, the sensory cortex, and the respiratory and cough centres, but other alkaloids (especially codeine, papaverine, narceine, noscapine, and thebaine) have stimulant action on the medulla and the spinal cord; papaverine and noscapine, in particular, relax intestinal muscle, thereby providing a modern explanation of raw opium's use since antiquity in the treatment of diarrhoeas.

Hellenistic and Roman medicine had many salves and ointments enriched with ingredients presumed to have – in the modern terminology – transdermal action, and such remedies incorporating opium have continued to be used through the centuries, even though some modern authorities deny their effectiveness.[79] Cooling oil of roses mixed with opium poppy's latex was presumed to be a good headache remedy:[80] the latex and rose-oil were used as an embrocation, applied as would be the usual liquid medicament prepared for external use. The petals of *Rosa* spp., of course, are still utilized to produce the famous volatile oil (Attar of Rose, or Oleum rosae),[81] which remains important in the perfume industry. By the early twentieth century, however, rose-oil had assumed a minor role in pharmacy and medicine, becoming a 'grateful perfume' added to alcoholic preparations for internal use, as well as to wax-salves (cerates) and ointments. 'It is both too expensive and too powerful for most pharmaceutic purposes.'[82] Dioscorides also recommends opium poppy latex (again in liquid form),[83] in combination with almond-oil, saffron, and myrrh as a remedy for earaches: one pours or instils the mixture into the ear. As an eye-salve (or *collyrion*: a term not used here by Dioscorides), opium latex was combined with saffron and baked egg-yolk, and again one meets opium latex (this time in vinegar) as a treatment for erysipelas. For gout (the Greek literally says 'for pains in the feet'), opium latex joined with 'a woman's milk' and saffron was deemed effective as an external remedy. And as his last suggestion among the most useful applications of the opium poppy's latex, Dioscorides writes, 'And applied to a finger and used like a suppository, the latex induces sleep.'[84]

Almond-oil is derived from the seeds of *Amygdalus communis* L., and this fixed oil is an excellent vehicle for oily injections,[85] but almond-oil's major physiological action (as a mild laxative) is irrelevant here. Saffron is the dried stigmas of the styles of the saffron crocus (*Crocus sativus* L.), and any drug – ancient or modern – which included this as an ingredient would be costly: '100,000 flowers are needed to produce 1 kg of saffron.'[86] Saffron-oil (from the stigmas and petals) contains up to thirty-four components, mainly terpenes, terpene alcohols, and esters, and the effect of these constituents as part of an ear instillation would combine with those of the opium latex. Opium tinctures with saffron remain in the pharmacopoeias, and Sydenham's Laudanum (a tincture made with opium, cinnamon, clove, and saffron) is listed in the Martindale *Extra Pharmacopoeia*, 28th edn of 1982.[87] Modern pharmacology employs saffron in combination with opium (Sydenham's Laudanum is adjusted to contain 1% w/v of anhydrous morphine, with recommended dosage of 0.25 to 2 ml), and it is probable that Greco-Roman pharmacologists understood the benefits of combining saffron with opium. It might be instructive to ascertain what pharmaceutical properties are presumed in modern earache remedies, and one could predict some parallels from ancient to modern.

The pharmaceutical properties of baked egg-yolk and human milk, used as external applications, do not appear in the professional literature, although 'alum curds' (eggs beaten with alum) were commonly employed as an astringent in the early twentieth century,[88] and a milk-soaked piece of bread applied to a boil remains a favoured folk remedy in many countries. Dioscorides' finger-coated opium suppository does, however, have its near-modern corollary: 'Suppositories of opium with lead have been used to relieve rectal and pelvic pain, and Gall and Opium Ointment is used for haemorrhoids.'[89] Modern literature and research on opium do not indicate any soporific effects, even though Dioscorides and his sources are quite certain of this result.

Myrrh is, of course, the famous oleo-gum-resin collected as reddish-brown lumps from natural cracks in the bark of *Balsamodendron myrrha* (= *Commiphora myrrha* (Nees.) Engl.) and related species of what Majno calls a 'scraggly, unfriendly tree of "crippled appearance"'[90] native to north-eastern Africa and southern Arabia. Greco-Roman medicine used myrrh in numerous manners,[91] but Dioscorides' ear-instillation of myrrh as combined with opium, almond-oil, and saffron had observed and reliable effects and benefits, especially if there chanced to be open sores or wounds in the external auditory meatus. Myrrh in solution (the lumps dissolve easily in water) is bacteriostatic against gram-positive bacteria, including the most 'typical wound bacterium, *Staphylococcus aureus*'.[92] If one considers the probable microbe-reducing properties in saffron now fused with specificity against gram-positive bacteria, and add the analgesic effects of opium, one ascertains what surely was a useful drug for ear troubles. Again Dioscorides is prescribing opium in a manner both cautious and helpful, and his combination of ingredients can elicit respect, even from modern pharmacologists. This short listing, moreover, of opium-remedies is all that Dioscorides recommends, indicating his care and painstaking observation throughout his career on what drugs 'do' and how they can be used safely.

Materia Medica, IV, 64. 5–7, takes up no further applications and uses of opium latex or any preparations of drugs from the opium poppy, but how to detect 'fake opium', followed by the short refutation of earlier Hellenistic authorities who had rejected opium in medical therapeutics; and finally (IV, 64. 7) is Dioscorides' description of how one harvests and prepares the opium poppy, both as a whole and as the latex alone; and if we recall that he has already specified an important 'when' for such harvesting – 'while [the poppy capsules] are still green' (*Materia Medica*, IV, 64. 2) – there is a hidden if very significant reason for this tradition of slitting or use of the whole capsule at this particular stage of its growth, a tradition 'explained' through modern chemistry. The centuries-old knowledge of the best time to harvest the latex, a knowledge gained by ancient farmers and botanists through a millennial trial-and-error, has received a remarkable confirmation from the study of biogenetics and phytochemistry.

The determination of the biogenesis of the opium alkaloids is, as one modern text puts it, 'a brilliant chapter in the history of phytochemical research'.[93] The first major alkaloid formed in the poppy capsule is thebaine, followed by an irreversible conversion to codeine, and then into morphine. The actual phytochemical process is, of course, far more complex than indicated by this simple summary, but one now perceives an answer to why ancient and modern harvesting of the opium latex occurs before the plant reaches full maturity. Ancient physicians and pharmacologists knew that the potency of opium latex had attained a certain level somewhat before the poppy capsule was fully ripened, and probably also understood that this particular level of potency suited medical employment within what we might call a margin of safety. One would welcome a future research project among phytochemists or pharmacologists which would demonstrate how much naturally occurring morphine is in the ripened poppy capsule: is the 20% morphine the greatest amount achieved (that is, the amount one finds when the capsules are slit while still green), or, is the more matured poppy capsule latex even more dangerous than the occasionally fatal substance widely utilized in Hellenistic and Roman medicine and pharmacy?

Comparison of harvesting techniques in a modern text,[94] with those given by Dioscorides in *c.* AD 70, shows little has changed over the centuries. Dioscorides' 'while still green' is a little more refined into when 'the colour is changing from green to yellow',[95] but even with more standard tools like scrapers, pan-receivers, and knives and multiple incision-makers,[96] there is little that marks a difference between modern Turkish or Indian latex gathering and the methods described by Dioscorides:

And it is not out of place to sketch out also the way in which they collect the juice [latex]; some, on the one hand, after beating the capsules with the leaves, squeeze it out through a press and pounding it in a mortar, they fashion lozenges: this as such is called *mēkōnion*, being less efficacious than the juice [latex]. But when extracting the latex, one ought to draw in the outline [*i.e.* cut] the 'little star' with a knife after the dew has evaporated, so that the incision does not perforate into the inside of the capsule, and to cut in from the top straight lines on the sides of the capsules, and to attach off the tear that comes out into a sea-mussel (*myax*) shell, and again to come back to this capsule after a short time; for there is to be found another congealed tear, and also another is to be found on the following day; one ought to pound it in a mortar and lay it up for storage when made into lozenges; and indeed in cutting the capsule for the latex one ought to stand back so that the latex is not attached to one's clothing.[97]

Drug fraud was common in Classical antiquity,[98] and detecting counterfeit opium was part of a physician's duty and skills. Dioscorides' methods are worthy of quotation in full, marked as they are by clarity and simplicity:

5. Best is the latex (*opos*) which is thick and heavy and soporific to the smell, bitter to the taste, easily diluted in water, smooth, white, neither rough nor full of lumps nor congealing as one passes it through [a sieve] as is [characteristic] of wax; set out in the sun and spreading, and being kindled by a lamp, it does not have a darkly coloured flame, retaining indeed its own particular odour. But they counterfeit it by mixing the juice of the horned poppy (*glaukion*) or acacia-gum (*kommi*) or the juice of the wild lettuce; that which is made from the juice of the horned poppy is like saffron in the solution, and that made from the lettuce loses its odour and is rougher, and that made from the acacia-gum is weak and translucent.

6. And some people are attended by so much madness so as to mix animal fat (*stear*) with it. And it is roasted in a new earthenware pot to make the eye-salves (*ta ophthalmika*) until it should appear soft and more tawny-orange.[99]

Modern opium remains an important item of illicit commerce, and it is not surprising that one finds the following in a contemporary reference on medicinal plants: 'The juice [of the horned poppy, *Glaucium flavum* Crantz] is used as a purgative, sedative and as an adulterant for opium',[100] and the gum from *Acacia* 'is light brown',[101] the latter showing why Dioscorides takes pains to write how the fake opium made from acacia is 'translucent' (*diaugēs*), and that the 'real stuff' is tawny-orange after roasting.

Finally, one can conclude with the role of opium in the famous theriacs of antiquity, especially the multi-ingredient drugs one reads in extensive quotation as given in the writings of Galen of Pergamon (AD 129–after 210). Much can be gleaned on the problems of theriacs and mithridatium in the book on the topic by Watson, but as a major ingredient of theriacs, opium is obscured in modern scholarship by assumptions that anyone who indulged regularly in opium-laced drugs would be as subject to addiction as twentieth-century dependants on heroin. In what may be a slip of the pen or perhaps rapid skimming of the texts of Galen – and finding what he expected to find – Watson
* writes 'Disconnected passages about Marcus [Aurelius] in [Galen's] writings, when pieced together, make a story of particular value, since it is the only case-record of a patron or addict of these fortifiers and remedies.'[102] That word 'addict' leaps out at any modern reader, and as such obliterates the context and sense of Galen's verbose account of exactly what the emperor Marcus Aurelius consumed and why he consumed it, presumably under Galen's direction.

Opium does figure as a major ingredient in the galene-poem by Andromachus the Elder,[103] and following the full quotation of this poem, Galen then lists the contents of a galene-formula by Andromachus the Younger which specifies 24 drachmas of opium.[104] A 'galene' to Galen is a broadly applied theriac: in addition to being a prophylactic against poisoning and the bites and stings of venomous animals, it was a kind of all-round, multi-ingredient preparation intended to promote a sense of well-being, comparable to modern anti-depressants (Andromachus the Younger's galene has just under sixty ingredients, with opium as number six, followed by oil of roses). Galen notes that he does, indeed, follow the formula of Andromachus (which of the two is not indicated) in his preparation of theriac (= ? galene) for the 'use of the royalty',[105] but Galen also writes that Marcus is taking as well a four-ingredient theriac (aristolochia, bitumen, rue, bitter vetch – to be taken in wine and oil (the drug first prepared as lozenges)) invented by Heras,[106] and there is no opium in the short formula.

Key passages on the question are in Galen's *Antidotes*, 1, 1,[107] and here one does read that Marcus Aurelius did consume daily the drug called Mithridatium in a dose measured to the size of an Egyptian bean.[108] And depending on whether Marcus wanted to sleep or to feel good about dealing with the day-to-day duties of being an emperor, the opium content was adjusted accordingly. Galen, moreover, points out that the emperor could distinguish high-quality theriac from that prepared from inferior ingredients,[109] suggesting not only that Marcus was well aware of particular effects from specific components but also that Galen shared with his royal patient exact and technical methodologies regarding the preparation of theriacs. Marcus Aurelius took his daily dose of Mithridatium with large quantities of honey,[110] and one can assume a 'sugar high' added to the elevated mood engendered by the opium in the theriac/galene.

One needs to recall that true addiction to opium requires greater and greater dosages to maintain the sensations of well-being,[111] and from the evidence teased from Galen's off-handed comments about how and when Marcus Aurelius used opium, the emperor was not addicted to opium. Marcus and his doctor knew exactly what they were doing and they used opium (among the many other ingredients in theriacs or galenes) carefully and with good control over physiological effects. One must infer from Galen's remarks that the emperor could 'cutback' on the opium as required in his function to perform his duties as ruler of the Roman Empire, and that on its own indicates Marcus Aurelius was not an opium addict. Perhaps we are afflicted with the negative nuances, currently in vogue regarding so-called 'addictive' substances, and one could easily make analogy to an 'addiction' (if so termed) to salicylates taken daily, even as physicians now recommend daily dosages of aspirin for the prevention of cardiac and vascular problems. Perhaps, too, as we peer and ponder the texts on opium and the anodynes commonly prepared from the latex of the opium poppy in Classical antiquity, we unwittingly reflect a common fear – exhibited by both lay persons and medical professionals – that opium's alkaloids are more dangerous than helpful. Physicians and their patients in Hellenistic and Roman times do not display this general unease, even as our shrewd ancestors were fully aware of the fatal consequences of opium overdoses. Perhaps we should always put 'addiction' in a context of interpretation, according to the social opinions which dominate a particular era.

NOTES

Unless otherwise specified, translations from the Greek or Latin are by the present author.

1 On this and related matters, see my 'The Pharmacology of Sacred Plants, Herbs, and Roots', in Christopher A. Faraone and Dirk Obbink, eds., *Magika Hiera: Ancient Greek Magic and Religion* (Oxford, 1991), pp. 138–74 (esp. pp. 139–42).

2 Homer, *Iliad*, VIII, 306–7; *Odyssey*, IV, 220–30.

3 Theophrastus, *Historia plantarum*, IX, 8. 2. See my 'Theophrastus on Herbals and Herbal Remedies', *Journal of the History of Biology*, 11 (1978), pp. 353–85.

4 E. Littré, ed., *Oeuvres complètes d'Hippocrate*, 10 vols. (Paris, 1839–61), x, p. 725 (index refs.: *pavot*).

5 Dioscorides, IV, 64. 6 = Max Wellmann, ed., *Pedanii Dioscuridis Anazarbei De materia medica*, 3 vols. (Berlin, 1906–14; repr. 1958), II, pp. 220–1.

6 In spite of Wellmann's confidence that Diagoras of Cyprus can be dated to the third century BC, there is great uncertainty regarding this physician, whose works are embedded in Pliny's *Natural History*, and against whom Dioscorides argues about opium. M. Wellmann, 'Diagoras (3)', in *Paulys Realencyclopädie der classischen Alterumswissenschaft* (= *RE*), V, pt 1 (Stuttgart, 1903), col. 311.

7 M. Wellmann, 'Andreas (11)', *RE*, I, pt 2 (Stuttgart, 1894), cols. 2136–7.

8 Dioscorides' citation of Mnesidimus is the single reference to this otherwise unknown Hellenistic physician, who appears to have been a noted authority on the opium poppy. K. Deichgräber, 'Mnesidemos (2)', *RE*, XV, pt 2 (Munich, 1901), col. 2275.

9 Nicander, *Alexipharmaca*, 433–64 = A. S. F. Gow and A. F. Scholfield, eds., *Nicander. The Poems and Poetical Fragments* (Cambridge, 1953), pp. 122–5.

10 W. G. Spencer, ed. and trans., *Celsus. De medicina*, 3 vols. (London, 1935–8), II, p. xlvi.

11 See John Scarborough and Vivian Nutton, 'The *Preface* of Dioscorides' *Materia Medica*: Introduction, Translation, Commentary', *Transaction and Studies of the College of Physicians of Philadelphia*, n.s., 4 (1982), pp. 187–227 (esp. 187–95).

12 John M. Riddle, *Dioscorides on Pharmacy and Medicine* (Austin, Tex., 1985), pp. 94–131.

13 Dioscorides, IV, 64. 6 (ed. Wellmann, II, p. 221).

14 Theophrastus, *Enquiry into Plants*, IX, 12. 4 = A. F. Hort, ed. and trans., *Theophrastus. Enquiry into Plants and Minor Works on Odours and Weather Signs*, 2 vols. (London, 1916), II, pp. 280–1.

15 See my 'Pharmacy in Pliny's *Natural History*: Some Observations on Substances and Sources', in Roger French and Frank Greenaway, eds., *Science in the Early Roman Empire: Pliny the Elder, his Sources and Influence* (London, 1986), pp. 59–85 (esp. 62 and 64).

16 Scarborough and Nutton, '*Preface* of Dioscorides' *Materia Medica*', p. 202.

17 Pliny, *Natural History*, XX, 200.

18 E.g. Oribasius, *Medical Collection*, V, 18–20 = J. Raeder, ed., *Oribasii Collectionum medicarum reliquiae*, 4 vols. (Leipzig, 1928–33), IV, pp. 132–6 (from the works of Galen and Philagrius).

19 Galen, *Compounding Drugs According to Place [on the Body]*, VII, 2 = C. G. Kühn, ed., *Claudii Galeni Opera omnia*, 20 vols. in 22 pts (Leipzig, 1821–33; repr. Hildesheim, 1964–5), XIII, pp. 38–47. In further citations, this edition of Galen's works will appear simply as 'K.,' with volume and page.

20 Asclepiades as cited may be Asclepiades of Bithynia (*fl.* in Rome *c.* 120 BC), but more likely Galen's source here is Asclepiades Pharmacion, a noted writer on drugs who lived in the reigns of Vespasian and Titus (AD 69–81). Cajus Fabricius, *Galens Exzerpte aus älteren Pharmakologen* (Berlin, 1972), p. 103. Galen, *Compounding Drugs According to Place*, X, 3 = K., XIII, p. 360, is a key passage for dating Asclepiades Pharmacion. Themison of Laodicea *fl.* in Rome under Augustus (31 BC–AD 14), and floats uncertainty as a 'pupil' of Asclepiades of Bithynia and one of the purported founders of the medical sect called

Methodists. For a cogent discussion of Themison's role in the development of Methodist theory, see now J. T. Vallance, *The Lost Theory of Asclepiades of Bithynia* (Oxford, 1990), pp. 141–2.

21 Galen, *Compounding Drugs According to Place*, VII, 2 = K., XIII, pp. 40–2. Servilius Damocrates *fl.* in the reigns of Nero and Vespasian (AD 54–79), and little of his writing is known except for quotations by Galen. M. Wellmann, 'Damokrates (8)', *RE*, IV, pt 2 (Stuttgart, 1901), cols. 2069–70. Fabricius, *Galens Exzerpte*, p. 189.

22 Soranus of Ephesus (*fl.* AD 98–117) wrote voluminously, but surviving in Greek are only his masterwork, *Gynecology*, and two shorter tracts *Signs of Fractures* and *On Bandages*, as well as a *Life of Hippocrates* = J. Ilberg, ed., *Sorani Gynaeciorum libri IV. De signis fracturarum. De fasciis. Vita Hippocratis secundum Soranum* (Leipzig, 1927). One knows of Soranus' writings on drugs solely through citations and quotations by Galen, E. Kind, 'Soranus aus Ephesos', *RE*, 2nd series, III, pt 1 (Stuttgart, 1927), cols. 1113–30 (esp. 1128–9). Criton (*fl.* AD 96–117) accompanied his royal patron on the Dacian campaigns, and became one of the ancient physicians who also wrote history. See my 'Criton, Physician to Trajan: Historian and Pharmacist', in John W. Eadie and Josiah Ober, eds., *The Craft of the Ancient Historian: Essays in Honor of Chester G. Starr* (Lanham, MD., 1985), pp. 387–405.

23 Heras of Cappadocia *fl.* in Rome *c.* 20 BC–AD 20, so Fabricius, 'Die Zeit des Heras' in his *Galens Exzerpte*, pp. 242–6. Quoted frequently by Galen, Heras investigated the properties of simples (Fabricius, *Galens Exzerpte*, pp. 209–12, lists the important ones), and became a widely used authority on drugs and compound medicines. Galen, *Compounding Drugs According to Place*, III, 1 = K., XII, p. 610, gives a formula for Heras' multiple-ingredient medicament 'For All Pains and Wounds in the Ear' quite similar to the recipe in Dioscorides, IV, 64. 4 (ed. Wellmann, II, 220). Heras includes the opium poppy, but adds frankincense to the portion of myrrh, and omits rose-oil, which Galen suggests one ought to reinclude (perhaps reflecting Dioscorides' formula).

24 Galen, *Compounding Drugs According to Place*, VII, 2 = K., XIII, pp. 43–5.

25 Dioscorides, IV, 64. 1 (ed. Wellmann, II, p. 218).

26 Cf. Galen, *Mixtures and Properties of Simples*, VII, 12. 13 = K., XII, pp. 72–4.

27 James A. Duke, *Handbook of Medicinal Herbs* (Boca Raton, Fla., 1985), p. 344. Paul G. Stecher *et al.*, eds., *The Merck Index*, 8th edn (Rahway, N.J., 1968), p. 850.

28 Duke, *Handbook*, p. 344.

29 E.g. Oribasius, *Medical Collection*, I = ed. Raeder, I, 4–27.

30 Cf. Duke, *Handbook*, p. 344.

31 Dioscorides, IV, 64. 1 (ed. Wellmann, II, pp. 218–19).

32 Galen, *Blendings*, III, 1 = G. Helmreich, ed., *Glaudius Galenus De temperamentis libri III* (Leipzig, 1894; repr. Stuttgart, 1969), p. 87. Galen, *Causes of Diseases*, III = K., VII, p. 14.

33 Dioscorides, IV, 64. 2 (ed. Wellmann, II, p. 219).

34 Duke, *Handbook*, p. 344.

35 R. G. Todd, ed., *Extra Pharmacopoeia Martindale*, 25th edn (London, 1967), p. 810.

36 *Ibid.*, p. 802, doubts the traditional use of opium liniments and lotions: 'There is no evidence of local analgesic action.'

37 Dioscorides, IV, 64. 2 (ed. Wellmann, II, p. 219).
38 *Ibid.*
39 James E. F. Reynolds and Anne B. Prasad, eds., *Martindale: The Extra Pharmacopoeia*, 28th edn (London, 1982), p. 1029 (No. 6260-y).
40 E.g. George Edward Trease and William Charles Evans, *Pharmacognosy*, 1th edn (London, 1978), p. 576.
41 Dioscorides, IV, 64. 2 (ed. Wellmann, II, p. 219).
42 E.g. Pliny, *Natural History*, XXVI, 49; Galen, *Affected Parts*, II, 9 = K., VIII, p. 114). Cf. Dioscorides, I, 97 (ed. Wellmann, I, pp. 87–9).
43 Soranus, *Gynecology*, I, 50. 3 (ed. Ilberg, p. 36).
44 Reynolds and Prasad, eds., *Martindale*, p. 949 (No. 5402-m).
45 William Charles Evans, *Trease and Evans' Pharmacognosy*, 13th edn (London, 1989), p. 373.
46 Susan Budavari *et al.*, eds., *The Merck Index*, 11th edn (Rahway, N.J., 1989), p. 11 (No. 10).
47 Wolfgang Schneider, *Lexikon zur Arzneimittelgeschichte*, 7 vols. in 9 parts (Frankfurt, 1968–75), V, pt 1, p. 419.
48 Dioscorides, I, 97. 2 (ed. Wellmann, I, pp. 87–8). Galen, *Mixtures and Properties of Simples*, VII, 10. 27 = K., XII, 27–8.
49 Oleg Polunin, *Flowers of Europe* (London, 1969), p. 61.
50 So Wellmann in apparatus criticus to line 10, Dioscorides, I, 87.
51 Dioscorides, I, 97. 2 (ed. Wellmann, I, p. 88).
52 Dioscorides, IV, 64. 3 (ed. Wellmann, II, p. 220).
53 Dioscorides, IV, 64. 3 (ed. Wellmann, II, p. 219).
54 Pliny, *Natural History*, XX, 199.
55 Albert F. Hill, *Economic Botany*, 2nd edn (New York, 1952), p. 279.
56 Duke, *Handbook*, p. 345.
57 Nicander, *Alexipharmaca*, 433.
58 *Ibid.*, 434.
59 *Ibid.*, 434–42. The translation is by Gow and Scholfield, *Nicander*, p. 123.
60 Nicander, *Alexipharmaca*, 460.
61 Sergio Sconocchia, ed., *Scribonii Largi Compositiones* (Leipzig, 1983), pp. vi–vii. Scribonius Largus accompanied Claudius in the Roman invasion of England in AD 43.
62 *Ibid.*, pp. 19–27.
63 *Ibid.*, pp. 28–31.
64 *Ibid.*, pp. 32 and 33.
65 *Ibid.*, p. 52.
66 *Ibid.*, p. 77.
67 *Ibid.*, pp. 85–93.
68 E.g. *ibid.*, pp. 112, 115, and 120.
69 *Ibid.*, p. 180.
70 'sinapi ex aceto tritum circumdatum pedibus cruribusque et a somni tempore prohibere'.
71 Pliny, *Natural History*, XX, 199–200. Tacitus, *Histories*, II, 53.
72 Pliny, *Natural History*, XXIV, 108.
73 Scarborough, 'Pharmacy in Pliny's *Natural History*', p. 67.
74 George Lenz *et al.*, *Opiates* (Orlando, Fla., 1986), p. 2.

75 Budavari *et al.*, eds., *Merck Index*, p. 6810 (No. 6809).
76 Ronald D. Mann, *Modern Drug Use. An Inquiry on Historical Principles* (Boston, Mass., 1984), p. 471.
77 Todd, ed., *Martindale*, p. 801.
78 Budavari *et al.*, eds., *Merck Index*, p. 6810 (No. 6809) with refs.
79 E.g. Todd, ed., *Martindale*, p. 802 (opium).
80 Dioscorides, IV, 64. 4 (ed. Wellmann, II, p. 220).
81 Trease and Evans, *Pharmacognosy*, p. 411.
82 Horatio C. Wood, Charles H. LaWall *et al.*, *The Dispensatory of the United States of America*, 22nd edn (Philadelphia, 1937), p. 773.
83 Dioscorides, IV, 64. 4 (ed. Wellmann, II, p. 220).
84 *Ibid.*
85 Trease and Evans, *Pharmacognosy*, p. 313.
86 George Usher, *A Dictionary of Plants Used by Man* (London, 1974), p. 183.
87 Reynolds and Prasad, eds., *Martindale*, p. 1022.
88 Wood and LaWall *et al.*, eds., *Dispensatory*, p. 805.
89 Todd, ed., *Martindale*, p. 802; dropped from *Martindale*, 28th ed.
90 Guido Majno, *The Healing Hand, Man and Wound in the Ancient World* (Cambridge, Mass., 1975), p. 212.
91 *Ibid.*, pp. 215–17, with refs.
92 *Ibid.*, p. 217.
93 Trease and Evans, *Pharmacognosy*, p. 561.
94 Evans, *Trease and Evans' Pharmacognosy*, p. 583.
95 Trease and Evans, *Pharmacognosy*, p. 570.
96 *Ibid.*, p. 571, with Fig. 170.
97 Dioscorides, IV, 64. 7 (ed. Wellmann, II, pp. 221).
98 See esp. Vivian Nutton, 'The Drug Trade in Antiquity', *Journal of the Royal Society of Medicine*, 78 (1985), pp. 138–45.
99 Dioscorides, IV, 64. 5–6 (ed. Wellmann, II, p. 220).
100 Usher, *Dictionary*, p. 275.
101 *Ibid.*, p. 12.
102 Gilbert Watson, *Theriac and Mithridatium* (London, 1966), p. 87.
103 Galen, *Antidotes*, I, 6 = K., XIV, pp. 32–42, esp. line 121 of the poem. Andromachus the Elder was physician to Nero (AD 54–68), and his son, Andromachus the Younger, also functioned as a court doctor in the reign of Nero. Fabricius, *Galens Exzerpte*, pp. 185–6.
104 Galen, *Antidotes*, I, 7 = K., XIV, pp. 42–4, esp. 42.
105 Galen, *Theriac to Piso*, 12 = K., XIV, p.262.
106 Galen, *Antidotes*, II, 17 = K., XIV, p. 201.
107 K., XIV, pp. 3 and 5.
108 Galen, *Antidotes*, I, 1 = K., XIV, p. 4.
109 Galen, *Antidotes*, I, 1 = K., XIV, p. 5.
110 Roman medicine included honey as a potent drug, employed in numerous manners, as one reads in many passages and sections of Galen's writings, e.g. *Mixtures and Properties of Simples*, VII, 12. 9 = K., XII, pp. 70–1. Dioscorides, II, 82 (ed. Wellmann, I, pp. 165–7) is probably the most concise summary of pharmaceutical properties, as understood in Hellenistic and Roman pharmacy. What

Dioscorides terms *sakcharon* in II, 82. 4 (Wellmann, I, p. 167) is, incidentally, one of our first references to sugar cane from India.

111 A classic description remains that in Solomon Solis-Cohen and Thomas Stotesbury Githens, *Pharmacotherapeutics* (New York, 1928), p. 263.

VIII

Roman Pharmacy and the Eastern Drug Trade

Some Problems as Illustrated by the Example of Aloe

AN IMPORTANT aspect of Roman drug lore and the prescription of pharmaceuticals in Roman medicine are plants and plant-products that are imported from the "East."[1] Some can be identified with fair assurance, since * they have long histories going back at least into Dynastic Egypt (viz. frankincense, myrrh),[2] and several 'spices' turn up as valued substances in the Linear B tablets of the Mycenaens.[3] Many of the drugs and simples that Dioscorides lists as "Indian" have origins in what we would know as Ethiopia and the wider areas encompassing the headwaters of the Blue Nile,[4] and we can discard many of the assumptions of Bretzl who sought to prove that many drugs were introduced into Greek pharmacy as a result of Alexander the Great's far-flung military expeditions into Bactria and India.[5] Crucial for such conclusions are the citations of "eastern" plants by Theophrastus, and except for several vague references to "Indian" locales, there is little to suggest a new Far Eastern pharmacopeia that enriched Greek pharmacy in the 4th century B.C.[6] Most of the herbs described by Theophrastus in Book IX of the *Historia Plantarum*, as well as other species in his *On Odors*, can be placed within "local" origins: the plants grew somewhere within the usual orbit of Greek contacts and trade in the eastern Mediterranean, as well as Egypt, Syria, Asia Minor through the lands of the Tigris and Euphrates, the littoral of the Black Sea, and north Africa's coastline as far west as the holdings of Carthage; Theophrastus and his sources also knew a good deal about the northern Balkans, which provides a solid context for the "exotic" drug derived from the iris.[7] One can, to take another example, explain the "exotic" nature of silphium from its specific growing areas in Greek Cyrene,[8] and also make note of the particular exceptions to this Greek-dominated commercial world with the examples of frankincense and myrrh, which had been imported from southern and eastern Arabia for many centuries.[9]

By the time that Dioscorides wrote his *Materia Medica* (*c.* A.D. 65), this limited scope had broadened considerably. Not only are the traditional spices and herbs listed–pharmaceuticals repeated from the listings of Theophrastus[10] and Apollodorus[11] (best known through Nicander's borrowing of botanical and toxicological data in the *Theriaca* and *Alexipharmaca*, composed late in the 2nd century B.C.[12])–but Dioscorides now includes a number of plants that are, indeed, imported from the east, beyond Roman territory and even farther east than the extent of the Hellenistic Greek kingdoms of Bactria and India. Yet not all of these plants, designated as "Far Eastern" by modern scholars, are from the "East" in Dioscorides' day: Sesame seeds and oil, assumed to be imported from India by Miller,[13] are known from Ptolemaic Egyptian papyri as a "cash crop" in the 3rd century B.C.;[14] cardamom likewise grew in Egypt,[15] so that one does not have to assume a Far Eastern origin for this herb in the early Roman imperial pharmacopeia;[16] and as Raschke has shown,[17] products called "Indian" in the sources do not necessarily come from the Asian subcontinent, *e.g.* the sweet flag or calamus, which grew in abundance along the marshy shores of the Red Sea.[18] Part of the problem, of course, lies in the designation of "India" in the Greek geographic documents,[19] and many "Indian" exports came from northeastern Africa, especially Ethiopia, Somaliland, and points along the western shore of the Red Sea. Another part of the problem resides in dating the Greek (viz. Ptolemaic Egyptian) discovery of the monsoon weather cycles, which enabled Greek (and later Roman) merchants and navigators to travel with relative ease to and from India and to ports farther east on the Asian coasts. Thus one must study the question of Far Eastern drugs in Roman pharmacy in connection with the history of navigation and seafaring as it developed in late Hellenistic times and in the early Roman Empire.

Unquestionably, pepper was brought from the East,[20] as were aloe,[21] frankincense,[22] myrrh,[23] ginger,[24] cloves,[25] spikenard,[26] cinnamon,[27] and the costus-root.[28] Cassia remains uncertain,[29] although extant evidence suggests origins in Arabia and east Africa,[30] and some doubt may be assumed about the Far Eastern origins of spikenard and the costus, since Theophrastus mentions them in vague terms that could suggest growth in areas of the upper Tigris-Euphrates, quite consistent with known botanical geography.[31] Each plant has particular problems of species-identity, pharmacological biochemistry as related to growth patterns and soil conditions, and the occasional question of a plant having a 'Far Eastern' name that becomes garbled or confused as it is transmitted into Greek. Attempts at transplanting exotic herbs were not generally successful in classical antiquity, as illustrated by Ptolemaic efforts to grow the frankincense tree in Egypt,[32] or the apparent reference by Dioscorides to the poor quality of aloe grown on Aegean Islands.[33] Pharmacologists in antiquity clearly recognized that several of these imported drugs could be grown only in particular places (*e.g.* silphium, aloe, frankincense, myrrh) so that the modern observer needs to resist the temptation to lump together the pharmaceutical qualities of a drug derived from a transplant with the properties described in the sources as characteristic of a "native" plant or drug. In fact, modern research has determined that the pharmaceutical properties of aloe in a transplanted state are far less than from the plant gained from its native locale.[34] Moreover, since aloe illustrates the interlocking aspects of the problems in considering the eastern drug trade and Roman pharmacy, specific examination of how aloe was used in Roman pharmacy, as well as species locality, can show why one must bring to bear an understanding of a number of related questions in studying eastern drugs as they appear in Roman pharmaceutical lists: Greek and Latin sources and their mention of the drug; species identity and geographic distribution; particular terms for the drug and possible confusion with other drugs; the history of commerce and trade by the Romans with the Far East; and approximation of the time of introduction of aloe into the West.

The Example of Aloe

In his *Materia Medica,* Dioscorides gives a prominent place to the plant he calls *aloē.*[35] Considered very useful in the treatment of skin irritations,[36] constipation,[37] and in medications to promote the healing of boils and wounds,[38] *aloē* also receives an important role in the pharmacy and pharmacology of Antyllus, Soranus, Aretaeus, Galen, and several other medical * writers of the 1st and 2nd centuries A.D.[39] The plant remained a staple of Byzantine pharmacy,[40] and retained a popularity in Arabic medicine, as indicated by its importance in the *Medical Formulary* of al-Kindī.[41] Among the Latin writers on medicine, only Celsus precedes Dioscorides in mentioning *aloē,* but Celsus' notice is oddly scrappy, with the plant listed only once in *De medicina* as a suggested laxative.[42] Pliny the Elder provides numerous references to *aloē* in his *Natural History,*[43] generally duplicating much of the information given by Dioscorides, suggesting that both had derived their data on *aloē* from a common source.[44] Details on the *aloē* were commonly available in the time of Dioscorides (*fl. c.* A.D. 65),[45] and Pliny the Elder (A.D. 23/24-79),[46] but, by contrast, relatively rare when Celsus composed his multi-subject encyclopedia, probably sometime during the reign of Tiberius (A.D. 14-37).[47]

Aloē does not appear in earlier Greek sources on medicine and pharmacy, although a number of 'new' plants are included by Theophrastus in the *Historia Plantarum.*[48] The plant does not occur in Nicander's famous collection of antidotes in his *Theriaca* and *Alexipharmaca,*[49] probably compiled late in the 2nd century B.C.,[50] nor do the Hippocratic writers mention *aloē* among the many drugs prescribed in such works as *Diseases of Women, Sterility, Regimen, Regimen in Acute Diseases, Fistula, Superfetation, Affections,* and others.[51] The plant called *aloē* in Greek is an addition to the Materia Medica of Greek and Roman pharmacy shortly before Celsus wrote *De medicina.* It is, of course, quite possible that *aloē* was known to the Hebrews by the 2nd century B.C., but the Septuagint translation of the *Song of Solomon* shows that the "aloe" included in the famous garden of herbs and spices is aloe-*wood,* not *aloē.*[52] Moreover, the aloe does not have an important place in Jewish medicine.[53]

From the description of *aloē* in Dioscorides and in later Greek and Latin sources,[54] one can determine that the plant is *Aloe perryi* Baker, the Socotrine aloe, from the island of Socotra, located in the Indian Ocean, 150 miles due east of Cape Guardafui (Somalia). Similar to other species of aloe – although with distinctive features – *e.g. A. ferox* Miller [the Cape aloe of South Africa], and *A. barbadensis* Miller [the Barbados aloe of the West Indies = *A. vera* L. = *A. vulgaris* la Marck], as well as several others,[55] the Socotrine aloe is a succulent liliaceous plant that forms clusters of very fleshy leaf blades which are normally prickly on the margins and tips; it is generally stemless, although occasional woody branching stems may occur, and the Socotrine aloe bears yellow-orange or red or white flowers on erect spikes with six-lobed, tubular perianths. *A. vera,* which occurs in southern Arabia and northeastern Africa, has become naturalized in Greece during recent centuries (although the derived drug lacks the potency of the 'true' or Socotrine aloe),[56] but medieval Arabic sources show that the favored species from Socotra remained the prime source for the 'best' aloe, and that Socotra continued to be the locale for the growth, gathering, and exportation of this particular species, so highly valued in Arabic, Syriac, and even more modern Persian and Arabic pharmacy.[57]

Nielsen doubts that the *aloē* of classical antiquity was the same drug that is known today,[58] but he is right only in terms of exact species. Most often used in aloe preparations is *A. vera* or *A. ferox,* the latter being of venerated employment by the Xhosa and Mfengu of South Africa.[59] *A. perryi* Baker from Socotra gives an inspissated juice that causes severe intestinal cramps,[60] and Dioscorides' statement about how *aloē* mixed with other medicines does not harm the stomach as much as the 'straight' product agrees remarkably with the modern ideas of the pharmacology of *A. perryi* Baker. Modern biochemistry has isolated a substance called aloin (barbaloin) from the plant, and aloin is a far milder laxative than the earlier preparations of the inspissated juice from the leaves of the plant. Veterinary medicine still employs aloe as a purgative for adult horses, cattle, sheep, and goats (and sometimes dogs), while milder derivatives (aloin and aloe-emodin [3-hydroxymethylchrysazin; rhubarbarone, also from various spp. of *Rheum*]) remain in the medical pharmacopeia as laxatives. Modern preparation of the drug follows procedures that were familiar to Dioscorides: leaves of the aloe are cut, placed in troughs, and the slowly exuding juice is collected; then the juice is placed in pans for evaporation of the volatile fractions, and the residue turns into a viscous, black mass which soon solidifies.[61] Antiquity knew this drug in its commonly-exported form, brittle and blackish-yellow shiny lozenges which could, in the case of the finest variety, be easily melted and combined with other drugs.[62]

DIOSCORIDES also provides the first detailed account of what is called *agalochon xylon,*[63] probably the aloe-wood of the *Song of Solomon,*[64] and which seems conflated with true *aloē* by both Celsus and Pliny.[65] This confusion may be due to the bitter taste noted for true *aloē* and the occasionally bitter taste of aloe-wood,[66] or from the garbling of the original names of both species which emerge from Sanskrit with 'aloe' being a slurred Semitic variant,[67] but Dioscorides specifically says that *agalochon xylon* is brought from India,[68] showing that drug lore in the early Roman Empire now included details about herbs and medicinals from the Indian subcontinent and probably farther east.[69] Unlike the clipped and vague references to 'Indian' plants that form part of Theophrastus' account, presumably reflecting Alexander's expedition into India and the Trans-Oxus in the 320's B.C.,[70] the data on drugs, herbs, and medical derivatives from India, Arabia, and the Far East in the pharmacopeia in the 1st century are succinct, ample, and doubtlessly mirror the increased traffic by trading vessels from the Red Sea to India.

This heavy trade in luxury items has been carefully studied by Warmington, Casson, and others,[71] but controversy attends the date when the monsoon patterns were discovered and exploited by Greek navigators. Once it became clear how the monsoon winds shifted fairly regularly by season – blowing from the northeast in the winter and from the southwest in the summer, in general – [72] merchants could tap directly the spice and herb markets of Arabia and India, as well as the eastern coast of Africa, as far south as Zanzibar.[73] The problem of dating the western discovery of the * monsoons is centered upon when Hippalus made his voyage(s), and the argument turns upon the interpretation of Strabo, II, 3. 4 (98).[74] Thiel asserts that Eudoxus and Hippalus should be considered more-or-less contemporaries,[75] and thus the original voyage to India by a Greek navigator-explorer, using the monsoons, occurred about 120 B.C. Other scholars have disagreed, and Rostovtzeff argues for a date of "common knowledge" of the monsoons of *c.* 70 B.C.[76] Tarn offers *c.* 100 B.C.,[77] and Cary and Warmington prefer the reign of Tiberius (A.D. 14-37).[78] Each modern authority admits that the ancient evidence for the 'original' voyage to India is subject to various interpretations, and that final conclusions on this question are impossible without further and explicit evidence from antiquity.

ONE can conclude that Indian spices, herbs, and medicinal plants became common in the pharmacy of the early Roman Empire from the accounts of Celsus, Dioscorides, and Pliny,[79] but the particular instance of *aloē* may aid also in narrowing the presumed time when the expanded trade in drugs coincided with common exploitation of the monsoon patterns. The choicest *aloē (A. perryi* Baker) is confined to the island of Socotra, and *A. vera* was exported to the West from Cana on the coast of Arabia, according to the author of the *Periplus of the Erythrean Sea.*[80] Both Cana and Socotra were logical ports of call for merchants "... going to and from India."[81] Dioscorides tells us that *aloē* grows in Asia, India, Arabia, and on "certain islands,"[82] with the implication that the juice derived from the *aloē* of Andros (perhaps naturalized from Arabia or Socotra in the 1st century) is far less potent than the product of "the other kind," viz. from another island, probably Socotra. Coupled with Galen's adaptation of the description of *aloē* by Heras of Cappadocia *(fl. c.* 25 B.C.),[83] the accounts of voyages from Roman Egypt to India and the data on *aloē* in Dioscorides show that the drug was new in Greco-Roman pharmaceutical lore, and, that *aloē* in some quantity had made its way to Rome early in the reign of Augustus (27 B.C. – A.D. 14). This suggests a date slightly after 30 B.C. for an expanded and heightened trade between India and Roman Egypt in the reign of Augustus, following a mid-century decline.[84] The introduction of *aloē* in large quantities is related to this growth in trade from the East, and, one may argue for an early date for the discovery of the monsoons (sometime before 100 B.C.), given this resurgence in commerce following a decline. Dioscorides may have borrowed his description of *aloē* from Heras of Cappadocia,[85] much as did Galen over a century later, but Celsus' mention of the plant indicates *aloē* was known in Rome shortly after its introduction into the pharmacy of the Greek east. One can assume that the fragments of Heracleides provide a check on the dating of Heras,[86] but the remnants of Heracleides' writings are woefully truncated and often lacking in context. Nonetheless, Heras of Cappadocia can be dated to *c.*

25 B.C., and his description of Socotrine *aloē* as borrowed by Dioscorides and Galen shows the introduction of the drug into western pharmacy, much as the history of *aloē's* exportation indicates a renewed employment of Socotra as a port of call to and from India.

Notes

1. Two recent studies concentrate on this aspect. J. Innes Miller, *The Spice Trade of the Roman Empire 29 B.C. to A.D. 641* (Oxford, 1969), and Manfred G. Raschke, "The Spice Trade" in *New Studies in Roman Commerce with the East* (in H. Temporini, ed., *Aufstieg und Niedergang der römischen Welt,* Vol. IX, part 2 [Berlin, 1978], pp. 605-1361), pp. 650-676.
2. Nigel Groom, *Frankincense and Myrrh* (London, 1981), 22-54. A. Lucas, "Notes on Myrrh and Stacte," *Journal of Egyptian Archaeology,* 23 (1937), 27-33.
3. *E.g.* cumin *(Cuminum cyminum* L.), fennel *(Foeniculum vulgare* Mill.), safflower *(Carthamus tinctoria* L.), pennyroyal *(Mentha pulegium* L.), and several others. L. R. Palmer, *Interpretation of Mycenaean Greek Texts* (Oxford, 1963), 271-273 [Nos. 166-168]. See also John Chadwick, *Documents in Mycenaean Greek,* 2nd ed. (Cambridge, 1973), 223-224, 228, and 231 [Nos. 103, 105, and 107], and Richard Janko, "Herbal Remedies at Pylos," *Minos,* 17 (1981), 30-34.
4. *E.g.* Dioscorides, I, 68, and V, 92 (ed. Wellmann).
5. Hugo Bretzl, *Botanische Forschungen des Alexanderzuges* (Leipzig, 1903) passim.
6. John Scarborough, "Theophrastus on Herbals and Herbal Remedies," *Journal of the History of Biology,* 11 (1978), 353-385.
7. Theophrastus, *Historia Plantarum,* I, 7. 2; *De causis plantarum,* VI, 11. 13.
8. Else Strantz, *Zur Silphionfrage* (Ansbach, 1909), 15-25. Shim'on Applebaum, *Jews and Greeks in Ancient Cyrene* (Leiden, 1979), 122-125.
9. G. van Beck, "Frankincense and Myrrh in Ancient South Arabia," *Journal of the American Oriental Society,* 78 (1958), 141-152. A. Grohmann, *Südarabien als Wirtschaftsgebiet* (Prague, 1930), 127-142 and 148-155. Groom, *Frankincense and Myrrh,* 22-37.
10. H. Stadler, "Theophrast und Dioscorides," *Abhandlungen aus dem Gebiet der klassischen Altertums-Wissenschaft: Wilhelm von Christ zum sechzigsten Geburtstag dargebracht von seinen Schülern* (Munich, 1891), 176-187.
11. Max Wellmann, "Das älteste Kräuterbuch der Griechen," *Festgabe für Franz Susemihl* (Leipzig, 1898), 1-31.
12. John Scarborough, "Nicander's Toxicology, I: Snakes," *Pharmacy in History,* 19 (1977), 3-23 [3-5].
13. Miller, *Spice Trade,* 87.
14. Papyrological reffs. collected by Raschke, "Spice Trade," 906 n. 1016.
15. *Pap. Cairo Zen.* II, 59292.
16. Miller, *Spice Trade,* 71-73.
17. Raschke, "Spice Trade," 651-652.
18. Strabo, XVI, 4. 9. *Cf.* Dioscorides, I, 18, and Pliny, *Natural History,* XII, 104.
19. M. Cary and E. H. Warmington, *The Ancient Explorers,* rev. ed. (Baltimore, 1963), 80-93.
20. *Piper longum* L. (northern India). *P. nigrum* L. (southern India). Reffs. collected in Miller, *Spice Trade,* 80-83.
21. Esp. *Aloe perryi* Baker. See nn. 54-62 below.
22. *Boswellia carteri* Birdw. (Somaliland). *B. serrata* Roxb. (northwest India).
23. Prob. *Commiphora abyssinica* (Berg.) Engl. (Somaliland, Ethiopia, Arabia).
24. *Zingiber officinale* Roscoe (southeast Asia). Miller, *Spice Trade,* 53-57.
25. *Eugenia caryophyllata* Thunb. =*E. aromatica* (Moluccas).
26. *Nardostachys jatamansi* DC (Himalayan region).
27. *Cinnamomum tamala* Nees (northern India). *C. iners* Blume (southern India). *C. zeylanicum* Blume (Sri Lanka). Miller, *Spice Trade,* 74-77.
28. *Saussurea lappa* C. B. Clarke (Kashmir).
29. Raschke, "Spice Trade," 652-653.
30. E. H. Warmington, *The Commerce Between the Roman Empire and India,* 2nd ed. (London, 1974), 185-187.
31. Theophrastus, *Historia Plantarum,* IX, 7. 3.
32. F. M. Hepper, "An Ancient Expedition to Transplant Living Trees," *Journal of the Royal Horticultural Society,* 92 (1967), 436-438, and "Arabian and African Frankincense Trees," *Journal of Egyptian Archaeology,* 55 (1969), 66-72.

33. Dioscorides, III, 22. 1-2.
34. Lily M. Perry and Judith Metzger, *Medicinal Plants of East and Southeast Asia* (Cambridge, Mass., 1980), 234.
35. Dioscorides, III, 22. 1-5.
36. Dioscorides, III, 22. 5.
37. Dioscorides, III, 22. 3.
38. Dioscorides, III, 22. 4.
39. Antyllus (*fl. c.* A.D. 130) on *aloe,* as quoted by Aetius of Amida, III, 24 (ed. A. Olivieri [CMG VIII 1, Leipzig, 1935, p. 280]). Soranus (*fl.* in the reigns of Trajan and Hadrian, A.D. 98-138) on *aloe: Gynecology,* I, 50. 2 and III, 41. 7 (ed. J. Ilberg [CMG IV, Leipzig, 1927, pp. 36 and 120]). Galen has many references to *aloe, e.g.* in *Blendings and Properties of Simples,* VI, 23 (ed. C. G. Kühn, Vol. XI [Leipzig, 1826], pp. 821-822), *That the Mental Faculties Follow the Bodily Constitution,* 2 (ed. I. Mueller, in J. Marquardt, I. Mueller, and G. Helmreich, Eds., *Claudii Galeni Pergameni Scripta Minora* [Leipzig, 1884-1893; 3 vols.], Vol. II, p. 34), and *Hygiene,* VI, 9. 16 (ed. K. Koch [CMG V 4, 2, Leipzig, 1923, p. 188]), among many. Aretaeus on *aloe: Acute Diseases,* II, 3. 13 (=VI, 3. 13) (ed. C. Hude [CMG II, Berlin, 1958, p. 129]), II. 4. 6 (=VI, 4. 6) (ed. Hude, p. 132) among several. Rufus of Ephesus on *aloe: Fragments of Rufus,* No. 71, "Treatment of *Melancholia*" (C. Daremberg and E. Ruelle, eds., *Oeuvres de Rufus d'Éphèse* [Paris, 1879] p. 359), No. 80, "Treatment of Jaundice," 17 (Daremberg-Ruelle, p. 386) among several.
40. *E.g.* Oribasius, *Medical Collection,* XIA32 [from Dioscorides] (ed. J. Raeder, *Oribasii Collectionum medicarum reliquiae* [Leipzig, 1928-1933; 4 vols.; CMG VI 1, 1 and 2, 2], Vol. II, p. 85); Alexander of Tralles, I, 16 (ed. T. Puschmann, *Alexander von Tralles* [Vienna, 1878-1879; 2 vols.], Vol. I, p. 579) among many; and Paul of Aegina, VII, 3 (ed. I. L. Heiberg, *Paulus Aegineta* [Leipzig, 1921-1924; 2 vols.; CMG IX 1 and 2], Vol. II, p. 191 [from Galen]). B. Langkavel, *Botanik der spaeteren Griechen* (Berlin, 1866), 115-116.
41. Arabic *sabr.* al-Kindi, *Aqrabadhin* (Aya Sofia MS 3603), fols. 124^r and 130^r. For an English rendition, see M. Levey, *The Medical Formulary or Aqrabadhin of al-Kindi* (Madison, Wisconsin, 1966), 162 and 186.
42. Celsus, *De medicina,* I, 3. 25-26 (ed. F. Marx, *A. Cornelii Celsi* [Leipzig, 1915; CMG I], p. 36): Qui deicere volet, primum cibis vinisque utetur is, qui hoc praestant; dein si parum illa proficient, aloen sumat. Other notices of 'aloe' in Celsus are to aloe-wood, *Aquilaria malaccensis* la Marck, imported from India, China, and Malaysia. Miller, *Spice Trade,* 34-36 and 65-67.
43. Esp. Pliny, *Natural History,* XXVII, 14-22.
44. Probably from Sextius Niger. Wellmann, ed., Dioscorides, Vol. II, p. 28 [apparatus criticus 1]. See also Max Wellmann, "Sextius Niger, eine Quellenuntersuchungen zu Dioscorides," *Hermes,* 24 (1889), 530-569, and Jerry Stannard, "Pliny and Roman Botany," *Isis,* 56 (1965), 420-425.
45. John M. Riddle, "Dioscorides," in C. C. Gillispie, ed., *Dictionary of Scientific Biography,* Vol. IV (New York, 1971), 119-123, and *Dioscorides* in F. E. Cranz and P. O. Kristeller, eds., *Catalogus Translationum et Commentariorum,* Vol. IV (Washington, D.C., 1980), 1-144 [esp. pp. 4-15]. M. Wellmann, "Dioskurides (12)," *Real-Encyclopädie der classischen Altertumswissenschaft,* Vol. V, part 1 (Stuttgart, 1903), cols. 1131-1142.
46. Ronald Syme, *Tacitus* (Oxford, 1958; 2 vols.), I, 60-63. John Scarborough, "Some Beetles in Pliny's *Natural History," Coleopterists Bulletin,* 31 (1977), 293-296.
47. Marx, ed., Celsus, Prolegomena, XIV-XVII. John Scarborough, *Roman Medicine* (London, 1969), 59-63. David Daube, "The Mediocrity of Celsus," *Classical Journal,* 70 (1974), 41-42.
48. Scarborough, "Theophrastus," *Journal of the History of Biology,* 11 (1978), 353-385.
49. A. S. F. Gow and A. F. Scholfield, eds., *Nicander: The Poems and Poetical Fragments* (Cambridge, 1953). Scarborough, "Nicander's Toxicology, I: Snakes," *Pharmacy in History,* 19 (1977), 3-23, and "Nicander's Toxicology, II: Spiders, Scorpions, Insects and Myriapods," *Ibid.,* 21 (1979), 3-34 and 73-92.
50. Gow-Scholfield, *Nicander,* 8.
51. See esp. Jerry Stannard, "Hippocratic Pharmacology," *Bulletin of the History of Medicine,* 35 (1961), 497-518, and Georg Harig, *Bestimmung der Intensität im medizinischen System Galens* (Berlin, 1974), 87-89, as well as "Anfänge der theoretischen Pharmakologie im Corpus Hippocraticum" in M. D. Grmek, ed., *Hippocratica: Actes du Colloque hippocratique de Paris 1978* (Paris, 1980), 223-245.
52. Septuagint, *Song of Solomon (=Canticles),* IV, 14. Cf. Septuagint, *Proverbs,* VII, 17.
53. Julius Preuss, *Biblical and Talmudic Medicine,* trans. by F. Rosner (New York, 1978), 185.
54. Dioscorides, III, 22. 1-3.
55. George Usher, *Dictionary of Plants Used by Man* (London, 1974), 35. Oleg Polunin, *Flowers of Europe* (London, 1969), No. 1598 (p. 492).
56. Polunin, *Flowers of Europe,* No. 1598. J. Berendes, *Des Pedanios Dioskurides aus Anazarbos Arzneimittellehre* (Stuttgart, 1902), 276-278.

57. E. A. Wallis Budge, ed. and trans., *Syrian Anatomy Pathology and Therapeutics or "The Book of Medicines"* (London, 1913; 2 vols.), I, p. 86 [Syriac text], and II, p. 93 [English translation]. Cyril Elgood, trans., "Tibb-ul-Nabbi or Medicine of the Prophet," *Osiris*, 14 (1962), 33-192 [94]: "Aloes is a plant which grows, is cut, shrinks, and is left to dry. The best aloes are brought from Socotra, an island off the coast of Yemen." M. Meyerhoff, ed. and trans., *The Book of the Ten Treatises on the Eye Ascribed to Ḥunain ibn Isḥāq (809-877 A.D.)* (Cairo, 1928), 197, 199, 204, and 211. D. Hooper and H. Field, *Useful Plants and Drugs of Iran and Iraq* (Chicago, 1937), 83.
58. Harald Nielsen, *Ancient Ophthalmological Agents*, trans. from the Danish by L. McBride (Odense [Denmark], 1974), 29.
59. John Mitchell Watt, "Magic and Witchcraft in Relation to Plants and Folk Medicine," in Tony Swain, ed., *Plants in the Development of Modern Medicine* (Cambridge, Mass., 1972), 67-102 [88].
60. Paul G. Stecher, et. al., eds., *The Merck Index*, 8th ed. (Rahway, New Jersey, 1968), 39-40. R. G. Todd, ed., *Extra Pharmacopoeia Martindale*, 25th ed. (London, 1967), 1268-1269. See also G. E. Trease and W. C. Evans, *Pharmacognosy*, 11th ed. (London, 1978), 394-399, and V. E. Tyler, L. R. Brady, and J. E. Robbers, *Pharmacognosy*, 8th ed. (Philadelphia, 1981), 60-63.
61. Albert F. Hill, *Economic Botany*, 2nd ed. (New York, 1952), 252. Trease and Evans, *Pharmacognosy*, 396-397.
62. Dioscorides, III, 22. 2. Pliny, *Natural History*, XXVII, 16.
63. Dioscorides, I, 22. Miller, *Spice Trade*, 35-36.
64. Miller, *Spice Trade*, 35 with reffs.
65. Celsus, V, 1 [for suppression of bleeding], V, 20B 2 [the famous lozenge of Polyeidus, for the clotting of wounds. Cf. Galen, *Compounding Drugs by Kind*, V, 12 (ed. Kühn, XIII, p. 834)], VI, 6. 5B [collyrium of Attalus], VI, 6. 6 [collyrium of Euelpides], VI, 6. 24 [collyrium of Hermon], and VI, 7. 2D [ear salve of Crato]. Cf. Pliny, *Natural History*, XX, 142; XXI, 76; and XXVI, 59 and 61.
66. Miller, *Spice Trade*, 36.
67. Miller, *Spice Trade*, 35-36.
68. Dioscorides, I, 22.
69. Miller, *Spice Trade*, 65-67.
70. Scarborough, "Theophrastus," *Journal of the History of Biology*, 11 (1978), 378-383.
71. Warmington, *Commerce Between the Roman Empire and India*, 180-234. Cary and Warmington, *Ancient Explorers*, esp. ch. 4. Lionel Casson, "Rome's Trade with the East: The Sea Voyage of Africa and India," *Transactions of the American Philogical Association*, 110 (1980), 21-36. Mortimer Wheeler, *Rome Beyond the Imperial Frontiers* (Baltimore, 1955), esp. chs. 9-13. One of the better summaries remains J. Oliver Thomson, *History of Ancient Geography* (Cambridge, 1948), esp. 173-177, 298-306, and 368-370. See also Miller, *Spice Trade* passim, and Raschke "Spice Trade" passim.
72. Casson, "Rome's Trade with the East," *Transactions of the American Philological Association*, 110 (1980), 24.
73. Wheeler, *Rome Beyond the Imperial Frontiers*, 138. Thomson, *Geography*, 229. Gervase Mathew, "The East African Coast until the Coming of the Portuguese," in Roland Oliver and Gervase Mathew, eds., *History of East Africa*, Vol. I (Oxford, 1963), 99-127 [95]. *Periplus of the Erythrean Sea*, 16 (ed. H. Frisk, *Le Periple de la Mer Erythrée* [Göteborg, 1927], p. 5).
74. J. H. Thiel, *Eudoxus of Cyzicus*, trans. from the Dutch by A. M. Bruin-Cousins (Groningen, 1966), esp. 29-43.
75. Thiel, *Eudoxus*, 44-55.
76. Michael Rostovtzeff, *Social and Economic History of the Hellenistic World* (Oxford, 1941; 3 vols.), II, 927-929, and III, 1556 n. 205.
77. W. W. Tarn, *The Greeks in Bactria and India* (Cambridge, 1951), 369-370 nn. 2-3 [369] and nn. 1-5 [370].
78. *Ancient Explorers*, 95-96 with n. 50.
79. Miller, *Spice Trade*, 65-97.
80. *Periplus*, 28 [along with frankincense]. Groom, *Frankincense and Myrrh*, 149-152.
81. Warmington, *Commerce*, 14.
82. Dioscorides, III, 22. 1-2.
83. Galen, *Compounding Drugs by Kind*, V, 2 (ed. Kühn, Vol. XIII, pp. 767, 775, and 779). Hans Gossen, "Heras (4)," *Real-Encylcopädie*, Vol. VIII, part 1 (Stuttgart, 1913), col. 529, as contrasted with the clipped notice by F. Kudlien, "Heras aus Kappadokien," *Der Kleine Pauly*, Vol. II (Stuttgart, 1967), col. 1053. The early notice of *aloe* by Celsus, I, 3. 25-26, also indicates an earlier date.
84. Suetonius, *Augustus*, 98. 2, shows this renewed activity.
85. Cajus Fabricius, *Galens Exzerpte aus älteren Pharmakologen* (Berlin, 1972), 209.
86. Karl Deichgräber, *Die griechische Empirikerschule*, 2nd ed. (Berlin, 1965), 186 and 188 (=Heracleides, Frgs. Nos. 196 and 203).

IX

PHARMACY IN PLINY´S **NATURAL HISTORY**: SOME OBSERVATIONS ON SUBSTANCES AND SOURCES

Very prominent in books XX through to XXXII of the **Natural History** are drugs and medicinals that appear to span the entire scope of pharmacy of classical antiquity. One is regaled with presumed quotations of sources, from the quasi-mystical Magi to straightforward writers who include Celsus and Sextius Niger, as well as obvious magical remedies that are part of a hoary folk tradition not limited to Italy, but which includes matter from around the mediterranean dominions of Rome. Moreover, if the reader performs the arduous task of counting varieties of plants, minerals, animal drugs and related substances employed as drugs - omitting the synonyms and repetitions - he emerges with an astounding array of over 900 substances, well over the nearly 600 remedies described by Dioscorides, the almost 550 species of plants contained in the works of Theophrastus, and even in excess of the 650 or so remedies assembled by Galen and the over 500 drugs listed by Paul of Aegina. The very bulk of Pliny´s data defies simple analysis, and it is clear enough that Pliny is quite proud of his collection of details on drugs and drug lore, as if he did not expect a reader to question either his sources or his substances: all were part of the natural world and its multitudinous wonders. This enthusiastic, breathless mood has endeared Pliny to centuries of readers, and the tumbling of facts, tales, stories told for amusement, anecdotes, legends and ´things heard´ carries us along as a good story should. One soon recognises, however, that embedded in this huge assemblage are underlying sources for the history of Greek and Roman pharmacy, now generally lost, and that untangling those sources would provide great insight into the development of pharmacy before Pliny´s day.

IX

Pharmacy in the Natural History

In the beginning of book XX Pliny tells us why he has decided to include medicinal plants in his gigantic pot-pourri of natural wonders and facts gleaned from voluminous reading and wide personal experience, and he begins where a Roman thought he should: in his garden or farm.

> **Maximum hinc opus naturae ordiemur et cibos suos homini narrabimus faterique cogemus ignota esse per quae vivat. Nemo id parvum ac modicum existimaverit nominum vilitate deceptus.**
> "Now we begin the greatest of Nature´s works and we will address foods for man, and compel him to admit that he is ignorant about how he lives. Let no one, deceived by the common quality of the names, think that this is of little value or of moderate importance." (**Natural History** XX.1)

This initial statement by Pliny about the forthcoming consideration of medicinals and healing substances is of crucial importance in understanding Roman concepts concerning pharmaceuticals, as well as in explaining why Pliny would speak of "foods" here, when he has given extensive coverage to cereals, the preparation of bread, garden vegetables and the like in books XVIII and XIX: drugs are to be understood as an integral part of the lore of food, and thereby an important emphasis throughout Pliny´s thinking about pharmacy would be in terms of medical dietetics. Foods and medicines are to be, at once, sources of wonder and admiration, and Pliny´s avowed devotion to the "old Roman ideal"(1) will lead him repeatedly to assert how plants - even the most common - can provide mankind with healing drugs, particularly those plants a Roman farmer or citizen of the numerous Italian towns would know from childhood.(2) This point needs to be stressed at the beginning of a brief overview of Pliny´s drug lore and the sources for that knowledge as they appear in the **Natural History**: in contrast to the twentieth-century ignorance of plants in the field, most of humanity in classical antiquity dwelled on farms or lived very close to the life of a non-urbanised countryside. Pliny´s account of drugs is bedecked with multitudinous quotations from "foreign authorities", and he is indeed fascinated by what he has found in the Greek treatises on medicine and pharmacy, but he also infuses these data with a native Italian knowledge of plants and herbs.(3) We may rightly call much of this ´folklore´ and many of the suggested remedies are in the purely magical or folkloristic class, but Pliny consciously separates them from his "Greek authors" as he culls information from all sources.(4) Noteworthy among his **auctores** - Roman authors - of works on drugs and medicinals are tracts by Sextius Niger(5) and Julius Bassus,(6) both of whom wrote in Greek. The context, however, of almost all the drugs in Pliny´s **Natural History** is one of the fullness of Roman Italy, and this setting lends a certain omnivorous cast to his writing, which is the result of his assumption that **all** aspects of human investigation of nature - from the completely magical to the absolutelv philosophical - are fit subjects for his encyclopedia.(7)

In some respects, Pliny is writing for an ´educated public´ in the middle of the first century, a public that would be curious about odd tales and local customs, peculiar animals of legend and Greek biology as well as what the ´latest thinking´ might be about Italian flora and fauna, and Pliny could assume a readership that would be as intelligent and curious as he was.(8) The **Natural History** met a need filled today by a comprehensive popular encyclopedia, and the pharmaceutical sections served the same purpose as seen today in the revival of books on herbal lore. One is struck at first by Pliny´s general lack of interest in diseases themselves, although there is ample citation of various names, gradations, and technical terms which can be grouped and classed according to Greco-Roman pathology;(9) but Pliny is far more interested in any drugs or remedies suggested for their cure, and one calls to mind similar approaches in modern handbooks of herbs, as by Grieve, Flück, and Schauenberg and Paris.(10) This does not make herbal lore any less useful or valid in its ancient Roman or modern versions,(11) but this emphasis on cure rather than disease (or perhaps more strictly medical theory) indicates the difference between a ´formal medicine´ and a more encompassing medicine ´practised´ by others than physicians.(12)

There is little doubt that Pliny is well aware of Greek medical writers, from Diocles and the Hippocratics to the Greek physicians of his own day, and many of the ´medical´ books in the **Natural History** are taken up with drugs and pharmaceuticals, drawn from a presumed large variety of sources in both Greek and Latin.(13) Yet there are many curious errors in the ´facts and observations´

about drugs, and Pliny's rampant and childlike curiosity led to a too rapid compilation of pharmaceutical data, shown by a lack of attention to specific detail and an apparent lack in cross-checking references and the omission of revisions. Some of these mistakes can be corrected through parallel readings in the Greek of Dioscorides, who used common sources cited by Pliny, particularly Sextius Niger's work on medicinal plants,(14) written in Greek.

Books XX-XXXIV of the **Natural History** are stuffed with herbal and medical lore, and Pliny's own listing of the raw numbers of details is in itself staggering: **medicinae** together with **historiae** and **observationes** in the fourteen books comes to a total (as I have added them) of 13,805 'facts'.(15) Not all of these data are pharmaceutical, but a good majority are concerned with remedies, purported powers and quoted sources on drug lore, so that Pliny is faced with an enormous task of classification. How would he draw together all these varied bits into a comprehensive and useful whole? Other medical writers wrestled with this problem, and in Latin, Celsus' methods of classification of drugs are probably the most streamlined in classical antiquity.(16) Yet there were as many ways of listing drugs as there were authors who compiled such remedies: the Hippocratic writers generally listed the diseases and then the drugs useful in treating those ailments;(17) Theophrastos left his herbal lore until book IX of the **Historia Plantarum** and attempted a poorly defined taxonomy of herbs while relying on the observations of the everyday **rhizotomoi**, who did not consider taxonomy as much as effects when a given drug was administered;(18) the pseudo-Aristotelian **Problems** seems to have attempted to class drugs according to their essential qualities, with an equally imprecise result;(19) Apollodorus chose toxic effect for his drug classifications,(20) and the obtuse poems of Nicander record the muddled nature of this attempt;(21) and Dioscorides - a contemporary of Pliny, but apparently unknown to him - invented a brilliant 'drugs-by-affinity' system,(22) which was to be completely ignored by pharmacologists in later centuries, including the polymatic and chalcenteric Galen.

It is curious that Pliny did not know the work of Scribonius Largus, whose **Conpositiones** was set down during the reign of Claudius, and the contrast between Scribonius' drug lore and that of Pliny is instructive. Scribonius, as noted by Rinne,(23) unites book-learning with experienced, practical knowledge of drugs, so that the **Conpositiones** records what a ´professional druggist´ would do in classification of medicinals:(24) one does get a kind of rough head-to-toe arrangement, but crucial to Scribonius is the prepared form of his drugs. Decoctions, infusions, plasters, salves, ointments, potions and so on provide the basic framework. Thus each of the 242 plants, 36 minerals, 27 animal products and eight poisons have specific methods of preparation in the **Conpositiones** - similar in many respects to a large portion of Galen´s huge compilation of drugs and drug recipes(25) - whereas Pliny´s drug lore has only a very loose classification by types of plants that yielded drugs, for example, book XX of the **Natural History** with **medicinae ex his quae in hortis seruntur**, XXI with **naturae florum et coronamentorum** (with drugs derived from the rose beginning at XXI.13), XXII as **continentur auctoritas herbarum** (as if Pliny were culling without worrying about classing his herbs, except that many in XXII are wreath-flowers, trailing in from XXI), XXIII **medicinae ex arboribus cultis**, and XXIV **medicinae ex arboribus silvestribus** (six drugs here (XXIV.10) from **loto Italica**) and so on. Thus Pliny´s drug lore is a medley of facts and details, taken both from his written sources and from current oral traditions, meshed with inaccuracies resulting from rapid reading and recording and an occasional blind eye to the ridiculous in his sources. One can of course simply argue that Pliny was giving an accurate account of such sources, but the self-contradictions suggest that he either did not notice variations in his written materials, or that his purpose was **not** to compile a well digested encyclopedia (as was the case with Celsus´ complete work) but a series of notes on intriguing aspects of nature that would be an inclusive record of knowledge of natural history as he had found it in his own time. Stannard has argued succinctly that Pliny´s command of botany, at least for Italian flora, is reasonably good,(26) and one may also suggest that Pliny´s acumen in recording his Greek sources is often rather high.(27) There are, however, numerous problems that exist in the texts of the **Natural History** that contain medical botany and pharmacology, and one has to approach the question of Pliny´s texts on two levels: his sources; and what are the actual species and substances within the huge gathering of materials on drug lore.

Some Sources for Pliny´s Drug Lore

One of the odd facts of early imperial Roman pharmacy is that both Dioscorides and Pliny published their respective works within two decades of one another, and neither seems aware of the other. Textual and historical evidence shows that Dioscorides´ **Materia Medica** appeared about 64 AD, and Pliny´s **Natural History** is firmly dated 77 AD. Thus any correspondence of specific description or details between Pliny´s drugs and those of Dioscorides emerges from both authors having independently employed common sources. This enables the modern scholar to make judicious comparisons between the two sets of quoted materials, and such an analysis becomes doubly valuable since it allows us to recover some sense of the contents of earlier works on pharmacy and pharmacology, which have disappeared except in quotations in Dioscorides, Pliny, Galen, Oribasius and other Roman and early Byzantine writers. The first document of importance in a comparative examination is the difficult **Preface** by Dioscorides to his **Materia Medica.**(28)

Unlike Pliny, Dioscorides was a physician - perhaps even an army doctor,(29) although our evidence is far from secure - with a special interest in medical botany and general pharmacology. Recent research has shown that Dioscorides most likely began his study of plants and medical botany at Tarsus,(30) which apparently functioned as a famous ´teaching centre´ for pharmacy. Various other and previously obscure names are now linked with this Tarsian tradition that reaches back at least several generations before Dioscorides´ own time.(31) It is clear also that Dioscorides has read deeply in the medical and pharmacological literature available to him in Greek, and even though the well known names of Hippocrates, Theophrastos and Nicander only appear rarely as cited authorities in the **Materia Medica,**(32) there is an indication that data from these three very famous writers have made their way into Dioscorides´ text. It is, however, in the short - but exceedingly difficult - **Preface** that Dioscorides tells us which authorities are before him, and why he believes that his work on medical botany and general pharmacology will be much better than all of the previous authorities: "...some of my predecessors did not give a complete survey, while others took most of their information from written sources".(33) Then he begins to name these predecessors:

> ...Iollas of Bithynia and Heraclides of Tarentum touched on only a small portion of the subject, entirely omitted the botanical tradition, and made no mention at all of metallic drugs and spices. Crateuas the Rootcutter and Andreas the Physician - who are apparently more precise in this aspect - omitted many exceptionally useful roots and a few herbs.
>
> However, one must admit that the older authors combined the paucity of their information with precision, in contrast to recent writers like Julius Bassus, Niceratus, Petronius, Niger, and Diodotus, all followers of Asclepiades.(34)

Areius, the individual to whom the **Materia Medica** is addressed, was a doctor and a pharmacologist in his own right,(35) but is not quoted directly by Dioscorides. Other authorities cited in the **Materia Medica** include Diagoras (IV.64), Erasistratus (IV.64), Iobas (III.82), Mnesidemus (IV.64) and Philonides (IV.148) and perhaps Thessalus (I.26) and Peteesius (V.98). This list of 19 sources is not necessarily complete, but does provide a convenient group of names which can be compared with the far less specific listings of sources given by Pliny. From Dioscorides we can learn the names of authors of works particularly devoted to pharmacy, which possibly can be correlated with the names and quotations in Pliny´s **Natural History**; then a comparison can be made of the quoted extracts in terms of some of the specific pharmaceuticals that are mentioned.

There are Greek sources used by Pliny which are not cited by Dioscorides, so that one must also consider quotations by Pliny from Apollodorus (as opposed to Apollodorus through Nicander), Aristophanes, Menander, Callimachus, Diocles and Xenocrates. After detailed consideration, it seems probable that Pliny employed one set of authorities for strictly pharmacological information (Sextius Niger, Erasistratus, Iollas, Diagoras, Mnesidemus (that is, Mnesides in Pliny), Heraclides of Tarentum and the Asclepiadeans Julius Bassus, Niceratus, Petronius, Diodotus and Philonides), and a second group of authors and works for the names of plants (the Hippocratic corpus, Diocles, Apollodorus and the poetry of Aristophanes, Menander, Callimachus and Nicander); the doxographical evidence, best seen in Athenaeus, shows a rich history of plant names in the "old Greek" poets.(36) A third kind of written authority, used by Pliny as an important part of his basic information on medical botany, would be represented by Xenocrates, whose **Peri tēs apo tōn phytōn ōphelias (Useful things from plants)**was based, in turn, on a number of occult and quasi-occult authors and works that included the **Physika** by Democritus Bolus, the "Magi" (Ostanes and Zoroaster), Agathocles' **Peri Diaites (Regimen),** and various Pythagorean and neo-Pythagorean writers.(37)

If one compiles further citations of authorities, as given by Pliny for his botanical, medical and pharmaceutical books, there results a lengthy listing. There is, however, something rather misleading about these long lists of authorities, which can be illustrated by a consideration of Pliny's handling of garden vegetables and herbs.(38) In addition to Sextius Niger and Xenocrates, there seems to be a third Greek source used by Pliny, indicated by a uniformity of repeated details from varied sources, a uniformity that corresponds to the quotations from Sextius Niger and Xenocrates. One may immediately suspect some kind of doxographical collection that would, indeed, include extracts from the Hippocratic corpus,(39) as well as the following: Philistion, Diocles, Chrysippus, Praxagoras, Pleistonicus, Dieuches, Medius, Simus, Cleophantus, Pythagoras, Glaucias, Dionysius, Apollodorus, Diodorus, Heraclides of Tarentum, Chrysermus, the followers of Erasistratus(40) as contrasted to the followers of Asclepiades,(41) Solon of Smyrna and probably Sosimenes and Tlepolemus. One could add the name of Theodorus(42) to this doxographical collection, but he is identified among the pneumatics by Athenaeus, so that Pliny gained this source through Xenocrates, not in the collection of extracts represented by the listing of previous names.(43)

Once these "names" have been linked to their respective passages in the **Natural History**, it is apparent that Pliny has consulted a collection of writings that summarised a medical botany that emphasised dietetics: Chrysippus,(44) Democritus joined to Diocles and Dionysius,(45) Democritus,(46) Hicesius(47) and Erasistratus.(48) In the **Natural History** XX.187-190, Pliny employs a characteristic phraseology(49) that links with the **sunt qui** in the closing section of XX.195, which smooths out the quotations - so it seems at first glance - from Evenor and Iollas.(50) Textual parallels, however, in Dioscorides, Galen, Symeon Seth(51) and others(52) show that the full block of material has come from Sextius Niger. Tlepolemus, along with Dalion, Sosimenes, Dieuches, Evenor and Heraclides of Tarentum are all cited alongside Sextius Niger,(53) but a section in Dioscorides shows that the information on the anise had been compacted by Niger, even though Pliny has recorded the names of the multiple authors, while Dioscorides has not.(54)

It appears, therefore, that Sextius Niger has in his turn consulted and extracted a collection of pharmacological opinions, particularly emphasising the medical botany of dietetics. Wellmann has proposed that this doxographical collection came from Hellenistic Smyrna,(55) which had a long tradition of medical figures who studied pharmacy and dietetics. The most likely candidate as the author of the Smyrna collection, which was the basis for Niger´s account, is Solon of Smyrna, known through Galen as the "dietician".(56) The key in identifying this doxographical source underneath Sextius Niger as employed in the **Natural History** is Pliny´s **sunt qui**,(57) and Solon appears clearly as a mingled part of a doxographical tradition.(58) As one reads **Natural History** XX.235,(59) it appears reasonably certain that Solon of Smyrna is the author of this third Greek source, heavily employed by Pliny in his herbal medicines in books XX through to XXVII. Animal drugs, that is, pharmaceuticals that are derived from animals,(60) come in large part from another work by Xenocrates of Cilician Aphrodisias(61) titled **Peri tēs apo tou Anthrōpou kai tōn Zōōn ōpheleias (Useful (things) for Man from Animals)**, as well as from the **Physika** of pseudo-Democritus.(62) Apollodorus and Nicander do appear in the listings of authorities for books XXVII - XXX, Nicander for XXXI -XXXII,(63) and the mysterious Licinius Macer for XXXII. Sextius Niger is listed for books XXVIII - XXX and XXXII.

Latin sources for the drug books in the **Natural History** are less troublesome. A major source of data for Pliny is the lost work by Valgius Rufus, as well as a tract by Antonius Castor,(64) but it seems clear that Pliny has excerpted much of his Latin medical botany from the expected writings available in his own time: Cato,(65) Varro and Celsus. One also finds quotations from an Asclepiades,(66) and these data are generally from the drugbooks of Asclepiades of Bithynia,(67) perhaps ocasionally conflated with the pharmacy of Asclepiades Pharmacion, known through fairly copious citations in Galen´s summary of drug lore.(68) Pliny borrowed heavily from Celsus´ botanical and herbal lore,(69) but one can also make the argument that Pliny did, indeed, have a text of Theophrastos before him as well.(70) One cannot, however, escape the impression that Pliny´s main sources for his pharmaceutical lore were either encyclopedic (for example Celsus) or doxographical (Solon of Smyrna, for example), with certain, nearly contemporary works that supplied not only masses of data, but also the names of quoted authorities, which would be duly recorded by Pliny amongst his sources. Sextius Niger, Xenocrates and Solon of Smyrna emerge as Pliny´s major references for many of the facts gathered from the Greek, and the traditional Latin lore assembled by Cato, Varro(71) and perhaps Valgius Rufus formed a core for Italian materials. Celsus,(72) of course, would give Pliny a conduit into both a native Latin tradition coupled with a shrewdly perceived Hellenistic drug lore, so that Celsus´ **De Medicina** looms as a far more important source for Pliny´s pharmaceuticals than has been previously assumed.

Given the evidence which indicates that Pliny most often used written sources of the first 75 years of the Roman Empire, one can assume that Solon of Smyrna´s compilation was in circulation some time after Celsus published his encyclopedia (during the reign of Tiberius), and that the works of Sextius Niger and Xenocrates were very nearly contemporary with Pliny himself. Xenocrates, however, is something of a problem: Pliny´s citations reveal either a confusion between an ´Elder´ and a ´Younger´, or his employment of some care in an attempt to distinguish between the ´stone books´ of Xenocrates of Ephesus and the ´medical books´ of Xenocrates of Aphrodisias. Fabricius(73) represents the current thinking among specialist scholars that Xenocrates of Aphrodisias lived in the second half of the first century, but Ullmann follows the earlier suggestion of Wellman that Xenocrates of Ephesus also lived during the reign of Nero,(74) and both would be contemporary with Pliny. If we believe the opinions of Galen, Xenocrates of Aphrodisias was something of a charlatan, even as he assembled a fat collection of quoted sources on drugs made from animals and animal parts. The firm dating of Fabricius and Kudlien seems supported by Galen´s statement that Xenocrates was alive "...during the time of our great-grandfathers",(75) putting Xenocrates of Aphrodisias´ **floruit** at about 50 AD. It is not impossible, as observed by Ullmann, that there might be two authors named Xenocrates (an ´Elder´ from Ephesus and a ´Younger´ from Aphrodisias), but it only adds to the complexity to assume two separate authorities called Xenocrates, both of whom wrote on medical topics at roughly the same time. Given the long fragment from Xenocrates´ **Food from Water Animals**, preserved by Oribasius,(76) and the notices by Galen of a tract called **Useful (Things, viz. Drugs) from Animals**,(77) as well as the ´medical nature´ of Xenocrates´ **Book on Stones**,(78) it appears far more reasonable to suppose that **a** Xenocrates was the author of a number of works, cited as part of a pharmaco-doxographic tradition by Pliny. Perhaps there has been confusion by various scribes in the textual history between "Ephesus" and "Aphrodisias", which might have been insignificant especially to copyists in the Latin West. Xenocrates´ writings were very important to Pliny, as the numerous citations suggest, and the fragments of the original Greek treatises show how the state of medical dietetics and medical zoology - and their relationship to pharmacology - had developed in Greek works on the topic during the first half of the first century. It may be noted, in passing, that Xenocrates apparently represented a long-lived tradition in medical dietetics that can be traced back to Aristotelian thinkers and Hippocratic physicians, and which was to claim much attention in the Hellenistic era, as seen in the remnants of the writings of Diphilus of Siphnos.(79)

Sources and Substances in Pliny´s Drug Lore

Even though Dioscorides does not often name specific written sources in his **Materia Medica**, there are numerous parallels in the **Materia Medica** with passages in Pliny´s **Natural History** which do bear the names of cited authorities. Since Solon of Smyrna probably underlies Sextius Niger´s account, and would therefore provide many of the ´names´ in Pliny´s extensive listing, one can conclude that the parallel passages in Pliny and Dioscorides are derived independently from Sextius Niger. Dioscorides has rejected the simple acceptance of his written sources on pharmacology, in favour of seeking the plants and testing them as drugs,(80) but there is clear evidence that he did, indeed, record data on drugs from his written sources, especially Sextius Niger. Thanks to Dioscorides´ care and precision, particularly as he confirms or denies statements found in his sources, we can gain insight into the way in which Pliny used his written materials to gain specifics on pharmaceuticals. It was very unlikely that direct use was made by Dioscorides of those he names as "recent writers",(81) except for Niger, given his ridicule for such sources as "...vain prating about causation".(82) Dioscorides shows that of all his sources, he had studied the work of Sextius Niger most closely, and says the following about his botanical, medical and compiling abilities:

> ...Niger, who seems to be the best (of the recent writers) says that spurge-resin is the juice from the olive-spurge (**Daphne oleoides** Schreb.) and that perfoliated St John´s wort (**Hypericum perfoliatum** L.) is the same as triangular St John´s wort (**Hypericum triquetrifolium** Turra); he says that bitter aloe (**Aloe perryi** Baker) is dug up in Judea and makes many equally wrong statements in defiance of manifest truth, which proves that he took his evidence not from his own eyes but from faulty secondhand written sources. Niger and the rest also made mistakes in the organization of their material, some throwing together incompatible properties, others using an alphabetic arrangement which splits off genera and properties from what most resembles them.(83)

These lines from the **Preface** (3) of Dioscorides´ **Materia Medica** show several characteristics of Sextius Niger´s writing on medical botany and pharmacy: he had based his account on earlier treatises, an aspect of Niger´s writing discerned in Pliny´s use of Niger and the underpinnings of Solon of Smyrna; Niger had compiled his works on drugs on an alphabetic arrangement, also seen in some of Pliny´s excerpts;(84) Niger had not sought the plants in the field, but relied on his written sources, which led to gross errors cited here (confusing the prepared form of aloe with a mineral),(85) confusing spurge-resin (derived from a North African shrub, **Euphorbia resinifera** Berg.)(86)

with the olive-spurge; and mauling the descriptions of the two different kinds of St John´s wort,(87) and dependence on a quasi-philosophical doctrine of properties ("Asclepiadean") that is also occasionally mirrored in Pliny.(88)

As contrasted to the murky state of our knowledge of the texts of Solon of Smyrna and Xenocrates, we can make some fairly assured judgements about the writings of Sextius Niger. Dioscorides has singled him out for major criticism, indicating that it was Niger´s "drug books" - compiled from many earlier works - that Dioscorides knew best of his predecessors, and the close approximation in many passages of the **Materia Medica** and the **Natural History** delineate how a skilled field pharmacognosist would employ the facts of Niger´s compilation, as compared with an encyclopedist making a new compilation based on older ones. Sextius Niger as quoted and used by both Pliny and Dioscorides provides us with specific substances, and a few selected corollary sections in the **Materia Medica** and **Natural History** will enable us to see how Pliny made use of specific details in one of his sources.

In his consideration of a plant called **epimedion**, Pliny (XXVII.76) says that it has a stem of moderate size and ten or twelve leaves that resemble those of the ivy. Moreover, he continues, the plant never bears flowers, has a thin black root, a heavy odour, a feeble taste and grows in humid soils.

> **Et huic spissandi refrigerandique natura, feminis cavenda. Folia in vino trita virginum mammas cohibent.**
>
> And this plant has thickening and cooling properties, and it should be avoided by women. Beaten up in wine, the leaves restrain the growth of the breasts in young women. (89)

The parallel passages on the **epimedion** in Dioscorides, **Materia Medica**, IV.19 would read in translation:

> **Epimedion:** it has a small stalk, ten or twelve leaves resembling ivy; it bears neither seed nor flower; the roots are thin, black, strong-smelling, and taste flat; it grows in wet places.
>
> The leaves pounded up with oil make a plaster for the breasts, applied so that they do not grow large. The root is contraceptive

> (**atokios**), and the leaves when pounded up in wine and drunk after the menstrual flow (five drachams for five days) prevent conception).(90)

The common source for the two accounts is Sextius Niger, but one looks with fascination at what Pliny has omitted from his text: the description of the contraceptive use of the plant. Pliny has also confused the "pounding with oil" of Niger (the breast plaster) with the "pounding in wine" (the post-menstrual contraceptive). The "thickening and cooling properties" is an addition by Pliny, which may have been inserted from one of his Hippocratic texts, but generally (except for the omission of the contraceptive prescription) Pliny has been quite faithful to his Greek original. The Latin text may bear the marks of scribal tampering, and the **feminis cavenda** could easily be an intentional interpolation by uneasy medieval copyists, since the rest of the passage reflects rather well what Dioscorides has also recorded in Greek.

This is one of those cases where Dioscorides has **not** verified the plant, since the description is poor, no matter how one interprets the Greek. Identification of **epimedion** is very uncertain,(91) but Pamphilus (Dioscorides, IV.19 RV) gives a series of synonyms for the plant that includes **erinos**, which would make it some kind of basil-like herb, shown by Nicander, Diocles and elsewhere in Pliny.(92) If **epimedion** is equivalent to **erinos**, then it is possibly **Campanula rapunculoides** L., the creeping bellflower, very poorly described. If Greco-Roman pharmacy had indeed prescribed contraceptive powers for **epimedion** as the supposed equivalent of **erinos**, such have dropped out of the descriptions recorded by Paul of Aegina.(93) It seems that ancient botanists did not observe the bellflower in July and August, the normal time for the blooming of its purple flowers. Pliny does not know the plant, and merely copies from his source, Sextius Niger.

Sextius Niger is the common source for Pliny, **Natural History** XXII.51-52, and Dioscorides, **Materia Medica** IV.24-25. Comparison of these two extant accounts can suggest further points in regard to Pliny's acquaintance with specific drugs and his employment of written sources. In translation, Pliny, XXII.51-52:

> There is another plant also, properly called

onochilon, named by some anchusa, by others archebion, by still others onochelis or rhexia, and most commonly enchrysa. It has a small stalk, a purple flower, rough leaves and branches, a root the colour of blood at harvest time, though black at other times, and it grows in sandy soils. It is an antidote for snakebite, especially poisonous snakes, both the root and the leaves being equally efficacious in food and drink. It has its properties (**vires**) at harvest time. When pounded, its leaves smell like cucumber. (52) It is given in doses of three cyathi for a prolapsed uterus. With marjoram (**hysopum**) it expels tapeworms, and for pains in the kidneys or liver, it is drunk in hydromel (**aqua mulsa**) if one has a fever, but otherwise, in wine. The root is smeared on freckles and psoriatic sores (**lentigini ac lepris radix inlinitur**). It is said that those who carry the root are not bitten by snakes. And there is another plant similar to this one, but smaller, with a red flower, and it is used in the same way as the other one (above); and they record that if it is chewed thoroughly and spat out on to a snake, it dies. (94)

In translation, Dioscorides, IV.25-25:

Another alkanet (**anchousa**), which some call Alkibiadeion or onocheiles. This differs from the previous one in that it has smaller leaves, but they are sharp like those of the previous plant; it has thin branches, on which is a flower that is reddish-purple, tending towards Phoenician purple; it has very long red roots, at harvest time having (in them) something like blood; it grows in sandy places.

Its property (**dynamis**) and of the leaves is to be an antidote for those bitten by wild animals, especially for those bitten by poisonous snakes (**echiodektois**); (the root and leaves) are eaten, or drunk, or hung about one´s neck. And if someone has chewed it well, he should spit it out into the mouth of the wild animal to kill it.

(25) And there is another plant, resembling the previous one, but having a smaller seed the colour of Phoenician purple: if someone chews up the seed thoroughly and spits it into the mouth of the snake (**herpeton**) it dies. The root

> being drunk with marjoram (**hyssopos**) and garden cress (**kardamon**) in the amount of an **oxybaphon** expels the tapeworm.(95)

The "other alkanet" is probably **Echium diffusum** Sibth.,(96) a bugloss in the Boraginaceae, and the "smaller one" may be **Lithospermum fruticosum** L.,(97) or **L. diffusam** Lag., both being gromwells also in the Boraginaceae. In this case Pliny´s framework is a text of Sextius Niger, but he has added bits from other sources on the crushed leaves smelling like cucumbers and on the use of the root as a liniment (an embrocation usually made with oil) to smear on freckles and scaly and red skin sores. Pliny has received the folk tradition of spitting the masticated leaves into the "snake´s mouth" to kill it, and he has modified it into the more ´sensible´ spitting the chewed leaves **on** the snake. Pliny has retained the marjoram (**Origanum vulgare** L.) to expel tapeworms, but he has omitted the garden cress (**Lepidum sativum** L.) in Niger´s prescription. Both plants are fairly common in Italy, so that Pliny´s omission has no real explanation, unless this is the result of a rapid skimming of the Greek text. In summary, in **Natural History**, XXII.51-52, Pliny has been fairly faithful to his Greek source with the exception of the garden cress.

Very similar employment of Sextius Niger by Pliny can be documented in numerous instances paralleled in Dioscorides,(98) and each is suggestive of the manner in which Pliny used his pharmaco-doxographical sources. The following are merely illustrative. **Natural History**, XXVII.74 (**elatine**) compared with Dioscorides, IV.40 (**elatine**) shows that Pliny has used a text by Sextius Niger, who is probably quoting Crateuas, and the plant is probably **Kickxia spuria** (L.) Dumort, the round-leaved fluellen,(99) used for ´rheumy eyes´ and diarrhoea. **Natural History**, XXVII.93 (**Ideae herbae**) compared with Dioscorides, IV.44 (**idaia rhiza**) again indicates that Pliny was using a text by Sextius Niger, probably quoting Crateuas, and the herb is most likely **Streptopus amplexifolius** (L.) DC, a mountain broom, used for loose bowels and for a woman´s excessive menstruation. **Natural History**, XXXXVI.132 (**Equisaetum hippuris Graecis dicta**) compared with Dioscorides, IV.46.1 (**hippouris**) again reveals that Pliny is quoting from a Greek text by Sextius Niger, quoting Crateuas, and the specific plant under consideration is one of the **Equisetum** species (horsetails, here probably **E. arvense** L., or perhaps **E. limosum** L. or **E.palustre** L.), used as a diuretic and as a styptic; but Pliny in **Natural History** XXVI.133 has switched to another source, and then returned to Sextius Niger at XXVI.134, as comparison with Dioscorides, IV.46.2 and 47 would suggest. Pliny´s rendition has carefully retained the species differentiation marked in the Greek original, although it seems that Pliny does not perceive too many variations in the various horsetails described.(100)

Natural History, XXVII.142 (**Herba tragos quam aliqui scorpion vocant**)(101) as compared with Dioscorides, IV.51.1,(102) is of interest beyond Pliny´s employment of Sextius Niger. The species is **Ephedra distachya** L.,(103), a joint-pine shrub employed (the seeds being pounded in wine) for diarrhoea and excessive menstruation (Pliny´s **sanguinem excreantibus** is not in Sextius Niger/Dioscorides). Ephedrine, the active principle derived from **Ephedra** spp. (especially **E. distachya** and Far Eastern species) remains in use as a treatment for the relief of asthma and hay fever due to its properties as a vaso-constrictor and sympathomimetic. Ephedras have about 0.5 - 2 percent alkaloids and (depending on species) ephedrine and its isomers are about 30 to 90 percent.(104)

There are instances in Pliny´s drug lore in which parallel sources seem to be piled one on another, so that definite assigment of a single source becomes impossible. For example, **Natural History,** XXIV.117-120 can be compared with Dioscorides, IV.37, and a presumed common source is Sextius Niger. The plant described is the blackberry (Pliny: **rubus**; Dioscorides: **batos**) **Rubus fruticosus** L. agg., used, according to Dioscorides and his source, as a hair dye, styptic and dessicant, as well as an anti-diarrhoeal agent, a drug to treat excessive menstruation, an antidote against the bite of poisonous animals, a general wound styptic, a treatment for haemorrhoids and as a general mouthwash. One can, however, detect traces of several other sources, especially in Pliny: Theophrastos (description of **batos**);(105) Zopyrus (**batos** as a standard astringent);(106) Celsus (various uses of **rubus**);(107) Nicander (flower of the **batos** useful against snakebite).(108) Another series of a mixed sequence of possible citations by Pliny can be seen by comparing **Natural History,** XXXII.33 with Dioscorides, II.79.2 and then noting the parallels in Galen (from Apollodorus),(109) Nicander **Theriaca** and **Alexipharmaca** (from Apollodorus)(110) and wondering which collection of medical opinions would have given Pliny **both** Nicander and Apollodorus, or perhaps supposing that Pliny had texts of the lost works on toxic animals and plants by Apollodorus before him, as well as texts of Nicander´s **Theriaca** and **Alexipharmaca.**

Pliny´s assessment of particular substances in his drug books of the **Natural History** closely follows his employment and understanding of his written sources in both Greek and Latin. In the case of his use of the Greek texts of Sextius Niger (who has, in his turn, compiled data probably based on Solon of Smyrna), Pliny shows a usual care with the particulars and an occasional lapse that may be due to his rapid methods of reading and compiling. More often than not, however, Pliny simply follows his sources verbatim, with slight variations as he knows them from other corollary sources, but it seems clear that he depended very heavily indeed on Sextius Niger for his drug lore. There is some indication also that Pliny may have had a text of Solon of Smyrna and the compilations by Xenocrates, but the **Natural History** rarely reflects the employment of pharmacological texts that predate Augustus. Exceptions may be the Greek texts of Theophrastos and Nicander, and perhaps Apollodorus, but Pliny´s drug lore from his Greek sources is generally derivative from a long tradition of pharmacological doxography, represented by both Sextius Niger and Solon of Smyrna. Pliny is not the best of medical botanists, although he does often mirror a common knowledge of herbal plants that would be well known in Italy: his truncation of Sextius Niger´s accounts of non-Italian plants continually suggests that Pliny did not understand the often subtle distinctions necessary to comprehend different species as they grew in the eastern Mediterranean. And as mentioned, there are signs of scribal meddling in the history of the Latin texts of the **Natural History,** which will further obscure those texts which cannot be checked against extant Greek sources.

NOTES

Abbreviations and short titles

Celsus: F Marx, ed., **A.Cornelius Celsi quae supersunt**, Leipzig, Teubner, 1915 (**CML I**)

CMG: Corpus Medicorum Graecorum

CML: Corpus Medicorum Latinorum

Diocles: M Wellmann, ed., **Die Fragmente der sikelischen Ärzte Akron, Philistion und des Diocles von Karystos**, Berlin, Weidmann, 1901 (Fragmentsammlung der griechischen Ärzte, I)
Dioscorides: Max Wellmann, ed., **Pedanii Dioscuridis Anazarbei De materia medica**, Berlin, Weidmann, 1906-1914; 3 vols., reprinted 1958
K.: C G Kühn, ed., **Claudii Galeni Opera Omnia**, Leipzig, Cnoblochius, 1821-33; 20 vols. in 22, reprinted Hildesheim, G Olms, 1964-65
Littré: E Littré, ed., and trans. **Oeuvres complète d´Hippocrate**, Paris, 1839-1861; 10 vols., reprinted Amsterdam, Hakkert, 1973-80
NH or Pliny, **NH**: various eds. of the volumes of the Budé edition (Paris: Société d´Edition ´les Belles Lettres´), viz.:

Jean Beaujeu, ed., **Pline l´Ancien Histoire Naturelle**, Livre I (1950)
Henri le Bonniec and Andre le Boeuffle, eds., **Pline l´Ancien Histoire Naturelle**, Livre XVIII (1972)
J André, ed., **Pline l´Ancien Histoire Naturelle**, Livre XIX (1964)
J André, ed., **Pline l´Ancien Histoire Naturelle**, Livre XX (1965)
Jacques André, ed., **Pline l´Ancien Histoire Naturelle**, Livre XXI (1969)
Jacques André, ed.,**Pline l´Ancien Histoire Naturelle**, Livre XXII (1970)
Jacques André, ed., **Pline l´Ancien Histoire Naturelle**, Livre XXIII (1971)
Jacques André, ed.,**Pline l´Ancien Histoire Naturelle**, LivreXXIV (1972)
Jacques André, ed., **Pline l´Ancien Histoire Naturelle**, Livre XXV (1974)
A Ernout and R Pépin, eds., **Pline l´Ancien Histoire Naturelle**, Livre XXVI (1957)
A Ernout, ed., **Pline l´Ancien Histoire Naturelle**, Livre XXVII (1959)
A Ernout, ed.,**Pline l´Ancien Histoire Naturelle**,Livre XXVIII (1962)
A Ernout, ed., **Pline l´Ancien Histoire Naturelle**, Livre XXIX (1962)
Alfred Ernout, ed., **Pline l´Ancien Histoire Naturelle**, Livre XXX (1963)
Guy Serbat, ed., **Pline l´Ancien Histoire Naturelle**, Livre XXXI (1972)
E de Saint-Denis, ed., **Pline l´Ancien Histoire Naturelle**, Livre XXXII (1966)

Oribasius: J Raeder, ed., **Oribasii Collectionum Medicarum Reliquiae**, Leipzig, Teubner, 1928-1933; 4

vols., reprinted Amsterdam, Hakkert, 1964 (**CMG** VI.1, 1-2, 2)
Paul of Aegina: I L Heiberg, ed., **Paulus Aegineta**, Leipzig, Teubner, 1921-1924; 2 vols. (**CMG** IX 1-2)
PH: Pharmacy in History
RE: Real-Encyclopädie der classischen Altertumswissenschaft

1. Pliny, **NH**, XXIX.14 (quoting Cato on Greek physicians). Alan E Austin, **Cato the Censor**, Oxford, 1978, pp. 170-171. "(Cato)...preferred to rely on traditional and familiar recipes, taking from the Greeks only a few herbal remedies similar in kind" (p.171). E.g., **NH**, XVIII.205

2. John Scarborough, **Roman Medicine**, London, 1969, pp. 63-65

3. E.g. **NH**, XXVII.131, as examined in J H Phillips, "Juxtaposed medical traditions", **Classical Philology** 76, 1981, pp.130-132. Cf. Celsus, V.26.35C and VI.7.1D

4. J Stannard, "Medicinal plants and folk remedies in Pliny, Historia Naturalis", **History and Philosophy of the Life Sciences** 4, 1982, pp. 3-23

5. Caelius Aurelianus, **Acute Diseases**, III.16.134 (ed. Drabkin, p. 386) says that Niger was a friend of Julius Bassus (n.6 below), which probably dates him to about 10-40 AD. Galen thinks well of him, as do Pliny and Dioscorides (independently). John Scarborough and Vivian Nutton, "The Preface of Dioscorides´ Materia Medica: introduction, translation, commentary", **Transactions and Studies of the College of Physicians of Philadelphia**, n.s. 4, 1982, pp. 187-227: 206, and Max Wellmann, "Sextius Niger. Eine Quellenuntersuchungen zu Dioskorides", **Hermes**, 24, 1889, pp.530-569

6. Julius Bassus **fl.** c. 10-40 AD. Scarborough and Nutton, "Preface", (n.5 above), p. 205

7. G E R Lloyd, **Science, Folklore and Ideology**, Cambridge, 1983, pp.135-149

8. W H S Jones, "Ancient documents and contemporary life", in: E A Underwood, ed., **Science, Medicine and History: Essays...in honour of Charles Singer**, London, 1953, 2 vols.; vol. 1, pp. 100-110: 106-108

9. Esp. eye diseases, skin ailments and rashes, various fevers, and the bites and stings of poisonous animals and insects.

10. M Grieve, **A Modern Herbal**, New York, 1931; 2 vols. Reprinted 1971. Hans Flück,

Medicinal Plants, trans. (from the German) J M Rowson, London, 1976. Paul Schauenberg and Ferdinand Paris, **Guide des plantes médicinales**, 3rd ed., Neuchâtel and Paris, 1977. Cf. Juliette de Baïracly Levy, **Herbal Handbook for Farm and Stable**, rev. ed., London, 1973

11. The range of modern approaches is merely suggested in the following volumes: G E Trease and W C Evans, **Pharmacognosy**, 11th ed., London, 1978; W H Lewis and M P F Elvin-Lewis, **Medical Botany**, New York, 1977; V E Tyler, L R Brady and J E Robbers, **Pharmacognosy**, 8th ed., Philadelphia, 1981; A F Hill, **Economic Botany**, 2nd ed., New York, 1952.

12. A Sofowora, **Medicinal Plants and Traditional Medicine in Africa**, New York, 1982, and T Swain, **Plants in the Development of Modern Medicine**, Cambridge, Mass., 1972 show the modern counterparts of this venerable tradition throughout the world. One may also cite the rich pharmacy and medical plant lore of pre-Columbian America suggested by Ralph L Roys, **The Ethno-Botany of the Maya**, New Orleans, 1931, reprinted Philadelphia, 1976

13. Jones, "Ancient documents" (n.8 above), p.109, puts it, "In Pliny pharmacology has swamped everything else".

14. Welmann, "Sextius Niger" (n.5 above) passim

15. **NH**, XX:1606. XXI:730. XXII:406. XXIII:1418. XXIV:1116. XXV:1292. XXVI:1019. XXVII:602. XXVIII:1682. XXIX:621. XXX:854. XXXI:924. XXXII:990. XXXIII:288. XXXIV:257 (**medicinae**)

16. Esp. Celsus, V.1-17: simples classed by pharmaceutical/physical properties, e.g. V.2: **glutinant vulnus** (19 substances)

17. **Vid.** e.g. the Hippocratic **Wounds**, 11-12 (ed. Littré, VI.410-417)

18. John Scarborough, "Theophrastus on herbals and herbal remedies", **Journal of the History of Biology** 11, 1978, pp. 353-385

19. John Scarborough, "Theoretical assumptions in Hippocratic pharmacology", in: F Lasserre and P Mudry, eds., **Actes de Colloque hippocratique Lausanne 1981**, Lausanne, 1983, pp.275-293: 276-280

20. Max Wellmann, "Das älteste Kräuterbuch der Griechen", in: **Festgabe für Franz Susemihl**, Leipzig, 1898, pp.1-31; and John Scarborough, "Nicander´s toxicology,I: snakes", **PH**, 19, 1977, pp.3-23: 3-4; and "Nicander´s toxicology, II:

spiders, scorpions, insects and myriapods", **PH**, 21, 1979, pp.3-34 and 73-9:4

21. Scarborough, "Nicander I" and "Nicander II" (n.20 above) passim

22. John M Riddle, **Dioscorides**, Austin, Texas, in press (1984) develops this thesis with precision. **Vid.** also Scarborough and Nutton, "Preface" (n.5 above) pp. 190-1

23. Felix Rinne, "Das Receptbuch des Scribonius Largus", **Koberts Historische Studien aus dem Pharmakologischen Institut der Universität Dorpat**, 5, 1896,1-99: 32, reprinted in **Historische Studien zur Pharmacologie der Griechen, Römer und Araber, Leipzig DDR 1968**

24. The basic modern edition is Georg Helmreich, ed., **Scribonii Largi Conpositiones**, Leipzig, Teubner, 1887, but Sergio Sconnochia, **Per una nuova edizione di Scribonio Largo**, Brescia, 1981, has announced preparation of a new text based upon fresh readings obtained from MS Toletanus 98,12.

25. Analysis of Galen´s "drug books" shows that he remained uncertain regarding the best method of pharmaceutical classification. The three major tracts by Galen on drugs are **Mixtures and Properties of Simples** in eleven books (XI.459-892, K. and XII.1-377. K.) **Compound Drugs arranged by Location of Ailment**, in ten books (XII.379-1007, K., and XIII.1-361, K.), and **Compound Drugs arranged by Kind**, in seven books (XIII.362-1058). **Mixtures** is a listing of about 440 plants (books I-VIII) and about 250 other substances in the remainder of the tract, and - along with a ´system of degrees´ - the organisation principle is an alphabetic arrangement. **Drugs by Ailment** was written down after **Mixtures** (XII.378, K. = **Drugs by Ailment**, I.1) and here Galen provides a crude ´head to toe´ ordering, with gout qualifying as the ´bottom´ tier. **Drugs by Kind** was written in response to criticism of his earlier drug works (XIII.363, K. = **Kind** I.1) and incorporates the venerated ´treatment by contraries´, with numerous earths, plasters, pills, etc., quoted from many authorities, esp. Andromachus.

26. J Stannard, "Pliny and Roman botany", **Isis**, 56, 1965, pp. 420-425

27. E.g., using Sextius Niger: **NH**, XXXII.26 compared with Dioscorides, II.62

28. The only sound Greek text is that ed. by Max Wellmann in vol. 1 of the **Materia Medica**, pp. 1-5. One may **not** trust the "translation" by John Goodyear (1655) in R T Gunther, ed., **The Greek**

Herbal of Dioscorides, Oxford, 1934, reprinted New York, 1959, pp. 1-4. **Vid.** translation (from the Wellmann text) by Scarborough and Nutton (n.5 above), pp.195-7

29. Dioscorides, **Preface, 4. Vid.** commentary by Scarborough and Nutton (n.5 above), pp. 213-217

30. Scarborough and Nutton (n.5 above), pp. 192-4

31. E.g. Philo of Tarsus, **fl.** 20 AD. **Vid.** refs. in Scarborough and Nutton (n.5 above) p. 193, n.24

32. Hippocrates: Dioscorides, III.59 and IV.168. Theophrastos: Dioscorides, III.74 and V.108. Nicander: Dioscorides, III.29 and IV.99. Comparison of Dioscorides, II.169.3 with Galen, **Properties of Foods**, II.63.2 (ed. G Helmreich, **Galeni De Alimentorum Facultatibus**, (Leipzig, 1923; in **CMG** V.4.2) p.326) and the Hippocratic **Diseases**, II.38 (ed. Littré, VII.54) with Pliny **NH** XXII.71 (all on mallow and asphodel) shows a deeply embedded and very ancient source for all four authors. It is significant that Galen, **Properties of Foods**, II.63.1 (ed. Helmreich, p.325) quotes from Hesiod, **Works and Days**, 41. The "old poets" were important doxographical sources in their own right for plant names. **Vid.** also n.36 below. Pliny, **NH** XXII.73, acknowledges this tradition specifically: **Asphodelum ab Hesiodo quidam halimon appellari existimavere, quod falsum arbitror**

33. Dioscorides, Pref.1, trans. Scarborough and Nutton (n.5 above) p.195

34. Dioscorides, Pref.1-2, trans. Scarborough and Nutton (n.5 above) p.195. **Vid.** commentary, ibid.,pp.202-208 for details on Iollas, Heraclides of Tarentum, Crateuas, Andreas, Bassus, Niceratus, Petronius, Niger, Diodotus and Asclepiades.

35. Ibid.,pp.198-9 (commentary)

36. Athenaeus, **Deipnosophistae**, quoting (for example) Aristophanes, Callimachus, Menander and Nicander. **Vid.** index entries in the standard modern edition of the Greek text of the **Deipnosophistae**, ed. Georg Kaibel, Leipzig, Teubner, 1889-1890; 3 vols.

37. Max Wellmann, "Beiträge zur Quellenanalyse des Älteren Plinius", **Hermes**, 59, 1924, pp. 129-156 esp. 129-132.

38. **NH**, XX, XXII, XXIV.124ff. and XXVI.82f.

39. Wellmann, "Plinius" (n.37 above) p. 135, n.7

40. **NH**, XX.85

41. **NH**, XIV.76, e.g. Hicesius. Cf. **NH**, XX.35. The Hicesius citation in **NH**, XXVII.31 (on the cabbage) stems, by contrast, from Xenocrates, and behind Xenocrates is probably the physician Aristagoras, listed **with** Xenocrates in the index of authorities for **NH**, XXIX and XXX.

42. **NH**, XX .103 and XXIV.186

43. Max Wellmann, **Die Pneumatische Schule bis auf Archigenes**, Berlin, 1895, p.13

44. **NH**, XX.17 (Chrysippus)

45. **NH**, XX.19 (Democritus, Dionysius, Diocles). Cf. Diocles, Frg. no. 156 (ed. Wellmann, p. 192), which Wellmann suggests comes to Pliny through Julius Bassus, quoting Dionysius. Cf. also Gargilius Martialis, XXV (ed. V Rose, **Plinii Secundi** quae fertur una cum Gargilii **Martialis Medicina**, Leipzig, Teubner, 1875, p. 173, on turnips, who either borrows directly from Pliny, **NH**, XX.19 or uses the same text (Julius Bassus?) employed by Pliny.

46. **NH**, XX.28 (Democritus)

47. **NH**, XX.35 (Hicesius). Cf. **NH**, XXVII.31

48. **NH**, XX.85, 113, 119, 185-195 (Erasistratus). Cf. **NH**, XIX.167 and Dioscorides, III.56

49. **NH**, XX.187: **laudatissimum.** XX.190: **utilissimum**

50. Evenor: **NH**, XX.187, 191. Iollas:NH, XX.187

51. Dioscorides, III.56 (on anise). Galen, **Mixtures and Properties of Simples**, VI.1.4 (XI.833 K.). **Simples**, VI preface (XI.797 K.) with Niger among many authors named: was Galen using the same pharmaco-doxographical collection? Symeon Seth, I: on the anise (ed. B Langkavel, **Simeon Sethi Syntagma De Alimentorum**, Leipzig, Teubner, 1868, pp. 23-4.

52. E.g. Oribasius, **Medical Collection**, XIV.45.1 (ed. Raeder, II, p.217), quoting from a collection of data by Zopyrus, and XIV.50.2 (ed. Raeder, II, p.223), again from Zopyrus. Cf. Celsus, II.31. The "anise" section in Paul of Aegina, VII.3 s.v. is derivative from Galen.

53. **NH**, XX.185 and 186 (Pythagoras). XX.191-194 (Tlepolemus). XX.193 (Heraclides).

54. **NH**, XX.189 compared with Dioscorides, III.56

55. Wellmann, "Plinius" (n.37 above). p.142

56. Galen (quoting Andromachus), **Compound Drugs arranged by Location of Ailment**, III.1 (XII.630 K.) and **Compound Drugs arranged by Kind**, VI.13 (XIII.928 K., viz. ed. Silon).

57. **NH**, XX.221. Cf. **sunt qui** XX.242 (Castor) and 231 (Niger). Cf. Dioscorides, II.119.

58. **NH**, XX.220: **miror quare difficulter in Italia nasci tradiderit id Solon Smyrnaeus.**

59. **NH**, XX.235: **adiecit Solo, ne quod omittamus.**

60. Generally **NH**, XXVII-XXXII

61. Max Wellmann, "Xenocrates aus Aphrodisias", **Hermes**, 42, 1907, pp. 614-629

62. **Vid.** the confused and confusing melange of "sources"for pseudo-Democritus in Franz Susemihl, **Geschichte der griechischen Literatur in der Alexandrinerzeit**, Leipzig, 1891-2; 2 vols., vol. I, pp. 483-4. Cf. the sage remarks by P M Fraser in **Ptolemaic Alexandria**, Oxford, 1972; 3 vols., vol.II, p.641 (n.536) and pp. 644-645 (n.548).

63. Esp. interesting for suggesting how the scholia on Nicander can occasionally help in understanding (and correcting) Pliny´s text is I Cazzaniga, "Note critico-filologiche, III: Plinio il Vecchio XXX 35 e la tradizione di Schol. Nicandro Ther. 372", **Studi Classici e Orientale**, 14, 1965, pp. 16-19

64. Wellmann, "Plinius" (n.37 above) pp. 143-156. Cf. M Geymonat, "Una prefazione in senari al trattato di Valgio Rufo sulle erbe?", **La Parola del Passato**, 29, 1974, 256-261

65. A Ernout, "La magie chez Pline l´Ancien", **Latomus**, 70, 1964, pp. 190-195

66. **Vid.** John Scarborough, "The drug lore of Asclepiades of Bithynia", **PH**, 17, 1975, pp. 43-57

67. Now firmly dated back to the second century BC. Elizabeth Rawson, "The life and death of Asclepiades of Bithynia", **Classical Quarterly**, n.s. 32, 1982, pp. 358-370

68. Cajus Fabricius, **Galens Exzerpte aus alteren Pharmakologen**, Berlin, 1972, pp. 192-198

69. J G Sprengel, **De Ratione, quae in Historia Plantarum inter Plinium et Theophrastum intercedit**, Marburg, 1890

70. L Renjes, **De Ratione, quae inter Plinium Naturalis Historia lib. XVI et Theophrastum libros de Plantis intercedit**, Rostock, 1893

71. Wellmann, **Pneumatische Schule** (n.43 above) p. 26, n.3 (cont. from p. 25)

72. H Stadler, **Die Quellen des Plinius im 19 Buch der Naturalis Historia**, Munich, 1891; Simon Sepp, **Pyrrhoneische Studien**, Freising, 1893, esp. pp. 53-58

73. Fabricius, **Galens Exzerpte** (n.68 above) p. 226, following F Kudlien, "Xenocrates, Nr.8", **RE**, 2nd ser., IX part 2, Stuttgart, 1967, cols. 1529-1531

74. Manfred Ulllmann, "Xenocrates Nr. 7", **RE**,, Supplementband XIV, Stuttgart, 1974, cols. 974-977: 975

75. Galen, **Mixtures and Properties of Simples**, X.1 (XII.248, K.)

76. Oribasius, II.58 (ed. Raeder, I.)

77. Galen, **Mixtures and Properties of Simples** X.2.4 (XII.261, K.)

78. Ullmann (n.74 above) col.976

79. John Scarborough, "Diphilus of Siphnos and Hellenistic medical dietetics", **J. Hist. Med.**, 25, 1970, pp. 194-201

80. Dioscorides, **Preface,** 5: "For I have exercised the greatest precision in getting to know most of my subject through direct observation, and in checking what was universally accepted in the written records and in making enquiries of the natives in each botanical region." trans. Scarborough and Nutton, (n.5 above), p. 196

81. Dioscorides, **Preface**, 2. **Vid.** also n. 34 above

82. Dioscorides, **Preface,** 2, trans. Scarborough and Nutton (n.5 above) p. 196

83. Dioscorides, **Preface,** 2, trans. Scarborough and Nutton (n.5 above) p. 196

84. For example, **NH** XXVII.4-142 (**aconitum** to **tragopodon**)

85. Scarborough and Nutton (n.5 above), pp. 210-212 (on aloe). **Vid.** also John Scarborough, "Roman pharmacy and the eastern drug trade: some problems as illustrated by aloe", **PH**, 24, 1982, pp. 135-143

86. Scarborough and Nutton (n.5 above) p. 209 (commentary on spurge-resin). **Vid.** Dioscorides, III.82

87. Scarborough and Nutton (n.5 above) pp. 209-210 (commentary on the two kinds of St John´s wort).

88. Scarborough and Nutton (n.5 above) pp. 206-208 (commentary on Asclepiades and the **anarmoi onkoi**).

89. ed. A Ernout, **NH**, XXVII.76 (pp.45-46). App. crit. p.45 suggests **gustu languido** for the lacuna (from Dioscorides)

90. ed. M Wellmann,II, p. 184

91. ed. A Ernout, **NH**, XXVII, p. 94: "Plante non identifée", following all dictionaries of Greek

and Latin.

92. Nicander, **Theriaca**, 647. Diocles, Frg. 149 (ed. Wellmann, p. 191). Pliny, **NH**, XXIII.131

93. Paul of Aegina, VII.3 s.v. (ed. Heiberg II, p. 211)

94. ed. Jacques André, **NH**, XXII.51-2 (pp.39-40)

95. ed. Wellmann, II, pp. 188-9

96. ed. André, **NH**, XXII, p. 93 (commentary)

97. Ibid., p. 94 (accepted with reservations).

98. Among a great number, e.g. Dioscorides, IV.86 and Pliny, **NH**, XXVII.23; Dioscorides, IV.88 and **NH**, XXV.160; Dioscorides, IV.89 and **NH**, XXV.161; Dioscorides, IV.90 and **NH**, XXV.162; Dioscorides, IV.91 and **NH**, XXV.159

99. This plant turns up in the papyrus Vindobonensis D. 6257 as the Demotic **ertyn**; the papyrus emerges from Roman Egypt, but records data from far earlier eras. Pap. Vinob. D. 6257 Bk. A, col. x+II, 24

100. **NH**, XXVI.134: **faciunt et aliam hippurim.**

101. Cf. **NH** XIII.116

102. Cf.NH, XXI.119

103. ed. Ernout, **NH**, XXVII, p. 115 (commentary)

104. Trease and Evans (n.11 above) pp. 565-7

105. Theophrastos, **Historia Plantarum**, III. 18.4

106. Oribasius, **Medical Collection**, XIV.61 (ed. Raeder, II, p. 231, from Zopyrus' **Astringents**).

107. Celsus, II.33.4 and III.19.2 (pounded leaves as powder + wine as repressant chest plaster); IV.23.2 (**rubus** + plantain as anti-diarrhoea medicine); and IV.26.8 (**rubus** decoction for anti-diarrhoea treatment: part of a section of drugs from orchard fruits).

108. Nicander, **Theriaca**, 839

109. Galen, **Antidotes**, II.14 (XIV.182, K.)

110. Nicander, **Theriaca**, 700-713, and **Alexipharmaca, 585.**

X

THE PHARMACY OF METHODIST MEDICINE

The evidence of Soranus' *Gynecology*

* The origins of the Methodist Sect probably will remain shrouded in controversy, even though the account by Celsus in *De medicina* suggests acquaintance with doctrines stemming from the sect's beginnings[1]. Drabkin and Edelstein are generally correct when they set Methodism in contrast to Dogmatism and Empiricism[2], showing that the origins of Methodism was in reaction to the radical scepticism of Empiricism and the conjectural physiology of the Dogmatics. Yet, as Rubinstein has lucidly demonstrated[3], one cannot presume that Celsus was an unbiased observer in recounting the approaches of the Methodist Medical Sect as it may have been applied by physicians in the first half of the first century in Rome[4]; Celsus himself apparently espoused a kind of 'Methodism' which was a new version distinct from the teachings of Asclepiades[5], or from Themison[6], presumably a 'follower' of Asclepiades and a member of this new sect. What can be noted, however, is that whenever the sect came into being, it has the trappings of a Roman reaction to Hellenistic theory, a context which fit admirably into Celsus' overall view of medicine, summed as an *ars coniecturalis* [7]. Carefully peeling away Celsus' purported objectivity, Rubinstein brilliantly teases into view an on-going dispute among medical philosophies and physicians in the reign of Tiberius (A.D. 14-37)[8], and shows - among many other specifics about Methodism - that Celsus' account reflects the fluid nature of Methodist doctrines.

Many textbooks assert that Asclepiades of Bithynia (fl. in Rome, c. 120 B.C.)[9] foresook drugs in his therapeutics, a statement that may

---

1Celsus, *De medicina*, proemium, 11. *Vid.* commentary in Philippe Mudry, *La Préface du De medicina de Celse* (Lausanne, 1982), 74-76. *Vid.* also Gary L. Rubinstein, *The Riddle of the Methodist method: Understanding a Roman Medical Sect* (Cambridge, 1985 [Diss.]), 11-14.

2I.E. Drabkin, "Soranus and his System of Medicine", *Bulletin of the History of Medicine*, 25 (1951), 503-518. Ludwig Edelstein, "Methodiker", *RE*, Supplementband VI (Stuttgart, 1935), cols. 358-373 = trans. by C. Lilian Temkin in Owsei and C. Lilian Temkin, eds., *Ancient Medicine : Selected Papers of Ludwig Edelstein* (Baltimore, 1967), 173-191 ("The Methodists").

3Rubinstein (n. 1 above), 16.

4Edelstein (n. 2 above), 176-177 [English trans.].

5Celsus, *De medicina*, I, 3. 6-7 and 18.

6Celsus, *De medicina* , III, 1. 5-6 viewed in conjunction with III, 4. 6 and 6. 13.

7Rubinstein (n. 1 above), 9-11.

8Edelstein (n. 2 above), 9-11.

9John Scarborough, "The Drug Lore of Asclepiades of Bithynia", *Pharmacy in History* , 17 (1975), 43-57 [45]. Elizabeth Rawson, *Intellectual Life in the Late Roman Republic* (London, 1985), 170-171.

result from a hurried reading of the relevant passages in Scribonius Largus' *Compositiones*[10]. Since the Methodists generally claimed Asclepiades as one of their forerunners, even while differing from him[11], it is important to note that Asclepiades certainly did suggest the use of many drugs[12], even while he prescribed the mildest treatments possible for a variety of diseases. Moreover, the remnants of Themison's tract *On Acute and Chronic Diseases* (one now assumes a date for Themison sometime in the late first century B.C. in view of Rawson's redating of Asclepiades[13]) demonstrate a full command of pharmaceutical therapeutics, although such are bereft of dosage-forms or specific measures[14], a characteristic of Soranus' drug-lore and generally that of Caelius Aurelianus. And if one includes Thessalus of Tralles (fl. in the reign of Nero [A.D. 54-68]) in the list of Methodist physicians preceding Soranus, one finds a very clear indication of a complicated pharmacy, albeit self-contradictory from time to time as noted by Soranus[15]. In addition, if the Thessalus of Tralles, who is the author of an extant tract *On the Powers of Herbs*[16] is the same person as the often-excoriated (by Galen) Thessalus of Tralles, 'Methodist physician'[17], then one also can document an aspect of methodist pharmaceutics which included herbal astrology and several layers of folkmedicine interwoven with literature under the name of Hermes Trismegistus[18]. If Thessalus, the Methodist physician, is the same as the

---

[10]Scribonius Largus, *Compositiones*, Epistula dedicatoria, 7 (Sergio Sconocchia, ed., *Scribonii Largi Compositiones* [Leipzig, 1983], p. 3), *Vid.* also Celsus, *De medicina*, V, prooemium 2.

[11]E. Kind, "Soranos aus Ephesos", *RE*, Zweite Reihe, Vol. III, pt. 1 (Stuttgart, 1927), cols. 1113-1130 [col. 1114].

[12]Scarborough, "Asclepiades" (n. 9 above), 46-55.

[13]Elizabeth Rawson, "The Life and Death of Asclepiades of Bithynia", *Classical Quarterly*, n.s. 32 (1982), 358-370; incorporated in Rawson, *Intellectual Life* (n. 9 above), 170-171.

[14]R. Fuchs, "Aus Themisons Werk ueber die acuten und chronischen Krankheiten", *Rheinisches Museum für Philologie*, N.F. 58 (1903), 67-114 [Greek texts with short introduction].

[15]Soranus, *Gynecology*, IV, 39 [88]. 4 (J. Ilberg, ed., *Sorani Gynaeciorum* [Leipzig, 1927 ; in *CMG* IV], p. 152).

[16]Hans-Viet Friedrich, ed., *Thessalos von Tralles griechisch und lateinisch* (Meisenheim am Glan, 1968 [*Beiträge zur klassischen Philologie*, ed. Reinhold Merkelbach, Heft 28]).

[17]Theod. Meyer-Steineg, "Thessalos von Tralles", *Archiv für Geschichte der Medizin*, 4 (1910), 89-108, collects the references. But cf. Rubinstein (n. 1 above), 38 with n. 6, and 46.

[18]A.J. Festugière, "L'expérience religieuse du médecin Thessalos" in *Hermétisme et mystique païenne* (Paris, 1967), 141-180 [rpt. of an essay first published in 1939]. *Vid.* also P. Boudreaux, ed., *Catalogus Codicum*

author of *Powers of herbs*, this may explain why Soranus (and Caelius Aurelianus much later) go to such lengths to comment on "superstition in therapy"[19], even while acknowledging the usefulness of such medicines of magical import to some patients. There are, of course, certain treatments openly rejected by Soranus, treatments which are patently magical, "...
* *which by their results are shown to be lies*"[20]. Yet it was Thessalus who first among the Methodist physicians made distinctions among diseases to be "*treated by drugs and surgery*"[21] as contrasted to illnesses which could be alleviated through regimen and diet[22].

* It was Soranus of Ephesus (fl. in reign of Trajan [A.D. 98-117]) who - in the phrase of Edelstein - "... *reinstated etiology and physiology in* [methodist] *medicine*" [23], refining the old Hippocratic formula of diagnosis, prognosis, and treatment without any hint of humoral pathology or even the underpinnings of pseudo-atomism characteristic of the 'Methodists' since Asclepiades. Drabkin suggests that Themison was inspired to formulate his idea of "*communities of diseases*" (*i.e.* κοινότητες, "*general states*") from Asclepiades' notions of atoms moving about in pores[24], and that illness resulted from a disturbance in this normal motion; from this followed that there were three basic kinds of illness:

1) an abnormally dry, or tense, or stringent state,
2) an abnormally fluid or relaxed state, and

Astrologorum Graecorum, Vol. VIII: *Codicum Parisinorum*, part 4 (Brussels, 1922), pp. 253-262 ["Thessalus medici de virtutibus herbarum ad Claudinum vel Neronem"].

19 E.g. Caelius Aurelianus, *Acute Diseases*, III, 16. 137 (I.E. Drabkin, ed. and trans., *Caelius Aurelianus: On Acute Diseases and On Chronic Diseases* [Chicago, 1950], pp. 386 and 388 [Latin text], and 387 and 389 [English translation]): on hyenas' hides used to 'cure' rabies).

20 Soranus, *Gynecology*, I, 63. 3 (ed. Ilberg [n. 15 above], p. 47): contraceptive amulets of mules' uteruses, mules' ear cerumen, etc. *Vid.* the parallel magical text (in Greek) as contained in the *Papyri Graeci Magicae*, ed. Karl Preisendanz and Albert Henrichs, 2nd ed. (Leipzig, 1973-1974: 2 vols.), Vol. II, p. 174 [*PGM* XXXVI, 320-332] = John Scarborough, trans., "A Contraceptive, the only one in the world", in Hans Dieter Betz, ed., *The Greek Magical Papyri in Translation including the Demotic Spells* , Vol. I: *Texts* (Chicago, 1986), p. 277; the last line reads (in translation), "Mix in also with the barley grains cerumen from the ear of a mule".

21 Galen, *Sects for Beginners*, 6 (G. Helmreich, ed. in *Claudii Galeni Pergameni scripta minora* [Leipzig, 1884-1893 ; 3 vols.], Vol. III, p. 15).

22 *Ibid.* (ed. Helmreich, p. 12).

23 Edelstein (n. 2 above), 190.

24 Drabkin, ed. and trans., *Caelius Aurelianus* (n. 19 above), xvii. Cf. Galen, *Sects for Beginners*, 6 (ed. Helmreich [n. 21 above], p. 12).

3) a disease which combined both states of abnormality.
It is little wonder that the Methodists highly refined differential diagnosis and details of symptomatology, but one also needs to be reminded that Soranus' aims in his medicine were based on a desire for practicality and simplicity, so that one cannot assume a tightly constructed doctrine for the Methodist Sect, even in the pages of its most gifted member. Caelius Aurelianus makes this vividly clear in his translation/adaptation of Soranus in the extant Latin texts of *Acute and Chronic Diseases*: ailments do, indeed, receive precise aetiologies, careful descriptions, and detailed treatments (along with refutations of alternative therapies), but except for the venerated concept of "treatment by contraries", there is no pre-determined classification in Soranus' drug lore, such as one finds in the complex pharmaceutical systematics elaborated by Galen on the basis of humoral doctrines combined with notions of qualities and elements[25]. By contrast, Soranus concentrated on the properties of drugs themselves, and in keeping with the generally-perceived "three states" of disease[26], therapies would be combinations of foods and mild drugs, possibly followed by differing regimens and harsher drugs if the condition were diagnosed as chronic. Once Soranus has made a diagnosis, he "... *knows the "quality" of treatment to employ - even if he does not yet know what strength of qualitative treatment to give. For this will depend on the course of the disease and thus affection*".[27] Pharmaceuticals are fundamental in this system, and Soranus' knowledge of drugs and their useful and harmful properties is evident throughout the *Gynecology* and certainly mirrored by Caelius Aurelianus in the *Acute and Chronic Diseases.*

The Role of Drugs in Methodist Therapies.

To illustrate how Soranus went about diagnosis and treatment of a disease, Rubinstein has chosen Soranus' account of amenorrhea[28], a most apt example since *Gynecology*, III, 6-16 (ed. Ilberg, pp. 97-104) provides not only a lucid sequence of how the Methodist physician arrived at his diagnosis, but also a carefully timed series of treatments, depending on the severity of the retained menses. First comes the "relaxing" stage, and Soranus writes:

---

[25] John Scarborough, 'Galen's Pharmacy' in "Early Byzantine Pharmacology", *Dumbarton Oaks Papers*, 38 (1984), 213-232 [215-221].

[26] Drabkin, ed. and trans., *Caelius Aurelianus* (n. 19 above), xix: "The terms *status strictus, status laxus*, and *status mixtus*, frequently used at a later time, are not found in Caelius".

[27] Rubinstein (n. 1 above), 148.

[28] *Ibid.*, 146-151.

> "After the pains have begun and have become fixed, or after the menstrual blood has been completely kept back, one ought to get the woman into a bed in a room which is comfortably warm and well-lighted, and one ought to ensure that she is awake but quiet and that she eats no food; one ought to press lightly on her extremities as well as those parts of her body which are in the graetest pain... If, however, the pain is not alleviated, one ought to apply also warmed objects and layers[29] either warm cloths, or linen strips and wool and warming-pans filled with hot water, or bladders filled with warm olive oil, or bags filled with moderately heated ground grain, or a sponge wrung out in boiling water and wrapped in a cloth, so that the parts may not be cooled by the moisture but gently soothed by the influence of the vapor. Then one ought to apply on the pubes and abdomen and - at the same time - on the loins and hips, a soft clean piece of wool soaked and wrung out in warm sweet olive oil... warm water is administered as a mouth-wash and for drinking"[30].

Gentle treatment, indeed. Soranus adds, almost parenthetically, that if the beginning stages of the affliction are not too severe, the doctor ought to let the woman sleep[31]. Thus far, one could not class this aspect of therapy for amenorrhea as harsh, or as having any links with a true drug therapy. Yet at the conclusion of his instructions for the "relaxing" phase of his treatment for amenorrhea, Soranus does include three very mild plasters (or poultices), as he advances from the completely harmless external therapies to the murky boundaries between a food and a drug:

> "Also one ought to employ linseed plasters, or plasters of bread kneaded in warm hydromel [water + honey], and sitz-baths[32] which will be described shortly; and at the beginning of the first three-day period [of treatment], one ought to administer a rub-down with an

---

[29]III, 10. 3 (ed. Ilberg [n. 15 above], p. 99, line 29): θερμάσματα. Usually θέρμασμα will mean "warm fomentation" (i.e. poultices or plasters), but Soranus does not use either, so that one can best render this as "warmed objects and layers" which would act like "fomentations".

[30]Soranus, *Gynecology*, III, 10. 2-4 (ed. Ilberg [n. 15 above], pp. 99-100). Cf. Owsei Temkin, trans., *Soranus' Gynecology* (Baltimore, 1956), p. 136 [adapted in parts].

[31]*Ibid.*, III, 10.4 (ed. Ilberg [n. 15 above], p. 100).

[32]τὰ ἐγκαθίσματα, "hip baths" with the woman sitting in a tub, legs outside. Dioscorides, III, 113. 2 (ed. Max Wellmann, *Pedanii Dioscuridis Anazarbei De materia medica* [Berlin, 1906--1914; 3 vols.], Vol. II, p. 126).

> ointment [unspecified]and provide a mouthwash [unspecified] and warm and simple food"[33].

Apparently, the herbal sitz-baths will be repeated again, after the end of a three-day wait, at which time the doctor is instructed in particular techniques of venesection[34], followed by the repeated sitz-bath; the sitz-bath is either warm olive oil, mixed with water, or made with a decoction[35] of fenugreek (*Trigonella foenum-graecum* L.)[36], or of linseed (presumably the oil), or of either garden-variety or wild mallow (either *Malva sylvestris* L., or *Althaea officinalis* L.)[37]. Important is Soranus' warning that successive stages of treatment be administered only after "the disturbance" from the preceding therapy "has subsided"[38] again in keeping with the overall Methodist notions of therapeutics, which may be expressed as treatment: rest, treatment: rest, etc., in increasingly severe therapies.

The second phase of therapy for amenorrhea begins on the third day, and - as noted above - the doctor performs some limited bloodetting, carefully specified to the left arm; one is to avoid venesection from the ankle[39]. Then comes the repeated sitz-bath, using fenugreek or linseed oil, or mallow, or olive oil and water, followed by:

> "The labia having been separated, one should pour in the same oil together with an egg, alone or with one of the decoctions mentioned, beaten up to the thickness of glue. One should next apply to the genitals a piece of soft wool soaked in the same fluids and should then put a piece of felt around. When the disturbance has subsided, one should give warm water for a mouthwash and as

---

[33] Soranus, *Gynecology*, III, 10.5 (ed. Ilberg [n. 15 above], p. 100).

[34] Soranus, *Gynecology*, III, 11. 1-3 (ed. Ilberg [n. 15 above], p. 100).

[35] *Ibid*., line 21: τὸ ἀφέψημα, the technical term used to describe a "boiling down" of a drug to obtain its concentrated form. Dioscorides, II, 107. 1 (ed. Wellmann [n. 32 above], Vol. I, p. 181).

[36] ἡ τῆλις. Theophrastus, *Historia plantarum*, III, 17. 2. Dioscorides, II, 102 (ed. Wellmann [n. 32 above), Vol. I, pp. 176-177.

[37] ἡ μολόχη (Dioscorides, II, 118 [ed. Wellmann (n. 32 above), pp. 191-192]) = ἡ μαλάχη cultivated: Theophrastus, *Historia plantarum*, VII, 7. 2 and 8. 1; wild (ἀλθαία): Theophrastus, *Historia plantarum*, IX, 15. 5; Diocorides [RV] III, 146 (ed. Wellmann [n. 32 above], Vol. II, p. 155). *Vid.* Jacques André, *Les noms de plantes dans la Rome antique* (Paris, 1985), p. 163.

[38] E.g. Soranus, *Gynecology*, III, 11. 3 (ed. Ilberg [n. 15 above), p. 100, line 19).

[39] Soranus, *Gynecology*, III, 11. 1-3.

> a drink in order to assuage the thirst and to facilitate the digestion of food. After the drink one should give a little simple light food, warm and in the form of a gruel, e.g. spelt prepared with water or with honey water boiled down moderately; or the spelt gruel made with honey or olive oil, dill, and a little salt; or bread soaked in water or else together with eggs that can be sipped. After a short interval following the meal, one should allow the patient to sleep"[40].

Two new ingredients have been added in the second part of this second stage of treatment of amenorrhea: dill (*Anethum graveolens* L.)[41], and "a little salt"[42]. Each of these substances has an important role in the gradually intensifying drug therapy, accompanied by increasingly drastic non-pharmaceutical treatments; it is significant that Soranus' carefully-worded description incorporates the technical form for "salt", always given in the plural when a medical preparation or use is intended[43].

Should the ailment not respond to the second phase of therapies (the patient having been kept on a restricted diet, with food on the second day), the third stage of treatments begins (after three days) with cupping followed by bloodletting using leeches[44]. Then comes a phase of treatment employing plasters with "relaxant properties"[45], which include kneaded bread combined with warm fat from a pig[46], or kneaded bread combined with finely-ground mallow roots (cultivated or wild not specified in this passage), or a poultice made with the best meal combined with linseed or fenugreek, or all three boiled together in olive oil, honey, and the decoction of mallow or fenugreek[47]. Added to the oil-soaked lint and linen applied to the wounds engendered by the cupping-vessels and leeches are these plasters applied to "the inflamed parts", plasters which have to be changed frequently. Helpful too, says Soranus, would be a rectal injection

---

40 Soranus, *Gynecology*, III, 11. 3-4 (ed. Ilberg, pp. 100-101). Trans. Temkin (n. 30 above), pp. 137-138.

41 τὸ ἄνηθον. Theophrastus, *Historia plantarum*. I, 11. 2. Dioscorides, III, 58 (ed. Wellmann [n. 32 above], Vol. II, pp. 70-71.

42 καὶ ὀλίγων ἁλῶν. Cf. Dioscorides, V, 109. 1 (ed. Wellmann, Vol. III, p. 79): ἅλς in plural for medical preparations.

43 *Ibid.*

44 Soranus, *Gynecology*, III, 11. 5-7 (ed. Ilberg [n. 15 above], p. 101).

45 Soranus, *Gynecology*, III, 11. 8: τοῖς χαλαστικοῖς χρηστέον καταπλάσμασιν (ed. Ilberg, p. 101, lines 17-18).

46 *Ibid.*, line 18: ὕεια. Dioscorides, I, 76. 2-4 (ed. Wellmann [n. 32 above]. Vol. I, pp. 151-152): how to prepare 'lard' (pigs fat).

47 Soranus, *Gynecology*, III, 11. 8 (ed. Ilberg [n. 15 above], p. 101).

of warm olive oil (as much as four *kyathoi* [c. 1/3 pint), as well as "simple pessaries"[48].

No new ingredients appear in this third stage of therapies, although the inclusion of pig's fat (i.e. "lard") is suggestive of a tradition for its medical employment recorded by Dioscorides[49]. One specifically used lard in treating burns and ailments *"...around the womb as well as on the buttocks"*, so says Dioscorides, and Soranus' incorporation of pig's fat among the ingredients of his "relaxing plasters" may indicate some acquaintance with Dioscorides' work, or at least the pharmacological tradition represented by Dioscorides. Additionally, Soranus now specifies the "roots" of the mallow, whereas previously no particular part of the herb was suggested. Again Dioscorides may be the source of this distinction, although he writes that the *"decoction of mallow is soothing for the uterus* [when made part of a] *sitting-bath"*[50] a particular previously included by Soranus; Dioscorides notes that mallow roots are useful as antidotes agains poisons.

Soranus' "simple pessaries" begin with "the best": a piece of wool soaked in warm, sweet olive oil[51]. He continues by listing wool which has been smeared with a mixture of fenugreek sap with boiled and separated goose or chicken fat[52], or linseed [oil] or mallow likewise compounded with goose or chicken fat. Other ingredients for pessaries - earlier defined by Theophrastus, and reiterated by Dioscorides, as *"a medicated plug of wool or lint to be used as an insert into the anus or vagina"*[53] - suggested by Soranus include triturated egg-yolk, triturated with the goose or chicken fat and fenugreek or linseed, fused into a single substance with strained honey[54]. Egg-yolks are recommended by Dioscorides as part of a recipe for treatment of anal inflammation and 'callous lumps' [hemorrhoids ?][55] along with melilot (prob. either

---

48 Soranus, *Gynecology*, III, 11. 9 : καὶ πεσσοῖς ἀπεριέργοις (ed. Ilberg, p. 101, line 27).

49 Dioscorides, I, 76. 18 (ed. Wellmann [n. 32 above], Vol. I, p. 157) : ὕειον δὲ ἀναλογεῖ τοῖς περὶ ὑστέραν καὶ ἕδραν καὶ πυρικαύτοις ἁρμόζει.

50 Dioscorides, II, 118. 2 (ed. Wellmann, Vol. I, p. 192).

51 Soranus, *Gynecology*, III, 13. 1 (ed. Ilberg [n. 15 above), p. 102, line 14).

52 στέαρ πρόσφατον χήνειον ἢ ὀρνίθειον. Cf. Dioscorides, II, 76. 1 (ed. Wellmann [n. 32 above], Vol. I, p. 151): στέαρ πρὸς μὲν τὰ περὶ μήτραν ἁρμόζει τὸ νεαρὸν χήνειον ἢ ὀρνίθειον.

53 Theophrastus, *Historia plantarum*, IX, 20. 4. Cf. Celsus, V, 21.

54 Soranus, *Gynecology*, III, 13. 1 (ed. Ilberg [n. 15 above], p. 102).

55 Dioscorides, II, 50 (ed. Wellmann [n. 32 above], Vol. I, p. 136).

Melilotus alba Desr., or *M. officinalis* [L.] Lam.)[56], a striking parallel to Soranus' next suggested pessary: a decoction of melilot in sweet wine[57]. The following pessary recommended by Soranus does, indeed, have another parallel in Dioscorides, but the employment of dates from the date palm (the fruits of *Phoenix dactylifera* L.)[58] have opposite effects: Soranus writes that peeled juicy dates boiled in sweet wine would make a good "relaxant" pessary, but Dioscorides says that dates are styptic and quaffed in neat wine are useful in stemming hypermemorrhea[59]. All of Soranus' suggested pessaries in treatment of amenorrhea are those, which he says are "gently relaxing"[60].

Soranus precedes his list of choice pessaries with his reasons for rejecting those simples of harsher properties with a carefully reasoned synopsis; in these passages (*Gynecology*, III, 12. 1-2), one receives a vivid capsule of Soranus' understanding of drugs and their use in the medical treatments of second century Rome:

> "For the ancients were wrong in prescribing so-called blood-drawing suppositories for bringing the blood down, and draughts producing the same result. They did not realize that the draughts harm and upset the stomach, while corroding suppositories ulcerate the uterus and thus produce deep ulcerations of an evil character which heal poorly, while over the ulcerations a scar forms which is thicker than any normal flesh, so that the menstrual catharsis may be retained. And in general all such draughts and suppositories, being of pungent power, act as irritants upon inflammation and thus double the pains and enhance the impediment to menstruation. For just as it is not good to use pungent collyria when the eyes are inflamed, nor irritating remedies in dysuria or difficult defecation, by the same token one should not use pungent things when the uterus is inflamed in very painful menstruation. For such are the

---

56 ὁ μελίλωτος. Cf. Theophrastus, *Historia plantarum*, VII, 15. 3. André, *Noms* [n. 37 above], p. 158. George Usher, *A Dictionary of Plants Used by Man* (London, 1974), p. 385. Oleg Polunin, *Flowers of Europe* (London, 1969), pp. 201-202 [nos. 573 and 575].

57 Soranus, *Gynecology*, III 13.1 (ed. Ilberg [n. 15 above], p. 102, line 19): μελίλωτον ἐν γλυκεῖ καθεψηθέν.

58 Here φοῖνιξ, but properly τοῦ φοίνικος ὁ καρπός, Herodotus, I, 193.

59 Soranus, *Gynecology*, III, 13. 1 (ed. Ilberg [n. 15 above], p. 102). Dioscorides, I, 109. 1 (ed. Wellmann [n. 32 above], Vol. I, p. 102).

60 Soranus, *Gynecology*, III, 12. 2 (ed. Ilberg, p. 102, lines 21-22).

remedies which among the ancients had a reputation for bringing blood... drugs which women have often used for abortion"[61].

Soranus gives four examples of those simples which he repudiates: the squirting cucumber (*Ecballium elaterium* Rich.)[62], black hellebore (*Helleborus niger* L.)[63], pellitory (*Anacyclus pyrethrum* DC)[64], and opopanax (*Opopanax chironium* [L.] Koch.)[65].

During this third stage of therapies, Soranus advises swinging in a hammock, as the treatments progress; after the menstrual flow has returned, there come a series of restorative therapies which include taking baths, eating varied foods, drinking wine (amount not specified), as well as walking, some active exercising of the body and full-body massages. These parts of a restorative regimen are accompanied by what Soranus considers restorative drugs[66], and the manner in which these substances are listed strongly suggests that someone other than the physician is compounding them, at least the cerates[67]:

---

[61] Ed. Ilberg, pp. 101-102, as translated by Temkin (n. 30 above), pp 139-140. Caelius Aurelianus, *Gynaecia*, 8 (ed. Miriam F. Drabkin and Israel E. Drabkin, *Caelius Aurelianus Gynaecia*/ *Fragments of a Latin version of Soranus' Gynaecia from a thirteenth century manuscript* [Baltimore, 151; supplements to the *Bulletin of the History of Medicine*, No. 13], p. 68), renders this last line as: *quibus abhortionibus faciendis utuntur mulieres.*

[62] ἐλατήριον. Theophrastus, *Historia plantarum*, X, 9. 4, and 14. 1. Dioscorides, IV, 150. 3-4 (ed. Wellmann [n. 32 above], Vol. II, pp. 294-295). André, *Noms* (n. 37 above), p. 93. John Scarborough, "Theophrastus on Herbals and Herbal Remedies", *Journal of the History of Biology*, 11 (1978), 353-385 [366 with nn. 84-85].

[63] ἐλλέβορος μέλας, Scarborough, "Theophrastus", 361-362.

[64] τὸ πύρεθρον. Dioscorides, III, 73 (ed. Wellmann [n. 32 above], Vol. II, p. 85).

[65] ὁ ὀποπάναξ, properly the gum of what is sometimes called Hercules' woundwort. Dioscorides, III, 48 (ed. Wellmann, Vol. II, p. 61). Scarborough, "Theophrastus" (n. 62 above), 363-364 with n. 69. Scarborough, "Asclepiades" (n. 9 above), 53. Caelius Aurelianus, *Gynaecia*, 8 (ed. Drabkin and Drabkin [n. 61 above], p. 68) : electerium, elleborum, nitrum, piretrum, opopance ; the scribe (or the Latin tradition itself) had added the fifth to the list, nitrum.

[66] Soranus, *Gynecology*, III, 14 (ed. Ilberg [n. 15 above], pp. 102-103). Caelius Aurelianus, *Gynaecia*, 10 (ed. Drabkin and Drabkin [n. 61 above], pp. 68-69).

[67] αἱ κηρωταί: these were unctuous solid preparations, generally harder than ointments or salves, containing just enough wax to prevent them from melting when applied to the skin. Wax-salves were very prominent in Roman

"One must, moreover, approve after scrutiny[68] cerates [wax-salves), [particularly those made with] oil of sweet marjoram (*Origanum majorana* L. [= *Majorana hortensis* Moench])[69], or oil of lilies (*Lilium candidum* L.)[70], or some similar oil-and-cerate compound; one should not only insert them but also one must smear them over the whole mouth and the neck of the uterus; also one must use very soft emollient pessaries, such as the one made with beeswax, resin of the terebinth tree (*Pistacia terebinthus* L.)[71] [viz. 'turpentine'], and bull's fat[72], combined with sufficient sweet olive oil or henna-oil (*Lawsonia inermis* L.)[73], so that the ingredients all become glutinous; one should also use the pessary prepared from plant-juices[74], and any pessary made from marrow[75], fat, and relaxing seeds; among these substances in the [drug] called "The Pain-Reliever"[76], which is compounded from marjoram. Very helpful also is a bath in olive oil[77]".

---

pharmacy, with a number of popular combinations, e.g. oil-of-roses cerates, etc. Dioscorides, I, 109. 4 (ed. Wellmann [n. 32 above], Vol. I, p. 103).

68 Soranus, *Gynecology*, III, 14. 3 (ed. Ilberg [n. 15 above], p. 103, line 5): δοκιμαστέον δὲ καὶ κηρωτάς.

69 τὸ σάμψυχον (viz., σαμψύχινον) . Usher, *Dictionary* (n. 56 above), pp. 426-427. André, *Noms* (n. 37 above), p. 225.

70 τὸ σοῦσον (viz., σούσινον) usually in Greek as τὸ κρίνον. E. Masson, *Recherches sur les plus anciens emprunts sémitiques en grec* (Paris, 1967), 58-59. André, *Noms*, p. 252.

71 ὁ τερέβινθος (viz.,τερεβίνθινος), usually written τέρμινθος (the resin as τερμίνθινος). Theophrastus, *Historia plantarum*, IX, 2.2.

72 Cf. Dioscorides, II, 76. 6-7 (ed. Wellmann [n. 32 above], Vol. I, p. 153).

73 ἡ κύπρος, Dioscorides, I, 95 (ed. Wellmann, Vol. I, p. 86). André, *Noms*, p. 95. Usher, *Dictionary* (n. 56 above), pp. 346-347.

74 ὁ διὰ χυλῶν πεσσὸς σκευαζόμενος. Soranus may have in mind drugs which contained frankincense, myrrh, aloe, among other substances which were made into lozenges. *Vid*. Galen, *Compound Drugs Arranged by Kind*, V, 11 (ed. C.G. Kühn, *Cl. Galeni Opera omnia* [Leipzig, 1821-1833; 20 vols. in 22 parts], Vol. XIII, p. 831 [among the lozenge-formulas recorded by Hierax of Thebes, as quoted in the *Lozenges* of Asclepiades]). *Vid*. also index entries under χυλίζεται in Dioscorides (ed. Wellmann [n. 32 above), Vol. III, p. 392).

75 Cf. Dioscorides, II, 77. 1 (ed. Wellmann, Vol. I, p. 158).

76 *Vid*. Dioscorides, III, 39. 2 (ed. Wellmann, Vol. II, p. 52).

77 Soranus, *Gynecology*, III, 14. 3 (ed. Ilberg [n. 15 above], p. 103.

Soranus' drugs are carefully chosen for their soothing and emollient properties, and as one follows the gradually increasing variety of pharmaceuticals prescribed for treating amenorrhea (here assumed to be the "acute" form), one perceives a painstaking sequence of mild substances slowly graded into those drugs somewhat stronger with the restorative stage. Soranus' drug lore is detailed and precise, much as would be expected of someone acquainted with Dioscorides' writings - and someone who apparently used them in formulating his own thinking in parts of the materia medica which appear in goodly numbers in the Greek text of Soranus' *Gynecology*. Yet Soranus was no field botanist and his semi-quotations of Dioscorides merely indicate that he - like Pliny before him[78], and Galen later in the century[79] - knew a formidable amount of pharmacy and pharmacology, gleaned from a commonly available number of drug-books, a "pharmacological doxography" purloined by every physician who took knowledge of pharmaceuticals as a precious aspect of the practice of medicine. This may explain why Soranus apparently assumes a general command of pharmacology on the part of his readers: he can, for example, take for granted we would know (without further explanation) "The Pain-Reliever" made from marjoram (this turns up in Dioscorides), or wax-salves and what they were intended to do as contrasted with ordinary salves and ointments, or exactly what a pessary or suppository might be, or just what any of the nine recommended herbs and herbal compounds suggested for amenorrhea might do (or, conversely the harm caused by the four rejected herbs): one knew these things, either from general experience in the practice of medicine, or from exposure to plants from childhood, or from the books which made up the pharmaceutical encyclopedias. As Temkin cogently reminds us, there was a *"... large body of pharmacological and surgical practices shared by most ancient physicians...*[and] *the sects differed mainly in the dietetic treatment on internal diseases"*[80].

If a woman's amenorrhea failed to be cured by the three-stage therapies as detailed in *Gynecology*, III, 6-14, the Methodist physician then proceeded into a *"metasyncritic cure"* for a chronic condition[81], and there are some harsh drugs prescribed, with a last resort making *"... the patient choke on white hellebore"*[82]. If *this* does not effect a cure.

---

[78] John Scarborough, "Pharmacy in Pliny's Natural History: Some Observations on Substances and Sources" in Roger French and Frank Greenaway, eds., *Science in the Early Roman Empire: Pliny the Elder, his Sources and Influences*, London, 1986, 59-85.

[79] Scarborough, 'Galen's Pharmacy' (n. 25 alove), 221.

[80] Temkin (n. 30 above), introduction, p. xxxvi.

[81] *Ibid.*, xxxv, for summary.

[82] Soranus, *Gynecology*, III, 16. 4 (ed. Ilberg [n. 15 above], p. 104, line 23).

"[we] must afterwards prescribe prolonged traveling, the use of natural waters, and, in general, diversion of the mind. For if by thus keeping on with the same things and adding more active ones the condition is relieved, menstruation becomes unimpeded"[83].

The pattern of interweaving pharmaceutical simples into a progressing series of therapies is generally followed throughout the *Gynecology*, whenever Soranus describes treatment for an ailment; likewise, the illnesses recorded in Caelius Aurelianus' adaptation of Soranus in *Acute and Chronic Diseases*, also have drugs interspersed with non -pharmaceutical treatments, so that one receives a clear impression of how the Methodist physician valued pharmacy as an integral part of his practice. Among the over 250 substances of plant, animal, and mineral origin mentioned in the *Gynecology*, Soranus tends to favor (and use repeatedly) about a dozen herbs or herbal preparations, suggesting a personal experience and some success with fenugreek, the oil of sweet marjoram, the oil of white lilies, various fats and marrows, wax-salve pessaries, henna-oil, melilot, dill, mallow, honey, and the ever-present olive oil. By contrast, the nearly 30 substances suggested by Soranus as having contraceptive properties[84], generally do not reappear in the pharmacy and pharmacology of the *Gynecology:* we may be reading a document which records the pharmaceutics, dosage-forms, and hopes gathered by Soranus in his practice - perhaps from midwives and prostitutes, and modern pharmacologists might be surprised at the biochemical and physiological properties (especially spermacidal) of such herbal preparations as oak gall, sumac, pomegranate, ginger and myrtle.

---

[83] Soranus, *Gynecology*, III, 16.4 (trans. Temkin [n. 30 above], p. 143).

[84] Soranus, *Gynecology*, I, 62-63 (ed. Ilberg [n. 15 above], pp. 46-47.

XI

Criton, Physician to Trajan: Historian and Pharmacist

Among the scattered listings of "famous doctors" of Roman times as given in the Byzantine Suda, a prominent name is that of Rufus of Ephesus,[1] well known from a number of important and extant Greek and Arabic texts.[2] The tenth-century Suda says that Rufus lived during the reign of Trajan (A.D. 98-117), a dating that is generally accepted by medical historians, since there is corroborating evidence from Galen and other sources.[3] But the Suda entry, "Rufus of Ephesus," continues by noting that Rufus not only lived during the reign of Trajan, but that Rufus was a doctor in the same era as someone named Criton, who was likewise a physician. Unlike Rufus of Ephesus, who has left us several lengthy tracts in Greek by which to assess his medical practice, Criton the doctor is known only through extracts quoted in Galen and in some Arabic traditions which tell us that a translation of Criton's Kosmētika (Arabic Kitāb az-Zīna) had been rendered by an unknown hand probably before the late ninth century.[4] Galen knows Criton as an important source for the compilation and quotation of drug formulas, but except for some vague mention of Criton's being attached to the "imperial house,"[5] Galen does not indicate either specific reign or emperor.

Other sources aid in dating Criton, apart from the often untrustworthy Suda. Martial, Epigrams, 11.60.6, mentions a Criton, who can cure satyriasis (viz. ulcus tendere),[6] whereas even Hygeia, the goddess of health, could not.[7] Criton was apparently a famous physician in Martial's time, and this particular epigram can be dated to December, A.D. 96,[8] some two years before Trajan became emperor. If the Suda associations reflect historical reality, it would appear that Criton became Trajan's personal physician shortly after the period of Trajan's command in Upper Germany.[9] An "aside" in John Lydus' Magistrates shows that a Criton accompanied Trajan on the Dacian campaigns (A.D. 101-106),[10] and that Criton had written an account of the Dacian Wars, which -- if the testimony of John Lydus is accurate -- was rhetorical and overblown, replete with exaggerations. The Getika of Criton survives in thirty-one lines as quoted by John Lydus, scholiasts on Lucian and Strabo, and five different entries in the Suda.[11] If Jacoby is correct, Criton's Getika probably underlies many of the lines on Trajan's Dacian Wars as found in Dio Cassius, and possibly Jordanes.[12] Pliny the Younger mentions that a friend, Caninius Rufus of Como, had written a long poem (in Greek) on the Dacian Wars,[13] but even though Pliny lavishes great praise on his friend's effort, the poem has vanished without a trace. Appian's account, called the Dakike, is also lost, so that our basic knowledge of the Dacian campaigns of Trajan emerges from Dio Cassius in the extant epitomes by Xiphilinus and Zonarus, the direct quotations of Criton in John Lydus, the scholiasts on Lucian and Strabo, and the Suda -- and, of course, the famous pictorial rendition on Trajan's Column.[14] In spite of the assumption that Dio's account may have been derived mainly from Appian,[15] it seems more reasonable to suppose that Appian's Dakike was, in turn, founded upon Trajan's journal or more probably on Criton's Getika, which had survived long enough to be excerpted directly by the Byzantine scribes who compiled the Suda. Except for Trajan's journal, represented by a single line quoted by Priscian of Caesarea,[16] there seems to be no other basic source for Trajan's Dacian campaigns that was extant for the use of both Appian and Dio, so that Criton's Getika probably was the major source for later accounts of these important campaigns into Dacia.[17]

Kind was rather hesitant in making "Criton the Physician" of the Suda the same person as "Criton the Historian, author of a Getika," lost except for fragments.[18] Context for Criton among late first- and second-century Roman physicians seemed secure,[19] and Wellmann pointed out that Criton was well aware of the works of several older physicians (especially Herodotus) of the "Pneumatic" medical philosophy,[20] but neither Criton nor Herodotus could be identified with the contemporary schools of historical or philosophical scepticism, as had been argued by Sepp.[21] Moreover, the medical texts themselves (especially those contained in the quotations by Galen), did not support linking Criton the Physician with Criton the Historian, even though one could argue the "historical" tendencies displayed by Criton's quotation of Herodotus.[22] The texts did, however, suggest the numerous links between Criton and Herodotus,[23] and it was clear that Criton was a member of some sort of medical "elite" in the last decade of the first century.[24]

Kind's caution was reasonable, since Criton is a common name, and since a doctor-as-historian had become a medical *topos* by the time of Ctesias.[25] Medical texts, from Galen to Aetius of Amida in the sixth century, did speak highly of Criton's status as a physician in the time of Trajan, but except for the mention of a Criton by Martial in a medical context, the evidence connecting the historian with the doctor of the same name was weak. The context fit, the era was right, but there was no explicit text that named "Criton, physician to Trajan, *and* author of the *Getika*."

With the discovery of several inscriptions from Ephesus, Heracleia Salbace in Caria, and elsewhere,[26] the likelihood has increased substantially that Criton the physician is indeed the Criton who wrote a history of the Dacian Wars. *SEG*, IV, 521[27] tells us that his full name was Titus Statilius Kriton, and that he was "chief physician" (*archiatros*) to Trajan.[28] Moreover, as Benedum demonstrates, Criton was part of a tradition of medical families in western Asia Minor,[29] and the term *epitropos* also applied to Criton suggests high honor from the Emperor,[30] if not the actual exercise of a procuratorship. The epigraphical texts show a great prominence for Criton, and later for other Statilii,[31] who apparently had inherited the imperial patronage. Given this added context, Criton the physician was almost certainly an important dependant of Trajan, and can now be securely assumed to be the historian of Trajan's Dacian campaigns.

Physicians as historians had a long pedigree in classical antiquity. One may begin with the traveling doctor Democedes.[32] Although Herodotus does not mention any historical writings by this doctor of the sixth century B.C., the striking details of his career as contained in the *Histories* suggest that there may have been some source that recorded his exploits, perhaps a personal journal. In the fifth century B.C., Ctesias of * Cnidus had traveled widely, doctored the rich and famous, and composed one of the first known Greek accounts of India.[33] Even if Ctesias did not actually fabricate many of the details he "recorded,"[34] he was certainly duped by local wonder tales. His abilities as historial writer may be safely presumed as less than his medical talents,[35] although specifics are lacking on his medical practice.

In the Roman Empire, Criton was not the first physician to receive royal honors as set down in extant inscriptions. C. Stertinius Xenophon, as physician to Claudius (A.D. 41-54), is commemorated in flowery language from Cos,[36] and Xenophon figures in one of the better examples of Tacitean irony -- this time at the expense of the medical profession.[37] Doctors as politicians appear in Roman and early Byzantine times,[38] and it does not seem to be unusual for physicians to double as public and political figures or as prominent writers.[39]

Both the medical and historical writings by Criton retained their importance for some centuries, even though our knowledge of the Kosmētika and Getika is founded upon embedded quotations in later authors. Criton's Getika apparently survived long enough to be quoted directly in the early tenth century by the compilers of the Byzantine Suda and Criton's medical works continued to be used as late as the sixth century, indicated by quotations in Aetius of Amida's Tetrabiblos. The Arabic translations -- now lost -- made of Criton's drug books, as well as a Pseudo-Criton tract On Stones,[40] were done in the ninth century. After the Suda, the Getika disappears as an independent text, and after the quotations by Aetius of Amida, the Greek texts of Criton's medical works seem to have faded away, except for those in the hands of Arabic translators in the ninth century.

Criton and the Dacian Wars

Although one cannot recover enough of Criton's Getika to delineate much more than a general outline, comparison of the extant fragments with the epitomes of Dio Cassius' account of the Dacian Wars is instructive. Dio, 68.14.4-5, tells the interesting story of how Decebalus had diverted the River Sargetia, dug a pit in the dry riverbed, put in it a good amount of gold and silver and other water-resistant precious objects, covered the large hole with stones and dirt, and then rediverted the river into its original course. "But his friend, Bicilis, who knew what had been done, was captured and he provided information about these things."[41] Unless the name is bogus, Bicilis must have been recorded by an eyewitness, and Criton is the most likely candidate.[42] The Romans apparently got the gold and silver out of the riverbed, as well as much other similar booty, since the "aside" in John Lydus' Magistrates, reads as follows:

> [Scythia] was first captured, together with Decebalus who was leader of the Getae, by the great Trajan; and [Trajan] brought to Rome

> 5,000,000 pounds of gold and twice that amount of silver, without counting the drinking-vessels and valuable implements which were beyond estimate, as well as herds of animals and arms and armor, and over 500,000 of the very brave [Dacian] soldiers along with their weapons, as Criton affirmed, being present during the war.[43]

Criton was impressed by the haul from Dacia, and it may be that the Column of Trajan illustrates the episode of Bicilis telling the Romans of the buried treasure under the river.[44] But Criton did more than record the results of Dacia's conquest, since he was following a model of military history that acknowledged the decency of an honorable enemy and provided justifications for a war against such a foe. A passage in Dio (67.7.4) which details the false triumphs and tribute paid by Domitian to Decebalus probably was based upon the beginning of Criton's Getika. Dio sought to put Trajan's actions in a favorable light, as did a scholiast to Lucian in his excerpt from Criton's description of Decebalus in the Dacian Wars waged by Trajan.[45] Moreover, the excerpt from Criton's Getika by the scholiast on Strabo mentions the distinctive pilophoroi,[46] probably felt hats or caps worn by the Dacian nobility, a detail that appears in Dio, 68.8.3 (Boissevain). This suggests also that Criton may have been one of the so-called ethnographic historians of Roman antiquity. Notably, Stephen of Byzantium's Ethnika employs Criton's Getika as a source.[47] Peter the Patrician must also have had Criton's Getika before him, because even more details are recorded about these curious Dacian felt caps:

> Decebalus sent felt-hat wearers as ambassadors to Trajan: these are the more honored men among [the Dacians]. Before that, Decebalus had been sending men with long hair, who are held in less esteem among [the Dacians].[48]

The Suda quotations from Criton's Getika function as glosses on peculiar employment of ordinary words, and the compilers of the Byzantine encyclopedia apparently were amused or perhaps puzzled by the unusual constructions they uncovered. These are more significant than one might assume from a first reading; for example, "they depart to have placed for themselves in completed deeds just now"[49] makes little sense, but if one presumes a "medical" vocabulary, the reading that emerges, "they prove to have been applied just now for completed transactions," is a little less opaque.[50] The Byzantine scribes were quoting Criton for the gloss on arti, and his use of artiōs, but the nuances of peraioumenos, apobainō, and epitithēmi (the last in an unusual passive infinitive) may reflect a specialized medical vocabulary employed for historical writing. But Criton's boōtia is a hapax legomenon for "arable land" or "ploughing," simply recorded by the Byzantine scribes,[51] and the peculiar "defenses" (erumata) of the Dacian farmlands under Decebalus as mentioned by Criton may be echoed in the ta erumata of Dio, 68.9.5. It is possible that Jacoby's Fragment 4 can be somewhat untangled by presuming an underpinning of medical vocabulary, but even the parallel texts from the Hippocratic corpus and Rufus of Ephesus do not improve comprehension substantially. Thus the Suda excerpts consist generally of odd constructions, unique uses of specific words, or sentences and phrases that struck the Byzantine scribes as unusual or perhaps simply mysterious.

It seems that although Criton's Getika underlies much of what we have in Dio's epitomized account of the Dacian Wars, the style and vocabulary may have doomed Criton's original to an almost immediate redaction. If we possessed Appian's lost account of the Dacian Wars, there might exist a more precise pattern of the original Getika and the modern scholar could trace more accurately just what happened to Criton's description of the Dacian Wars in its initial stages of absorption into the Roman historical traditions of the second and third centuries. The short segments that have come down to us relatively intact show a narrative of events of Trajan's Dacian Wars by Criton, replete with specific names connected with particulars, a narrative that could only have been compiled by someone on the scene who could speak to eyewitnesses and participants. Yet Criton may have been one of many such on-the-spot reporters, whose style and odd verbosity caused chuckling among readers, similar to reactions to Callimorphus' History of the Parthian War. Not insignificantly, Callimorphus was also a doctor; this is what Lucian has to say about his Parthian War and similar histories written by physicians in the second century:

> Another of them has compiled a bare record of the events and set it down on paper, completely prosaic and ordinary, such as a soldier or craftsman or merchant following the army might have put together as a diary of daily events. This beginner, however, was not all that bad: it was very apparent at the start of his account what he was, and his writing has provided

> the materials for some future historian of taste and ability. I fault his work on this alone: he wrote more pompously than his treatises deserved -- "Callimorphus, Physician of the Sixth Kontophoroi [Lancers], History of the Parthian War," followed by the number of each book. And -- by Zeus -- even his preface was too formal, being as follows: it was fitting for a physician to write history, because Asclepius was the son of Apollo, and Apollo was the leader of the Muses and lord of all cultural matters; and after beginning his work in Ionic, he suddenly shifted to the Greek vernacular (koinē) -- for a reason I do not comprehend -- using anyway [the Ionic] for "medicine," "attempt," "how many," and "diseases," but the other [terms] from common speech and most of them from the language of the crossroads [vulgar speech].[52]

From the remnants of the Getika, one cannot accuse Criton of being pompous, but he does seem to have mixed his terminologies as Lucian charges Callimorphus had done in the Parthian War. Lucian's remarks about medical "Ionisms" in Callimorphus' historical writing would apply equally well to Criton's Getika, if the fragments of the work are representative. This is an expected trait in the medical works of the Roman Empire composed in Greek, since many doctors sought to emulate the "style" of the great Hippocrates, whose purported works were almost always in the Ionic.[53] It should be added that Lucian is an able critic of medicine and medical works in his day (ca. A.D. 120-180),[54] so that his observations on doctor-historians would not simply reflect matters of style, vocabulary, and form, but also the content of such works. It may be remotely possible that along with Callimorphus, Lucian may have in mind Criton's Getika as he begins this section of How to Write History, when he says "another of them has compiled a bare record of events...completely prosaic and ordinary,"[55] but unlike Criton's work on the Dacian campaigns under Trajan, Callimorphus' account of Trajan's Parthian War is unknown except for this notice by Lucian.[56] Criton's Getika probably was rated as one of the better "amateur efforts," while Callimorphus' work could be pilloried as one of the worst.

Criton's Pharmacology

When one turns to Galen's quotations from Criton's drug books, one is struck by the respect paid by Galen to a rather large mass of compiled recipes, drawn together by Trajan's physician. Criton had become famous enough by A.D. 96 to be mentioned by Martial,[57] and it seems clear that Criton was part of a circle of prominent, socially respectable physicians just before and during the reign of Trajan. Links with Ephesus are established through the inscriptions summarized above, and connections between Criton and Asclepiades Pharmacion, as well as Lucius, and probably Archigenes and Herodotus, are all indicated in the quotations from Criton's works in Galen.[58] If one totals the extant remains of Criton's medical and pharmaceutical writings in Galen's compilations of earlier recipes, there are about fifty Teubner-size pages of text from Criton. Galen is not the only medical writer to quote Criton: we have shorter citations and excerpts in Oribasius, Paul of Aegina, and Aetius of Amida.[59]

Criton assembled four books on _Kosmētika_ (probably more accurately rendered as "Art of Dress and Ornament" than simply "Cosmetics"), summarized by Galen according to subject matter.[60] The _Kosmētika_ included more than the "cosmetic drugs" which were used to enhance natural beauty through simples and mixtures of drugs in face packs and other means,[61] but also the matters that would come under the category of _kommōtikē_, the "Art of Embellishment," which sought through artistic arrangement of face and body ornaments to increase the attractiveness of one's natural appearance.[62] We can detect the wishes of the imperial household behind Criton's composition of his _Kosmētika_,[63] and can also easily envision the ladies and gentlemen of the court being advised seriously by Criton regarding the best hair dyes, the finest face packs, the safest treatments that would prevent hair loss, the least risky depilatories, ways to arrange jewelry, and the like. The _Kosmētika_ was, however, no frivolous tract, composed to amuse the fops of Trajan's court: it was a solid collection of many recipes for plasters, hair dyes, and similar concoctions that had known and beneficial properties, and Criton drew on the best pharmaceutical authorities he could find,[64] including Dioscorides.[65] Other known authorities turn up in Criton's second work in five books,[66] called either _Peri tēs tōn pharmakōn syntheseōs_ (_Compound Drugs_),[67] or _Peri tōn haplōn pharmakōn_ (_Simples_).[68]

If Galen has recorded the form and contents of Criton's Kosmētika accurately, we know that Criton had begun his account of drugs first of all, not only to "preserve hair," (as the quotation from the Preface of Book I of Criton's Kosmētika shows),[69] but also that he had lifted recipes on the treatment of hair loss from noted authorities on the subject. In Book I, he had excerpted eight recipes taken from the earlier works of Heracleides of Tarentum,[70] and one from Andromachus the Younger.[71] Galen writes that Criton had, in the first book of his Kosmētika, described from his own experience the use of drugs for the treatment of lice in the hair and scalp,[72] which Galen warns are dangerous in the hands of unpracticed doctors but notes that a physician is often called upon to use them as safely as possible. Having said this about Criton's delousing drugs, one would then expect Galen to provide examples from Criton's list of lice-killers, but instead, Galen gives five recipes for depilatories (psilōthra) from Book I of Criton's Kosmētika.[73] Two are listed as Criton's formulas, one is called "the Paris" (perhaps "the Depilatory of Paris," the name of a prominent actor of the day),[74] another is simply given as "another recipe" (following "the Paris"), and the fifth recipe is quoted from the writings of Heracleides of Tarentum.

The Greek is peculiar, and it is apparent that Galen has excerpted and summarized more than Criton's formulas for hair removers, but the first recipe reveals much about Criton's acquaintance with the best earlier authorities on pharmacology, as well as his consideration of the people undergoing a rather risky treatment:

> Depilatories: the Work by Criton. [1]. Take seven or ten scruples[75] of golden orpiment, and an equal amount of quicklime, two ounces[76] of fine meal, one ounce of the earth called by the Romans "Selinisian." Having pounded and sifted everything through a sieve with very small holes, put it away for storage. When using [the preparation], taking as much of the drug as is strong enough, let it take effect [mixed] in water; then it is to be smeared on as an ointment, and he advises that one pay close attention so that it will not burn [the skin].[77]

Depilatories had a long history before Criton,[78] but the use of yellow orpiment (arsenic trisulfide, As_2S_3; Greek arsenikon, here with chrysizonton) is rather unusual in ancient formulas for hair removers. Among the Greek and Roman medical authors who mention arsenic trisulfide, only Dioscorides before Criton suggests orpiment as a depilatory.[79] This strongly implies that Criton was well acquainted with Dioscorides' Materia Medica, and that -- as Dioscorides urged -- the drugs were "tested" before they were used.[80] On the other hand, Dioscorides does not recommend quicklime (asbestos) as a depilatory,[81] nor do other pharmacological writers who mention asbestos.[82] One may suppose that Criton had employed quicklime in his depilatories and found it to be quite effective, if somewhat caustic, as indicated by Galen's summary in the last line of his first quotation from Criton's listing (lexis) of hair remover formulas. The fop or actor might, indeed, be rather uneasy about this application, if he knew about the substances involved, but Galen's afterthought that Criton "advised close attention to the treatment" so that it would not become a harmful experience shows that Trajan's doctor was very much aware of the ointment's effectiveness and the latent danger of this strong combination. Not unexpectedly, modern preparation for the removal of hair from skins of animals includes the application of arsenic trisulfide.[83]

"Selinisian Earth" is mentioned by Dioscorides,[84] but except for the summary of "earths" by Galen,[85] which is very similar to the classifications and uses given by Dioscorides, this form of natural chalk does not seem to reappear in Greco-Roman drug lists. Again it is reasonable to suppose that Criton knew of this "earth" which took its name from Selinus in Sicily, through the works of Dioscorides, who had written that Selinisian Earth is white, brittle, and extremely water soluble ("...quickly dissolved should it receive water").[86] This particular property would, indeed, make it ideal for the prepared form of the depilatory ointment, signaled by Criton's unusual use of epichriō,[87] also in Dioscorides.[88] It may be, moreover, significant that Galen's quotation of Criton's arsenikon-asbestos depilatory includes the rare meaning of anakoptō, here "take effect" as employed otherwise by Herodotus, the older contemporary of Criton.[89]

The remnants of Criton's drug lore show that he was an astute pharmacologist who knew the best written sources of his time,[90] and who was careful with his patients and shrewd in his preparations of drug recipes. Association with other well-known physicians of his day also indicates the probability of firsthand observations of formula preparations -- and perhaps employment on patients. And there is enough evidence to suggest a fame for Criton, not only from his drug lore but also from his treatment of satyriasis,[91] a condition that worried Martial and his readers as well as numerous medical writers including the Latin adapter of Soranus, the fifth-century Methodist physician Caelius Aurelianus.[92] Trajan may have decided to make Criton his own personal physician after his reputation as an excellent doctor with a special skill in compounding drugs had reached the future emperor's ears. The post offered Criton an opportunity to pursue his historical interests as well.

Notes

1. Suda, P, 241 (Ada Adler, ed., Suidae Lexicon [Leipzig, 1928-1938; repr. Stuttgart, 1971; 5 vols.], vol. IV, 301-2).

2. The basic collection of Greek texts (with French trans.) remains Ch. Daremberg and Ch. Emile Ruelle, eds., Oeuvres de Rufus d'Éphèse (Paris, 1897; repr. Amsterdam, 1963). Recent texts re-edited from a fuller manuscript tradition include Alexander Sideras, ed. and trans. (German), Rufus von Ephesos: Über die Nieren- und Blasenleiden (Berlin, 1977 [Corpus Medicorum Graecorum III 1]) and Hans Gärtner, ed., trans. (German), and commentary, Rufus von Ephesos: Die Fragen des Arztes an den Kranken (Berlin, 1962 [Corpus Medicorum Graecorum, Suppl. IV]). Unknown except for its Arabic version is Rufus' "Case Histories," now available in a printed Arabic text and German translation: Manfred Ullmann, ed., Rufus von Ephesos Krankenjournale (Wiesbaden, 1978). This tract does not appear in the list of Rufus' writings in the Suda (ed. Adler, IV, 302 [n. 1 above]).

3. Fridolf Kudlien, "Rufus of Ephesus," in C.C. Gillispie, ed., Dictionary of Scientific Biography, vol. XI (New York, 1975), 601-3.

4. Fuat Sezgin, Geschichte des arabischen Schrifttums, vol. III: Medizin -- Pharmazie -- Zoologie -- Tierheilkunde (Leiden, 1970), 60-61.

5. Galen, Compound Drugs Arranged by Location of Ailment, I, 3 (ed. C.G. Kühn in Claudii Galeni Opera omnia [Leipzig, 1821-33; repr. Hildesheim, 1964-65; 20 vols. in 22], vol. XII, 445).

6. J.N. Adams, The Latin Sexual Vocabulary (London, 1982), 40-41.

7. M. Wellmann, "Herodots Werk," Hermes 40 (1905), 580-604 [esp. 581-83] shows that satyriasis was considered a major disease by Archigenes and Herodotus, older contemporaries of Criton.

8. F.E. Kind, "Kriton (7)," RE, XI, part 2 (1922), cols. 1935-38 [1935].

9. Cf. Historia Augusta: Hadrian, 2.5-6. Ronald Syme, Tacitus (Oxford, 1958; 2 vols.), I, 11 n. 3, and 34 nn. 3-4.

10. John Lydus, De magistratibus, II, 28.2 = FGrH 200 F 1. Cf. Syme. Tacitus, I, 52-53.

11. FGrH 200: Kriton. Eight fragments.

12. Ibid., Kommentarband.

13. Pliny the Younger, Letters, 8.4. Syme, Tacitus, I, 221 n. 4.

14. I.A. Richmond, "Trajan's Army on Trajan's Column," Papers of the British School at Rome 13 (1935), 1-40. Lino Rossi, Trajan's Column and the Dacian Wars, Eng. trans. rev. J.M.C. Toynbee (London, 1971).

15. Bernard W. Henderson, Five Roman Emperors (Cambridge, 1927), 294.

16. Ibid., 252.

17. Syme, Tacitus, I, 221: "There were certain impediments, however, to the delineation of the campaigns in Dacia. Too much material, perhaps, and too many experts at hand to help or criticize...The subjugation of Dacia was slow work and hard work. The pictured scroll on Trajan's column exhibits Roman warfare as routine and engineering, not battle and splendour and glory."

18. Kind, "Kriton," col. 1935.

19. Max Wellmann, Die Pneumatische Schule bis auf Archigenes (Berlin, 1895 [Philologische Untersuchungen 14]), 20.

20. Ibid., 14 n. 7.

21. Simon Sepp, Pyrrhonëische Studien (Freising, 1893), 120-21.

22. Kind, "Kriton," col. 1938.

23. Aetius of Amida, 15.14 and 17 (ed. S. Zervos, Aetiou Amidinou logos dekatos pemptos in Athēna 21 [1909], 1-144 [61 and 103-5]). Cf. Galen, Compound Drugs Arranged by Kind, V, 3 (ed. Kühn [n. 5 above], XIII, 786-94).

24. Galen, Compound Drugs by Location, I, 3 (ed. Kühn [n. 5 above], XII, 443). Juvenal, 6.236 [Archigenes as fashionable doctor]. Wellmann, Pneumatische Schule, 20 n. 10.

25. Truesdell S. Brown, "Suggestions for a Vita of Ctesias of Cnidus," Historia 27 (1978), 1-19.

26. Jost Benedum, "Kriton (7)," RE, Suppl. XIV (1974), cols. 216-20, and Benedum, "Titos Statilios Kriton. Ein Beitrag zur medizin-historischen Epigraphik der Antike," Clio Medica 7 (1972), 249-58.

27. = E. Mary Smallwood, Documents Illustrating the Principates of Nerva, Trajan and Hadrian (Cambridge, 1966), no. 175 (71-72).

28. SEG, IV, 521, line 5. See also Vivian Nutton, "Archiatri and the Medical Profession in Antiquity," Papers of the British School at Rome 45 (1977), 191-26 (221, no. 40, with refs. to further literature).

29. Benedum, "Kriton," cols. 218-19.

30. SEG, IV, 521, line 5.

31. Nutton, "Archiatri," 221, nos. 40-42. Jost Benedum, "Statilios Attalos. Ein Beitrag zur medizinhistorischen Numismatik der Antike," Medizinhistorische Journal 6 (1971), 264-77.

32. Herodotus, 3.129-37. Dio Chrysostom, Discourses, 77/78 [Envy], 10-11.

33. Truesdell, S. Brown, The Greek Historians (Lexington, Mass., 1973), 77-86.

34. Ibid., 77-78 nn. 3-11 reviews some of the ancient and modern literature. Representative of the negative view (both omitted by Brown) are Lucian, True Story, 1.3, and Ronald Syme, Emperors and Biography (Oxford, 1971), 263 nn. 1-7. More succinctly, Syme writes, "The faking of history can serve for guidance, with Ctesias as the primordial exhibit" (Ronald Syme, "Fraud and Imposture" [Geneva, 1972] repr. in Historia Augusta Papers [Oxford, 1983], 9).

35. Jacoby, FGrH 688, collects 74 fragments from Ctesias' lost writings, but only two (F 67-68) are related to his medical practice. F 67 (in Galen [ed.

Kühn, n. 5 above], XVIII, part 1, 731) shows that Ctesias apparently was acquainted with the Hippocratic work On Joints, and F 68 (quoted in Oribasius, Medical Collection, VIII, 8 [J. Raeder, ed., Oribasii Collectionum medicarum reliquiae (Leipzig, 1928-33; 4 vols.; Corpus Medicorum Graecorum VI 1, 1-VI 2, 2), vol. I, 261]) is an extract of Ctesias' work on medical plants, here the black hellebore.

36. IG Rom., IV, 1086 = Dittenberg. SIG, 804 = E. Mary Smallwood, Documents Illustrating the Principates of Gaius, Claudius and Nero (Cambridge, 1967), no. 262 (p. 74). Nutton, "Archiatri," 196 and 223-24 (nos. 68A and B).

37. Tacitus, Annals, 12.67.2. John Scarborough, Roman Medicine (London, 1969; repr. 1976), 96.

38. Scarborough, Roman Medicine, 112-13. Nutton, "Archiatri," 220 no. 27) and Nutton, "L. Gellius Maximus, Physician and Procurator," Classical Quarterly n.s. 21 (1971), 262-72. See also Barry Baldwin, "Beyond the House Call: Doctors in Early Byzantine History and Politics" and Vivian Nutton, "From Galen to Alexander: Aspects of Medicine and Medical Practice in Late Classical Antiquity" in John Scarborough, ed., Byzantine Medicine (Washington, D.C., 1984 [Dumbarton Oaks Papers, vol. 38, in press]).

39. E.g. Callimorphus the physician, author of a History of the Parthian War. Lucian, How to Write History, 16.

40. Sezgin, Geschichte, 60.

41. Dio, 68.14.5.

42. Cf. Dio, 68.12.1-5. In the affair of Longinus details appear to have been gathered on the spot or from participants or from eyewitnesses; one would like to know exactly what sort of poison (here simply pharmakon) Longinus used to commit suicide (68.12.3-4). Criton most likely gave the name of the particular drug, and so probably did Dio's original.

43. John Lydus, Magistrates, II, 28.2 = FGrH 200 F 1.

44. Rossi, Trajan's Column, 200 with refs.

45. FGrh 200 F 2.

46. Ibid., F 3.

47. Stephen of Byzantium, Ethnika, s.v. Getia (ed. A. Meineke, Stephani Byzantii Ethnicorum [Berlin, 1849; repr. Graz, 1958].

48. Peter the Patrician, frag. 5 (in C. Müller, ed., Fragmenta Historicorum Graecorum [Paris, 1841-70; 5 vols.], vol. IV, 185, col. 1).

49. Suda, A, 4035 (ed. Adler [n. 1 above], vol. I, 368) = FGrH 200 F 4.

50. Using readings as found in Rufus of Ephesus, Anatomy of the Parts of the Body, 64 (ed. Daremberg and Ruelle [n. 2 above], 183 [peraioumenos]); the Hippocratic Coan Prognostics, II, 405 (ed. E. Littré, Oeuvres complètes d'Hippocrate [Paris, 1839-61; 10 vols.], vol. V, 676 [apobainō]); and the Hippocratic Sterility, 214 (ed. Littre, vol. VIII, 414 [epitithēmi]).

51. Suda, B, 388 (ed. Adler [n. 1 above], vol. I, 480) = FGrH 200 F 5.

52. Lucian, How to Write History, 16. The last words in the passage (ek triodou) are literally "from where the three roads meet." Such spots were apparently frequented by sleazy drug panderers and less-than-respectable would-be doctors. Galen, Crisis Days, I, 11 (ed. Kühn [n. 5 above], IX, 823) and Method of Medicine, XI, 15 (ed. Kühn, X, 786).

53. Modern scholars generally believe that no work we have under the "name" of Hippocrates is actually by him. G.E.R. Lloyd, "The Hippocratic Question," Classical Quarterly n.s. 25 (1975), 171-92. But see Wesley Smith, The Hippocratic Tradition (Ithaca, N.Y., 1979), 60-63, who argues that the Hippocratic Regimen is "genuine," an argument critiqued by John Scarborough in a review of Smith in American Journal of Philology 103 (1982), 340-44.

54. Barry Baldwin, Studies in Lucian (Toronto, 1973), 36-40. Scarborough, Roman Medicine, 127-28.

55. Lucian, How to Write History, 16, lines 1-3.

56. Yet some kind of medical underpinning is apparent in Xiphilinus' epitome of Dio, 68.33.2-3 (on the illness and death of Trajan). Callimorphus? Criton? See the discussion -- and resultant quandaries -- in F.A. Lepper, Trajan's Parthian War (London, 1948), 199-200.

57. Martial, Epigrams, 11.60.6.

58. See nn. 19, 20, and 24 above.

59. Cajus Fabricius, Galens Exzerpte aus älteren Pharmakologen (Berlin, 1972), 190-92 [Galen]. Oribasius, Synopsis for Eustathius, IX, 61, chap. addit. (extant in a Latin translation only), in U.C. Bussemaker and Ch. Daremberg, eds., Oeuvres d'Oribase (Paris, 1851-76; 6 vols.), vol. VI, 397-402: "Ad eos qui sanguinem per urinam faciunt: Criton in libro tertio." Aetius of Amida, 15.14 and 17 (ed. Zervos [n. 23 above]). Aetius, 6.64 (in Alexander Olivieri, ed., Aetii Amideni libri medicinales V-VIII [Berlin, 1950; Corpus Medicorum Graecorum VIII 2], 210-211) is derivative from Galen. See also Paul of Aegina, 1.46 (Criton and Archigenes), 3.1.4 (Criton on baldness and hair growth), 4.7.1-2 (Criton on the removal of stigmata, perhaps both tattoos and/or scars, and blemishes of the skin), and 7.13.19 (Criton's two formulas for smegmata, probably soaps) in I.L. Heiberg, ed., Paulus Aegineta (Leipzig, 1921-24; 2 vols.; Corpus Medicorum Graecorum IX 1 and 2), vol. I, 30, 130, and 328-29; and vol. II, 326-27. On soap in antiquity, see John Scarborough, "Roman Medicine and Public Health," in T. Ogawa, ed., Public Health (Tokyo, 1981), 33-74 [esp. 39-40 nn. 58-83].

60. Galen, Compound Drugs by Location, I, 3 (ed. Kühn [n. 5 above], XII, 446-50).

61. Peter Green, "Ars gratia cultus: Ovid as a Beautician," American Journal of Philology 100 (1979), 381-92, with refs. Scarborough "Public Health," 39.

62. Galen, Compound Drugs by Location, I, 2 (ed. Kühn [n. 5 above], XII, 434-35).

63. Ibid., I, 2-3 (esp. XII, 434-35, 443, and 445).

64. Kind, "Kriton," col. 1936. 36-58.

65. Galen, Compound Drugs Arranged by Kind, II, 11 (ed. Kühn [n. 5 above], XIII, 515-17); cf. Dioscorides,

Simples, I preface (in Max Wellmann, ed., Pedanii Dioscuridis Anazarbei De materia medica...Liber De simplicibus [Berlin, 1906-14; repr. 1958; 3 vols.], vol. III, 151).

66. Galen, Compound Drugs by Kind, IV, 6; V, 3; and VI, 1-2 (ed. Kuhn [n. 5 above], XIII, 708-16, 786-801, and 859-82).

67. Ibid., V, 3 (XIII, 786).

68. Ibid., VI, 1 (XIII, 862).

69. Ibid., Compound Drugs by Location, I, 2 (XII, 435).

70. Ibid., (435-39). Heracleides of Tarentum was active in the first quarter of the first century B.C., and was one of the most famous of the Empiricist physicians. John Scarborough and Vivian Nutton, "The Preface of Dioscorides' Materia Medica: Introduction, Translation, Commentary," Transactions and Studies of the College of Physicians of Philadelphia n.s. 4 (1982), 187-227 [203 with refs.].

71. Galen, Compound Drugs by Location, I, 2 (ed. Kühn [n. 5 above], XII, 438-39). Andromachus the Younger fl. ca. A.D. 70, and may have been a physician of Nero, along with his father "the Elder." Andromachus the Younger composed three books on pharmacy and drugs, according to Galen, Compound Drugs by Kind, II, 1 (XIII, 463): one was on external medicines, the second considered drugs taken internally, and the third was a short booklet on drugs for eye diseases.

72. Galen, Compound Drugs by Location, I, 4 (ed. Kuhn [n. 5 above], XII, 450).

73. Ibid. (453-55).

74. Suetonius, Domitian, 3.1. Martial, Epigrams, 11.13.7. Juvenal, 6.87.

75. This is an approximation of the peculiarly corrupted Greek text (ed. Kühn, XIII, 453).

76. That is, Roman ounces (ounkiai, normally abbreviated -- as here -- γο).

77. Galen, Compound Drugs by Location, I, 4 (ed. Kühn [n. 5 above], XII, 453-54).

78. Among many references: Theophrastus, *Historia Plantarum*, 9.20.3. Nicander, *Theriaca*, 902. John Scarborough, "Theophrastus on Herbals and Herbal Remedies," *Journal of the History of Biology* 11 (1978), 353-85 (382 n. 160), and Scarborough, "Nicander's Toxicology, II: Spiders, Scorpions, Insects and Myriapods," *Pharmacy in History* 21 (1979), 3-34 and 73-92 (91 n. 367).

79. Dioscorides, *Materia Medica*, V, 104.2 (ed. Wellmann [n. 65 above], vol. III, 74).

80. Scarborough and Nutton, "Preface" [n. 70 above], 199-202 and 218.

81. Dioscorides, *Materia Medica*, V, 155 (ed. Wellmann [n. 65 above], vol. III, 85-86).

82. E.g. Lycus in Oribasius, *Medical Collection*, VIII, 25.16 (ed. Raeder [n. 35 above], vol. I, 279).

83. E.S. Dana, *A Textbook of Mineralogy*, 4th ed., rev. W.E. Ford (New York, 1949), 408.

84. Dioscorides, *Materia Medica*, V, 155.2 (ed. Wellman [n. 65 above], vol. III, 105).

85. Galen, *Mixtures and Properties of Simples*, IX, 1.4 (ed. Kuhn [n. 5 above], XII, 180).

86. Dioscorides, V, 155.2 (ed. Wellmann [n. 65 above], vol. III, 86).

87. Cf. Zopyrus in Oribasius, *Medical Collection*, XIV, 58.1 (ed. Raeder [n. 35 above], vol. II, 228).

88. Dioscorides, *Materia Medica*, III, 22.5 (ed. Wellman [n. 65 above], vol. II, 30).

89. Robert Fuchs, "Anecdota medica graeca," *Rheinisches Museum* 58 (1903), 67-102 [92]. Cf. Wellmann, "Herodots Werk," 581.

90. Kind, "Kriton," col. 1936.

91. Martial, *Epigrams*, 11.60.6.

92. Wellmann, "Herodots Werk," 581-84.

XII

Pharmaceutical Theory in Galen's Commentaries on the Hippocratic Epidemics: Some Observations on Roman Views of Greek Drug Lore

Galen of Pergamon (A.D. 129-after 210) wrote a number of commentaries on Hippocratic works, intending – so he believed – to improve understanding of the Father of Medicine. In fact, Galen formulated a "Hippocratism" that suited his own ideals of what a doctor should be, and this Hippocratic ideal became the basis upon which western medicine founded its memory of Hippocrates and the Greek medicine of the 5th century B.C. But as Temkin[1], and more recently Wesley Smith have demonstrated[2], Galen's "Hippocratism" was, in many cases, derived from a self-induced desire by Galen to create a medical ideal, and was not founded upon any particular "genuine" works by Hippocrates. Moreover, the current majority opinion among scholars of ancient medical history indicates that we have no actual works by a Hippocrates in the corpus of writings under his name[3], but rather we possess a collection of medical treatises and data from about the middle of the 5th century B.C. to perhaps as late as the 1st century A.D. Once this opinion is assumed, we may be able to derive fruitful insights into the evolution of Greco-Roman medicine, especially if we see this medicine as a continually changing series of doctrines as contrasted with fossilized dogmas that were merely passed on for almost six centuries.

An important part of Roman medicine was pharmacy, generally in the form of medical botany, although Roman pharmacology (like its Greek and Hellenistic predecessors) had many medical uses for various minerals, insects, and animal products.[4] Galen recognized the value of drugs in the practice of medicine, but he was baffled by the multiplicity of prescriptions he found in the written sources of his day, and he was constantly frustrated by the usual lack of precision both in terms of species identity in medical botany and the wildly varying suggestions for dosages as prescribed by his written authorities. A perusal of Galen's "drug books" shows him at his least effective as he attempts, through lengthy excerpts of earlier sources, to gain a concise organization for the almost 700 pharmaka known to

1 Owsei Temkin, Geschichte des Hippokratismus im ausgehenden Altertum, Kyklos 4 (1932) 1–80, and Galenism (Ithaca, New York: Cornell Univ. Press, 1973), 10–50.

2 Wesley D. Smith, The Hippocratic Tradition (Ithaca, New York: Cornell University Press, 1979), 61–176.

3 Vid. e.g. G. E. R. Lloyd, The Hippocratic Question. Classical Quarterly, n.s. 25 (1975) 171–192. But vid. Smith, Hippocratic Tradition, 44–60, who argues for the genuineness of the Hippocratic Regimen.

4 Vid. e.g. John Scarborough, Some Beetles in Pliny's Natural History. Coleopterists Bulletin 31 (1977) 293–296, and Nicander's Toxicology, II: Spiders, Scorpions, Insects and Myriapods. Pharmacy in History 21 (1979) 3–34 and 73–92.

Greco-Roman medicine. In his Properties and Mixtures of Simples[5], Galen undertakes a simplified alphabetical listing which is more confusing than helpful, thus verifying Dioscorides' warning against such alphabetical compilations of drugs.[6] In his Compound Drugs Arranged by Location of Ailment[7], and in his Drugs by Kind[8], Galen simply borrows large swatches of material from the earlier recipe-compilations by Andromachus, Asclepiades Pharmacion, Criton, and others.[9] There is a muddling of drug lore, only gradually corrected by later Byzantine pharmacologists, who did not generally take Galen as the ultimate blueprint for pharmacy.[10]

In his Commentaries on Hippocrates' Epidemics, Galen also shows how he views such pharmaceuticals in the broader theory and practice of medicine, and he uses the Hippocratic texts to make comment on what drugs would or would not be useful. Within the scope of his Commentaries on Epidemics, Galen discloses that he has employed some kind of "canon" of Hippocratic works compiled by a Dioscorides (not the pharmacologist from Anazarbus).[11] Galen not only believes that Dioscorides "the Editor of Hippocrates" was quite wrong in a number of judgments regarding what was and what was not "genuine Hippocrates,"[12] but also that the ignorance of this Dioscorides about the theory of pharmacy and the drugs in the Hippocratic texts was abysmal. Galen says he will dismiss the Hippocratic works as edited by Dioscorides[13], especially noting that Dioscorides' errors in editing badly obscure Hippocrates' true meaning and intent. Galen writes that he will be able to explicate Hippocrates on drug lore, particularly regarding the famous dictum of treatment by contraries.[14] As a general example of how he will discern a clearer interpretation of Hippocrates' words, Galen offers a multiple definition of purgative, which can not only include a drug that purges the bowels but also a treatment that cleanses humors, including bloodletting – founded upon the basic assumption of the concept of the humors, and how humors can best be evacuated in given treatments.[15] But

5 XI 789–XII 377 Kühn.

6 Dioscorides, Preface, 3. John Scarborough and Vivian Nutton, The Preface of Dioscorides' Materia Medica: Introduction, Translation, Commentary. Transactions and Studies of the College of Physicians of Philadelphia, n.s. 4 (1982) 187–227 [196: translation; 212–213: commentary].

7 XII 378–XIII 361 Kühn.

8 XIII 362–1058 Kühn.

9 Cajus Fabricius, Galens Exzerpte aus älteren Pharmakologen (Ars medica II 2), Berlin: de Gruyter, 1972. For Criton, vid. John Scarborough, Criton. Physician of Trajan: Historian and Pharmacist, in: J. Eadie and J. Ober, eds., Festschrift Chester Starr (Washington, D.C.: University Press of America, 1985) [in press]

10 John Scarborough, Early Byzantine Pharmacology, in: Dumbarton Oaks Papers 38 (1984), 213–232.

11 Galen, Commentary on Epidemics III 2.60 Wenkebach [CMG V 10,2,1]. Cf. Smith, Hippocratic Tradition [n. 2 above], 237–238.

12 Smith, Hippocratic Tradition [n. 2 above], 235–236.

13 Galen, Commentary on Epidemics VI 2,9. 69 Wenkebach and Pfaff [CMG V 10,2,2].

14 Ibid., lines 12–14.

15 Ibid., pp. 69–70.

possibly the clearest and most definitive commentary proffered by Galen on Hippocratic drug lore in the Epidemics occurs when he reaches Epidemics, VI 6. The Hippocratic Epidemics, VI 6,3, reads:[16]

> *To cleanse the bowels and [relieve] the nearest [parts] from pains, and to open the bowel of blood: cautery, use of the knife, application of fomentations (viz. warming drugs), and cooling (i.e. application of cooling drugs), sneezes, humors of the plants which have the property, and kykeon; for bad pains, milk, garlic, boiled wine, vinegar, salt.*

In beginning his remarks on these lines[17], Galen notes that there is a list of remedies for large and small pains, as in his commentary on the Aphorisms of Hippocrates on pains in the eyes. Hippocrates had written, *Pains of the eyes are removed by drinking undiluted wine, by bathing, by vapor baths, by bloodletting, or by purging*[18], and Galen says that *others* have added remedies inappropriate for pains in the eyes.[19] And in spite of his declaration that he will be commenting on Hippocrates Epidemics VI 6,3, Galen proceeds to rephrase points he has made in his remarks on the Aphorisms of Hippocrates:

> *... cleansing [katharsis] is denoted in the Aphorisms by 'liquid-drug' or potion. I have taught you that Hippocrates used the word "drug" in many passages in his writings, and moreover means the drug which purifies the body through diarrhea or vomiting or something of this kind. Here he has added: "One must clean the nearest hollow space," i.e. the nearest extensive place in which sits the pain ...*

And then Galen links this with his comments on Epidemics VI 6,3:

> *... after he has mentioned the cleansing, he writes "the crack of a hollow space for blood." With this he means bleeding in a large vein. Afterwards he mentions cautery and the use of the knife. In the treatment of the eyes, he says nothing about this. Essentially he says nothing about it. Afterwards then he says "the warming."*[20]

In his critique of Hippocratic drug theory in Epidemics VI 6, Galen's underlying criticism is that earlier Greek pharmacy had a broad vagueness, a set of "sliding definitions" that could not only include the large number of purgatives and emetics but also cautery. He acknowledges the basic definition of "cleansing" would encompass bloodletting as well as emetics and purgatives, and he buttresses this Hippocratic notion by emphasizing how important is the theory of humors, which thereby would be cleansed. But Galen must dispose of the curious problem of overlapping distinctions among definitions of pain that appear in the Hippocratic text:[21] this he does neatly by calling attention to the large blood vessels anatomi-

16 ed. Manetti and Roselli, p. 126 = V 324 Li.
17 Galen, Commentary on Epidemics VI, 6,3. 333 Wenkebach and Pfaff [CMG V 10,2,2].
18 Aphorisms, 6,31.
19 Galen, Commentary on Epidemics VI, 6,3. 333, 24–25 Wenkebach-Pfaff [CMG V 10,2,2].
20 Ibid., p. 334.
21 Ibid., pp. 335–336.

cally obvious as seats of great pains[22], which must have been what Hippocrates meant all along. Hippocrates' "cautery" causes Galen little hesitation: this is easily interpreted as sometimes the use of white-hot irons for burning, and sometimes the use of ***burning drugs*** (*φάρμακα καυστικά*).[23] Therefore, Hippocrates indicates that he well understood the differences among application of a soft sponge to the eye, the prescribing of sharp foods for afflictions of the chest, and the bad practice of applying fomentations on the eye with poultices and plasters.[24] Galen continues by mentioning the custom of sprinkling oil on the body and hot water on the limbs, which then logically illustrates Hippocrates' dual cooling and warming treatments: thus doctors employ fomentations (θάλψεις) since ... *the warming* [*substance*] *stretches and relaxes, completely evacuates and* [*thereby*] *cools.*[25] Galen's subtle and deft casuistry has salvaged an apparent internal contradiction in Hippocrates' theory of drug actions, but once Galen performs this act of intellectual gymnastics, he is forced to abandon any pretence that he is commenting on the pharmaceutical theory and drugs found in Hippocratic works. It seems that as Galen sought a supporting theory that might underpin Hippocrates' employment of various drugs, he found few indications that Greek pharmacy had formulated such theories, although examination of Theophrastus' Historia plantarum (especially Book IX) suggests the beginnings of a Greek drug theory[26], and a comparison of the Pseudo-Aristotle Problems with the Hippocratic Wounds, Fistulas, Diseases III, and other Hippocratic tracts[27], also indicates an incorporation of the theories of elements and humors into some aspects of Hippocratic pharmacology. A basic, comprehensive underlying theory, however, would not be found for drug action in the Hippocratic treatises that Galen is examining. He would, therefore, "interpret" Hippocratic drug theory according to his own rather elaborate, seven-part system of medicine, adapted and modified from Hippocrates, Aristotle, Plato, and the Stoics.[28] An important fact of this complicated adaptation by Galen is the theory of humors[29], openly 'borrowed' from Hippocrates.[30]

Galen's comments on "Hippocrates' drug theory" are very important, because they indicate how pharmaceutical theory had changed and become consolidated by

22 Ibid., pp. 336–337.
23 Ibid., p. 338, lines 6–9.
24 Ibid., lines 14–17.
25 Ibid., lines 21–23.
26 John Scarborough, Theophrastus on Herbals and Herbal Remedies. Journal of the History of Biology 11 (1978), 353–385.
27 John Scarborough, Theoretical Assumptions in Hippocratic Pharmacology, in: F. Lasserre and P. Mudry, eds., Formes de Pensée dans la Collection hippocratique: Actes du Colloque international hippocratique, Lausanne ... 1981 (Geneva: Droz, 1983), 307–325.
28 John Scarborough, The Galenic Question. Sudhoffs Archiv 65 (1981), 1–31 [esp. 13–16].
29 Ibid., 15 with n. 76. Cf. Karl Deichgräber, Hippokrates De humoribus in der Geschichte der griechischen Medizin (Wiesbaden: Franz Steiner, 1972 [Abh. Akad. Wissensch. u. Lit. Mainz, Geistes- und sozialwissenschaft. Klasse, Nr. 14]), 33–55.
30 E.g. Galen, Natural Faculties, 1,2. II 5–6 Kühn = A. J. Brock, ed. and trans., Galen: On the Natural Faculties [London: Heinemann, 1916], 4–13).

the 2nd century A.D. Galen can state, given his assumptions about κρᾶσις, qualities, elements, and humors[31], that cooling is therapeutic[32], since it results from the dispersal of the scattered qualities of the hot which exist alone in an imbalance (δυσκρασία).[33] This, in turn, explains the headaches in both heatstroke (enkausis)[34] and fever. Thus pouring oil of roses over the patient's head would be curative for these afflictions[35], according to the signs and symptoms. Likewise, so Galen continues, physicians can cure the pains of erysipelas, gout, and a bilious discharge which would be, by definition, results of an excess of heat.[36]

Once these definitions and examples are in place, Galen can turn to the cryptic Hippocratic line, "the humors of the plants which have the property (dynamis)."[37] This allows Galen to presume *humor* (χυμός) must have been the same as "juice" (χυλός) to Hippocrates, somewhat supported by passages in the Hippocratic Regimen.[38] And "juices" can certainly be interpreted broadly. Among the humors-juices, used in medicine as drugs, the first place is held by olive oil[39], which has many applications in treating pains engendered by an excess of heat, but other fundamental simples (modern pharmacology would call them 'essential oils') that would make a basic listing for alleviation of such pains are oil of the bay (or laurel, usually the berries), cedar oil (or juniper oil), castor oil, mustard oil, and oil of radishes[40] – all *fluids* (ὑγρά). These "fluids" are thicker than some others (which Galen does not name) but less thick than the *resins* (ῥητίναι), especially those called *self-flowing* (αὐτόρρυτοι), which includes the *deadly carrot* (θαψία), the spurge (εὐφόρβιαν), all of the various juices of σίλφιον (viz. Cyrenaic, Parthian, and the Median)[41], and sagapenum juice. As Galen extends the list of drugs, which he says are implied by Hippocrates' "humors of the plants which have the property," one wonders how many actually appear as part of the drug lore of the Hippocratic corpus.

The bay (Laurus nobilis L.) is, indeed, found in the pharmaceutical listings of Hippocratic works, but all save two of the eighteen Hippocratic references to oil or other preparations of drugs from bay are in the gynecological books of the corpus. In Diseases, II 2 (13),3. 146 Jouanna, an unguent is to be made from bay leaves and the oil of bay berries (plus other ingredients including myrrh and pig's fat) for the treatment of skin rashes. Superfetation 29,4. 86 Lienau prescribes bay lea-

31 Scarborough, Galenic Question [n. 28 above], 13–15.

32 Galen, Commentary on Epidemics VI 6,3. 338, 27. Wenkebach-Pfaff [CMG V 10,2,2].

33 Ibid.

34 Dioscorides 5,13.

35 Galen, Commentary on Epidemics VI 6,3. 338, 28–30 Wenkebach-Pfaff [CMG V 10,2,2].

36 Ibid., lines 30–32.

37 "Property" seems a better translation of δύναμις when applied to drugs, than the traditional "power" or "faculty." Scarborough and Nutton [n. 6 above], 191–192.

38 Regimen II 42,3 and 54,8. 43 and 53 Joly.

39 Galen, Commentary on Epidemics VI 6,3. 339,5 Wenkebach-Pfaff [CMG V 10,2,2].

40 Ibid., lines 7–8.

41 Cf. Dioscorides 3,80, and Galen, Mixtures and Properties of Simples, 8,15, 12. XII 90–91 Kühn.

ves in wine and as part of a vapor bath for the treatment of prolapsed uterus, and Superfetation 41.96 Lineau suggests green bay leaves as a portion of a smoke-fumigation treatment for opening the womb. Internal Affections 52. VII 298 Li., advises that bay leaves beaten up and applied as a poultice would be useful against tetanus. Nature of Woman 6 and 14. VII 320 and 332 Li. has two preparations of bay leaves to treat a displaced uterus, and Nature of Woman 109. VII 426 Li. lists a concoction of twenty bay berries beaten up in 1/2 oxybaphon (c. 1/16 pint = c. 28 grams) of hartwort (Torydylium apulum L.)[42], to be drunk as an emmenagogue. Nature of Woman 33. VII 368 and 370 Li. suggests bay berries and elder berries pounded in wine as a uterine injection, and also has a vague prescription to employ bay (the part of the plant is not specified) in a drink to be given to the woman if she is bilious. Thus, except for the oil of bay in Diseases II 2(13),3, the Hippocratic use of Laurus nobilis has little resemblance to Galen's assertions that this is what Hippocrates "really means." A clear reference to oil of bay occurs in Theophrastus. Odors 28, and Dioscorides, Materia Medica 1,40. I 40–41 Wellmann lists δάφνινον as a significant medicinal oil. As revealed by the Hippocratic references. bay is an important pharmaceutical ingredient in the armory of drugs used by the midwives. and this can be paralleled with the fairly frequent occurrence of bay in the magical papyri.[43] Furthermore, the Hippocratic Diseases of Women I has five references to the employment of bay: bay berries and leaves (among other substances including olive oil) as an injection for post partum pain (I 51. VIII 111 Li.) bay [leaves?] in fumigation for cleansing phlegm from the uterus (I 58. VIII, p. 116 Li.): bay berry and olive oil as part of a multi-ingredient emmenagogue pessary (I 74. VIII 160 Li.); ten black bay berries, three δραχμαί (c. 3/8 oz. = c. 11 grams) of frankincense. and a little cumin mixed with honey to help a woman conceive (I 75. VIII 170 Li.); and bay berries as part of a pessary with oil of roses to help speed up delivery (I 77. VIII 172 Li.). Diseases of Women II 131.278 Li. suggests a vapor bath with bay to treat a displaced uterus, and Diseases of Women II 147. VIII 324 Li. green bay leaves in a drink (or perhaps a watery salve) as a treatment for ulcers and a dropped uterus. And the Hippocratic Sterile Women 242. VIII 456 Li. says that bay leaves are part of a recipe for an anti-abortifacient.

In Galen's other fairly numerous accounts of drugs that include bay[44], the oil is almost always the specific "bay" drug, and except for the implications here in his Commentary on the Epidemics VI, he calls the oil of bay warming and drying in its

42 Cf. Theophrastus, Historia Plantarum 9, 15,5, and Dioscorides 3,54. Scarborough, Theophrastus [n. 26 above], 374 with n. 124. Usher, 579. Polunin, Flowers, No. 904. Baumann, Pflanzenwelt, 122 with plate 224.

43 E.g. Papyri Graecae Magicae, I, 264; II,75; III,291; IV,2206, 2647, and 2679; V,199, 370, and 453; VII,802; and XIII,103 (Karl Preisendanz and Albert Henrichs, eds. and trans., Papyri Graecae Magicae: Die griechischen Zauberpapyri, 2nd ed. [Stuttgart: Teubner, 1973–1974; 2 vols.]; cited by 'papyrus-book' and printed line number). Vid. also Marie-Hélène Marganne, Inventaire analytique des papyrus grecs de medecine,Geneva, 1981, 170 and 248 (two instances of Laurus nobilis in the non-magical medical papyri).

44 E.g. Galen, Mixtures and Properties of Simples 2,35, and 6,5,4. XI 530 and 871 Kühn.

properties. The oil of bay is a fixed oil from the fresh fruit of Laurus nobilis, chiefly the lauryl alcohol esters of lauric, stearic, and other acids and a volatile oil. The so-called laurel camphor is greenish, fatty, and fairly solid, with the green color due to the presence of some chlorophyll. The Hippocratic and Galenic suggested uses for bay have only some analogies in modern pharmacy: the Swiss pharmacopoeia lists the dried ripe berries of the bay, which are reputed to have carminative, emmenagogue, and diuretic properties; and the Austrian, Czech, Dutch, and Portuguese pharmacopoeias suggest the use of the expressed oil (Oleum lauri) in stimulating liniments.[45]

Galen's knowledge of bay bears little likeness to the evidence one finds on Laurus nobilis in the Hippocratic corpus. Apparently, Galen has not employed specific texts deemed Hippocratic to make his pronouncements on bay oil, and it is Roman imperial pharmacy one sees, not any exact analysis of Greek drug lore as it might have existed in the 5th century B.C. or even in Hellenistic pharmacy down to the time of Dioscorides of Anazarbus (fl. c. A.D. 65). The earliest datable reference to the oil of bay is in Theophrastus, Odors 28, and in the 4th or early 3rd centuries B.C., this oil was one of the "fruit perfumes" (along with the myrtle and quince). The first clearly medicinal use of bay oil is in Dioscorides, Materia Medica 1,40, so that Galen's assumptions about the employment and properties of this particular oil derive not from earlier Greek pharmacy, but from the wealth of pharmaceutical handbooks available in the 1st and 2nd centuries of the Roman Empire.[46]

Laurus nobilis is, of course, only one species mentioned in Galen's listing of what Hippocrates must have intended with the "humors of the plants which have the properties." An examination of some of the remaining drugs in this short catalogue in Galen's Commentary on Epidemics VI may reveal similar patterns of his imposition of Roman pharmacy upon a purported Hippocratic foundation. Oil of cedar occurs only twice in the entire Hippocratic corpus[47], and Erotian believes it unusual or obscure enough to give a definition.[48] Aristotle mentions cedar oil[49], and Theophrastus notes it as a 'product' of a given tree[50], but gives it no medical quality or property. It is Dioscorides who provides the first full description of the preparation and use of cedar oil:[51] it is prepared by boiling the pitch and placing a fleece over the boiling resin, and the fleece pulls out the oil which is very helpful against sores and ulcers of the skin. Dioscorides adds that combined with pepper[52], cedar berries are a very good emmenagogue. By contrast with his presumably "cooling" property for cedar oil implied in his Commentary on Epidemics VI 6.3, Galen

45 Martindale, 1531. Usher, 346. Merck Index, 199 and 610. Trease and Evans, 296. North Africa, 116. Schauenberg and Paris, Guide, No. 307.

46 Scarborough, Criton [n. 9 above] passim.

47 Diseases of Women I 78. VIII 184 Li. Nature of Woman 33. VII 368 Li.

48 Erotian K 73 p. 56 Nachmanson.

49 Aristotle, Historia Animalium 583c23.

50 Theophrastus, Historia Plantarum 1,9.4.

51 Dioscorides 1,77,3–4.

52 Ibid., 77,4.

normally writes that cedar oil is even "hotter" than bay oil, as in Mixtures and Properties of Simples 6.4.4. XI 871 Kühn.[53] Oil of cedar remained in Byzantine pharmacy[54], and is the extract from cedar resin of either the Greek juniper (Juniperus excelsa Bieb.) or the common juniper (J. communis L.).[55] From the ancient evidence, one can observe that oil of cedar is an addition to the pharmacopoeia of late Hellenistic times, and Erotian's judgment that this specific substance required special comment as one studied the Hippocratic writings is telling proof against Galen's direct reading of *κέδρινον* in the works of Hippocrates.

Galen's inclusion of *κίκινος*, the oil derived from the castor oil plant (Ricinus communis L.)[56], is explicitly revealing of his ignoring specifics in the Hippocratic texts. Although Hippocratic writers do mention *κάστορος*, the "castor" gained from the preputial follicles of the beaver[57], there is no instance in the Hippocratic corpus of *κίκινος*. The first reference to this name for the oil from the castor oil plant is in Herodotus 2.94, followed by Plato, Timaeus 60a. It is Theophrastus, however, who shows why Galen's term for the castor oil will not be found in the Hippocratic corpus, since it is called *κροτών* in the Historia plantarum 1,10.1, and 3.18.7. Theophrastus lists the plant in a morphological comparison of leaves and does not give any medical uses. Dioscorides provides the first account of the preparation methods of the castor oil and its employment as a pharmaceutical[58], and he also tells us that *κροτών* = *κίκι*.[59] According to Dioscorides, castor oil (*κίκινον ἔλαιον*) is useful for the treatment of a displaced uterus[60], and this does link nicely with two references to *κροτών* in the Hippocratic corpus. In Diseases of Women II 201. VIII 386 Li., the author advises the use of the root of the castor oil plant for treatment of the "wandering womb,"[61] in combination with several other ingredients, all to be given a drink. It is of interest that these passages in Diseases of Women II 201, also record a clear distinction between the use of beaver-castor and the employment of castor oil plant (VIII 384 Li.; two instances of *καστόριον*), so that the Hippocratic writers know of both incredibly rancidly smelling extracts which do resemble one another. The Hippocratic Nature of Woman 32. VII 358 Li. prescribes the *κροτών* root as a remedy in a drink for hysteria. These two passages in the Hippocratic corpus are the only ones which suggest the medical employment of the castor oil plant, and Galen's use of *κίκι* (*κίκινος* would be the oil) shows he is unaware that the Hippocratic authors called the plant *κροτών*. Galen gained his

53 Cf. Papyri Graecae Magicae [n. 43 above], LVII,6.
54 Aetius 1,190. 85 Olivieri.
55 Schauenberg and Paris, Guide, No. 306. Hill, Botany, 450. Usher, 329. Martindale, 856. Trease and Evans, 425.
56 North Africa, 86. Hill, Botany 200–201. Trease and Evans, 316–317. Martindale, 866–867.
57 Martindale, 1513, John Scarborough, The Drug Lore of Asclepiades of Bithynia. Pharmacy in History 17 (1975), 43–57 [51].
58 Dioscorides 1,32,1–2.
59 Ibid., 32,1.
60 Ibid., 32,2.
61 Cf. Papyri Graecae Magicae [n. 43 above], VII, 260–271.

term from a late Hellenistic source, not from any known work that could be classified as "Hippocratic."

A second instance of Galen's uncritical presumption that a pharmaceutical term he knows would be the same as in Hippocratic (Ionic) Greek occurs when he lists oil of mustard as one of the important drugs meant by Hippocrates among the "humours of plants." Σινάπινον is the same as σιναπέλαιον[62], and is the oil of mustard (Sinapis alba L. = Brassica alba [L.] Boiss.)[63], quite common in Roman pharmacology.[64] The term, however, does not occur in early Attic or Ionic Greek, but mustard is called napu, seen in Theophrastus, Historia Plantarum 1, 12,1, and in three passages of the Hippocratic corpus: Diseases III 15,9.86 Potter; Diseases III 16, 17.92 Potter; and Diseases of Women I 13. VIII 52 Li. In this last reference, the Hippocratic writer prescribes mustard in a fumigation-recipe for the 'opening of the uterus' to ensure the reception of the sperm during coitus. Galen has not consulted a text on mustard earlier than the 1st century A.D.

When Galen names oil of radishes as one of Hippocrates' 'intended pharmaceutical humors," he is ignorant of the fact that htere is but a single reference to this oil in the Hippocratic corpus (Diseases of Women II 133. VIII 296 Li.). an indication that Hippocratic physicians did not value it in their drug lore. Galen's Ῥαφάνινον is the same as ῥαφανέλαιον, so a scholiast on Dioscorides tells us[65], and radish oil appears quite frequently in the drug listings of the Roman Empire.[66]

Quite peculiar is Galen's classification of the *self-dripping* (*αὐτορρυτοί*) resins, which he makes into a subcategory of the "Hippocratic humors" that have just included the various oils as well as the large class of resins. He implies that Hippocrates would have incorporated θαψία, εὐφόρβιον, and "all the juices" (viz. the various types of σίλφιον) in this subcategory. Θαψία is Thapsia garganica L., the so-called deadly carrot[67], and occurs only once in the Hippocratic corpus. In Epidemics VII 79. V 346 Li., it is suggested as a purgative for phrenitis. It is mentioned by Aristotle and Theophrastus[68], but it is Dioscorides again who provides the first complete description we have of the preparation and medical use of θαψία. In Materia Medica 4,153. II 298–300 Wellmann he writes that the juice from the root is obtained by cutting it, and then gathering the exudation the following day, or, by beating the root and straining out the juice and drying it in the sun (4,153, 1–2. II 298 Wellmann), Εὐφορβιον is a spurge, probably Euphorbia resinifera Berg.,[69] and does not occur in the drugs of the Hippocratic corpus. The herb was

62 Schol. Dioscorides 1,38 (ed. Wellmann, I, p. 39, app. crit. to line 5).

63 Usher, 541. Martindale, 279. Merck Index, 706. North Africa, 73. Trease and Evans, 524. Polunin, Flowers, No. 362.

64 E.g. Galen, Mixtures and Properties of Simples 6,5,4. XI 870 Kühn. But cf. Galen, Mixtures and Properties of Simples 2,34. XI 528 Kühn.

65 Schol. Dioscorides 1,37 (ed. Wellmann, I, p. 39, app. crit. to line 9).

66 E.g. Galen, Mixtures and Properties of Simples 5,14. XI 750 Kühn.

67 North Africa, 187–188 and 191. Usher, 573. Scarborough, Theoprastus [n. 26 above], 359 and 382 with nn. 39 and 162.

68 [Pseudo] Aristotle, Problems, 864a5. Theophrastus, Historia Plantarum 9,9,1 and 6.

69 Usher, 246. North Africa, 83. Martindale, 691. Scarborough and Nutton [n. 6 above], 209.

named, so our sources say, for the physician of King Juba II (c. 50 B.C.–c. A.D. 15), and Juba had written a short tract on the medical properties of *εὐφορβιον* which he had discovered in the Atlas Mountains.[70] Dioscorides gives the first complete description of *εὐφορβιον* (perhaps based on Juba), and Galen's "self-flowing" or "self-dripping" characteristic of euphorbion juice is quite at variance from Dioscorides' precise account of gathering techniques: the sap of Euphorbia resinifera was considered so very pungent and so hot that one pierced its stalk from a distance with long knives, and the juice was collected in sheep stomachs previously bound to the stem.[71] This is not the *self-dripping* plant as Galen asserts.[72] *Σίλφιον* remains one of the "mystery drugs" of classical antiquity, although *σίλφιον* may be an extinct member of the genus Ferula, or quite possibly the living Ferula narthex Boiss.[73] The Hippocratic corpus does have a large number of passages in which *σίλφιον* is suggested for various ailments[74], but Galen's "brand name" list for *σίλφιον* probably is based on Dioscorides.[75] Whatever species was *σίλφιον*, Dioscorides' account of collecting its juices indicates that both the root and stem were cut, and the sap gathered (Dioscorides does not say how).[76] Moreover, the supposition that Galen is taking part of his "Hippocratic list of humors" from Dioscorides is buttressed by the next *self-dripping* herb, sagapenum, which occurs in Dioscorides' Materia Medica immediately following *σίλφιον*.[77] Galen's *σαγαπηνός* is the exudation of Ferula persica Willd.[78], and excision of the stem produces a gum still employed to treat lumbago and rheumatism[79], analogous to some of the suggestions by Dioscorides. The exudate of F. persica, like other species of Ferula, is in the form of greyish white or yellow tears that have a strong garlicky odor and an extremely bitter taste[80], but Galen's usual mention of this drug is in the form of its "juice,"[81] as opposed to the clearly defined "gum" of Celsus, Scribonius Largus, Dioscorides, and Pliny.[82] The Hippocratic corpus has a single mention of sagapenum: according to the author of Diseases of Women I 78. VIII 184 Li., beaver-castor can be used as a substitute for sagapenum.

Continuing with his "Hippocratic" humors-as-drugs, Galen lists juice of *τιθυμάλ*-

70 Pliny, Natural History, 25, 77–79. Dioscorides 3, 82.2.
71 Dioscorides 3,82,1.
72 Cf. North Africa, 83–86.
73 Usher, 253, simply calls F. narthex "silphium." Vid. also Else Strantz, Zur Silphionfrage, Ansbach, 1909, esp. 174–183.
74 Littré, X, 792 [index listings].
75 Dioscorides 3,80. Cf. Galen, Commentary on Epidemics VI 2,5, and 6,3. 64 and 341,21–24 Wenkebach and Pfaff [CMG 10,2,2], and Philo in Galen, Drugs by Place of Ailment 9,4. XIII 270–274 Kühn.
76 Dioscorides 3,80.2.
77 Dioscorides 3,81.
78 Usher, 253. Merck Index, 104.
79 Usher, 253.
80 Martindale, 223–224. Hill, Botany, 173. Trease and Evans, 465.
81 E.g. Galen, Drugs by Kind, 3,2. XIII 367 Kühn.
82 Celsus 5,23. 3A, Scribonius Largus 69. Dioscorides 3,81. Pliny, Natural History 20,197.

λος, the kind of juice of All-Heal called ὀποπάναξ, and χαλβάνη.[83] and *all the rest as I have taught in my Properties of Simples,* which would likewise be within the Hippocratic drugs-as-humors. If, Galen writes, one can assume ὀπός and χυλός are parts of what can be derived from humors, one can then presume that all such "juices" from resins and perfumed saps to the wide variety of oils and medical juices-can be called humors, and such are produced from the full range of vegetation, whether trees, shrubs, or plants. This is what is meant by Hippocrates' clipped statement[84], and one may also extend Hippocrates' distillation of drug lore into all forms of pharmaceutics, including minerals, antidotes, and animal products.[85] After all, says Galen, the Father of Medicine had incorporated milk, garlic, boiled wine, vinegar, salt, κυκεών[86] among his drugs.

***

Several preliminary conclusions can be drawn from Galen's verbose commentary on a few terse lines regarding drugs in the Hippocratic Epidemics VI. (1) Galen's drugs and drug lore, which is meant presumably to elucidate and delineate Greek pharmacy in Hippocratic times, is not founded upon medicinal knowledge as known by Greek physicians and pharmacologists before Dioscorides; (2) those "Hippocratic" drugs mentioned by Galen most often appear in the gynecological books of the Hippocratic corpus, suggesting that the richest collection of data on drugs dating from Hippocratic times emerges from the lore of midwifery, not from "formal" medicine, and this may be corollary to the agricultural medical lore recorded in part by Theophrastus and later by Nicander[87]; (3) Galen's terms for specific drugs or extracts reflect late Hellenistic traditions, generally encapsulated by Dioscorides in the important Materia Medica, but also mirrored in Galen's other

83 Τιθύμαλλος is another spurge, probably Euphorbia peplus L. Theophrastus, Historia Plantatum 9,8,2, and 11,8. Scarborough,Theophrastus [n. 26 above], 368. Dioscorides 4,164 (seven kinds of spurge). Polunin, Flowers, No. 675. 'Οποπάναξ is a fetid gum-resin obtained from the roots of Opopanax chironium (L.) Koch, a yellow-flowered umbelliferous plant that resembles the parsnip. Scarborough, Asclepiades [n. 57 above], 53. Usher, 424. Hill, Botany, 174. Dioscorides 3,48. Heraclides of Tarentum in Galen, Antidotes 2,14. XIV 186–187 Kühn. Χάλβάνη is the gum resin of the Syrian Ferula galbaniflua Boiss. and Buhse. Usher, 253. Trease and Evans, 465. Scarborough, Asclepiades [n. 57 above], 53. Theophrastus, Historia Plantarum 9,7,2. Dioscorides 3,83. Cf. Andromachus in Galen, Antidotes 1,6. XIV 41 Kühn, and Nicander, Theriaca 52 and 938.

84 Galen, Commentary on Epidemics VI 6,3. 339, 19–20 Wenkebach-Pfaff [CMG V 10,2,2].

85 Ibid., pp. 344–345.

86 Κυκεών seems to have been various combinations of barley meal with honey, wine, oil, and other liquids, prepared for a number of traditional rituals and ceremonies. Vid. the Hippocratic Regimen II 41,1. 42 Joly for some medical uses. Vid. Armand Delatte, Le Cycéon, Breuvage rituel des mysteres d'Eleusis, Paris 1955 [in: Collection d'Etudes anciennes ... l'Association Guillaume Bude]), 715–716 and 726 for discussion of the Hippocratic and Galenic passages on κυκεών the booklet has pp. numbered 690–752, with four end leaves of plates).

87 Esp. in Theophrastus, Historia Plantarum 9, and Nicander's Theriaca and Alexipharmaca. Scarborough, Theophrastus [n. 26 above], Nicander's Toxicology, I: Snakes. Pharmacy in History 19 (1977), 3–23, and "Nicander's Toxicology, II" [n. 4 above].

written sources on pharmacy, openly revealed in the lengthy quotations from earlier Roman compilers of recipes in Galen's Mixtures and Properties of Simples, Drugs by Location of Ailment, and Drugs by Kind[88]; and (4) Galen's knowledge of Hippocratic drug lore is shadowy at best, and his criticism of Dioscorides the Editor of Hippocrates on this matter is quite hollow. Concerning Galen's interpretation of the "humors-as-drugs," it is probable that he may have recalled in a garbled fashion the Hippocratic equivalence between chylos and chymos as seen in Hippocrates' Regimen II 42,3 and 54,8. 43 and 53 Joly. A fuzzy recollection of these passages could explain why Galen would also expound upon the medical properties of foods, signalled by the discussion of kykeon and milk in Regimen II 41. 42 Joly, the chapter immediately preceding the passage about the humor (chymos) of boiled wheat meal.

***

As a postscript, one can compoare John of Alexandria's comments on this section of the Hippocratic Epidemics VI pp. 296–297 Pritchet. John is much less inclusive, writing that *Hippocrates says that humors also include the juices of plants and their gums* (Commentary VI 141a. 296 Pritchet). And even though John asks, *Just what is a juice?,* he limits his definition of "juice" (succus) to milk, olive oil and various other oils, and wine. In spite of the apparent parallels to Galen's Commentary on Epidemics VI[89], John's remarks are distinguished by a cautious good sense and a reluctance to display either a learned verbosity or wide reading in pharmacology. Palladius also shows a commendable incisiveness regarding this Hippocratic equivalence of "juice" with "humor,"[90] perhaps indicating that Byzantine commentators in Alexandria during the 6th and 7th centuries understood their Hippocratic texts of Epidemics VI 3, far better than had Galen, who chose to ignore the careful strictures laid down in the words of his ideal physician.[91]

ABBREVIATIONS AND SHORT TITLES EMPLOYED: TEXTS

Aetius: Alexander Olivieri, ed., Aetii Amideni Libri medicinales I–IV. Leipzig: Teubner, 1935 [CMG VIII 1]

CMG: Corpus Medicorum Graecorum

Dioscorides: Max Wellmann, ed., Pedanii Dioscuridis Anazarbei De Materia Medica. Berlin: Weidmann, 1906–1914. 3 vols. rptd. 1958.

88 Particularly prominent are Apollonius the Herophilean, Heras, Andromachus the Younger, Damocrates (who contributes much medical poetry), Criton, Asclepiades Pharmacion, Archigenes, Asclepiades of Bithynia, Philo of Tarsus, and Heraclides of Tarentum. Fabricius, Galens Exzerpte [n. 9 above], 180–199, 200–202.

89 App. crit. to John of Alexandria 141a. 296–297 Pritchet.

90 Palladius in F. R. Dietz, ed., Scholia in Hippocratem et Galenum (Königsberg, 1834; 2 vols. rptd. as one vol. Amsterdam: Hakkert, 1966), II, p. 161.

91 Other passages in Galen's Commentaires on the Epidemics on "Hippocratic" drug theory simply reiterate similar theories and repeat similar impositions of Roman pharmacy on Greek drug lore, e.g. Galen, Commentary on Epidemics II 5,82. 194–195 Wenkebach and Pfaff [CMG V 10,1], and Commentary on Epidemics III 2,13, and 3,79. 101 and 173 Wenkebach [CMG V 10,2,1].

Erotian: Ernst Nachmanson, ed., Erotiani Vocum Hippocraticarum collectio cum fragmentis. Göteborg/Uppsala: Eranos/Appelberg, 1918.

Galen, ed. Kühn: C. G. Kühn, ed., Claudii Galeni Opera omnia. Leipzig: Cnblichius, 1821–1833. 20 vols. in 22. rptd. Hildesheim: Georg Olms, 1964–1965.

Galen, Commentary on Epidemics I and II: Ernst Wenkebach and Franz Pfaff, eds., Galeni in Hippocratis Epidemiarum libros I et II. Leipzig: Teubner, 1934 [CMG V 10.1]

Galen, Commentary on Epidemics III: Ernst Wenkebach, ed., Galeni in Hippocratis Epidemiarum librum III. Leipzig: Teubner, 1936 [CMG V 10,2.1]

Galen, Commentary on Epidemics VI: Ernst Wenkebach and Franz Pfaff, eds., Galeni in Hippocratis Epidemiarum librum VI commentaria I–VIII, 2nd ed. Berlin: Academiae litterarum, 1956 [CMG V 10,2,2]

Hippocrates, ed. Littré: E. Littré, ed. and trans., Œuvres complètes d'Hippocrate. Paris, 1839–1861. 10 vols. rptd. Amsterdam: Hakkert, 1973–1982.

Hippocrates, Diseases II, ed. Jouanna: Jacques Jouanna, ed. and trans., Hippocrate. Tome X. 2e partie: Maladies II. Paris: Société d'Edition 'Les Belles Lettres,' 1983 [Collection ... l'Association Guillaume Budé]

Hippocrates, Diseases III, ed.Potter: Paul Potter, ed. and trans., Hippokrates Über die Krankheiten III. Berlin: Akademie-Verlag, 1980 [CMG I 2,3]

Hippocrates, Epidemics VI, ed. Manetti and Roselli: Daniela Manetti and Amneris Roselli, eds. and trans., Ippocrate Epidemie libro sesto. Florence: La Nuova Italia, 1982 [Biblioteca di Studi Superiori, Vol. LXVI, Filosifia Antica]

Hippocrates, Regimen, ed. Joly: Robert Joly, ed. and trans., Hippocrate Du régime. Paris: Société d'Edition 'Les Belles Lettres,' 1967 [Collection ... l'Association Guillaume Budé]

Hippocrates, Superfetation, ed. Lienau: Cay Lienau, ed. and trans., Hippokrates Über Nachempfängnis, Geburtshilfe und Schwangerschaftsleiden. Berlin: Akademie-Verlag, 1973 [CMG I 2,2]

John of Alexandria, ed. Pritchet: C. D. Pritchet, ed., Iohannis Alexandrini Commentaria in sextum librum Hippocratis Epidemiarum. Leiden: Brill, 1975.

Scribonius Largus, ed. Sconocchia: Sergio Sconocchia, ed., Scribonii Largi Compositiones. Leipzig: Teubner, 1983

OTHER ABBREVATIONS AND SHORT TITLES:

Baumann, Pflanzenwelt: Hellmut Baumann, Die griechische Pflanzenwelt. Munich: Hirmer, 1982

Hill, Botany: Albert F. Hill, Economic Botany, 2nd ed. New York: McGraw-Hill, 1952

Martindale: R. G. Todd, ed., Extra Pharmacopoeia Martindale, 25th ed. London: The Pharmaceutical Press, 1967

Merck Index: Paul G. Stecher, et al., eds., The Merck Index, 8th ed. Rahway, New Jersey: Merck & Co., 1968

Polunin, Flowers: Oleg Polunin, Flowers of Europe. London: Oxford University Press, 1969

North Africa: Loutfy Boulos, Medicinal Plants of North Africa. Algonac, Michigan: Reference Pub. Inc., 1983

Schauenberg and Paris, Guide: Paul Schauenberg and Ferdinand Paris, Guide des plantes médicinales, 3rd ed. Neuchâtel: Delachaux & Niestlé, 1977

Trease and Evans: George Edward Trease and William Charles Evans, Pharmacognosy, 11th ed. London: Balliere Tindall, 1978

Usher: George Usher, A Dictionary of Plants Used by Man. London: Constable, 1974

***

XIII

EARLY BYZANTINE PHARMACOLOGY

Introduction

The study of Byzantine drug lore presents the modern scholar with several problems. At first glance, it would appear that Oribasius, Aetius of Amida, Alexander of Tralles, and Paul of Aegina have simply replicated data and nomenclature found in the works of Dioscorides, Galen, and other earlier Greek and Roman accounts of herbs and herbals, medicinal minerals, and animal products employed in the manufacture of drugs. Yet when one investigates carefully the Greek texts of all four of these major so-called compilers in the history of early Byzantine medicine, one soon discovers that there are indeed duplications from Greco-Roman authorities in consideration of drugs and drug lore, but that the theory of drug-action has shifted in an important manner, and also that substances used in pharmacy have been augmented, both in number and in kind. This new theory of pharmacology, based firmly upon scattered statements from a wide range of Galenic writings, can be nicely illustrated with the lengthy prologue by Aetius of Amida to his *Medical Books* (the *Tetrabiblon*).[1] Moreover, when one compares "borrowing" by Oribasius, Aetius, Alexander, and Paul, from Galen and earlier authorities, one discerns significant variations in syntax and, most importantly, a clear consideration of medicinal substances in their own right, rather far removed from the copyist epithet often given to these early Byzantine medical writers. Oribasius and Alexander, in particular, submit drug recipes that show a command of the ancient texts and personal experience with pharmaceuticals.

We are also fortunate in being able to link the allegedly formal aspects of early Byzantine drug lore with data that the non-physician might know—at least in late Roman and Byzantine Egypt. Many papyri, especially those contained in the collection called the *Papyri Graeci Magicae*,[2] show how drugs and pharmaceuticals were used in numerous non-medical contexts, but of great importance among these papyrological citations is the assumption of common knowledge of the *kyphi* and *krisma* recipes, also significant in the formal works by Byzantine physicians on pharmacology. Early Byzantine pharmacy drew upon classical heritages—from the Hippocratics through Galen—but it also shows a clear development of its own, seen best in a reworked drug theory and in the augmentation of particular substances employed as pharmaceuticals. This sophisticated pharmacy is also paralleled in the papyri,[3] but these documents are, of course, shorn of theory, which may or may not have penetrated into the ranks of Egyptian priests, soothsayers, and purported experts in magic.[4]

The Historical Background of Greek and Roman Pharmacy to Galen

Drug lore is the first aspect of Greek medicine that can be documented, since spices and presumed pharmaceuticals turn up in the Linear B tablets of Mycenaean Greece and Crete.[5] After the

[The reader is referred to the list of abbreviations at the end of the volume.]

[1] Aetius I *prooemium* (ed. Olivieri [*CMG* VIII 1], pp. 17–30).

[2] See esp. *PGM*, IV, 2307–9; XII, 401–45; XXXVI, 322–32.

[3] Marie-Hélène Marganne, *Inventaire analytique des papyrus grecs de médecine* (Geneva, 1981). Magical papyri are excluded.

[4] E.g., *PGM*, XII, 401–45. Cf. H. Harrauer and P. J. Sijpestein, *Medizinische Rezepte und Verwandtes* (Vienna, 1981); K. Sudhoff, *Ärztliches aus griechischen Papyrus-Urkunden* (Leipzig, 1909); H. I. Bell, A. D. Nock, and H. Thompson, *Magical Texts from a Bilingual Papyrus in the British Museum* (London, 1931 [Proceedings of the British Academy, Vol. XVII]). Unfortunately, the rich lore and medical equivalencies in E. A. E. Reymond, *From the Contents of the Libraries of the Suchos Temples in the Fayyum*, Part I: *A Medical Book from Crocodilopolis P. Vindob. D. 6257* (Vienna, 1976), cannot be trusted. A new edition with translation and commentary of P. Vindobonensis D. 6257 is in preparation at the Oriental Institute of the University of Chicago.

[5] See esp. L. R. Palmer, *Interpretation of Mycenaean Greek Texts* (Oxford, 1963), Nos. 163–168 [pp. 269–73], and J. Chadwick, *Documents in Mycenaean Greek*, 2nd ed. (Cambridge, 1973), Nos.

passing of the Mycenaeans, there is good indication of a common knowledge of *pharmaka* (at least those that were involved in application of simples for minor wounds, and those that were deemed potent in spells and incantations) in Homer's epics,[6] so that drug lore probably flourished among the Greeks of the Homeric Age, much as it would later.[7] Lyric poetry has left us with some isolated mentions of drugs and salves,[8] and there is firm evidence that certain drugs were well known among the Greeks in the fifth century B.C., suggested by puns in Aristophanes and other non-medical writers.[9] It is not until the fifth and fourth centuries B.C. that a separate study of medical plants was made a part of formal medical practice, and the Pseudo-Aristotelian *Problems* probably mirror the same sources for drugs and drug theory that appear also in several books of the Hippocratic *corpus*.[10] Diocles of Carystos (a contemporary of Aristotle)[11] studied plants for their pharmaceutical properties, and the study of botany received a canonical form in Theophrastus' *Historia plantarum* and *De causis plantarum* (both c. 300 B.C.);[12] Book IX of *Historia plantarum* is our first extant herbal in Greek.[13] Theophrastus carefully classifies plants by their leaves, roots, seeds, stems, and growing season, and the methodologies of his master, Aristotle, show brilliantly in the taxonomy and morphology.[14]

Although there is good evidence for the study of pharmacy in the Hellenistic era, our available texts for the period consist of fragmentary remains of the drug lore of Apollodorus (*fl.* c. 250 B.C.),[15] and such notables as Herophilus and Erasistratus (both *fl.* 270–260 B.C.),[16] as well as the two poems on toxicology by Nicander of Colophon (*fl.* c. 130 B.C.) called *Theriaca* and *Alexipharmaca*.[17] Nicander stole his data from the lost works of Apollodorus, who had made a detailed study of toxic substances, poisonous snakes, scorpions, spiders, and insects,[18] apparently in the manner of Peripatetic natural history,[19] but it would be Nicander's obtuse poems that became standard "textbooks" in toxicology, employed by almost all medical authorities from his own time through the European Renaissance.[20]

Theophrastus struggled with the problem of how drugs were to be classified, and he provides an extremely muddled system in *Historia plantarum* IX.[21] Much of his data is derived from a professional class of *rhizotomoi*, whose firsthand experience Theophrastus records in several instances.[22] Yet the definition of *poa* ("herb") remains hopelessly vague, since Theophrastus' overriding methodology demanded first attention to morphology and taxonomy, not to the medical properties of any particular plant or drug made from a plant. A foggy notion

103, 105, and 107 [pp. 224, 228, and 231]. A few, scattered studies have begun to appear on these texts and similar ones, e.g., Anna Sacconi, "La mirra nella preparazione degli unguenti profumati a Cnosso," *Athenaeum*, n.s. 47 (1969), 281–89; C. P. W. Warren, "Some Aspects of Medicine in the Greek Bronze Age," *Medical History*, 14 (1970), 364–77; and R. Janko, "Un 1314: Herbal Remedies at Pylos," *Minos*, 17 (1981), 30–34.

6 E.g., Homer, *Odyssey* X, 304–6, 316–17, and 391–94, among many references.

7 Cf. Homer, *Iliad* VIII, 306–8, with Dioscorides IV, 64.1 (ed. Wellmann, II, p. 218).

8 When Sappho, Frg. 96 (var. eds., trans. D. A. Campbell, *Greek Lyric*, I [Cambridge, Mass., 1982], p. 120 [Loeb]), writes "the dew is shed in beauty, and roses bloom and tender chervil and flowery melilot," one immediately perceives a long-lived close acquaintance with herbs and flowers. Sappho, Frgs. 105, 143, 189, and 210 (Campbell, pp. 132, 156, 180 and 192) mention hyacinth, chick peas, nitrum, and fustic. Cf. Theognis 537 and 1193 (squill and spiny broom); Simonides 10 (myrtle); Hesiod, *Works* 41 (asphodel), etc., among many references.

9 E.g., Aristophanes, *Lysistrata* 89, and *Peace* 712 (puns on the uses of the pennyroyal [*Mentha pulegium* L.]). Discussion in Scarborough, "Nicander II," 74–75 with nn. 239–54.

10 J. Scarborough, "Theoretical Assumptions in Hippocratic Pharmacology," in F. Lasserre and P. Mudry, eds., *Formes de pensée dans la collection hippocratique: Actes du IVe Colloque international hippocratique (Lausanne . . . 1981)* (Geneva, 1983), 307–25.

11 W. Jaeger, *Diokles von Karystos*, 2nd ed. (Berlin, 1963), 186–236. The fairly extensive fragments of Diocles' writings are collected in M. Wellmann, ed., *Die Fragmente der sikelischen Ärzte Akron, Philistion und des Diokles von Karystos* (Berlin, 1901), 117–207.

12 F. Egerton, ed., *Edward Lee Greene: Landmarks of Botanical History* (Stanford, California, 1983; 2 vols.), I, 128–211.

13 J. Scarborough, "Theophrastus on Herbals and Herbal Remedies," *JHB*, 11 (1978), 353–85.

14 Egerton, ed., *Greene* (n. 12 above), I, 169–89. O. Regenbogen, "Theophrastos," *RE*, Supplementband VII (Stuttgart, 1940), cols. 1354–1562, esp. 1435–79 (botany).

15 M. Wellmann, "Apollodorus (69)," *RE*, Vol. I, part 2 (Stuttgart, 1894), col. 2895, and (same author), "Das älteste Kräuterbuch der Griechen," in *Festgabe für Franz Susemihl* (Leipzig, 1898), 1–31. J. Scarborough, "Nicander's Toxicology, I: Snakes," *PH*, 19 (1977), 3–23 (3–4, with nn. 8–19).

16 P. M. Fraser, *Ptolemaic Alexandria* (Oxford, 1972; 3 vols.), I, 353, and II, 519 n. 116, and 627 n. 472 [Herophilus]. R. Fuchs, "Eine neue Receptformel des Erasistratos," *Hermes*, 33 (1898), 342–44.

17 Nicander (ed. and trans. Gow and Scholfield) is the best edition available, with a translation quite often based on shrewd guesswork—openly admitted by the editors.

18 Scarborough, "Nicander's Snakes" (n. 15 above), 3–4, and (same author), "Nicander II" *passim*.

19 Scarborough, "Nicander II," 5–6. Wellmann, "Kräuterbuch" (n. 15 above), 28.

20 E.g., a late Greek manuscript (Bologna, Bibl. Univ. Codex 3632, esp. fol. 417) of the late fifteenth or early sixteenth century. Scarborough, "Nicander II," 4, with nn. 4–8.

21 Egerton, ed., *Greene* (n. 12 above), I, 180–81. Scarborough, "Theophrastus" (n. 13 above), 356–57.

22 Theophrastus, *HP* IX, 8 *passim*; 11.7 and 9; 15.2; 16.3; 18.3 and 10; and 20.4.

of toxicology does appear in Book IX of *Historia plantarum*,[23] but Theophrastus and his sources seem unaware of a basic theory that would explain the differences among drugs. Some hints of an embryonic theory of toxicology do, indeed, appear in the Pseudo-Aristotelian *Problems*, as well as certain tracts of the Hippocratic *corpus*, but there is more of an attempt to collect data than to propose a logical and careful hypothesis about how and why drugs "work" as they do. Nicander's poems also reflect this attention to the collection of details, and the lack of a cohesive theory to link them together, and the fragments of other Hellenistic pharmacologists likewise suggest a haphazard and often erroneous set of prescriptions, or—in the cases of Herophilus and Erasistratus—an attempt to set down specific treatments for particular ailments, in the classic manner of the Hippocratic writers.

Dioscorides of Anazarbus (*fl.* c. A.D. 65) attempted to change the chaos of pharmacology into an ordered system.[24] He seems to have invented a "drug affinity" methodology for the study of pharmaceuticals, quite similar to the modern concepts underlying pharmacognosy, but this non-alphabetical, non-humoral theory demanded precise observation of plants in their varying growing seasons as well as extreme accuracy in the physician's observations concerning which drugs were useful against which specific ailments and diseases. Dioscorides' *Materia medica* certainly became a classic handbook, quoted by almost all later writers on pharmacy (both Greek and Latin, as well as Arabic) for nearly 1800 years.[25] He includes nearly 600 species of plants in the *Materia medica*,[26] compared with approximately 450 species in the Hippocratic *corpus*,[27] the 550 species recorded by Theophrastus,[28] and the 300 plant names given by Nicander.[29] Dioscorides' listings encompass many drugs introduced into Greco-Roman pharmacy from the Far East,[30] showing the expansion of trade and geographic knowledge in the Hellenistic era and in the first decades of Roman imperial rule in the eastern Mediterranean.[31] His rejection, however, of both the poetic form of relating knowledge of drugs (illustrated by the difficult hexameters of Nicander) and also the apparently standard manner of listing simples in alphabetical order,[32] led in turn to the discarding of Dioscorides' classification system by later pharmacologists, including the chalcenteric Galen.[33] Dioscorides' drug lore tapped not only the formal sources of pharmacology, as they might be found in earlier written records, but also folk medicine, acknowledged from time to time in the *Materia medica*.[34] Moreover, he insists that the would-be pharmacologist has to know his plants, not from book-learning, but by patient and lengthy observation of herb growth as they changed form, shape, and color through differing seasons in various geographic locations as he knew them generally in the eastern Mediterranean litoral.[35] Added to the demand of painstaking observation of reaction to drugs by actual patients, these two requirements by Dioscorides soon led to modifications, including a return to alphabetical listings and pharmaceutical poetry.[36] While respecting Dioscorides for his obvious learning and meticulous attention to botanical details, Galen rejected the "drug affinity" system, while retaining (at least he says he does) Dioscorides' admonition to know the plants from personal experience. And it would be Galen, not Dioscorides, who would provide the beginning models for Byzantine drug lore.

Galen's Pharmacy

Galen of Pergamon (A.D. 129-prob. 210) looms as one of the most influential writers in the entire history of medicine.[37] His summary of all aspects

[23] Theophrastus, *HP* IX, 16.4–7. Scarborough, "Theophrastus" (n. 13 above), 376–77 with nn. 131–35.

[24] Scarborough and Nutton, "Preface," 189–90. J. M. Riddle, "Dioscorides," *DSB*, Vol. IV (New York, 1971), 119–23. Riddle's *Dioscorides* (Austin, Texas [in press]) explicates in brilliant detail Dioscorides' "drug affinity" system.

[25] J. M. Riddle, "Dioscorides" in *Catalogus* IV, 1–143. Scarborough and Nutton, "Preface," 187–88.

[26] J. Stannard, "Byzantine Botanical Lexicography," *Episteme*, 5 (1971), 168–87 [171].

[27] My "count" differs sharply with that of Stannard (*ibid.*), who suggests about 225 spp. [p. 170].

[28] Regenbogen, "Theophrastos" (n. 14 above), col. 1467. Egerton, ed., *Greene* (n. 12 above), I, 96 gives 500 as his "count."

[29] Based on Nicander, ed. and trans. Gow and Scholfield.

[30] E.g., ginger (*Zingiber officinale* Roscoe) among several. J. I. Miller, *The Spice Trade of the Roman Empire* (Oxford, 1969), 53–57.

[31] J. Scarborough, "Roman Pharmacy and the Eastern Drug Trade," *PH*, 24 (1982), 135–43.

[32] Scarborough and Nutton, "Preface," 212–13.

[33] *Ibid.*, 190–91.

[34] *Ibid.*, 189 with nn. 10 and 13.

[35] Dioscorides, *Preface* 7 (ed. Wellmann, I, p. 4; trans. Scarborough and Nutton, "Preface," 196–97).

[36] E.g. the medical poetry of Damocrates (quoted by Galen) and most of the drug lists by Galen.

[37] The literature on Galen is enormous, but only a few works are based securely on the Greek texts. Recommended are: V. Nutton, "The Chronology of Galen's Early Career," *CQ*, n.s. 23 (1973), 158–71, and [same author], "Galen and Medical Auto-

of medicine and related matters, including philosophy and pharmacology, exerted a heavy sway over physicians and medical commentators well into the nineteenth century,[38] and one may gauge his prolixity and learning by the simple task of counting the volumes (20) represented by the Kühn edition of Galen.[39] Since his drug lore influenced later writers, especially in the Byzantine East, so heavily, one necessarily must consider Galen's pharmacology in some detail in order to perceive how early Byzantine drug theory might be similar to and different from the presumed blueprints laid down in several of his treatises which consider pharmaceuticals in particular.

Galen's drug lore is scattered throughout the massive number of works left under his name, but much of his approach to pharmacology, herbs, and treatments through pharmaceuticals is concentrated in *Mixtures and Properties of Simples*,[40] *Compound Drugs Arranged by Location of Ailment*,[41] *Compound Drugs Arranged by Kind*,[42] *Antidotes*,[43] and similar tracts, some of which may be spurious.[44] Galen quotes from dozens of earlier Greek and Roman pharmacologists—including Dioscorides—and although Galen insists one had to know plants and drugs personally,[45] many of the recipes, prescriptions, and treatments are filched from earlier authorities,[46] most often through previous collections of recipes compiled by Andromachus (physician to Nero [A.D. 54–68]), Asclepiades the Pharmacist (prob. *fl.* c. A.D. 50), and Criton (physician to Trajan [A.D. 98–117]). He includes all of the famous simples, known from the time of Theophrastus, but adds no new herbs to the varieties already known to Dioscorides.

In *Mixtures and Properties of Simples* I–V,[47] Galen sets out in an incredibly verbose fashion his composite theory of drug action, based upon degree of cold and hot, moist and dry, with subtle subclassifications generally measured according to the senses of taste, touch, and smell. Not surprisingly, these 329 Kühn pages will not form the foundation of Byzantine adaptation of Galen's drug theories, as will be suggested below with the consideration of the Preface to Aetius' *Medical Books*. Galen proposes his arguments upon what he says are the "best authorities," and *Simples* I–V is replete with name-dropping of the worthies of the pharmaceutical past, from Diocles, Hippocrates, and Theophrastus, through Dioscorides and Asclepiades. What emerges in this involuted summary is the famous "drugs by degrees" system,[48] which would retain its hold on western pharmacy until the nineteenth century. Only in the beginning of Book VI of *Simples* does Galen speak in specific about drugs, and then only after a Preface to Book VI in which he warns against misleading authorities (for example, Pamphilus)[49] who were not experts in plants, and in which he re-lists the reliable sources (a long list that includes Dioscorides)[50]—but Galen lets us know that none of his predecessors understood drugs as well as he does. Then follows the listing of drugs, beginning with "On Shrubby Wormwood and Absinthe and their Particular Kinds."[51] Unlike the extreme clarity of Dioscorides, we read a muddled catalogue of properties generally based on locale. *Simples* VI, 2[52] is "On Agnus Castus," *Simples* VI, 3 is "On Dog's Tooth Grass" [*agrōstis*],[53] VI, 4 is "The Four Kinds of Alkanet" [*anchousa*],[54] VI, 5 is "The Agaric 'Root'"

biography," *Proceedings of the Cambridge Philological Society*, 18 (1972), 50–62; J. Scarborough, "The Galenic Question," *SA*, 65 (1981), 1–31, and (same author), "Galen and the Gladiators," *Episteme*, 5 (1971), 98–111; J. Ilberg, "Aus Galens Praxis," *Neue Jahrbücher für das klassische Altertum*, 15 (1905), 276–312 (rptd. in H. Flashar, ed., *Antike Medizin* [Darmstadt, 1971], 361–416); J. Mewaldt, "Galenos (2)," *RE*, Vol. VII, part 1 (Stuttgart, 1910), cols. 578–91; F. Kudlien and L. G. Wilson, "Galen," *DSB*, Vol. V (New York, 1972), 227–37; W. D. Smith, *The Hippocratic Tradition* (Ithaca, New York, 1979), 61–176; J. Kollesch, "Galen und die Zweite Sophistik," in Nutton, ed., *Galen: Problems*, 1–12; and—above all—Temkin, *Galenism*, 10–50 ("The Portrait of an Ideal").

[38] Temkin, *Galenism*, 134–92 ("Fall and Afterlife").

[39] The texts of Galen in *CMG* are a small proportion of the works contained in the Kühn ed., which is badly marred by corruptions. To the listing in H. Leitner, *Bibliography to the Ancient Medical Authors* (Bern, 1973), 38–39, can now be added: Nutton, ed., *Galen On Prognosis*; and De Lacy, ed., *Galen On the Doctrines of Hippocrates and Plato*.

[40] Ed. Kühn, XI, 379–892, and XII, 1–377 (in 11 books).

[41] Ed. Kühn, XII, 378–1007, and XIII, 1–361 (in 10 books).

[42] Ed. Kühn, XIII, 362–1058 (in 7 books).

[43] Ed. Kühn, XIV, 1–209 (in 2 books)

[44] *Theriac to Piso* (ed. Kühn, XIV, 210–94 [possible]), *Theriac to Pamphilus* (ed. Kühn, XIV, 295–310 [certainly spurious]), *Easily-Obtained Drugs* (ed. Kühn, XIV, 311–581 in 3 books [certainly spurious]).

[45] Galen, *Mixtures and Properties of Simples* VI, preface (ed. Kühn, XI, 797). Scarborough, *Medicine*, 128–30.

[46] Fabricius, 62–100.

[47] Ed. Kühn, XI, 459–788.

[48] See discussion of Aetius with nn. 149–68 below.

[49] Ed. Kühn, XI, 793–94.

[50] *Ibid.*, 794 and 797.

[51] *Simples* VI, 1 (ed. Kühn, XI, 798–807). Scarborough and Nutton, "Preface," 225–27 (wormwoods).

[52] Cf. Dioscorides I, 103. This is *Vitex agnus-castus* L. (ed. Kühn, XI, 807–10).

[53] Scarborough and Nutton, "Preface," 219 (dog's tooth grass: *Cynodon dactylon* [L.] Pers.). ed. Kühn, XI, 810–11.

[54] Ed. Kühn, XI, 811–13. Cf. Dioscorides IV, 23. This is *Anchousa tinctoria* L.

[*agarikos*],[55] and so on, so that by the end of Book VI of *Simples*, Galen has reached *iota* in what has become an alphabetical listing of simples (all plants) with some properties given according to "heating" and "cooling." Books VII and VIII[56] complete the alphabetical listing of herbs and their properties by their classes of heating and cooling qualities. *Simples* IX, 1.1–4 is "Earths,"[57] IX, 2.1–21 "Stones,"[58] and "Things Mined as Drugs" [*metallika pharmaka*] is *Simples* IX, 3.1–40.[59] Most of these substances are in alphabetical order, with some exceptions suggesting possible corruptions in the Greek texts. *Simples* X is what we would call "animal products," and much as had Dioscorides often prescribed blood for various ailments, so too does Galen extrapolate on this "humor" as a drug along with a number of other materials presumably classed with blood because they emerge from animals; the listing in and of itself is instructive, not so much for what Galen recommended, but for the substances he found listed in his sources (Xenocrates seems to be a major authority).[60] After listing various animal bloods (dove, bat, rabbit, deer, rooster, male goat, lamb, bear, bull, green frog, crocodile and lizard),[61] one reaches a "dairy product" listing (milk, cheese, butter, rennet, seal rennet),[62] followed by biles, perspiration, urine, saliva, and various kinds of animal and bird dungs and manure.[63]

In Book XI of *Simples*, Galen lists other "animal products,"[64] ranging from the flesh of poisonous snakes, marrow, and the liver of a mad dog,[65] to spider webs, blister beetles, cicadas, castor, brains of various animals, eggs, and charred crabs.[66] *Simples* XI, 2 is a collection of oddments that could be labeled "products of the sea useful in medicinals,"[67] and here are sponges, garum, coral, various sorts of salts and salt products including *asphaltos*.[68] Unlike the herbs and plants of *Simples* VI–VIII, which are given alphabetically, Galen's animal products and sea-medicines seem entered according to another pattern, perhaps ultimately derived from Dioscorides or earlier data found in some of the Hippocratic texts. In sum, Galen lists about 440 different plants in his accounting of herbs in *Simples* I–VIII, and about 250 other substances in the remaining books as useful in making drugs. Indeed, there are caustic remarks concerning the drugs of Xenocrates, especially the varieties of dung, but Galen *does* list them, and one can presume that such materials had long standing in ancient pharmacology, verified by a comparison with medicinals suggested by writers in the Hippocratic *corpus*, Dioscorides, as well as the magical papyri.[69]

Once the alphabetical and non-alphabetical listings of drugs are completed in *Simples*, Galen apparently decides to approach pharmaceutical lore in another way in the ten books we have as *Compound Drugs Arranged by Location of Ailment*.[70] These ten books were written after Galen had put down the *Method of Healing*,[71] whereas the *Simples* predates it.[72] Galen's struggle with drugs—and how to classify them—can be discerned through the successive attempts he made to provide lucid catalogues: first is his *Properties of Cleansing Drugs*, writ-

[55] Ed. Kühn, XI, 813–14. As this is a shelf-fungus, the passage shows Galen's ignorance. G. Maggiulli, *Nomenclatura micologica latina* (Genoa, 1977), 85–87. Cf. Dioscorides III, 1.

[56] Ed. Kühn, XII, 1–158.

[57] *Ibid.*, 165–92.

[58] *Ibid.*, 192–208.

[59] *Ibid.*, 208–44.

[60] *Simples* X, preface (ed. Kühn, XII, 245–53).

[61] *Simples* X, 2–6 (ed. Kühn, XII, 256–63).

[62] *Simples* X, 2.7–12 (ed. Kühn, XII, 263–75).

[63] *Simples* X, 2.13–29 (ed. Kühn, XII, 275–308). *Simples* X, 2.15 (ed. Kühn, XII, 284–88) ends with Galen noting that "drinking the urine of a prepubescent boy is not recommended," and *Simples* X, 2.16 (ed. Kühn, XII, 288–90: on salivas) has a rare direct quotation from Nicander (*Theriaca* 86). *Simples* X, 2.17 (ed. Kühn, XII, 290) summarizes why one uses such materials. Cf. Paul of Aegina VII, 3, *s.v.* κόπρος (ed. Heiberg, II, 228).

[64] Ed. Kühn, XII, 310–77.

[65] *Simples* XI, 1.1 (snakes, esp. the *echidnē*: Scarborough, "Nicander's Snakes" [n. 15 above], 7–8); XI, 1.3 (marrow); and XI, 1.10 (rabid dog's liver). ed. Kühn, XII, 311–23, 311–33, and 335.

[66] *Simples* XI, 1.23 (spider webs); XI, 1.44–45 (blister beetles); XI, 1.36 (cicadas); XI, 1.15 (castor); and XI, 1.31 (brains, kidneys, and eggs). Ed. Kühn, XII, 343, 363–64, 360, 337–41, and 349–55. Charred or burned crabs, or more accurately the ashes of crabs, are prescribed in *Simples* XI, 1.24 (ed. Kühn, XII, 356–59). See J. Scarborough, "Some Beetles in Pliny's Natural History," *Coleopterists Bulletin*, 31 (1977), 293–96 ("Spanish Fly" and beetles of Lyttinae) and (same author), "Nicander II," 13–14, 20–21, 73–80 with nn. 134–45, 215–30, and 237–325 (blister beetles, descriptions, and purported remedies for the ingestion of "Spanish Fly" in classical antiquity); and (same author), "The Drug Lore of Asclepiades of Bithynia," *PH*, 17 (1975), 43–57 (51: castor).

[67] Ed. Kühn, XII, 369–77.

[68] *Simples* XI, 2.11 (sponges); XI, 2.12 (garum); XI, 2.3 (coral); and XI, 2.5–10 (salts and salt products). Ed. Kühn, XII, 376, 377, 370–71, and 372–75. For garum, see R. I. Curtis, "In Defense of *Garum*," *CJ*, 78 (1983), 232–40, and [same author] "The Garum Shop of Pompeii," *Cronache Pompeiane*, 5 (1979), 5–23. For sponges, see J. Théodoridès, "Considerations on the Medical Use of Marine Invertebrates," in M. Sears and D. Merriman, eds., *Oceanography: The Past* (New York, 1980), 734–49 (esp. 734–36).

[69] Cf. *PGM*, I, 224–25; IV, 1439–40, 2574–75, 2585, 2651; VII, 486; XII, 410, 414.

[70] Ed. Kühn, XII, 378–1007, and XIII, 1–361.

[71] *Drugs by Location* I, 1 (ed. Kühn, XII, 378).

[72] Ilberg, *Schriftstellerei*, 89.

ten before A.D. 169;[73] then Galen wrote the second of his "drug books," *Simples*, probably in the 170s, number six on the list of the works as suggested by Ilberg, after Galen's return to Rome in 169;[74] *Location* was written sometime in the period between A.D. 180 and 193, preceded by *Compound Drugs Arranged by Kind*.[75] Even though Ilberg shows that *Drugs by Kind* was composed before *Drugs by Location*, the Kühn edition places *Location* previous to *By Kind*, so that the following synopsis proceeds according to the unfortunately erroneous order (which has become traditional) set down in the Kühn volumes. Both *Drugs by Location* and *Drugs by Kind* indicate Galen's continual efforts to obtain clarity in description of medicinals, and Ilberg rightly notes that these two collections of drug lore came from Galen's pen very close to one another in time, perhaps in the two or three years preceding the fire in the Temple of Peace in A.D. 192.[76]

The arrangement of drugs in *Location*, so Galen writes,[77] is inspired by the example of Hippocrates, and would seem to show an order of the simplest sort: a beginning with affections of the head would lead, naturally enough, to ailments to be treated as one proceeds down from the head through other parts of the body (each with its own malfunctions: *tou kamnontos krasis hē te tou paschontos moriou physis*[78]), a manner called in the later Latin tradition, *a capite ad calcem*. What follows in *Drugs by Location* is a series of suggestions for various problems, indicative more of an "upper class" practice and a culling of beauty-care manuals than of Galen's original intent to organize drug lore in a logical head-to-toe pattern. Titles of the sections delineate the subject matter of *Drugs by Location*, almost in contradistinction to what Galen has said he wants to do in the short preface: "Alopecia," "On Hair Loss," "On the Coloring of Hair," "Drugs for Broken Hair," "Thin Hair," "On Hair that is Dying," and "Dandruff."[79] Much of this material comes from quoted extracts of Criton's books on drugs,[80] in turn extracting earlier sources on pharmaceuticals under the names of Archigenes, Cleopatra, and Apollonius.[81] Book II of *Drugs by Location* has recipes from a number of sources on "illnesses of the head,"[82] but most of the prescriptions for ear and nose problems are in Book III,[83] and the list of "authorities" has expanded to include Damocrates (recipes in poetry), Heras, Apollonius, Archigenes, Andromachus, Xenocrates, Harpalus, Harpocrates, Solon the Dietician, Zoilus the Ophthalmologist, Asclepiades, Charixenus, Antonius Musa, Heraclides of Tarentum, etc.[84] Eye diseases and numerous *kollyria* recipes comprise *Location* IV,[85] and more "beauty aids" for eye-bruises and black eyes begin *Location* V,[86] followed by lachrymal fistulas,[87] and salves, ointments, and plasters for the forehead, along with a great number of mouthwashes, dentifrices (Damocrates' poems) and treatments for various tooth problems.[88] Stomach soothers and gargles form Book VI,[89] congestion relievers and arteriaces are Book VII,[90] but *Drugs by Location* IX contains a melange of remedies, including internal treatments for jaundices and affections of the spleen, followed by hemorrhoids, priapism, anal suppositories, and finally a recipe for the treatment of "uterine suffocation."[91] Book X provides recipes for the treatment of kidney problems, gout, sciatica (*ischias*), and arthritis,[92] and at one point where a poem of Damocrates is being quoted for a cure of sciatica, there is clear indication that an illustrated text has been consulted.[93] *Compound Drugs Arranged by Location of Ailment* does not emerge as a complete and coherent tract on drug lore, but seems to be a potpourri of recipes collected and loosely grouped by external parts, emphasizing the head, with sections on gout, sciatica, and the like that might formally qualify the work as a "head-to-toe" treatise.

The third of Galen's massive pharmaceutical

[73] Ed. Kühn, XI, 323–42. Ilberg, *Schriftstellerei*, 77.

[74] Ilberg, *Schriftstellerei*, 89.

[75] *Ibid.*, 20–23 and 84.

[76] *Ibid.*, 84.

[77] *Drugs by Location* I, 1 (ed. Kühn, XII, 381).

[78] *Ibid.* (ed. Kühn, XII, 378).

[79] *Drugs by Location* I, 2–9 (ed. Kühn, XII, 381–497).

[80] On Criton, physician to Trajan (A.D. 98–117), see E. Kind, "Kriton (7)," *RE*, Vol. XI, part 2 (Stuttgart, 1922), cols. 1935–38, and J. Benedum, "Kriton," *RE*, Supplementband XIV (Stuttgart, 1974), cols. 216–20.

[81] Fabricius, 198–99 (Archigenes), 180–83 (Apollonius).

[82] Ed. Kühn, XII, 498–598.

[83] *Ibid.*, 599–695.

[84] Fabricius, 189–90 (Damocrates), 183–85 (Heras), 180–83 (Apollonius), 198–99 (Archigenes), 185–89 (Andromachus the Younger), etc. M. Wellmann, "Beiträge zur Quellenanalyse des Älteren Plinius," *Hermes*, 59 (1924), 129–56 (140–42; Xenocrates; 142–43: Solon).

[85] Ed. Kühn, XII, 696–803.

[86] *Ibid.*, 804–93.

[87] *Ibid.*, 820–22.

[88] *Ibid.*, 889–93 (Damocrates' poems).

[89] Ed. Kühn, XII, 894–1007.

[90] Ed. Kühn, XIII, 1–115.

[91] *Ibid.*, 228–320. "Uterine Suffocation": *Location* IX, 10 (ed. Kühn, XIII, 319–20). Cf. *PGM*, VII, 260–71, and Soranus, *Gynecology* III, 50 (ed. Ilberg, pp. 127–28).

[92] Ed. Kühn, XIII, 321–61.

[93] *Ibid.*, 351.

works is titled *Compound Drugs Arranged by Kind.*[94] It seems that Galen had been attacked by other physicians for his earlier writings on drugs,[95] which had omissions and faulty principles of organization; it also seems apparent that he wrote *Drugs by Kind* late in life, after the fire at the Temple of Peace in A.D. 192.[96] He will stick by his "system of degrees" as developed in the *Simples*, but he has shifted somewhat as he begins to write this "third approach" to drugs, taking up the venerated "treatment by contraries."[97] What follows in the seven books of *Drugs by Kind* is compilation accompanied by commentary, interspersed by recipes, and the remedies "work" according to the theory of treatment by contraries. An odd sort of fuzziness characterizes the initial chapters of *Drugs by Kind* I, but there is a greater care with sources than one finds in Galen's earlier treatises on pharmacy, illustrated by the subtitles: "A White [Plaster] from [White] Pepper, as Compounded by Attalus and Heras," followed by "Attalus, as Quoted by Andromachus, on the Compounding of a White [Plaster] for a Small Wound by a Rabid [Dog] and for Wounded *Neura*."[98] Heras was an authority on rabies,[99] but Galen is concentrating his attention in Book I of *By Kind* on the white color of the plasters under discussion, and he ends the book with a quotation from Damocrates' medical poem, "On the White Plaster."[100] Green plasters occupy Galen in *By Kind* II, 2–4 (Kühn, XIII, 470–99), but *By Kind* II, 3 (Kühn, XIII, 496) shows that Galen is *not* arguing that the similarities of color give certain "related" plasters their effectiveness, but that their similarity of properties (*dynameis*) provide their usefulness—even though he condemns Andromachus for taking color as a guide. *By Kind* II, 5 (Kühn, XIII, 499–503) is "Drugs That Can be Wiped Away Quickly," and here are salves and oily ointments as cited (without specific recipes) from Criton, Heras, Archigenes, Philip, Menecrates, and other authorities. *By Kind* II–IV contain a large number of suggestions on plasters, drugs for wounds of the *neura*, and drugs for promoting the healing of wounds and ulcerations, as well as plasters and ointments that helped form scar tissue (cicatrization), culled from a number of sources.[101] Book V of *By Kind* (Kühn, XIII, 763–858) might be titled "Multi-Purpose Drugs," and Galen gives a dazzling display of his purported knowledge of pharmaceuticals—or at least his command of the written sources that have recorded such multiple-use drugs. In *By Kind* V, 1 (Kühn, XIII, 763–65), Galen restates his basic, underlying theory of drugs by describing them all, in the first place, as characterized by the hot, the cold, the dry, and the wet, and then, consequently, considering the compounding from simples of these drugs according to their dominant quality; this, in turn, would indicate how these compound medicinals would perform according to their "thinning" properties, "thickening" properties, "promotion of scarring" properties, induction of flesh-growth properties, and so on. Only in this way, Galen insists, can one comprehend why drugs work as they do. Formulas abound. Authorities appear in a rapid blur, and the list of names cited in Book V of *By Kind* indicates which sources Galen had at his disposal, and will provide part of the pattern through which Byzantine medical writers would use *their* sources—whether through Galen or independently.[102]

Book VI of Galen's *Compound Drugs Arranged by Kind* (Kühn, XIII, 859–945) takes up the subject of multi-use plasters. First comes a "Preface" (*By Kind* VI, 1 [Kühn, XIII, 859–62]) in which Galen notes that the previous book of *By Kind* has considered the plasters called *poluchrēstoi*, designated as

[94] Ed. Kühn, XIII, 362–1058 (in 7 books).

[95] *By Kind* I, 1 (ed. Kühn, XIII, 363).

[96] *By Kind* I, 1 (ed. Kühn, XIII, 362).

[97] *By Kind* I, 1 (ed. Kühn, XIII, 367).

[98] *By Kind* I, 13–14 (ed. Kühn, XIII, 414–27).

[99] *By Kind* I, 16 (ed. Kühn, XIII, 431–42: Heras on hydrophobia, accompanied by Xenocrates).

[100] *By Kind* I, 19 (ed. Kühn, XIII, 455–57).

[101] Ed. Kühn, XIII, 503–762.

[102] Heras of Cappadocia, Epigonus, "from the Temple of Hephaestus at Memphis" (a plaster made from dittany [Kühn, XIII, 778–80]), Hicesius, Criton quoting Heras, Criton quoting Hicesius, Andromachus, Criton quoting the recipe of the "Medicine of Machairon" for the healing of all kinds of wound (Kühn, XIII, 796–97), Criton quoting Damocrates, Asclepiades (*By Kind* V, 4 [Kühn, XIII, 801–2] along with a recipe compounded by Galen), Phylacus quoting Diophantus the surgeon, Andromachus on green plasters (quoting Evagrius, Epicurus, Alcimonius or Nicomachus), Heraclides of Tarentum quoting Hicesius, Philoxenus, Damocrates' poem on making a plaster from dittany (*By Kind* V, 10 [Kühn, XIII, 820–23]), Asclepiades quoting Aristarchus of Tarsus (V, 11 [Kühn, XIII, 824–25]), Andronius, Terentius, Areius, [Scribonius] Largus (Kühn, XIII, 828), Threptus, Hierax of Thebes, Lucius, Magnus of Philadelphia, Gaius of Naples, Agathinus, Mnesitheus, Apollophanes. Nicolaus, Petronius, Agathocles, Achilla (Kühn, XIII, 834), Isidorus, Alcimion quoting Apollonius Archistrator on the "pill that acts like a scalpel" (Kühn, XIII, 835), Glaucius, Tiberius Caesar, Phanius, Antipatrus, Publius, Philinus, Melitonus, Apollonius of Tarsus, Asclepiades quoting Marcellus, Xenocrates from his work *Drugs from Vetch* (Kühn, XIII, 846), a recipe of Serapis "set up on metal plates: a fleshmaker" (Kühn, XIII, 847), Tryphon, Heliodorus, Ptolemy, Eunomus, Theotropus quoting Areius, Apelles, and Cleobulus. Galen has gained most of these names and recipes through the collections of Andromachus, Asclepiades, and Criton.

those preparations to be "laid on" for treatment of open sores, ulcers, and the like, either to cause them to heal rapidly, or to cause them to remain open, according to the course of therapy prescribed by the physician. Galen says he has observed the compounding of such drugs during his frequent travels, and how he will, now, record some further "wide-use" plasters, but only after he has verified their efficacy in his own experience with patients. These plasters are those which are employed for flesh that is rotting or semi-putrified, and he will begin with plasters made from herbs. But instead of a formula designated by some geographic location, Galen starts his account by quoting Criton's "Plaster from Herbs" (*By Kind* 2 [Kühn, XIII, 863–64]), with measurements. One wonders what happened to Galen's gathered drug lore, presumably recorded from his travels, when he proceeds to explain why *Criton's* formula would contain poppies (*mēkōn*: *Papaver* spp.), black henbane (*hyoskyamos*: *Hyoscyamus niger* L.)—these would give the "cold"—and the scarlet pimpernel (*anagallis*: *Anagallis arvensis* L.), which would provide the "drying property." Following in *By Kind* VI, 1 (Kühn, XIII, 869–73) is a "Squill Plaster" (*skilla*: *Urginea maritima* [L.] Baker), again probably from Criton's collection, and Galen commends this formula provided one tempers it with wax (Kühn, XIII, 871). After discussing further recipes from Criton and Andromachus,[103] Galen proceeds to the vexed question of weights and measures: after his valuable discussion of how weights and measures are calculated in Italy, Greece, Alexandria, and Ephesus, it seems clear enough that Galen is rather frustrated by the inexactitude of the formulas he has received in the pharmacological sources, and especially by the inexact equivalences that seem to thwart his reproducing the formulas to his satisfaction.[104] Adromachus continues to supply Galen with the listed plaster recipes, until one reaches "A Tyrian Plaster" (*By Kind* VI, 12; [Kühn, XIII, 915–23]), which turns out to be another medical poem by Damocrates, not an original formula from Phoenician Tyre as might have been recorded by Galen.[105] The confused nature of Galen's drug formulas in *By Kind* may be illustrated by an example from the listings of *malagmata*, "emollient" or "soft" plasters. *By Kind* VII summarizes *malagmata* with an apparent strained classification system, as Galen tries to distinguish them from other plasters,[106] and Galen's quotation from Heras on a compound called the *kērelaion* shows how Galen's written sources had confused the specific names of these drugs—and by implication why the best of the Byzantine writers on pharmacy did *not* use Galen as an exact blueprint:

> *Kērelaion*: Praised by Heras above all among Drugs. "Take freshly defibered clear fat, 44 [Roman] ounces, 24 ounces of beeswax, 6 ounces of cerussite,[107] 6 ounces of massicot,[108] and dissolve together the dry ingredients, and shortly they will become congealed." Heras said "the beeswax and the clear fat are the softening properties." Thus if some beeswax would be mixed with a little oil, you will make what is called by the doctors a *kērelaion*, a wax-oil.[109] But clearly the oil ought not to be called either the squeezings of unripe grape [*to omphakinon*] or oil of unripe olives,[110] nor should one assume the addition of the oil of palm leaves.[111]

The remainder of *By Kind* VII[112] continues in this confusion, with numerous quotations from Damocrates, Andromachus, Asclepiades (probably the "Younger," or Pharmacion), and other names now familiar from other Galenic drug books. One may suspect textual corruptions in the Kühn Greek, but interpolations do not explain away the rampant disorder in drug classifications, except for the broad categories of plasters, emollients, earths, herbal simples, and the like. Even though Galen has a reasonably clear theory of drug action, it is smothered by the numerous and often contradic-

[103] Of interest in terms of preparation technique is "A Plaster from a Whetstone," i.e., a powdered compound rubbed on a whetstone (ed. Kühn, XIII, 874–82; cf. Dioscorides I, 98). Criton also provides Galen with a formula from Heras (*By Kind* VI, 3 [Kühn, XIII, 882–83]), another by Serapion (*By Kind* VI, 4 [Kühn, XIII, 883–84]), and another by Andromachus (*By Kind* VI, 5 [Kühn, XIII, 884–85]). Galen seems to take some data directly from Andromachus (quoting Isidore of Antioch) on a plaster for gangrene (*By Kind* VI, 6 [Kühn, XIII, 885–86]). Then Galen tells us he will take up other sorts of plasters, arguing at some length that one ought not to be ignorant of the good data at one's fingertips—unlike so many in his day (*By Kind* VI, 7 [Kühn, XIII, 889]), and then we receive a formula (again from Andromachus) for the Egyptian *Phaia*[?] Black[?] Plaster (*By Kind* VI, 8 [*Kühn*, XIII, 890–91]), a good example of an excellent compound ignored by physicians (Kühn, XIII, 891).

[104] Ed. Kühn, XIII, 895–97.

[105] *By Kind* VI, 12 (Kühn, XIII, 915–23).

[106] *By Kind* VII, 1 (Kühn, XIII, 946–51).

[107] $PbCO_3$, lead carbonate, or "white lead" (*Psimythion*). Preparation of white lead: Theophrastus *On Stones* 56. Preparation of white lead salves: *Geoponica* XVII, 7.2; XVIII, 15.3; and VII, 15.18 (ed. Beckh, pp. 473, 494 [from Didymus], and 203 [from Sotion]). Cf. Dioscorides V, 82 and 88.

[108] PbO, lead monoxide (*lithargyros*). Cf. *PGM*, XII, 194; Nicander *Alexipharmaca*, 594; Galen, *Drugs by Kind* I, 5: "Plasters Made from Lead Monoxide" (Kühn, XIII, 394–98).

[109] This is Galen's "cooling wax salve" in *Hygiene* VI, 14.8 (ed. K. Koch, *Galeni De sanitate tuenda* [Leipzig, 1923; in *CMG* V 4, 2], p. 195).

[110] Theophrastus, *On Odors* 15. Dioscorides I, 30.

[111] *By Kind* VII, 2 (Kühn, XIII, 952–53).

[112] *By Kind* VII, 4–16 (Kühn, XIII, 958–1058).

tory quotations from earlier sources, and Galen's attempts to "explain" why various drugs might be included in the works of Criton, Andromachus, Damocrates, and others, are often surprisingly feeble. Galen generally has not actually sought out the drugs he prescribes—as he likes to boast—but has availed himself of a rich doxographical tradition in Greco-Roman pharmacy, a tradition that was exploited earlier by Criton in the reign of Trajan,[113] and by Dioscorides in the middle of the first century. Unlike Dioscorides, however, Galen did not simply survey his predecessors' work,[114] but excerpted those tracts in large swatches. Once the early Byzantine pharmacologists had analyzed Galen's "Drug Books," they were forced to rearrange, streamline, and "edit them" rather heavily, even though Galen remained a venerated fountainhead of drug lore. It is very significant that Byzantine medical writers, from Oribasius through Paul of Aegina, quite frequently sought out the "original" writings on drugs from earlier Greco-Roman antiquity, and did not continue the pharmaceutical doxography illustrated by Galen's summaries in the late second century.

Oribasius and Pharmacology

Oribasius functioned as court physician to the Emperor Julian (A.D. 361–363), but he had been friend and confidant of Julian before the eventful months of 360 and 361 that led to his elevation to the undisputed possession of the imperial purple. Oribasius had prepared a synopsis of Galen's works at Julian's request, while the future emperor served Constantius as Caesar in Gaul.[115] In 360—again at the request of Julian—he compiled a second work that summarized not only Galen but also many other medical authorities, and we have forty books plus a number of fragments of the original seventy in this *Medical Collection*. From the *Medical Collection*, one may gauge how Galen's pharmacology was employed by Oribasius, and one may also discern some skillful rearrangements, reclassifications, and fresh juxtapositions as Galen is quoted directly. In many respects, Oribasius' use of Galen's works provides a reasonable measure of what tracts by Galen were known in the mid fourth century, and the numerous quotations from all three of Galen's massive pharmacological books show that they all should probably be included within the "genuine" Galenic corpus. *Antidotes* is also excerpted,[116] but not to the extent that Oribasius uses Galen's *Mixtures and Properties of Simples* (593 citations), *Drugs by Location* (206 citations), and *Drugs by Kind* (62 citations). *Theriac to Piso* does not appear among the quoted extracts.

These raw numbers (almost 600 extracts from Galen's *Simples*, just over 200 from *Location*, and 62 from *By Kind*) may suggest a basic pattern for Oribasius' adaptation of Galenic pharmacology. In the first place, Galen's *Simples* had laid down a fairly precise theory of drug "properties," and this tract also included almost all of the listed medicinals known to Greco-Roman pharmacy; secondly, since Oribasius does not quote Damocrates' medical poems (nor any medical poetry at all), this would suggest that Oribasius valued *Location* and *By Kind* (in which Damocrates' poems bulk large) less than *Simples*, or, that medical poetry had fallen out of fashion by Oribasius' day; third, since Galen had given a fairly complete listing of pharmaceuticals in *Simples*, first listed alphabetically (the plants) and then "classed" by source (animals, minerals), Oribasius apparently assumed Galen's *Simples*, combined with the rearranged alphabetical listing of drugs taken from Dioscorides' *Materia medica*,[117] would provide the important substances used in pharmaceutical therapy; Galen's two other books on drugs (*Drugs by Location* and *By Kind*) did not offer a significant improvement in perceptions of drug lore. Moreover, Galen's *Location* and *By Kind* merely repeated the substances (using other authorities) previously listed in his simples, so that there was no quantitative improvement in Galen's nearly 450 drugs contained in his *Simples* that could not be gained by the more streamlined listing of pharmaceuticals from Dioscorides. Oribasius can thus assume his pharmacology would include all of the over 600 "standard" drugs by a judicious combination of Galen and Dioscorides, as well as careful quotations from other authorities directly from their works. Oribasius' arrangement of drugs most likely resulted from the requirements of an active and personal practice of medicine—particularly seen in the quotations of Galen's *Simples* in *Medical Collection* XV—and his adaptation of drug lore became a standard method in medical botany and

[113] See n. 80 above, and J. Scarborough, "Criton, Physician to Trajan: Historian and Pharmacist," in J. Eadie and J. Ober, eds., *Festschrift Chester Starr* (Washington, D.C., 1984) in press.

[114] Scarborough and Nutton, "Preface," 190.

[115] Oribasius, *Medical Collection* prooemium 1–2 (ed. Raeder, I, 4).

[116] Raeder, IV, 327 (nine citations).

[117] Oribasius, *Medical Collection* XI–XIII (ed. Raeder, II, 80–180).

pharmacology still followed in modern times.[118]

Galen's *Simples* had developed a tight theory of pharmaceutical action, based upon primary "qualities" (viz. properties) of particular classes of drugs, followed by a second set of secondary "qualities," and then a third classification of tertiary properties.[119] Galen had argued that the Hot, Cold, Wet, and Dry were common to all substances, and that changes came to matter through either active or passive influences.[120] This, in turn, explained the effects of all drugs.[121] Following from this premise, Galen can then argue for "secondary" properties and "tertiary" properties from the pharmaceutical effects derived from combinations and mixtures of the "primary" properties, as such would be perceived by the senses.[122] There is, however, a vagueness to Galen's "tertiary" qualities/properties, and Harig has shown that Galen meant merely "local effects" in his "tertiary level," that is, local effects of the "secondary qualities."[123] Thus in the beginning of Book V of *Simples*, Galen can make the statement that it is better to classify pharmaceutical compounds by their *eidē* ("species" or "kinds"),[124] apparently meaning their "useful effects" in pharmacy as they are perceived by the senses. By way of illustration, Galen writes that it is more accurate to say that wheat-meal plaster is a balance between the Wet and Hot,[125] rather than to list the plaster's qualities/properties as pus-producing, soothing, cathartic, and relaxing.[126]

Oribasius does some very significant things with Galen's drug theory, and the following can only be suggestive. In quoting from Galen's *Simples* V, 2,[127] Oribasius merely excerpts what Galen has to say about the "utility of drugs" (*peri chreias tōn pharmakōn*), the basic statement of how one understands drug action. Oribasius has, in effect, extracted exactly those passages from Galen's verbose description of drug properties which are precise and clear: "The utility of drugs among men is often from this alone: the heating, cooling, drying, and the moistening, or from the combination of effects as produced [by these properties]." Oribasius includes Galen's assumptions that such physical properties as condensation of drugs, rarifaction, and so on, would also be explained by the underlying theory of *stoicheia/dynameis*, but the repetitive passages following line 5 (Kühn, XI, 707) are not quoted. *Medical Collection* XIV, 4 (Raeder, II, 184–85), is not a continuation of Galen's *Simples* V, but begins with an excerpt from *Simples* III, 11 (Kühn, XI, 564–65), titled by Oribasius "How One Determines the Elementary Property of the Full Compound by Comparison with an Exactly Balanced Substance." *Simples* III, 11 is employed here because Galen has defined a "moderate *krasis*" (a "balancing," or in archaic English, a "temperament"), and such is determined by the sense of touch. *Medical Collection* XIV, 4.1–3, is extracted from Galen's *Simples* III, 11, but *Medical Collection* XIV, 4.4 is from *Simples* III, 13 (Kühn, XI, 571). Oribasius again has skipped an incredibly verbose and repetitive section of Galen's *Simples*, and extracts exactly those passages which summarize precisely what Galen means in terms of his mid-way *krasis*, after Galen has provided an excellent illustration of the cooling properties of rose oil in *Simples* III, 11. Oribasius has shown his shrewd adaptation and rearrangement of Galen, and the *Medical Collection* becomes an attempt to give Galen a clarity—using his own words—lacking in the original texts. Oribasius also has digested an enormous quantity of Galen's writing, no mean feat in itself, and has simplified Galen's tripartite "intensity theory" of drugs so that the original notion is preserved for the employment of future physicians and pharmacologists. In fact, as Harig has argued, Oribasius' quotations of Galen's *Simples* ensured the preservation of the most essential parts of Galen's theory, shorn of the vague and generally unsatisfactory extension of the theory into a "tertiary" level of effects.[128]

Oribasius exhibits great care in citing his sources. One would expect him to cite materials as he had found them quoted in earlier compendia of recipes, such as are found in Galen's *Drugs Arranged by Location of Ailment* and *Drugs Arranged by Kind*. A few examples of sources cited by name, compared to the sloppy manner of Galen's use of recipe col-

[118] G. Harig, "Die Galenschrift "De simplicium medicamentorum temperamentis ac facultatibus" und die "Collectiones medicae" des Oribasios," *NTM*, 7 (1966), 1–26 [4].

[119] See G. Harig, *Bestimmung der Intensität im medizinischen System Galens* (Berlin, 1974), *passim*.

[120] Galen, *Elements According to Hippocrates* I, 9 (ed. Kühn, I, 485), and *Commentary on Hippocrates' On the Nature of Man* I, 7 (ed. J. Mewaldt, *Galeni In Hippocratis de natura hominis* [Leipzig, 1914; in *CMG* V 9, 1], p. 22).

[121] Galen, *Simples* I, 8 (ed. Kühn, XI, 397).

[122] Galen, *Simples* III, 13, and V, 2 (ed. Kühn, XI, 573 and 709–10).

[123] Harig, *Intensität* (n. 119 above), 110–15.

[124] Galen, *Simples* V, 1 (ed. Kühn, XI, 704–6).

[125] Galen, *Simples* V, 2 (ed. Kühn, XI, 712).

[126] Galen, *Simples* V, 2 (ed. Kühn, XI, 711–12).

[127] Oribasius, *Medical Collection* XIV, 3 (ed. Raeder, II, 184) = ed. Kühn, XI, 706–7.

[128] Harig, "Oribasius" (n. 118 above), *passim*.

lections by Criton, Andromachus, and Asclepiades the Pharmacist, will suggest Oribasius' meticulous care and insistence on quoting *directly* from the original work. It will be recalled that Galen cites Xenocrates for a number of animal-derived drugs,[129] and one would, presumably, expect Oribasius to pick up these citations and record them somewhere in the *Medical Collection*. Except, however, for some scholia recording parallel passages from Xenocrates, Galen, and Dioscorides,[130] and one fragmentary quotation (twenty-one lines) from Xenocrates' "Plasters Made from Whelk [*kēryx*] and murex [shellfish],"[131] Xenocrates appears only in a lengthy, direct quotation from *Foods from Water Animals*,[132] which fits neatly into Oribasius' "elementary" books on preparation and recommendation of healthy foods. Here are how one classifies fish and shellfish,[133] and a catalogue of agreeable and disagreeable fish in the diet. No bloods, rennets, or dungs appear in Oribasius' quotations from Xenocrates, and one is again struck by the display of good judgment in the employment of an earlier source, quoted directly and not through an intermediary. Other quoted authors receive similar treatment (for example, the obscure Heraclas),[134] so that Oribasius has "gone to the sources," unlike his verbose model, Galen.

There is ample evidence throughout Oribasius' writing—*Medical Collection*, [*Medical*] *Synopsis for Eustathius*, and [*Medical*] *Books for Eunapius*—not only that he had read and assimilated the writings of many authorities of medicine in the Greco-Roman tradition, but also that his medical practice included much personal knowledge of pharmaceuticals, which he was pleased to share with his son, and with his friend Eunapius. A few examples will illustrate. *Medical Collection* IX, 27 (= *Synopsis for Eustathius* III, 79 [Raeder, II, 30, and Raeder, ed., *Synopsis*, 89]) is "Plasters from the Husks of Wheat." He tells us that one can use the "leftovers" of the wheat by pounding the husks, and the plaster (made from combining the pounded husks with a honey-vinegar mixture and a gum ammoniac [here probably *Ferula communis* L. or *F. marmarica* Asch. & Taub.; less likely *Dorema ammoniacum* D. Don.]) would be useful as a warming plaster for various skin ailments as well as liver and spleen problems. No source is discernable here, and there is only a slight resemblance to the mention of gum ammoniac by Dioscorides;[135] the suggestions by Dioscorides for *ammōniakon* in *Materia medica* III, 84 (Wellmann, II, 100–102) overlap with those by Oribasius only in terms of being useful for ailments of the liver and spleen (*Materia medica* III, 84.3 [Wellmann, II, 102]), but there is no combination with pounded husks of wheat. It is signifcant that Aetius borrows this account of the plaster of pounded wheat husks directly from Oribasius.[136] Thus, it is apparent that Oribasius was a skilled drug compounder in his own right, also shown by other adapted and "original" medicines.[137] Characteristic of Oribasius' command of drug compounding is his direct simplicity and general avoidance of complicated mixtures that might require exotic ingredients.

Oribasius was also well acquainted with Dioscorides' *Materia medica*, but he—like Galen before him—decided that Dioscorides' precise and difficult system of drug affinities was either too cumbersome for practical use,[138] or too diffuse as it stood. *Medical Collection* XI–XII (Raeder, II, 81–159) is an alphabetized listing of the simples in Dioscorides' *Materia medica* (456 substances, including some of Dioscorides' "animal products," for instance, *stear* ["fat"]), and *Medical Collection* XIII (Raeder, II, 160–80) is "From Dioscorides on the Properties [*Dynameis*] of 'Mined' Drugs [*Metallika*] and their Preparation" (88 medicinals, including various stones and earths). Oribasius has carefully alphabetized 544 pharmaceuticals as contained in Dioscorides' *Materia medica*, and there is, indeed, a succinct clarity that would be absent in Dioscorides' original tract. One can suppose that Oribasius drew up this listing, or one may assume that he took a previously-compiled alphabetical listing and simply reproduced it. Given Oribasius' normal habit of citing almost all of his sources by name, it seems unlikely that he had borrowed the alphabetical register of

[129] Galen, *Simples* X preface (ed. Kühn, XII, 245–53).

[130] Oribasius, *Medical Collection* XI A 54, and XV (ed. Raeder, II, 89, 293, and 296).

[131] Oribasius, *Medical Collection* XV, 3 (ed. Raeder, II, 296–97.).

[132] Oribasius, *Medical Collection* II, 58 (ed. Raeder, II, 47–57).

[133] Oribasius, *Medical Collection* II, 58. 11–13 (ed. Raeder, II, 48).

[134] Oribasius, *Medical Collection* XLVIII, 1–18 (ed. Raeder, III, 262–68). See also C. L. Day, *Quipus and Witches' Knots: The Role of the Knot in Primitive and Ancient Cultures, with a Translation and Analysis of "Oribasius De Laqueis"* (Lawrence, Kansas, 1967), 107–31.

[135] Dioscorides III, 48.3 (ed. Wellmann, II, 62). Cf. Pseudo-Dioscorides, III, 84 (ed. Wellmann, II, 101).

[136] Aetius III, 178 (ed. Olivieri [*CMG* VIII 1], p. 350).

[137] E.g., Oribasius, *Synopsis for Eustathius* III, 77 (Raeder, p. 88) = *Medical Collection* IX, 25 (Raeder, II, 28–29): "A Plaster Made from Beer-Yeast."

[138] Scarborough and Nutton, "Preface," 190.

Dioscorides from an unknown source, and the accuracy of the quotations would indicate that Oribasius had performed this onerous task himself. If so, it may be quite probable that Oribasius' alphabetical text of Dioscorides is the archetype of many later manuscripts of the Greek "alphabetical" Dioscorides, including the justly famous Vienna text of A.D. 512.[139]

From Oribasius to Aetius

Although it can be argued that Theodorus Priscianus' *Euporiston* could be included in the scope of early Byzantine medicine (Priscianus was court physician in the reign of Gratian [A.D. 375–383]), the text was written in Latin, as befitted the court of a western Roman emperor.[140] Moreover, the fascinating farrago of drugs and folklore that make up the *De medicamentis* by Marcellus Empiricus (*fl.* as *magister officiorum* under Theodosius I [A.D. 379–395]),[141] will not be considered here, since the work is in Latin, and belongs more to the history of pharmacy in early medieval western Europe. Caelius Aurelianus (*?fl.* c. A.D. 450) has left us a masterpiece of compression—also in Latin—of the best of the Methodist physicians, and the drug lore of Soranus of Ephesus assumes a major importance.[142] And the compendium of Cassius Felix, called *De medicina*, was published in A.D. 447, with the *a capite ad calcem* therapeutics of Galen summarized in Latin guise.[143] One would like to know more about Hesychius of Damascus (*fl.* A.D. 430 in Byzantium), the father of Psychestrus, Asclepiodotus, and Palladius,[144] but as important as were these medical practitioners in the fifth century, we learn about them through isolated quotations in later authors and from summaries as contained in the *Suda* and Photius' *Library*.[145] Alexander of Tralles (V, 4 [Puschmann, II, 163]) gives us a tantalizing bit about Psychestrus' therapy using a "liquifying diet,"[146] and all of these names, excepting Alexander of Tralles, were associated with some residence or study at Alexandria, which continued to be a famous center for medical education of many varieties.[147] It is only with Aetius of Amida, who had indeed spent time in Alexandria,[148] in the early sixth century that one again can assess the next stages of development in early Byzantine pharmacology.

Aetius of Amida

Drug theory begins Aetius' account of medical practice. In fact, the lengthy *Preface* to Book I of Aetius' *Medical Books* (Olivieri, I, 17–30) is entirely devoted to theoretical pharmacology. The complete *Preface* emerges from Galen, but in a deftly arranged manner from several different Galenic passages, generally from *Mixtures and Properties of Simples*, with the first eighteen lines quoted from *Simples*, prooemium VII (Kühn, XII, 2–4). Even in English translation, one is able to detect Aetius' subtle yet crucial modulations of Galen's original, as well as the important reorganization of vital passages from Galen's pharmacological theory, so that clarity could replace imprecision:

> The variations of the individual effects of drugs are due to each of them being to a certain sufficiency [*tō epi tosonde*: "to a certain degree" is the modern expression] hot or cold or dry or wet, or each having fine [or "small"] or coarse [or "large"] particles [or "parts"]. The extent/measure of the degree, however, of the attachments [lit. "fastenings-together"] in each of the drugs cannot be expressed with truthful accuracy. But we have attempted to encompass and characterize them with adequately clear terms and definitions for use in medical practice [*eis tēn cheian tēs technēs*]. We are demonstrating that there is one kind [*hen genos*] of drugs which is [*aphiknoumenon*: lit. "arriving at" or "coming into"] a same *krasis* as our bodies, when it has received some *archē* of both change and alteration [*alliōsis*] from the hot in this kind of drugs, and, that there is another kind of drugs which is hotter. From this, it seems to me that four orders [*taxeis*] can be made: the first is indistinct [*asaphē*] to the senses, [and] detecting it necessarily comes through pure reason [*logos*]; the second is distinct and perceivable to the senses; the third is rather hot, but not to the point of burning; the fourth and last is the corrosive or caustic kind of drugs.[149] Likewise also for the cooling kind of drugs, the first order must come from pure reason in demonstrating its coldness, the second is cooling detectable by the senses, the third is rather cold, and the fourth causes

[139] Vienna, Österreichische Nationalbibliothek MS Gr. 1.

[140] V. Rose, ed., *Theodori Prisciani Euporiston* (Leipzig, 1894).

[141] Marcellus (ed. Liechtenhan).

[142] Caelius Aurelianus (ed. and trans. Drabkin).

[143] V. Rose, ed., *Cassii Felicis De medicina* (Leipzig, 1879).

[144] Hunger, "Medizin," 292. Temkin, "Byzantine Medicine," *DOP*, 16 (1962), 100 = *Double Face of Janus*, 205–6.

[145] On Jacob Psychestrus: R. Asmus, *Das Leben des Philosophen Isodorus von Damaskios aus Damaskos* (Leipzig, 1911), esp. 72–75.

[146] Cf. Alexander of Tralles, ed. Puschmann, I, 74, and reffs. Puschmann, II, 162 n. 1.

[147] Hunger, "Medizin," 292. Temkin, "Byzantine Medicine," 101–2 = *Double Face of Janus*, 206–7.

[148] Aetius I, 131, and II, 3 (ed. Olivieri [*CMG* VIII 1], pp. 65 and 154).

[149] *Pharmaka kaustika*. Galen, *Simples* V, 15 (ed. Kühn, XI, 754). Zopyrus in Oribasius, *Medical Collection* XIV, 57.1 (ed. Raeder, II, 226).

necrosis.[150] Analogous in these definitions are also the wetting and drying drugs.[151]

Galen (*Simples* VII, 10.1) then proceeds to speak of catnip (*kalaminthos*: *Nepeta cataria* L.),[152] writing "catnip is basically of small particles and has a hot and dry *krasis*, and is from the third order with both qualities."[153] Aetius, however, does not continue with *Simples* VII: the next twelve lines in the *Preface* to Book I of the *Medical Books* come from Galen, *Simples* III, 13 (Kühn, XI, 571–72):

> Thus let there be set down a clear instruction of these very degrees [or sufficiencies]: in the first order [*taxis*] of cooling drugs would be placed rose oil or the rose (*Rosa gallica* L., and related spp.) itself; in the second would be placed rose-juice [*ho to rhodou chylos*]; and in the third and fourth orders we would include—for good reason—the very cold drugs: hemlock (*kōneion*: *Conium maculatum* L.), the juice of the opium poppy (*mēkōneion*, viz. opium from *Papaver somniferum* L.), mandrake (*mandragoras*: either *Mandragora officinarum* L. [mandrake], or *Atropa belladonna* L. [deadly nightshade]), and black henbane (*hyoskyamos*: *Hyoscyamus niger* L.). Concerning the hot drugs, dill (*anēthon*: *Anethum graveolens* L.) and fenugreek (*tēlis*: *Trigonella foenum-graecum* L.) are in the first order; the drugs which appear next to them are in the second order; and in the third and fourth orders we would include the caustic and corrosive drugs. And in the same manner in regard to the wetting and drying drugs, one begins with a drug of moderate and proportionate [*krasis*], [and] we will make orders [*taxeis*] one after the other until the farthest extremes [*akroi*]. For some use of such knowledge is not unimportant in the medical practice [*methodos*].

Aetius now drops Galen's *Simples* III, 13 (which goes on to grumble about the general ignorance of doctors in such matters), and switches to an adaptation of *three lines* from Galen's *Simples* IV, 4 (Kühn, XI, 632), in which Aetius writes: "One should also use the sense of taste, and retain in the memory the peculiarity of each quality of the juices" (Olivieri, I, p. 18, lines 15–17); and then Aetius shifts again to four, slightly modified lines from Galen, *Simples* I, 39 (Kühn, XI, 453), ". . . as, for example, when such a substance [*sōma*: lit. "body"] is laid on the tongue, it greatly dessicates, contracts, and deeply roughens it, such as unripe wild pears (*achrades aōroi*: probably *Pyrus pyraster* Burgsd., or *P. amygdaliformis* Vill.), Cornelian cherries (*krana*: *Cornus mas* L.), and the like; every such substance is called sour [or "astringent": *stryphnon*] since it is intensely bitter [*austēron*]" (Olivieri, I, p. 18, lines 17–20). With some slight syntactical adaptations, Aetius has provided a lucid account of Galen's basic pharmacological theory, using Galen's own words and phrases, but judiciously selected and rearranged so that the reader understands (as best as he would be able) this system of drug classification "by intensity" or "by degree." What has been muddled, scattered, and often repeated in Galen's original texts, has now been compacted, edited, and streamlined. The remainder of Aetius' *Preface* to Book I of his *Medical Books* shows a similar ability, and Galen's enormously influential classification of drugs "by degrees" has emerged in the form in which it would be used by countless physicians and pharmacists until well into the eighteenth and nineteenth centuries.

Once Aetius has completed his redaction of Galen's drug theory, he then proceeds to list alphabetically 418 medicinals of plant origin, almost all quoted from Galen, but with an occasional passage from Rufus, Dioscorides, and Oribasius.[154] Book II lists, in part alphabetically, 195 medicinals,[155] an occasional clipped, simplified recipe of drugs derived from metals (lit. "things mined"), stones, earths, and a wide spectrum of "animal products" (from milk to insects); most entries are quoted from Galen, Oribasius, and Dioscorides, but there are a few citations from Rufus, Antyllus, and Theophrastus. Book II, 196–271 returns to the "drugs by degrees" system[156] and now "fits" the 613 substances into the various grades of heating, cooling, drying, and moistening medicinals, followed by a discussion of the properties (*dynameis*) of foods.[157] Then Aetius turns his attention again to the definition of Galen's puzzling "large" and "small" particles as they relate to the properties of foods,[158] but the source is Oribasius, not Galen. With Book III,[159] Aetius begins to list formulas and recipes for cathartics and similar drugs, and his arrangement of simples in the first two books is explained: one has to be acquainted with the basic components—and the theory of how such ingredients would "work"—before the pharmacologist-physician could

[150] Galen, *Bloodletting* 4 (ed. Kühn, XI, 265).
[151] Aetius I *prooemium* (first eighteen lines) (ed. Olivieri [*CMG* VIII 1], pp. 17–18).
[152] A rare form. Cf. Nicander, *Theriaca* 60.
[153] Ed. Kühn, XII, 4.

[154] Aetius I, 1–418 (ed. Olivieri [*CMG* VIII 1], pp. 30–146.
[155] Aetius II (ed. Olivieri [*CMG* VIII 1], pp. 147–255).
[156] Ed. Olivieri (*CMG* VIII 1), pp. 223–55.
[157] Aetius II, 239 (ed. Olivieri [*CMG* VIII 1], pp. 237–38).
[158] Aetius II, 240–241 (ed. Olivieri [*CMG*, VIII 1]), 237–40.
[159] Ed. Olivieri (*CMG* VIII 1) pp. 256–355.

proceed into prescription of pharmaceuticals by a combined class of action. In Book IV,[160] Aetius takes up formal dietetics, quoting heavily from Galen's *Hygiene*,[161] and one also reads the expected admonitions about exercise and a generally healthy regimen to maintain a healthy body. His earlier discussion of the properties of foods now "fits," as he can suggest which foods would do the best service in the diet, according to the theoretical constructs laid down in Book II, 239–241.[162]

Books V and VI take up diagnostics and the venerated theory of the humors,[163] and some common diseases that can be elucidated through these theories. Only occasional pharmaceuticals appear as they are appropriate to the discussions, but Aetius' major sources have shifted to lengthy quotations from Aretaeus of Cappadocia as well as Galen and Oribasius. Book VII is one of the finest accounts of ophthalmology written in ancient and medieval times,[164] and the discussion is replete with collyria recipes drawn mostly from Galen and Oribasius. Although Aetius does not mention cataract couching, there are clear descriptions of sixty-one eye diseases, showing close acquaintance with the essential anatomical structures.[165] Book VIII is a mixture of materials on inflammations, various plasters, and the like, with many details drawn from Galen's *Compound Drugs Arranged by Place of Ailment*. And although Aetius' complete *Medical Books* are in sixteen books (hence the traditional title of *Tetrabiblon* of the *Biblia iatrika hekkaideka* from the customary division in manuscripts into four *tetrabibloi* to every four *logoi*), one lacks competent modern, well-edited Greek texts,[166] and therefore the pharmacy that teems in the last eight books cannot be accurately assessed. Famous, of course, is Book XVI with its splendid summary of gynecology and obstetrics, but the most often cited Ricci translation is based on the Cornarius *Latin* translation of 1542,[167] and the most recently edited Greek text suffers from a number of inadequacies.[168]

Alexander of Tralles

As Aetius of Amida had carefully redacted earlier pharmacology, so also Alexander of Tralles re- ∗ worked much of the earlier data into a lengthy compendium of suggested treatment of diseases by their symptomatology, explained through a general pathlogy that assumed a causation of illness from morbid humors. Alexander was born in A.D. 525, and was the son of a physician named Stephen. Our main data for Alexander's family comes from Agathias' *Histories* V, 6.3–6,[169] and Stephen had fathered five sons, all of whom became prominent in their professions: Anthemius, the architect-engineer who designed the magnificent St. Sophia; Olympius, a gifted lawyer; Metrodorus, a pre-eminent grammarian; Dioscurus, a doctor, "... who lived out his life in his native city in which he carried on the practice of medicine with great success;"[170] and Alexander, who "lived in Rome, summoned to hold high position."[171] Agathias implies that Alexander's fame had not reached the ears of Justinian, whereas both Anthemius and Metrodorus were well known to the emperor. After much travel and experience, Alexander settled in Rome and died in A.D. 605.

Of all the Byzantine physicians, Alexander of Tralles has exercised the greatest attraction for modern medical historians, due to his direct experience with the practice of medicine, vividly and frequently recorded in his extant books on various aspects of medical treatment. Two relatively modern translations (in French and German) of Alexander's works have been produced, and both Puschmann and Brunet are impressed by what they perceive as the "strikingly modern" approach by Alexander to medicine and pharmacy.[172] Alexander does represent a sharp contrast to the arid scholasticism of Aetius, but both Oribasius and Paul of Aegina were clearly practicing physicians, and

[160] Ed. Olivieri (*CMG* VIII 1) pp. 356–408.

[161] E.g., Aetius IV, 1 (ed. Olivieri [*CMG* VIII 1], pp. 358–59), and Galen, *Hygiene* I, 1 (ed. Koch [n. 109 above], p. 3); and Aetius, IV, 36 (ed. Olivieri, pp. 378–79) and Galen, *Hygiene* III, 3 (ed. Koch, pp. 85–86).

[162] Ed. Olivieri (*CMG* VIII 1), pp. 237–40.

[163] Ed. Olivieri (*CMG* VIII 2), pp. 1–249.

[164] Ed. Olivieri (*CMG* VIII 2), pp. 250–399.

[165] See Emilie Savage-Smith, "Byzantine Ophthalmology" (above in this volume), esp. nn. 61–69.

[166] Barely serviceable "modern" texts of various books of Aetius' *Tetrabibloi* include: G. A. Kostomiris, ed., *Aetiou Logos dōdekatos* (Bk. XII) (Paris, 1892); S. Zervos, ed., *Aetio Amidēnou Logos dekatos kai tritos ē Aetiou Amidēnou Peri daknontōn zōōn kai iobolōn* (Bk. XIII) in *Athēna*, 18 (1905), 241–302; and S. Zervos, ed., *Aetiou Amidinou* [sic] *Logos dekatos pemptos* (Bk. XV) in *Athēna*, 21 (1909), 3–144. Bk. XI is in the Daremberg and Ruelle edition of Rufus, pp. 85–126.

[167] J. V. Ricci, trans., *Aetios of Amida: The Gynaecology and Obstetrics of the VIth Century A.D.* (Philadelphia, 1950).

[168] S. Zervos, ed., *Aetii Sermo sextidecimus et ultimus* (Leipzig, 1901).

[169] R. Keydell, ed., *Agathiae Myrinaei Historiarum* (Berlin, 1967; *CFHB*, II), p. 171.

[170] *Ibid.*

[171] *Ibid.*

[172] Alexander (trans. Brunet), Vol. I. Puschmann, ed., Alexander, I, 75–87, 287–88.

their writings show a sense of the clinic as do those by Alexander. It will not, however, be accurate to describe Alexander of Tralles as a "modern" any more than to designate Galen as such; but Alexander is, indeed, humane and conscientious in his practice, meticulous in his prescriptions, and careful with his command of earlier authorities in medicine. Drugs are scattered throughout Alexander's books, given as recipes for the treatment of specific diseases, usually through the long-lived "treatment by contraries." The occasional complexity of Alexander's drug prescriptions (using 495 different pharmaceuticals) are justified by conflicting symptoms, and many medicinals are recorded as efficacious as verified by personal observation and experience. A critical attitude toward his numerous written sources is characteristic throughout Alexander's works, illustrated by the following, which appears in Book V, 4, "On Viscous Humors and Thick Masses Found in the Lung:"

> This is a true statement by Galen on Archigenes:[173] "He was but a man and it would be difficult for him not to make mistakes in many things, being completely ignorant, making bad judgments, and who provided carelessly written accounts." And I would not have said this about such a learned man, unless Truth itself had not inspired me and urged me on, and did I not believe that keeping silent was sinful. For a doctor who does not speak his opinion commits a great sin and through his silence is greatly to be condemned. But one ought to follow that which Aristotle says he has stated: "Plato is my friend, but the Truth is also my friend; between the two, one must choose the Truth."[174]

Alexander does not devote any of his tracts specifically to drugs, but pharmaceutical therapy is very prominent throughout the various subdivisions, for example, fevers, headaches, what we would call "nervous diseases," melancholia, ophthalmology, the rightly famous "Letter on Intestinal Worms," lung diseases, cholera, gout,[175] and so on. Many of the drug recipes seem original, although the particular ingredients have all been used and defined in Greek, Roman, and earlier Byzantine pharmacy. There are occasionally "new names" applied to certain substances, and this can be illustrated by Alexander's "Armenian Stone," which is part of a recipe in *On Fevers* VII [Quartans] (Puschmann, I, 429). Earlier Greek sources—including the *Papyri Graecae Magicae* XII, 201—had noted the use of *ios chalkou* ("verdigris," or copper oxyacetate, approximately $[C_2H_3O_2]_2Cu{\cdot}Cu[OH]_2{\cdot}5H_2O$), but Alexander's *Armeniakos lithos* has taken the place of *ios chalkou*. This "new" substance had been foreshadowed in Dioscorides, *Materia medica* V, 90, and if we understand the geological chemistry the "Armenian Stone" is a combination of copper oxyacetate, azurite ($2CuCO_3{\cdot}Cu[OH]_2$), and malachite ($CuCO_3{\cdot}Cu[OH]_2$).[176] Roman and Byzantine pharmacy could substitute one "kind" of copper oxyacetate for another, and it is probable that Alexander knew the "Armenian Stone" in the same role as had been played by verdigris in earlier prescriptions. The remainder of the recipe "On the Armenian Stone" suggests that Alexander's "new" pharmacy consisted of rearrangement of ingredients according to his experience:

> The stone, which is called "The Armenian," given washed or unwashed in a dosage of 4 *keratia* [c. 800 mg./12 grains] works well for all forms of quartan fever, since it [performs] as no other for the evacuation of black bile. Washed in water, it completely purges the lower bowels, but unwashed it is an emetic which does not cause too much heating, unlike the others. But if some [of your patients] regard the solution of "the stone" with disgust, make little pills using the following ingredients:
>
> 4 *grammata* [c. 4.6 grams/4 scruples/80 grains] of *pikras* [an aloe-honey mixture][177]
> 3 *grammata* [c. 3.5 grams/3 scruples/60 grains] of *epithymon* [lesser dodder, *Cuscuta epithymum* (L.) Murr.][178]
> 1 *gramma* [c. 1.2 grams/1 scruple/20 grains] of *agarikon* [prob. a tree mushroom of *Boletus* spp.][179]
> 1 *gramma* of *Armeniakos lithos*
> 5 "berries" of *karyophylla* [cloves, *Eugenia caryophyllata* Thunb.; here the sun-dried, unopened flowerbuds][180]
> 5 *grammata* [c. 5.9 grams/5 scruples] of *skammōnia* [scammony, *Convolvulus scammonia* L.][181]

[173] More-or-less Galen, *Drugs by Location* II, 1 (ed. Kühn, XII, 535).

[174] Alexander (ed. Puschmann), II, p. 155; French trans. by Brunet, III, 124–25.

[175] Alexander (ed. Puschmann), I, 290–439 (fevers; in 7 books); I, 465–507 (headaches); phrenitis, lethargy, epilepsy, etc. (I, 508–91); melancholia (I, 591–612); ophthalmology (II, 2–70); intestinal worms (II, 586–600); lung diseases (II, 146–244); cholera (II, 320–34); gout (II, 500–86).

[176] Cf. D. Goltz, *Studien zur Geschichte der Mineralnamen in Pharmazie, Chemie und Medizin von den Anfängen bis Paracelsus* (Wiesbaden, 1972; *SA* Beiheft 14), 146–47.

[177] Juvenal VI, 180, and Galen, *Hygiene* VI, 10.19 (ed. Koch [n. 109 above], p. 188).

[178] Dioscorides IV, 177 (ed. Wellmann, II, pp. 326–27). Galen, *Hygiene* VI, 7.18 (ed. Koch [n. 109 above], p. 182).

[179] Maggiulli, *Nomenclatura* (n. 55 above), 85–88.

[180] Paul of Aegina VII, 3 (ed. Heiberg, II, 211). A. F. Hill, *Economic Botany*, 2nd ed. (New York, 1952), 445–46. J. W. Purseglove, E. G. Brown, C. L. Green, and S. R. J. Robbins, *Spices* (London, 1981; 2 vols.), I, 237 ("fruits").

[181] Theophrastus, *HP* IV, 5.1, and IX, 1.3. Nicander, *Alexipharmaca* 565. Dioscorides IV, 170 (ed. Wellmann, II, 318–19).

Mix with juice of *kitrion* (citron, *Citrus medica* L.),[182] or with *krokomēlon* (a jam made from quince [*Cydonia oblonga* Mill.] and saffron [*Crocus sativus* L.]), or with *rhodomēlon* (a jam made from roses [*Rosa gallica* L.] and quince),[183] or with *rhodomeli* (rose-honey mixture). The dose is 2 *grammata* [c. 2.4 grams/2 scruples/40 grains].[184]

* It is significant that an alchemical papyrus from late Roman or Byzantine Egypt also has the combination of water and verdigris,[185] so that Alexander has recorded a common association of "washing" the "green rust" that is copper oxyacetate. The remaining substances in the recipe are known from earlier Greco-Roman sources, and even though the cloves appear exotic, they were known in Roman pharmacy in the first century,[186] but with the close links in the traditions between Cosmas Indicopleustes and Alexander,[187] it seems that this peculiar *hapax legomenon* may reflect a special connection with the spice trade from the Far East. The text of Alexander, *On Fevers* VII [Quartans] (Puschmann, I, 429 and 431) shows a careful assessment of drugs in the context of the ancient humoral pathology, and it appears that this recipe—and many others by Alexander—was compounded after a lengthy experience with patients who exhibited quartan fever. Alexander's pharmacy indicates that Byzantine drug lore was anything but repetitive and static: it shows a continual attempt by the best of the early Byzantine physicians to utilize the traditional pharmacopoeia in new patterns, while retaining the theoretical context of Hippocratic and Galenic medical theory.

Theophilus Protospatharius and Paul of Aegina

Before considering the lucid summary of pharmacology by Paul of Aegina (*fl.* in the 640s in Alexandria),[188] the works of Theophilus Protospatharius should be mentioned. Although there has been debate concerning the century in which Theophilus practiced medicine,[189] the dating by Krumbacher seems to have stood up to scrutiny; we may thus continue to assume that Theophilus lived during the reign of Heraclius (A.D. 610–641). Whenever one dates Theophilus, there can be little doubt about his masterful conglomeration of the ancient medical classics with the Byzantine Christian outlook, nicely exemplified by his *On the Structure of the Human Body*,[190] which fuses Galen's demiurge and teleology in *Use of Parts* with a continually emphasized *ho demiourgos theos hēmōn*.[191] Of interest for Byzantine pharmacy is the short fragment of Theophilus' *On Excrements*,[192] indicating a continued use of dungs in medicinals. And of fundamental interest in the fresh approaches of Byzantine medical practice and diagnosis is Theophilus' *On Urines*,[193] which became the probable ancestor of so many Byzantine works on the topic.

The seventh of Paul's *Seven Books* is devoted solely * to drugs and pharmaceuticals and represents a culmination of the Greek, Roman, and early Byzantine search for clarity in drug lore. In the first six books, Paul does indeed give a great number of prescriptions as treatments for diseases, but in the seventh, he gathers all of the 600 plants and 80 non-botanical ingredients into a crisply clear alphabetical catalogue. First, he pens a precisely worded introduction to drug theory, adapted from Oribasius and Aetius:

On the Mixtures [*kraseis*] of Substances as Indicated by Their Tastes. It is not adequate to judge from the smell concerning the *krasis* of things perceived by the senses. Substances without odors are made up of large particles, but it is not clear whether they are hot or cold. And things which do have an odor, to a certain extent, are made up of small particles and are hot. But the degree of the smallness of their parts, or of their heat, is not apparent, because of the inequality of their substance. And still more uncertain it is to judge them according to their colors, since with every color are found hot, cold, drying, and wetting substances. In tasting, however, all parts of the substances undergoing tasting come into contact with the tongue and stimulate the sense of taste, and thus one can judge clearly their properties in their *kraseis*. Astringents, therefore, contract, obstruct, condense, dispel, and thicken; and added to all of these properties, they are cold and drying. That which is acidic cuts, divides, thins, removes obstructions, and cleans without making heat; but that which is acrid is like the acidic in being thinning and purging, but it differs from it: the acidic is cold, and the acrid is hot; moreover, the acidic repels, but the acrid attracts, consumes, dissolves, and promotes scab [or scar] formation. Similarly, that which is

[182] Dioscorides I, 115.5 (ed. Wellmann, I, 109). Galen, *Simples* VII, 12.19 (ed. Kühn, XII, 77).

[183] Cf. Alexander (ed. Puschmann), I, 479, 503, 523, 613, and II, 371, 495, 567 [further reffs. to the rose-quince jam]; and cf. Alexander, I, 327, 383, 415, 613, and II, 61, 275, 371, 591, 593 [further reffs. to rose-honey].

[184] Alexander (ed. Puschmann), I, 429 and 431 (Greek text).

[185] *PGM*, XII, 193–201.

[186] Pliny, *Natural History* XII, 30.

[187] The "Cosmas," to whom the *Fevers* is dedicated (Puschmann, I, 289) is probably Cosmas Indicopleustes, whose father was an early medical teacher of Alexander (Puschmann, I, 83, following Meyer, *Botanik*, II, 384).

[188] Hunger, "Medizin," 302.

[189] *Ibid.*, 299.

[190] Ed. Greenhill.

[191] Hunger, "Medizin," 299.

[192] Ideler, I, 397–408.

[193] Ideler, I, 261–83.

bitter cleans the pores, is cleansing and thinning, and cuts the thick humors without any heat perceived by the senses. What is wet is cold, thick, and promotes condensation, contraction, blockage, necrosis, and torpidity. By contrast a salty substance contracts, strengthens, preserves as in pickling, and dries without detectable heat or coldness. What is sweet relaxes, "cooks" [viz. promotes "coction"], softens, and lessens density; and what is oily moistens, softens, and relaxes.[194]

On the Orders and Degrees of the *Kraseis* [adapted from Oribasius and Aetius]. A moderate drug is of the same *krasis* as that to which it is applied, so that it does not dry, moisten, cool, or heat, and it should not be called dry, wet, cold, or hot. But that which is drier, moister, hotter, or colder, is thereby known from its dominant property [*dynamis*]. It will be satisfactory to make—for practical use—four orders [*taxeis*] according to the dominant property, naming the substance hot as appropriate to the first order, when it would heat indistinctly and it would require reason to demonstrate its property; likewise this would be true for the cold, dry, and wet, when the dominant property requires reason to demonstrate its existence, and it has no strong or apparent property as perceived by the senses. And such substances as are clearly those having drying, wetting, heating, and cooling properties may be said to be in the second order. Such substances which have these properties, but not to an extreme degree even though they are strong, may be said to be in the third order, but such substances as those which are hot enough to cause scarring or burning are in the fourth order. Similarly, such substances as those which are so cold as to cause necrosis are also in the fourth order. Nothing, however, is found drying in the fourth order that does not burn: for that which dries to an extreme degree [*akrōs*] also always burns, for example, chalcopyrite [prob. $CuFeS_2$],[195] rock alum [a ferrous sulfate],[196] and quicklime [CaO].[197] But a substance may be in the third order of dessicants without being caustic, such as those substances which are sharply astringent, *e.g.* the juice of unripe grapes, sumac [*Rhus coriaria* L.],[198] and alum [prob. a potash alum: $KAl(SO_4)_2 \cdot 12H_2O$].[199]

Comparing this concise summary with the attempts by Galen to bring some sort of order and clarity into the chaos of drug lore delineates the Byzantine ability in choosing essentials and explicating them with great precision. Galen had posed questions and—having rejected the brilliant "drugs-by-affinity" system of Dioscorides—attempted an ordering for pharmaceuticals; but Galen had failed to provide a satisfactory method, even though he perceived three separate approaches evinced in his *Simples*, *Drugs by Location*, and *Drugs by Kind*. Oribasius had excerpted much of Galen, and had shown a method of extraction of drug theory.[200] Aetius of Amida had further refined the attempts by Galen to comprehend medicinals by a "system of degrees," but even though there is a judicious care in the lengthy preface on drugs and drug lore in Aetius, *Medical Books* I, there remains a muddled character and a somewhat jagged result from the painstaking juxtaposition of the carefully chosen extracts of Galen's drug theory. Alexander knows his Galen, but chooses to concentrate on the practical aspects of drug lore, so that one does not find a specific "book" on pharmaceuticals either in Alexander's separate tracts on fevers, or in his extant Twelve Books on Medicine: the theory of drugs is embedded in the recipes recorded. Paul's distillation of classical drug theory has finally captured the essence, and it has the characteristics of filtration and the reworked theory seen earlier in Oribasius and Aetius. Paul is also deeply learned in the medical classics, but his compilation bears the marks of an age skilled in ensuring that adaptation accompanied a creative synthesis borne of direct clinical experience combined with venerated assumptions applied to the "modern" age of Heraclius and the Arab invasions of Egypt, Palestine, Syria, and beyond. In the broader historical and cultural context, the early Byzantine physicians should be viewed as part of the same tendencies which produced the brilliant compactions of Roman law from the *Codex* of Theodosius through the *Institutes*, *Digest*, and *Novella* of Justinian.

Appendix: The Papyri and Byzantine Medicine on Multi-Ingredient Incense. *Kyphi* and *Krisma*

Among several hundred medicinals mentioned in the collection of Greek and Coptic papyri known as the *Papyri Graecae Magicae*,[201] occur the names

[194] Paul of Aegina VII, 1 (ed. Heiberg, II, p. 185).

[195] Dioscorides V, 74 and 100. *PGM*, XII, 195 and 399. Goltz (n. 176 above), 156–57 (μίσυ).

[196] Χαλκῖτις most often $Fe_4(OH)_2(SO_4)_5 \cdot 18H_2O$, as in the χαλκῖτις στυπτηρίη of the Hippocratic *Wounds* 14 (ed. Littré, VI, p. 416); ἄνθος αἰγυπτίη χαλχοῦ ὀπτὸν, στυπτηρίη αἰγυπτίη ὄπτη. Dioscorides V, 99. Goltz (n. 174 above), 154–55.

[197] Here τίτανος, as contrasted to the usual ἄσβεστος. Goltz (n. 176 above), 171.

[198] Theophrastus, *HP* III, 18.3. Dioscorides I, 108 (ed. Wellmann, I, pp. 101–2).

[199] Here the common στυπτηρία, as in Aristotle, *Historia Animalium* 547a20.

[200] E.g., Oribasius, *Medical Collection* XIV, 5 and 11 (ed. Raeder, II, 185–86 and 193), extracted from Galen, *Simples* I, 38, and V, 26–27 (ed. Kühn, XI, 450–51, and 785–87). Behind Oribasius, *Medical Collection* XIV, 5.1–2 (ed. Raeder, II, 185)—as quoted by Galen—are Plato, *Timaeus* 65B-66C, and Theophrastus, *De causis plantarum* VI, 4.1.

[201] My "count" is 425 different herbs, minerals, insects, dungs, etc. An English translation of the entire *PGM*, with commentar-

of two kinds of multi-ingredient incense, *kyphi* and *krisma*.[202] The anonymous writers apparently presume that their readers would know the ingredients for these two incenses, much as they have assumed a knowledge of the numerous medicinal plants, insects, minerals, and other animals employed in a curious mixture of rational and irrational medical-cum-magical prescriptions.[203] These papyri generally emerge from late Roman and Byzantine Egypt, and one may be sceptical of claims that Greek medicine had made its way into the everyday traditions of the native Egyptians, but it also must be recalled that a common knowledge of plants and animals among ancient peoples would be "taken for granted,"[204] a factor often ignored by modern scholars, who presume a constant specialized expertise, analogous to modern medicine and pharmacy. The magical papyri, however, afford a rare glimpse into the actual "medicine of the masses" (at least in Roman and Byzantine Egypt), and this medicine has great affinity to the religious/magical medicine explicated by Gary Vikan in this collection of essays.[205] If, however, the "upper class" pharmaceutical sources had not recorded the exact names of plants and herbs,[206] one would be reduced to learned speculation concerning ingredients, particularly in the cases of drugs compounded from a number of substances. *Kyphi* and *krisma* show a sophistication of both compounding drugs among the so-called common folk, and they also indicate a developing history of their own, destroying the accepted mythology of modern medical historians that ancient medicine developed to a certain point, and then remained utterly static for countless centuries. By contrast to this assumption, the Greek texts show that Egyptian priest-physicians—and their non-Egyptian Greek, Roman, and Byzantine medical counterparts—were in a continual process of "improving the product." One is able to trace *kyphi* from the first century through the mid seventh century, and the mentionings in the magical papyri indicate that such compounds were available far beyond the urban centers of the Roman and Byzantine Empires.

Dioscorides is well acquainted with Egypt, and his *Materia medica* has the first Greek record of *kyphi*, a multi-ingredient incense that not only was to be burned for its heavy and pungently aromatic odor, but which also was an effective medicinal salve—one could even eat it for presumed benefits. Dioscorides writes that in the Egypt of his day (the mid first century) there were many formulas for *kyphi*, and that he is setting down only one of them (*Materia medica* I, 25 [Wellmann, I, pp. 28–29]), and he lists ten ingredients with measures: ½ *xestēs* [c. ½ pint] of nut grass [*kyperos*: *Cyperus rotundus* L.]; ½ *xestēs* of ripe juniper berries [*Juniperus communis* L.]; 12 *minae* [c. 11 lbs.] of raisins, "the seeds having been removed"; 5 *minae* [c. 4.5 lbs.] of purified pine resin [*rhētinē apokekatharmenēs*]; 1 *mina* [c. 15 oz.] of sweet flag [*kalamos arōmatikos*: *Acorus calamus* L.]; 1 *mina* of camel's thorn (oil) [*aspalathos*: *Alhagi camelorum* Fisch.]; 1 *mina* of camel grass (oil) [*schoinos*: *Cymbopogon schoenanthus* Spreng.]; 12 *drachmai* [c. ¾ lb.] of myrrh [*smyrna*: *Commiphora* spp.]; 9 *xestai* [c. 9 pints] of old wine; and honey as part of the preparation instructions, viz.:

> Having removed the seeds from the raisins, pound and triturate them with the wine and the myrrh, and having pounded and sifted the rest of the ingredients, combine them all to soak for one day; then, having boiled the honey until it has a glutinous consistency, mix it carefully with the melted pine resin, and then having carefully pounded together the rest of the ingredients, put up for storage [this incense] in an earthenware vessel.[207]

Dioscorides does not say if other *kyphi* recipes in his time were more complicated, or if they had more ingredients, but Plutarch, *Isis and Osiris* 383E(80)–384C lists a *kyphi* formula with sixteen ingredients. Ten are the same as in Dioscorides' recipe (honey, wine, raisins, nut grass, pine resin, myrrh, camel's thorn oil, two sizes [large and small] of juniper berries, and sweet flag), but Plutarch's list adds six more ingredients: hartwort (*seselis*: *Tordylium officinale* L.), mastic (*schinos*: *Pistacia lentiscus* L.), Dead Sea bitumen (*asphaltos*: $C_nH_{2n}O_n$ + V, Ni, Mo [traces]), rush (*thryon*: *Juncus glaucus* Sibth.), spinach dock (*lapathon*: *Rumex patientia* L.), and cardamon (*kardamōmon*: *Elettaria cardamomum* [L.] Maton.). Unlike a similar recipe, reduced to a medical poem by Damocrates,[208] Plutarch provides no measures, nor does he give any instructions for the preparation of the *kyphi*. He simply writes that "the ingredients

ies, will shortly appear (ed. H. D. Betz, and a team of a dozen scholars), to be published by the University of Chicago Press.

[202] *PGM*, IV, 1313–14, 2971; V, 221; VII, 538, 873.

[203] Paralleled in the Greek texts known as the *Cyranides*. Dimitris Kaimakis, ed., *Die Kyraniden* (Meisenheim am Glan, 1976).

[204] G. E. R. Lloyd, *Science, Folklore and Ideology* (Cambridge, 1983), 119–35.

[205] See G. Vikan, "Art, Medicine and Magic in Early Byzantium" above in this collection of essays.

[206] Esp. Theophrastus in *HP* and *De causis plantarum*, and Dioscorides in his *Materia medica*.

[207] Dioscorides I, 25 (ed. Wellmann, I, pp. 28–29).

[208] Damocrates in Galen, *Antidotes* II, 2 (ed. Kühn, XIV, 117–19).

are not compounded haphazardly, but whenever the drug-preparers [*myrepsoi*] are mixing these substances, sacred writings are read to them."[209] Since the *Suda* mentions a work by Manetho called *Preparation of Kyphi-Recipes*,[210] Plutarch probably gained his listing of the sixteen ingredients from this lost book,[211] which suggests that Dioscorides' first-century *kyphi* recipe represented a pared-down version of earlier Ptolemaic Egyptian listings for *kyphi*, in turn derived from very ancient Egyptian origins.[212] "They use *kyphi* in both drinks and ointments,"[213] so Plutarch says, and even though he gives some farfetched speculation on why this incense should have been so valued as a drug, Plutarch has recorded an important detail: *kyphi* was commonly consumed in a drink.

Paul of Aegina VII, 22.5 (ed. Heiberg, II, p. 394) mentions a *kyphi*, called "the lunar" (*kyphi selēniakon*), which is termed *chrisma selaniakon* in the papyri.[214] Paul writes that, in addition to being used to give a pleasant (if heavy) odor, it is to be rubbed into the forehead as a salve. Oribasius had recorded a formula for a "lunar kyphi" with twenty-five ingredients,[215] while Paul's detailed recipe for the "lunar incense-salve" has twenty-eight ingredients.[216] Some of the ingredients overlap with those given by Dioscorides and Plutarch quoting Manetho, and the anonymous authors of the magical papyri indicate that by the fourth century, some *kyphi* recipes had become known by the more specific *chrismata*, perhaps to suggest their medical use as oily unguents and incenses, but not as drinks or an "edible" drug.[217] Yet the compiler of the papyrus can assume his reader would "know" the ingredients of this complicated incense-salve, and Oribasius and Paul seem to presume an equivalence of *kyphi* with *krisma*, which may indicate that the *kyphi* label had, indeed, become the more "Hellenic" *krisma* outside Egypt. The function, however, of the late Roman and early Byzantine *kyphi-chrismata* generally followed the hallowed Egyptian pattern, while adding an ever more impressive array of ingredients, exotic and local. Paul VII, 22.5, is illustrative:

> Another incense-salve of 28 ingredients, called "the lunar"
> 7 *ounkiai* [c. 191 grams] of *bdellion*: bdellium, either the aromatic gum of the Haddi tree, or, the bdellium of the Mukul "myrrh" tree (*Commiphora erythraea* Engl. var. *glabrescens* Engl., or, *C. mukul* Engl.)
> 7 *ounkiai* of *helenion*: either calamint [= basil thyme], or elecampane [= horseheal] (either *Satureja calamintha* [L.] Scheele, or *Inula helenium* L.)
> 2 *ounkiai* [c. 55 grams] of *schoinos*: camel grass (*Cymbopogon schoenanthus* Spreng.)
> 5 *ounkiai* [c. 136 grams] of *sphagnos*: horehound [= false dittany] (*Ballota acetabulosa* [L.] Bentham)
> 50 small juniper berries (*arkeuthides mikrai*): *Juniperus communis* L.
> 5 *ounkiai* of *kardamōmon*: cardamon (*Elettaria cardamomum* [L.] Maton.)
> 7 *ounkiai* of *aspalathos*: camel's thorn oil (*Alhagi maurorum* Medik.)
> 5 *ounkiai* of *kassia syrinx*: cassia "quill" (*Cinnamomum cassia* Blume.)
> 2 *ounkiai* of *nardostachys*: spikenard oil (*Nardostachys jatamansi* DC)
> 5 *ounkiai* of *kyperos*: nut grass (*Cyperus rotundus* L.)
> 4 *ounkiai* [c. 109 grams] of *asphodelos rhiza*: asphodel root (*Asphodelus ramosus* L.)
> 4 *ounkiai* of *brathu*: savin (*Juniperus sabina* L.)
> 3 *ounkiai* of *kyparissos* (*sperma*): cypress seeds (*Cupressus sempervirens* L.)
> 3 *ounkiai*. [c. 82 grams] of *nardos Keltikē*: valerian (*Valeriana celtica* L.)
> 3 *ounkiai* of *malabathron* (*meta tōn phyllōn*): Indian cassia + leaves (*Cinnamomum tamala* [Buch.-Ham] Nees. & Eberm.)
> 3 *ounkiai* of *rhoda xēra*: dried roses (prob. *Rosa gallica* L.)
> 2 *ounkiai* of *kostos*: costus (*Saussurea lappa* C. B. Clarke)
> 2 *ounkiai* of *krokos*: saffron crocus (*Crocus sativus* L.)
> 7 *ounkiai* of *ladanon*: gum labdanum (*Cistus ladaniferus* L.)
> 7 *ounkiai* of *symrna*: myrrh (*Commiphora myrrha* [Nees.] Engl.)
> 2 *litrai* [c. 655 grams] of *staphis* (*enkigartistheisos*): pitted, dried grapes = raisins (prob. *Vitis vinifera* L.)
> 2 *litrai* of *ischas liparos*: dried, fat figs (*Ficus carica* L.)
> 8 *ounkiai* of *strobilos*: kernels of the stone pine (prob. *Pineus pinea* L.)
> 1 *litra* [c. 327 grams] of *terebinthinē*: Chian turpentine from terebinth (*Pistacia terebinthus* L.)
> 7 *ounkiai* of *styrax*: storax gum (*Styrax officinalis* L.)
> 1 *litra* of *phoinikoi liparoi*: dates of the date palm (*Phoenix dactylifera* L.)
> 5 *litrai* of *meli*: honey [c. one and two-thirds kilograms]
> *oinos euōdes to akroun*: fragrant wine as is sufficient

Oribasius' "lunar salve" has almost all of the same ingredients and measures as seen here in Paul's

[209] Plutarch, *Moralia: Isis and Osiris* 383E(80).

[210] *Suda*, M no. 142 (ed. Adler, Vol. III, p. 318).

[211] Thus this is Frg. no. 87 in W. G. Waddell, ed. and trans., *Manetho* (Cambridge, Mass., 1940 [Loeb: in vol. *Manetho. Ptolemy: Tetrabiblos*], pp. 202–5).

[212] G. Ebers, "Ein Kyphirecept aus dem Papyros Ebers," *Zeitschrift für ägyptische Sprache und Altertumskunde*, 12 (1874), 106–11. Further reffs. in J. G. Griffiths, ed., with trans. and comm., *Plutarch's De Iside et Osiride* (Cambridge [for Univ. Wales Press], 1970), 569 n. 4.

[213] Plutarch, *Moralia: Isis and Osiris* 384B(80): τῷ δὲ κῦφι χρῶνται καὶ πώματι καὶ χρίματι.

[214] *PGM*, VII, 873.

[215] Oribasius, *Synopsis for Eustathius* III, 220 (ed. Raeder, p. 121).

[216] Paul of Aegina VII, 22.5 (ed. Heiberg, II, p. 394).

[217] Cf. Galen, *Hygiene* VI, 4.6 (ed. Koch [n. 109 above], p. 177).

recipe: Paul has added only the gum labdanum, saffron crocus, and the Indian cassia. One can presume that once mixed, this salve-incense would be doled out carefully and would have lasted for several months.

Paul VII, 22.1 (ed. Heiberg, II, p. 393) makes it clear that early Byzantine pharmacy placed the *kyphi* among perfumes, but he also tells us that the aromatic function is a minor one for especially the *kyphi*: one uses them as drugs, to be taken internally for the production of accumulation of mucus, and as preventative measures during times of epidemics, as well as for freeing up the lungs and for liver ailments caused by cold. Following are four recipes: perfume of roses, perfume of lilies, the "Great *Kyphi*, called 'The Solar'" (36 ingredients), and the 28-ingredient "lunar *kyphi*" given above in detail. Dioscorides had been one of the first Greco-Roman physicians to recognize the usefulness of the traditional Egyptian multi-ingredient incense recipes, and the *kyphi*/*krismata* soon occupied an important place in Roman pharmacy, as evinced by Damocrates' poem as quoted by Galen. And Paul, in the seventh century, probably indicates why these curious, quasi-folkloric incenses should have been regarded as very useful by formal pharmaceutics: *kyphi* occupied a place between drugs prepared as lozenges to be dissolved in the mouth, and those drugs thought to be true antidotes.[218]

[218] Paul of Aegina VII, 22.1 (ed. Heiberg, II, p. 393).

XIV

Herbs of the Field and Herbs of the Garden in Byzantine Medicinal Pharmacy

Among scholarly studies of Byzantine gardens are a number that provide details about what plants were grown and why they were cultivated as a common practice. Yet little attention has been paid to the botanical and pharmacal particulars of Byzantine garden lore. Moreover, even less well known are the all-season plant gatherers of the Byzantine Empire, plant collectors who continually augmented the herbal drugs of the monasteries. By focusing on some aspects of the gathering of wild specimens, which were, in many ways, "taken for granted," one receives a rather different picture of Byzantine botanical lore than if research depends solely on evidence drawn from gardens.

An interested student or scholar wishing to inquire about the essentials of herbalism in the Byzantine Empire likely will be led into the Greek texts on gardens, well illustrated by the Christian "dream garden" as published in Greek, with a French and now English translation, by Margaret Thomson.[1] Within are, indeed, the expected fruits and vegetables, sweet smelling and pleasantly verdant, along with some descriptions of "how to plant a garden." Presumably technical names, however, are not intended as a guide for the reader, but rather suggest how an ideal garden would appear. For example, in Thomson's text is the "knowledge of *smilax*,"[2] and one reads an ethereal account of the possible shapes of such a tree, but nothing one could designate as "practical." Thomson's notes on *Jardin,* 21, indicate biblical allusions, but nothing concerning botanical, agricultural, or medical utility. *Smilax* here is a tree (*to dendron*), so that one need not bother to consider other plants with the same name, for example, the cowpea or cherry bean as described by Dioskorides,[3] or the European sarsaparilla first noted by Pliny the Elder and Dioskorides,[4] probably drawing information

[1] M. H. Thomson, ed. and trans., *Le jardin symbolique* (Paris, 1960); and *The Symbolic Garden: Reflections Drawn from a Garden of Virtues. A XIIth Century Greek Manuscript* (North York, Ont., 1989).

[2] *Le jardin symbolique,* 68–77; *The Symbolic Garden,* 86–95.

[3] *Vigna unguiculata* L. = V. sinensis Endl., the cowpea or cherry bean, as in Dioskorides, *Materia medica,* 2.132 and 146 (Greek text ed. M. Wellmann, *Pedanii Dioscuridis Anazarbei De materia medica,* 3 vols. [Berlin, 1906–14; repr. Berlin, 1958], 1:132 and 146).

[4] *Smilax aspera* L., Dioskorides, 4.137 and 142 (ed. Wellmann, 2:282–83 and 285–86). Pliny the Elder, *Natural History,* 16.163 and 24.82–83. The common source is probably the lost tract on medical botany by Sextius Niger (fl. probably early 1st century).

from a common source; nor does one need to posit the infamous scammony (occasionally called *smilax*) with its well-known cathartic resin.[5]

Two trees are possible: *Taxus baccata* L., the so-called English yew, renowned in medieval Asia Minor for its heavy and hard, yet elastic, wood (thus the English "yew-bow" of folklore[6], and, second, the ever-popular tree of an enchanted grove, the holm oak (*Quercus ilex* L.),[7] with its prickly, hollylike sucker-shoot leaves. Centuries earlier, Theophrastus had remarked that the name is "Arcadian," and since Thomson's text leaves little doubt about the fairy-tale purpose of the anonymous writer, it seems clear enough that this famed "dream garden" manual is just that: an imaginary world of fragrances and wafting breezes, of pruned shapes and colorful flowers and equally colorful fruits edible only with the nose and eyes. Thomson attributes this "garden of the imagination" to the eleventh century,[8] and there is an ancestry in similar tracts of pagan antiquity, such as those published by A. Delatte in the *Herbarius.*[9] Delatte's texts retail the plants of medical astrology, with seven major kinds of plants linked with planets also of extremely important ceremonial use and prominence in mythology.

Yet this genre of the "dream garden" manual represents only one facet of Byzantine garden lore and herbalism. Too often, moderns ignore other types besides this religio-mystical "symbolism" of specific plants: Thomson herself had called attention to other and varying traditions of more practical utility in her seldomly cited *Textes grecs inédits relatifs aux plantes,*[10] texts in themselves supplementary to those on botany (and other topics) as edited and published earlier by Delatte.[11] Important is Thomson's section of Greek texts (with French translations) of botanical lexicography,[12] paralleled by Delatte's fifteen botanical glossaries,[13] only slightly emended by J. Stannard.[14] Delatte's glossaries include one by a Pseudo-Galen,[15] nine by anonymous authors, one by a Pseudo-Symeon Seth,[16] and one each by Neophytos, Nikomedes, and Nicholas Hieropais, followed by Thomson's Greek text of a "Lexicon of Arabic Plant Names,"[17] leading into several more tracts of similar content and with the obviously intended purposes of pure lexicography. These are not the vaguely perceived or

[5] *Convolvulus sepium* L. is the most common, cosmopolitan species of scammony, still used in Greece, Turkey, and Syria as a powerful cathartic. In some botanical guides, the plant bears the name *C. scammonia*. Why *Smilax,* in ancient Greek botanical nomenclature, should sometimes take the place of *skammonia* is a lexicographical mystery. The scammony's main pharmaceutical action is its properties to cause large amounts of bodily fluids to be evacuated, which explains why many modern herbal manuals describe it as a "diuretic."

[6] Dioskorides, 4.76 and 79 (ed. Wellmann, 2:88–89 and 92–93). Pliny the Elder, *Natural History,* 16.51.

[7] Theophrastus, *Historia plantarum,* 3.16.2; Pliny the Elder, *Natural History,* 16.19.

[8] Thomson, *Le jardin symbolique,* 10–11; *The Symbolic Garden,* 10–11.

[9] A. Delatte, *Herbarius: Recherches sur le cérémonial usité chez les anciens pour la cueillette des simples et des plantes magiques* (Paris, 1938).

[10] Paris, 1955.

[11] A. Delatte, ed., *Anecdota Atheniensia et alia,* vol. 2, *Textes grecs à l'histoire des sciences* (Paris, 1939).

[12] Thomson, *Textes grecs,* 125–77.

[13] Delatte, *Anecdota,* 273–454.

[14] J. Stannard, "Byzantine Botanical Lexicography," *Episteme* 5 (1971): 168–87.

[15] Delatte, *Anecdota,* 385–92.

[16] Ibid., 339–60.

[17] Thomson, *Textes grecs,* 139–67; Delatte, *Anecdota,* 279–318, 331–39, and 393–417.

fancifully aromatic plants of the symbolic garden: rather these spare listings show repeated attempts at precision in nomenclature, attempts forecast quite early by the multilingual synonyms provided by Dioskorides and later scholiasts,[18] augmented first by an obscure Pamphilus about a century after the original *Materia medica* appeared,[19] and by the "Synonym Lists" of drugs circulating by the second century, illustrated by the Galenic tract under this title.[20]

The Greek tracts published by Delatte and Thomson are ample evidence of an herbalism among the Byzantines, an herbalism rather far removed from the redolently imaginary gardens of pagan and Christian myth. Such treatises also tell us immediately that doctors, pharmacologists, herbalists, *and* farmers not only were very interested (and literate), but also required information about wild as well as cultivated plants: some were used as medicinals, others for the manufacture of ointments and perfumes (especially the numerous "oil plants"), others as food sources on a seasonal basis, still others as condiments, and, of course, as sources of the species transplanted and carefully tended in the well-known gardens of both the Byzantine East and medieval Latin West, with similar and carefully cultivated gardens also characteristic of the Islamic world.[21]

Yet even a short survey of this kind of modern study, representing excellent scholarship and detailed command of the texts and multilingual sources, shows the predominance of an "ideal garden," when a scholar considers medicinal plants or potherbs (e.g., J. Stannard, G. Keil, and C. Opsomer-Halleux in the 1986 *Medieval Gardens*).[22] This tendency is widespread

[18] Most of the presumed synonyms are set below the text of Dioskorides in the Wellmann edition, with the clear designation RV, in turn given parallel readings in other sources by the editor as part of the apparatus criticus.

[19] M. Wellmann, "Pamphilos," *Hermes* 51 (1916): 1–64.

[20] Often cited as "Galen, *Glossary*," the first set of synonym lists in the Galenic corpus appear in C. G. Kühn, ed., *Claudii Galeni Opera omnia,* 20 vols. (Leipzig, 1821–33; repr. Hildesheim, 1964–65), 19:62–157. The second set of exegetical references and synonyms are in the same volume, 721–47; the first of the pair is devoted to explicating "puzzling" words and definitions of Galen's ideal, Hippocrates; the second tract (if either is genuine: some scholars believe both are Renaissance forgeries) provides a set of "quickie" remedies in a kind of "Substitution List," not synonyms. Apparently whoever compiled this "Substitution List" was well aware that many drugs as listed in the Greco-Roman "Galenic" texts were not available locally from time to time, so such "substitution of drug B for the usual recommendation of drug A" became a model for later Byzantine Greek, classical Arabic, and medieval Latin glossaries of this sort. Unhappily, many scholars have confused Galen's *Glossary* (best read as a series of explications of earlier medical terminologies, including those from the Hippocratic corpus) with the *Substitutions,* so that the novitiate may gain a reference from the *Glossary,* when in actuality it emerges from *Substitutions.* Much of this confusion is nicely laid to rest by R. J. Durling, *A Dictionary of Medical Terms in Galen* (Leiden, 1993), to which an interested scholar should first resort, especially for the sometimes more-than-obscure terms of pharmacology.

[21] Illustrative are the following: A. Watson, *Agricultural Innovation in the Early Islamic World: The Diffusion of Crops and Farming Techniques, 700–1100* (Cambridge, 1983); E. B. MacDougall and R. Ettinghausen, eds., *The Islamic Garden* (Washington, D.C., 1976); D. N. Wilber, *Persian Gardens and Garden Pavilions,* 2d ed. (Washington, D.C., 1979); E. B. MacDougall, ed., *Medieval Gardens* (Washington, D.C., 1986). For Muslim Spain, one of the better studies is L. Bolens, *La cuisine andalouse: Un art de vivre, XIe–XIIIe siècles* (Paris, 1990).

[22] J. Stannard, "Alimentary and Medicinal Use of Plants," in MacDougall, *Medieval Gardens,* 69–92; G. Keil, "Hortus Sanitatis: Gart der Gesundheit. Gaerde der Sunthede," ibid., 55–68; and C. Opsomer-Halleux, "The Medieval Garden and Its Role in Medicine," ibid., 93–114.

in the specialist literature, and particularly characteristic (perhaps appropriately) of the numerous books on medieval English botanical lore, exemplified by the work of Teresa McLean.[23] One can, to be sure, argue that humankind's occupation and cultivation of Europe and the Near East had consumed millennia, and thereby truly feral areas were unusual (unlike the New World in 1492, which was almost *all* wild, with the exceptions of certain Amerindian cultures that flourished and passed away long before the arrival of Europeans), so that "wild" herbs were presumably unimportant in the pharmacal lore of classical antiquity and the Middle Ages.

Our texts, however, demonstrate vividly that physicians in ancient Greece, the Hellenistic world, the Roman Republic, and the successor empires of the Roman and Byzantine centuries, knew and valued *both* wild and cultivated plants, employed as drugs; such are fully attested in the works of many Byzantine physicians and pharmacologists, ranging from Alexander of Tralles to John Aktouarios. In fact, Byzantine concepts of what *was* herbal medicine were fundamental in the teaching of herbal pharmacology in the medical schools of Renaissance Europe; many of these teaching institutions boasted of their own "teaching gardens" that incorporated traditionally cultivated potherbs along with "wild herbs" gathered from local countrysides (with information on the curative powers of these plants also derived from local folklore); soon added to these often beautiful and scrupulously planned teaching gardens were the ever-increasing numbers of "new and wild" botanicals from the New World, Africa, and Asia.[24] And as one would expect, culinary arts overlapped pharmacy in the discussions of plant properties (or "virtues" as they were often termed), so that foods and foodstuffs became part of herbalism in almost all eras.[25] The Byzantines valued such expertise, and some recent scholarship has begun to explore how Portuguese, Spanish, and English, alongside long-term Venetian, trading ventures came to improve the Byzantine diet.[26]

Medical botany is quite prominent in Byzantine medicine, and, as I have indicated elsewhere,[27] early Byzantine pharmacy occupies a central role in how the doctor treats disease, in company with how the physician perceives the "properties" (here usually *dynameis* in the Greek as one explicates how drugs "work"). Our written texts, from Oribasios to Paul of Aegina, repeatedly show how the Byzantine philosopher-physicians (and those sometimes known as iatrosophists) reworked, streamlined, augmented, and clarified the medical and pharmacological texts of the Greco-Roman era. Dioskorides' great *Materia medica* (ca.

[23] *Medieval English Gardens* (London, 1981).

[24] There is an enormous bibliography on the "introduction" of new species into the pharmacal lore of Europe in the Renaissance. For a summary and collection of references, see J. Scarborough, "Botany, Pharmacy, and the Culinary Arts," in A. C. Crombie and N. Siraisi, eds., *The Rational Arts of Living* (Northampton, 1987), 161–204.

[25] This interplay is well demonstrated in two monographs (among many): R. Howard, *La bibliothèque et le laboratoire de Guy de la Brosse au jardin des plantes à Paris* (Geneva, 1983), and W. T. Stern, *Botanical Gardens and Botanical Literature in the Eighteenth Century* (Pittsburgh, 1961).

[26] Most recently (among the welcome interest in "food history" by classicists and medievalists), one may consult with profit A. Dalby, "Biscuits from Byzantium," *Siren Feasts* (London, 1996), 187–211.

[27] J. Scarborough, "Early Byzantine Pharmacology," *DOP* 38 (1984): 213–32.

A.D. 70) had become *the* basic treatise on all aspects of pharmacology and pharmacognosy, and pure botany continued to be represented by Theophrastus' rightly honored *Inquiry into Plants* and *Causes of Plants* (both ca. 300 B.C.). It is, however, Galen of Pergamon (A.D. 129–after 210) who became the absolute authority on all facets of medicine in the Eastern Roman Empire, especially after Oribasios of Pergamon (ca. A.D. 325–400) had performed probably the first known of many attempted truncations, summaries, and rearrangements of Galen's often massive, self-contradictory, and presumably all-inclusive works on medicine (the often-cited edition by C. G. Kühn [Leipzig, 1821–33; repr. Hildesheim, 1963–64] occupies four linear feet on one of my bookshelves).

This overriding authority is further attested by the "Seven Physicians" folio of the A.D. 512 Vienna manuscript of Dioskorides (fol. 3v),[28] which, accompanied by the previous "seven physicians" of folio 2v, provides a pictorial "history of medical authorities" in the early sixth century (notably absent is Hippocrates of Cos). Galen sits top and center on folio 3v, flanked by Dioskorides and Krateuas, the former the major author of this beautiful, alphabetical version of Dioskorides' *Materia medica.* And although one admires the occasionally magnificent (and one growls at some of the paintings, which are dreadful) illuminations of Dioskorides' plants, Nicander of Colophon's poisonous creatures, and some other topics including a manual of ornithology by an otherwise unknown Dionysius, *all* are but

[28] Regarding the famous Vienna codex (properly cited as Codex Vindobonensis med. gr. 1 der Österreichischen Nationalbibliothek), two reproductions of what constitutes 485 folios (weighing 14 lbs.) have appeared in the 20th century: the first was published in Leiden in two volumes by A. W. Sijthoff (1906), with the first volume of descriptive commentary and the second of black and white reproductions of the folios; useful in its day, this *De codicis Dioscuridei Aniciae Iulianae, nunc Vindobonensis Med. Gr. I* (with commentary by A. de Premerstein, C. Wessely, and J. Mantuani), has been completely superseded by the full-color, full-sized reproduction (five volumes, with a sixth containing commentary and listings by H. Gerstinger) published by the Akademische Druck- u. Verlagsanstalt (Graz, 1970). Unlike the 1906 Leiden edition, the 1970 reproduction has full commentary on the other works represented (other than a shortened, alphabetical version of Dioskorides): an anonymus *Poem on the Properties of Herbs* (fols. 388–392); two paraphrases of Nicander's *Theriaka* and *Alexipharmaka* by an otherwise unknown Euteknios (fols. 393–459 [many illuminations scattered here and there in the margins, with many accurate renderings—especially of the blister beetles—and many purely imaginary images of the poisonous creatures retailed by Nicander of Colophon]); a paraphrase of Oppian's *Book on Fishing,* again by Euteknios (fols. 460–473 [the illuminations, however, seem more intended to accompany pseudo-Oppian's lengthy poem, *On Hunting*]); and, finally, a paraphrase of an *Ornithology* (Grk. *Ixeutika*) by an (again) otherwise unknown Dionysios (fols. 474–485 [fol. 483v shows twenty-four birds, quite vividly painted from life]). Most large libraries have copies of the Graz reproduction volumes; I apologize to my readers for my inability to gain permission to reproduce relevant folios from Vienna in time for publication. One can, however, peruse the selection of illuminations, reproduced in full color and size, in O. Mazal, *Pflanzen, Wurzeln, Säfte, Samen: Antike Heilkunst Miniaturen des Wiener Dioskurides* (Graz, 1981), a volume held much more commonly in university libraries. It is interesting to speculate about the first illuminated folio, showing a peacock (male, with feathers spread in the "courting" position), presumably the family's animal (a kind of 6th-century coat of arms), and reflect how this peacock precedes the famous two folios of famous physicians, not to mention the portrait folio 6v, showing the princess Anicia Juliana and her attendants. The tale of how this magnificent manuscript survived to be deposited in the Hapsburg collection in the 16th century is a tale worth telling in itself, perhaps best summarized by G. Sarton, "Brave Busbecq," *Isis* 33 (1942): 557–75. Anicia Juliana was known as a generous benefactor in her day, as suggested by M. Harrison, *A Temple for Byzantium: The Discovery and Excavation of Anicia Juliana's Palace Church in Istanbul* (London, 1989). On this manuscript, see also Leslie Brubaker, "The Vienna Dioskorides and Anicia Juliana," in this volume, 189–214.

selections from the complete works; but those that do appear give us a reasonable guide to which plants were deemed useful in early sixth-century Byzantine pharmacology. It is important likewise that one have in hand the complete, nonalphabetical Greek text of Dioskorides (last and best edited by Max Wellmann in 3 vols. [Berlin, 1906–14; repr. 1958]), so that one can gain a clear impression of which plants were deemed useful in sixth-century Byzantine pharmacology including plants gathered in the wild and those emerging from one of the countless gardens, so appropriately recapitulated and condensed in several books in the tenth-century *Geoponika*. Sometimes what is omitted in the Vienna text of Dioskorides (admittedly our earliest medical manuscript in Greek) is surprising, but inclusion of a plant per se suggests a reader may be presumed to have "known" a more complete account: that the 14-pound codex was not intended as a "field manual" should be apparent, but even as a "royal gift" fit for a princess, the codex is a valuable guide to what plants were thought valuable for a household in the highest levels of the ruling class of the Byzantine Empire in the sixth century.

One example will serve to illustrate the question of "herbs in the field" and "herbs of the garden" as would be depicted in the Vienna manuscript: the opium poppy (*Papaver somniferum* L.).[29] Folio 221v gives a reasonably accurate painting of the opium capsules in the various stages of growth (the leaves are not well depicted, but at least the pinnate edges receive emphasis; the *P. somniferum* does not have multilobed, pinnated leaves as here represented by the unknown artist), and the root stock is somewhat of the "generic" type.

Here is what Dioskorides, 4.64 (ed. Wellmann, 2:218–21; my trans.) has to say about this famous and presumptive analgesic:

> 1. [The opium] poppy. Some is cultivated and grown in gardens, from which the seed is made into bread, and becomes part of a healthy diet; and with honey, they use the poppy seed in place of the sesame seed, and thereby it is called the "common poppy," which has a longish head and a seed that is white. Another kind that is wild has a capsule head that droops, a seed that is black, and is called the "corn poppy," and some term this "rhoias" on account of the juice flowing from it. But there is a third kind of these poppies, much less cultivated, and it is smaller and more useful as a drug; this type has a longish capsule.

Then follow medical and pharmaceutical uses, and Dioskorides makes explicit the variations between the "cultivated" and "wild" poppies (4.64.5 [ed. Wellmann, 2:221; my trans.]):

> Best is the latex (or "juice," = *opos*) which is thick and heavy of the wild kind; it is soporific to the person who smells it, bitter to the taste, easily diluted in water, smooth, white, neither rough nor full of lumps, nor does it congeal as it is passed

[29] For a discussion of both ancient and modern views of opium, see J. Scarborough, "The Opium Poppy in Hellenistic and Roman Medicine," in R. Porter and M. Teich, eds., *Drugs and Narcotics in History* (Cambridge, 1995), 4–23.

> through a sieve as would be characteristic of wax; and set down in the sun and allowed to spread out while melting [identifies it as genuine]; and set alight from an oil lamp, it does not have a darkly colored flame, retaining indeed the odor of its own particular property. Some, however, counterfeit it by mixing the juice of the horned poppy or acacia gum or the juice of the wild lettuce.

This is the text readers and viewers of the famous Vienna codex of the *Materia medica* would have known and consulted; Dioskorides has warned previously (4.3 [ed. Wellmann, 2:119]) that too much of the wild latex can kill, so that the physician-pharmacologist had to use great care in its employment. Several points are important, even in this short account of the opium poppy: some poppies are, indeed, part of garden plots, and would remain so from Roman times through the twentieth century (many botanical gardens today proudly display their specimens of this famous plant, sometimes with a guard closely observing the visitors); those poppies that are cultivated are raised for their oilseeds, and they remain a staple in the production of breads (the ancients were well aware that there are no narcotic properties in the seeds); and, as Dioskorides and the Vienna version make clear enough, it is the *wild* variety that is gathered for the ill-famed soporific and occasionally for its death-dealing properties. These uses were well known to Nicander of Colophon (fl. ca. 130 B.C.) and his sources,[30] so that wild and cultivated poppies are part of the long history of classical and Byzantine gardening culture, as well as the lore of gathering the latex from the maturing plant in the field.

It is unlikely that the artist who rendered the opium poppy on folio 221v of the Vienna codex has painted from life, but he *has* captured the four basic stages of the life cycle of the capsules' development (harvesting the best latex is detailed in Dioskorides, 4.64.7 [ed. Wellmann, 2:221]), and except for some slightly more sophisticated knives and collection pans, the methods of modern harvesting of the *P. somniferum*'s latex from the capsules *just before they ripen* (almost exactly what Dioskorides records) remain almost identical. Moreover, ancient pharmacologists and their Byzantine successors were well aware that there were several varieties of poppies, ranging from a truly "wild" kind (Vienna codex, fol. 222) through less potent varieties (fols. 223v, 224v, and 225v). The scholia on poppies in the text of Dioskorides are not particularly revealing of Byzantine gardeners' or physicians' experiences that might have varied from the textual tradition, so that it would seem that later doctors and pharmacologists found that Dioskorides was essentially correct. That same textual tradition, beginning in the second century, suggested that repeated employment of the opium poppy latex thus generally verified the account of Dioskorides, confirmed as one examines parallel passages, condensed by Oribasios, or elaborated by Alexander of Tralles, and a few others, conveniently listed in Wellmann's apparatus criticus.

Yet the Byzantine scribes did not simply parrot their classical texts in medicine and related matters, and one can choose no better example than that selected by John Riddle, in

[30] Scarborough, "Opium Poppy," 11.

his fine essay of 1984,[31] to illustrate two matters: (1) additional information by later and obviously experienced gardeners and physicians; and (2) parallel traditions accompanying the texts of the *Materia medica,* in this instance an almost exact match with a series of passages in the *Geoponika.* When Riddle submitted his essay for inclusion in the published collection of papers resulting from the 1983 Dumbarton Oaks Symposium on Byzantine Medicine, I was happy to augment his arguments on asparagus with the *Geoponika,* and I think it quite appropriate here to call attention to these again.

Dioskorides, 2.125 (ed. Wellmann, 1:198; my trans.), had written that "some" (in his usual manner of giving a report that he has heard but did not necessarily believe) "have set down that if someone were to bury rams' horns broken into small pieces, asparagus grows." A scribe, sometime before the fourteenth century, flatly denied this, saying in his scholiastic comment, "this appears incredible to me," and, as Riddle notes, this *emoi de apithanon* appears in at least ten variant manuscripts of Dioskorides' discussion of this common garden vegetable. And although Riddle did not make particular note of Dioskorides' account of the utility of the asparagus, it is clear (again) that both wild and garden-grown varieties are included: the feral sort grows in rocky soils, the cultivar as one would expect in the soils prepared for other vegetables (medicinal uses are those well known in many folk traditions: bowel softener, diuretic, treatment for sciatica and jaundice, as a remedy for toothache, and as an antidote for the bites of poisonous spiders). Perhaps the gardener is attempting to duplicate the "rocky" soil for his asparagus plot (a tricky and long-term vegetable to grow as any modern gardener all too well knows), but of importance is the parallel passage in the tenth-century *Geoponika* (last edited by H. Beckh as *Geoponica sive Cassiani Bassi scholastici De re rustica eclogae* [Leipzig, 1895; repr. Stuttgart, 1994]),[32] which reads: "If one wishes to produce an abundance of asparagus, chop up horns of the wild ram into small pieces, throw them into the asparagus beds, and water them. Some [others] say that it is better if the whole rams' horns are bored with holes and then put down into the soil, they will produce asparagus" (*Geoponika,* 12.18.2–3 [ed. Beckh, p. 365; my trans.]).

Quite puzzling in this passage is its description of technical details: is the would-be gardener being advised to put rootstocks (or crowns) of old asparagus into the holed rams' horns? Growing edible asparagus from seeds gives poor yield, but crown-growth from permanent beds can yield annually (after the third year); the tender shoots of springtime (in temperate climes) can be harvested repeatedly for up to twenty years. One is, however, struck by the *Geoponika* extract that both a "wild" and a "cultivated" sort are known and used. The extract (if we can rely on the copyists of the tenth century) is quoted from a Didymus, probably the Didymus of Alexandria known to have written a fifteen-book *Georgika* in the fifth century, and if Wellmann is right,[33] Didymus was a physician of some repute. The mix of agricultural and pharmacological data remains explicit, and the passage in Dioskorides neatly interlocks with that of Didymus as quoted in the tenth-century *Geoponika.*

[31] J. M. Riddle, "Byzantine Commentaries on Dioscorides," *DOP* 38 (1984): 95–102.

[32] On this text, see also Robert Rodgers, "Κηποποιΐα: Garden Making and Garden Culture in the *Geoponika,*" in this volume.

[33] M. Wellmann, "Didymus," *RE,* vol. 9 (Stuttgart, 1903), 445.

The Byzantine text is incorporated into the book "on" gardens (e.g., 12.2 [ed. Beckh, pp. 349–50]), quoted from an otherwise unknown Florentinus, and headed "How to make a garden," with a preceding "gardening calendar" (12.1.1–2 [ed. Beckh, pp. 347–49]): January through December, with each month specified with plantings "as is suitable for the climate of Constantinople." As one reads through the accounts of the particular vegetables and foodstuffs (asparagus, lettuce, beets, cabbages, and so on), one notes again and again that there are "wild kinds" also to be harvested, and one again can use the exemplar of the asparagus: *Geoponika* 12.18.4 and 5 (ed. Beckh, p. 365) tells us that in order to have asparagus year-round, one is to take the seeds [?: such are really more akin to "berries"] and weed around the surface roots, a description that can match only what one finds in the growth patterns of the still common "wild asparagus" of Turkey; its underground stem grows horizontally, which then produces the spring shoots that are very tender and tasty, the so-called turions. Gathering asparagus, for both medical and culinary purposes, thus includes garden lore as well as a common knowledge of how this vegetable favors sandy soils. Modern California's January "asparagus spears," so horribly expensive in a Wisconsin winter, are, in some respects, quite like those gained by herbalists in fifth-century Alexandria and tenth-century Constantinople. And these were gathered and marketed by professional "herbalists," not gardeners of the town. These "herbalists" were indeed "farmers" addressed and assumed to be literate, an assumption by the compilers of the text we have as the *Geoponika*. This manner of mixing the cultivars with the gathering of "wild" species, for the sake of (one presumes) freshness, could be illustrated by several accounts in *Geoponika* 12 and in other books of the same compilation that address plants and their employment as drugs, foods, or condiments.

My last example of the continual intermeshing of farm and field with the geometrically pleasing "ideal gardens," so common in medieval times from England to Bombay, had more to do with veterinary practices than with vegetables, but will illustrate the same point: knowledge flowing both ways, from city to countryside and back again, perhaps "corrected" or "refined" for the city slickers. We have to keep in mind that most people lived in the country in those days, with a few making a living knowing the plants to be gathered, while the great majority tilled the fields of one or another overlord, living out their years as had their forefathers before them. Life in the country, however, was not without its special realms of pure knowledge. Country dwellers (*pagani* in Latin) "knew" the plants: they did not "name" them, a habit that reaches back as far as Mycenaean times and Homeric Greece, if not to the beginnings of our species somewhere in northeastern Africa some many millennia ago.

Alongside the domestication of wheat, rice, barley, oats, and several other food plants came the domestication of animals. We do not know "when" these processes were firmly in place, but with the creation of urban centers in Mesopotamia, China, India, Egypt, and elsewhere after about 7000 B.C., we find animals side by side with the plants on the farms (by whatever name) most of the human population tilled. From the very beginnings, people and animals transferred illnesses to one another, but, except for the worst of the plagues, it would seem that most of what today we would call illnesses went unnoticed, as a part of normal life. Even so, as we learn in the late texts we know as the *Geoponika* and the collection of excerpts from the same era which we call the *Corpus hippiatricorum Graecorum,*[34] farmers and horsemen had many problems with parasites on and in their animals, and I have chosen one very intriguing passage in the *Geoponika* that indicates Byzantine sheep herders *did* deal with ticks and other irritating pests. Indeed, the modern world is coming back to something like these natural insecticides or vermicides, since there would be, by definition, very few (if any) "side effects" or long-term damage to either the environment or to the productive capability of the sheep and their prized wool. *Geoponika* 17.16 is headed "Concerning lice. From Didymus," and one reads (ed. Beckh, p. 495; my trans.):

> 1. If sheep have ticks or lice, pound thoroughly some maple tree roots and boil this mash in water; part the wool on the sheep from head to the end of the spinal column, and then pour this liquid on while still warm, so that it finds its way over the whole animal's body. Some use cedar oil in the same way.
> 2. Some others likewise in a similar fashion prepare mandrake root for this use, but one must ensure that the animals do not ingest this mandrake root wash, since it is poisonous to them.
> 3. Others prepare likewise in a similar fashion a decoction of cyperus root and wash the sheep with it.[35]

From the modern vantage, the phytochemistry and the "logic" of using a maple root wash and its tannin as an excellent flea- and tick-repellent, makes good sense, but the cyperus root's chemical properties remain obscure. At this juncture, however, I wish to emphasize the curious appearance of mandrake as a "delouser" for sheep.

Mandrake (*Mandragora officinarum* L. or *M. autumnalis* Spr.), among the six species known in ancient and modern times, contains goodly amounts of hyoscyamine, a powerful narcotic, especially in the famous "manlike" roots. The narcotic properties of the mandrake were famous among laypersons and professional medical practitioners, and its fame reached even into a well-known scene in Apuleius' *Golden Ass,*[36] where the physician and those listening to his testimony *both* knew of the generally safe anesthetic properties of mandrake. Mandrake leads us immediately back to the Vienna codex of Dioskorides: widely known is folio 5v, depicting three figures doing three things with the mandrake root (and *this* painting of the root [twice] is not replicated elsewhere in the codex); on the right is Dioskorides reading the account of the plant and its properties (4.75 [ed. Wellmann, 2:233–37]); in the center Epinoia holds the root in her hands extended in front of her to ensure that the

[34] E. Oder and C. Hoppe, eds., *Corpus hippiatricorum Graecorum,* 2 vols. (Leipzig, 1924–27; repr. Stuttgart, 1971). Most recently, a third compilation of this sort from the mid-10th century on toxicology has been documented by Sibylle Ihm, ed., *Der Traktat Peri tōn iobolōn thēriōn kai dēlētēriōn pharmakōn des sog. Aelius Promotus* (Wiesbaden, 1995).

[35] I suspect that *kypeiros* is not galingale, but either the edible cyperus (*Cyperus esculentus* L.), or perhaps a turmeric (*Curcuma longa* L.), known as early as Dioskorides, whose *Materia medica,* 1.5, seems to be the first mention of this Indian rhizome, today used as a condiment in curries.

[36] Apuleius, *Golden Ass* (or *Metamorphoses*), 10.11.

viewer sees exactly its color and shape; and on the left of the full-page folio is the artist depicting the plant while he looks at Epinoia, not Dioskorides. Mandrake is, in effect, the first medicinal plant in the codex, and Dioskorides' full description of the properties and uses of mandrake root parallels its employment today in many folk medical systems from Spain to India: it is an excellent purgative and emetic, with narcotic properties particularly valuable in treatment for asthma, hay fever, and coughs, since the alkaloidal phytochemistry in the "natural" drug acts as vasodilators. There are numerous references in the medical sources of classical antiquity, as well as those of the Byzantine era: mandrake was the narcotic of choice, or, as Dioskorides puts it, "The physicians use this whenever they are about to begin cutting [i.e., surgery], or when they are cauterizing [a wound] shut" (4.75.7 [ed. Wellmann, 2:237; my trans.]).

Garden plant or wild? Evidence shows (again) both. In the text "On the Mandrake," printed by Thomson in her *Textes grecs inédits* (pp. 84–87; numbered texts 5, 3, and 4), it is clear that this is indeed an herb raised and used against leprosy and eye diseases and as a remedy for raging diarrhea, among other afflictions. Older traditions (e.g., Theophrastus, *Historia plantarum,* 9.9.1 and Dioskorides as above) indicate that mandrake was brought into market by ever-present and expert *rhizotomoi* ("root cutters").

Throughout the centuries, there is little doubt that anyone could obtain mandrake in just about any season, as would be true of the opium poppy and its hardened latex, easily remelted as needed. Among the Byzantines, one gains the sure impression from Alexander of Tralles' directions for the preparation of pastilles for specific treatment of quartan fevers characterized by yellow bile,[37] that *all* ingredients are commonly obtained and that many are "garden cultivated": one reads about the saffron crocus, licorice, anise, castor (a plant in this instance), henbane (if this, indeed, is what *hyoskyamos leukos* means), and likely enough the three grams of mandrake "bark" (the outer layers of the root) that end the preparation formula. Alexander of Tralles is recording what he considered "tried and true" pharmaceutical recipes sometime at the very end of the sixth century or, at the very latest, the beginning years of the seventh. A principle of his practice and its written summary is almost always a direct simplicity, a characteristic especially true of his botanical or medicinal pharmacy. The opium poppy is an "ordinary" drug, much as is mandrake (whether its "apples" or juice or rind or stem or roots). Alexander's long career and extensive travels (he died in Rome in A.D. 605) enabled him to compose several medical masterpieces, including the *Book on Fevers,* the *Twelve Books on Medicine,* and the *Letter on Intestinal Worms* (this last tract is the first western treatise on parasitology and deserves careful translation and commentary). He has carefully selected drugs readily obtained from feral areas and then brought to the marketplace, or, as one would expect, from the common herb gardens; such cultivated plots included well-known poisons like aconite, the two hellebores, henbane, and the ever-infamous hemlock, not to mention the commonly employed female contraceptives, pennyroyal and rue. In both pharmacy and cooking, in the manufacture of perfumes or the flavorings of

[37] Alexander of Tralles, *Book on Fevers,* 7 (ed. T. Puschmann, *Alexander von Tralles,* 2 vols. [Vienna, 1878–79; repr. Amsterdam, 1963], 1:426–29, especially formulas and measures, 429).

wine, "fresh" was a mark of quality, so that "out of season" would engender the ordinary assumption of the continual activity of farmers and the *rhizotomoi* (who were in all likelihood farmers too) who gathered herbs for the market stalls, so nicely recorded by Pollux in the second century.[38]

In summary, even a short study reveals food and medicinal sources in the Byzantine Empire rather well balanced by city and countryside. Wheat, barley, and other long-cultivated staples continued to be planted and harvested by the traditional farmer, and his stock (whether pigs, chickens, and so on) contributed the major part of each Byzantine city's food supply. Herb gardens existed almost in all cities in great numbers, but much of what we know of Byzantine drugs, condiments, perfume production, and several other "luxury" products (e.g., wine flavorings), and the frequently ignored production of the best grapes for the finest wines, remained (obviously) products of the country dwellers. In medicinal pharmacy, Byzantine root gatherers and farmers at large provided specific herbs, especially "out of season," suggested by the examples of asparagus, the opium poppy, and mandrake.

[38] Pollux, *Onomasticon*, 5.132 (ed. E. Bethe, *Pollucis Onomasticon*, 3 vols. [Leipzig, 1900–1937; repr. Stuttgart, 1967], 1:297).

ADDENDA AND CORRIGENDA

I. The pharmacology of sacred plants, herbs, and roots

Since the appearance of my 1991 "Sacred Plants," there has been a veritable quantum increase in the scholarly literature on the roles of ancient magic, astrology, and the kindred approaches we call pseudo-science (our Greek, Roman and Byzantine predecessors certainly did not regard them as anything but 'true' sciences). In many respects, this fresh interest by classicists and historians of medicine and science, is far more honest than the formerly dominant "Sartonian" view, that denied alchemy, magic, astrology, and the like, were "sciences" in any era. As I have argued, magical beliefs in classical antiquity were "rational" in their own right, in that they "explained" given phenomena in the natural world in terms following "cause and effect," as well as the given presumptions that incantations and spells could shape the future. Lynn Thorndike in his *History of Magic and Experimental Science* (New York: Columbia University Press, 1923–58; 8 vols) asserted consistently that the methodologies of magic were the matrices of experimental science, and since the volumes are replete with close readings from Greek and Latin texts, as well as huge numbers of manuscripts, one was forced to debate Thorndike on the basis of sources, not according to any twentieth century school of thought. This point of view is stated succinctly by Thorndike in his "The True Place of Astrology in the History of Science," *Isis* 46 (1955), 273–8, echoed in part by Paul T. Keyser, "Science and Magic in Galen's Recipes (Sympathy and Efficacy)," in Armelle Debru, ed., *Galen on Pharmacology* (Leiden and New York: E.J. Brill, 1997), pp. 175–98, especially 178: "Galen's…stance can be both magical and rational." I think the return to this healthy position by many modern scholars is most welcome: our texts demonstrate not merely the curiosity displayed by scientists and physicians among the Greeks, Romans, and Byzantines, but also the multiple beliefs – ranging from pure magic to gleaming theories founded on fully rational constructs – that existed side-by-side in the intellectual cosmos of antiquity; sometimes there was vituperative quarreling, but most often our ancestors easily encompassed in a single world-view the rational with the irrational with little discomfort.

The following are merely samples of the recent and large literature on magic, astrology, dream lore, alchemy, and kindred pursuits, amalgamated with 'rational' approaches to health and disease, the questions of 'how drugs work,' how human interactions connect with the larger universe as a whole, and each study can lead anyone into further scholarship through the usually extensive bibliographies. I suggest:

Tamsyn Barton, *Ancient Astrology*. London and New York: Routledge, 1994. A welcome survey, non-technical enough that a beginner can comprehend general principles.

Tamsyn S. Barton, *Power and Knowledge: Astrology, Physiognomics, and Medicine under the Roman Empire*. Ann Arbor: University of Michigan Press, 1994. Focusing on the careers and practices of Galen, Vettius Valens, and Polemo of Laodicea (among a number of professionals), Barton shows how the three "sciences" intermingled both in a social context as well as in the continual intellectual tussles characteristic of physicians, astrologers, and physiognomists. Of value is the "Introduction" which summarizes the main lines of the George Sarton "school" in the History of Science, as well as more contemporary shifts away from the hyperrationality demanded by Sartonians of all stripes.

Franck Collard and Evelyne Samama, eds, *Le corps à l'Epreuve: Poisons, remèdes et chirurgie: aspects des pratiques médicales dans l'Antiquité et au Moyen-Âge*. Langres-Saints-Geosmes: D. Guéniot, 2002. Ten essays that take up a number of facets of ancient toxicology, pharmacology, and surgery, with learning and skill. Of special interest are Evelyn Samama, "Empoisonné ou guéri? Remarques lexicologiques sur les *Pharmaka* et venena," Véronique Boudon, "La thériaque selon Galien: poison salutaire ou remède empoisonné?," and Marie-Hélène Congourdeau, "Les abortifs les sources byzantines."

Glen Michael Cooper, *Galen's "On Critical Days:" Greek Medicine in Arabic*. New York: Columbia University, 1999 [diss.]. Galen's *Critical Days* (esp. Book III) is medical astrology "writ large." Modern physicians and students of 2nd century medicine who choose to deny Galen's employment of "irrational" sciences should study this tract very carefully.

Brian P. Copenhaver, trans., *Hermetica. The Greek Corpus Hermeticum and the Latin Asclepius in a New English Translation*. Cambridge and New York: Cambridge University Press, 1992. These woolly tracts that intertwined pseudo-Egyptian learning with a patina of Greek philosophical principles had a deep and long-term influence, attested by some important Renaissance thinkers. Copenhaver's lengthy "Introduction" is one of the best synopses of a complicated topic.

Matthew W. Dickie, *Magic and Magicians in the Greco-Roman World*. London and New York: Routledge, 2001. Male and female sorcerers and magicians often provided healing rituals, prostitutes and courtesans frequently used erotic magic in their professions (e.g. Socrates' conversation with Theodote [Xenophon, *Memorabilia*, III, 11. 1–5]), and magicians haunt the erstwhile rationality of Hippocratic physicians. In his meaty 380 pages, Dickie teases out the ever-present sorcerers, sorceresses, witches, and magicians among the Greeks and Romans from Homer's day through the later Roman Empire.

Esther Eidenow, *Oracles, Curses, and Risk among the Ancient Greeks*. Oxford and New York: Oxford University Press, 2007. Here is a book that sets out very clearly, indeed, how professional and non-professional alike presumed the rationality of supernatural events as they were calculated according to risk and benefit. See esp. the *defixiones* ("binding curses") in Ch. 7, "Curses!."

Christopher A. Faraone, *Ancient Greek Love Magic*. Cambridge, Mass., and London: Harvard University Press, 1999. "What plants do" forms a theme in Ch. 3, "Spells for Inducing Affection (*Philia*)." Here are the would-be aphrodisiacs explained through modern pharmacology and Greek myth.

John G. Gager, *Curse Tablets and Binding Spells from the Ancient World*. Oxford and New York: Oxford University Press, 1992. Many *defixiones* + readings from the *Papyri Graecae Magicae* show how common were these (usually) leaden objects that illustrate "...the potential harm to the entrenched reputation of classical Greece and Rome, not to mention Judaism and Christianity, as bastions of pure philosophy and true religion" (p. 3).

Maud W. Gleason, *Making Men. Sophists and Self-Presentation in Ancient Rome*. Princeton and Chichester [England]: Princeton University Press, 1995. The "Second Sophistic" among Roman imperial intellectuals in the 2nd century AD certainly incorporated a revival of a supposedly "true" Greek of a Demosthenes or an Aeschines, but it also featured a quasi-scientific approach to "what was a man," and what was not; important were the physiognomic details of a man's appearance (eyes, complexion, carriage, hair-color, general deportment) coupled with skills in oratory and rhetoric. Galen wanders in and out of Gleason's readable account (albeit with some skepticism for the "science" of appearances), as do Aelius Aristides (the classic hypochondriac), and other physicians, but the focus is on Favorinus (a squeakily voiced eunuch) and Polemo, the most famous of the rhetorical physiognomists of his day. Readers familiar with 19th century medical notions may be reminded of the faddish dominance of phrenology, a theory that proposed that one's intelligence could be measured by bumps on the skull.

Fritz Graf, *Magic in the Ancient World*, trans. from the French by Franklin Philip. Cambridge, Mass., and London: Harvard University Press, 1997. Perhaps the best general introduction to the subject available in English. See esp. index entries "Medicine and Apuleius" and following.

Margaret Hirt Raj, *Médecines et maladies de l'Egypte Romaine*. Leiden and Boston: E.J Brill, 2006 (*Studies in Ancient Medicine*, Vol. 32). Interspersed among the legal provisions in the papyri are the amulets and magical spells that marked a particular 'Egyptian' medicine of great antiquity. Hirt Raj, however, puts to rest the old canard of a millennial, unchanging medical practice in Egypt before the coming of Islam.

Wolfgang Hübner, *Raum, Zeit und soziales Rollenspiel der vier Kardinalpunkte in der antiken Katarchenhoroskopie*. Munich and Leipzig: K.G. Sauer, 2003. Picking up where Frederick H. Cramer left off in his 1954 *Astrology in Roman Law and Politics*, Hübner delineates a common expertise among educated Romans, regarding the details of astrology in everyday life, politics, and social relations.

Sarah Iles Johnston, *Ancient Greek Divination*. Malden, Mass., and Oxford: Wiley-Blackwell, 2008. Prominent was the "healer-seer" (*iatromantis*) in Greek life and society, a professional linked, in turn, with the famous oracles (Delphi, Dodona, Claros, Didyma, and others). Johnston's book is quite suitable for beginners, seeking a lucid introduction to an often ignored – if important – aspect of Greek thinking.

D.R. Jordan, "New Greek Curse Tablets (1985–2000)," *Greek, Roman, and Byzantine Studies,* 41 (2000), 5–46. A handy catalogue of known *defixiones*.

Paul Magdalino and Maria Mavroudi, eds, *The Occult Sciences in Byzantium*. Geneva: La Pomme d'or, 2006. Eleven essays on the multiple topics incorporated under the 'occult,' including alchemy, astrology, demonology, and related. Mavroudi's "Occult Science and Society in Byzantium: Considerations for Future Research" is a splendid introductory survey of the texts and sources (many in manuscripts, still unpublished), and medicine's connections with astrology and the easy cross-cultural exchanges with the Muslim centers of scientific research, are illuminated by Symeon Seth and others in the 11th century. "Graeco-Egyptian Alchemy in Byzantium" by Michèle Mertens is also a most worthy contribution

Patricia Cox Miller, *Dreams in Late Antiquity*. Princeton and Chichester [England]: Princeton University Press, 1994. Featured are Galen, Artemidorus, Aelius Aristides, Lucian, Macrobius, and many more texts and sources, which infuse the deep traditions of oneirocritica inherited by Christian intellectuals. Moderns need to be reminded that ancient dream lore did the opposite of what we expect today (dreams reveal aspects of our personal pasts, or sometimes suggest solutions to current problems, or reveal the truths of deeply seated opinions): Greeks, Romans, and Byzantines used dreams to predict the future.

Steven M. Oberhelman, *Dreambooks in Byzantium: Six Oneirocritica in Translation*. Aldershot [England] and Burlington [Vermont]: Ashgate, 2008. "Diagnostic dreams" had a lengthy and deep history in classical antiquity, illustrated by the famous Asclepian incubation slumbers taking place at the numerous shrines; Galen composed an important "Diagnostics from Dreams" (lost except for fragments), and Oberhelman provides good translations of the dream manuals of Daniel, Nicephorus, Astrampsychus, Germanus, Michael II Paleologus, and one anonymous tract titled "An Additional [Dreambook] Drawn from the Experience of the Wise." All these are "ordinary stuff," taken for granted by commoners and emperors alike; Oberhelman's "Dreams in Graeco-Roman Medicine," in Wolfgang Haase, ed., *Aufstieg und Niedergang der römischen Welt*, Teil II: *Principat*, Vol. 37, 1 (Berlin and New York: Walter de Gruyter, 1993), pp. 121–56, is one of the better overviews of the subject.

Daniel Ogden, *Magic, Witchcraft, and Ghosts in the Greek and Roman Worlds. A Source- book*. Oxford and New York: Oxford University Press, 2002. What the title says it is: sources in translation. Quite comprehensive, with lengthy sections devoted to Apuleius, Lucian, Ovid, Philostratus, and dozens more. The range is from Homer to Aetius of Amida, and Ogden gathers snippets on necromancy, sorcerers, witches, curses, werewolves, magicians (male and female), erotic spells, magical incantations, legal texts, and related topics. Several of the texts are medical (e.g. the Hippocratic *Sacred Disease* on magicians' "cures" for epilepsy, Aetius of Amida on lycanthropy).

Nicoletta Palmieri, ed., *Rationnel et irrationnel dans la médecine ancienne et médiévale. Aspects historiques, scientifiques et culturels*. Saint-Etienne: Université de Saint-Etienne, 2003 (Centre Jean Palerne *Mémoires* XXVI). Sixteen essays elucidating the recurrent mix of sturdy theories, founded on experiential data, combined with a usually accepted and assumed set of beliefs we might term 'irrational.' Several studies focus on Galen (e.g. Heinrich von Staden, "Galen's Daimon: Reflections on 'Rational' and 'Irrational'," and Isabelle Boehm, "Décrire les odeurs ou rationnaliser les sensations? Comment Galien conçoit le functionnement de l'odorat"), but the majority of the papers take up magic and related in Latin sources. Of interest are Joëlle Jouanna-Bouchet, "Scribonius Largus et Marcellus, entre rationnele et irrationnel," Valérie Gitton-Ripoli, "Les pratiques magiques dans le *Traité de médecine vétérinaire* de Pélagonius," and Muriel Pardon, "Œil de lynx pour œil de taupe. Les ingredients d'origine animale dans la pharmacopée ophtalmologique impériale."

Mladen Popovic, *Reading the Human Body. Physiognomics and Astrology in the Dead Sea Scrolls and Hellenistic-Early Roman Period Judaism*. Leiden and Boston: E.J. Brill, 2007. That astrology, magic and physiognomy pervaded many cultures and religions in antiquity, is vividly demonstrated by some of the famous Dead Sea Scrolls (Hebrew and Aramaic). Taking horoscopes were apparently ordinary and quite common among members of the sect, and Popovic's net is broad enough and finely woven to capture facets of intertwining magical and astrological assumptions about drugs, plants, animals, and people.

Catherine Rider, "'My Lady Knows Impious Things:' Impotence Magic in the Ancient World" in *Magic and Impotence in the Middle Ages* (Oxford and New York: Oxford University Press, 2006), pp. 14–28. The magic of anaphrodisiac spells, incantations, curse tablets, and witches' brews find reflection among the poets (esp. Ovid) and medical writers (Serenus Sammonicus, Pliny the Elder, Dioscorides, Marcellus Empiricus, "Sextus Placitus," others); sometimes the women use actual substances, sometimes the impotence follows invocation of demons and supernatural beings.

Simon Swain, ed., *Seeing the Face, Seeing the Soul: Polemon's Physiognomy from Classical Antiquity to Medieval Islam.* Oxford and New York: Oxford University Press, 2007. The lead essay, "Physiognomy and Ancient Psychological Theory" by George Boys-Stones, discusses views brought to bear on physiognomy by Plato, (Pseudo) Aristotle, Posidonius, the Hippocratic writers, "Post-Hellenistic Platonism," and Galen's careful assessment of the claims of physiognomists in his own times. On Galen, Boys-Stones concludes, "However much theoretical interest physiognomy might have in certain contexts, it could not have significant diagnostic value even for Galen" (p. 109). Five new edited texts with translations (pp. 329–636) complete the volume, of interest to those desiring immediate access to the primary texts of physiognomy in Greek, Roman, and Byzantine times, as well as classical Islam: Robert Hoyland, "New Edition and Translation of the Leiden Polemon" (Arabic); Antonella Ghersetti, "The Istanbul Polemon (TK Recension): Edition and Translation of the Introduction" (Arabic); Ian Repath "The *Physiognomy* of Adamantius the Sophist" (Greek), and "Anonymus Latinus *Book of Physiognomy*" (Latin), and Simon Swain "Appendix: Ps. Aristotle, *Physiognomy*" (Greek). Polemon's "straight" declamations do not receive attention in Swain's volume; for this aspect, see William W. Reader and Anthony J. Chvala-Smith, *The Severed Hand and the Upright Corpse: The Declamations of Marcus Antonius Polemo* (Atlanta: Scholars Press, 1996 [Society of Biblical Literature, *Texts and Translations,* 42, *Graeco-Roman Series,* 12]).

Katharina Volk, *Manilius and his Intellectual Background.* Oxford and New York: Oxford University Press, 2009. The most famous of the Latin sources on astrology, explicated with consummate understanding. Readers can also follow contextual discussions by using the English translation that accompanies the Latin text in G.P. Goold, ed. and trans., *Manilius: Astronomica* (London and Cambridge, Mass.: William Heinemann and Harvard University Press, 1977 [Loeb Classical Library]).

II. On medications for burns in classical antiquity

Dermatology has not attracted much interest from ancient medical historians, although there have been occasional articles by professional dermatologists, e.g. Willard L. Marmelzat, "History of Dermatologic Surgery: From the Beginnings to Late Antiquity," *Clinics in Dermatology,* 5 (1987), 33–43. In many respects, one still depends on the thorough research represented by Paul Richter, *Geschichte der Dermatologie* (Berlin: Julius Springer, 1928) in the extensive *Handbuch der Haut- und Geschlectskrankheiten* (Vol. 14, part 2), esp. pp. 20–84 ("Die Dermatologie der Griechen," "Die byzantinische Dermatologie," and "Die Griechenmedizin in Rom").

III. Theoretical assumptions in Hippocratic pharmacology

Few studies in the enormous literature on Hippocratic medicine have focused on the rich pharmacology found in a number of the works in the *corpus*, especially *Diseases of Women, Nature of Women, Diseases II* and *III, Fistulas, Wounds, Hemorrhoids*, and the second book of *Regimen*. There is now an English translation of *Diseases of Women I* and *II*, as well as *III* (*Sterility*), by Kathleen Whiteley (*I*: MA Thesis, University of South Africa, 2003; *II*: unpublished 2006; and *Sterility*: unpublished 2008), rendered from the Greek texts in Emile Littré, ed., *Oeuvres complètes d'Hippocrate* 8 (Paris, 1853; rptd. Amsterdam: Hakkert, 1982), pp. 10–463; Whiteley does not attempt to identify in modern nomenclatures the plants, minerals, and animal products used as drugs, but her translation is reasonably accurate as far as the Littré texts permit. The most inclusive tabulation of Hippocratic pharmacology (before Totelin's monograph [below]) was Rudolf von Grot, "Ueber die in der hippokratischen Schriftensammlung enthaltenen pharmakologen Kenntnisse," [*Kobert's*] *Historische Studien aus dem Pharmakologischen Institute der Kaiserlichen Universität Dorpat,* 1 (1889), 58–133. Among the handful of recent studies on the drug lore in the Hippocratic treatises:

Monique Moisan, "Les plantes narcotiques dans le *Corpus hippocratique*," and Marie Christine Girard, "L'hellébore: Panacée ou placebo?," in Paul Potter, Gilles Maloney, and Jacques Desautels., eds, *La maladie et les maladies dans la Collection hippocratique. Actes du Vie Colloque International Hippocratique (Québec, du 28 septembre au 3 octobre 1987)* (Québec: Les Editions du Sphinx, 1990), pp. 381–92 and 393–405. Moison summarizes the subtle distinctions among the anesthetic and analgesic effects of mandrake, hyoscyamus, and others, concluding that in some instances, these natural substances were quite beneficial. Girard notes the common occurrence of the hellebores in the pharmaceutical suggestions by the Hippocratic writers; occasionally there was little effect from the administration of hellebore, but the usual prescription of the plant indicated that it was a most effective laxative – if rather hard on the patient.

Moisan (in collaboration with Giles Maloney and D. Grenier) published the *Lexique du vocabulaire botanique d'Hippocrate* (Québec: Sphinx, 1990), based upon some of Littré's suggested nomenclatures, as well as the very problematic entries in the Liddell-Scott-Jones *Greek-English Lexicon*, 9th ed. (Oxford: Clarendon Press, 1940). The compilers would have been better served by Jacques André, *Les noms de plantes dans la Rome antique* (Paris: Les Belles Lettres, 1985); André provides not only the Latin terms, but also the transliterated Greek equivalents, so that *Les noms* functions as a good, bi-lingual guide to ancient botanical names.

Superseding von Grot is Laurence M.V. Totelin, *Hippocratic Recipes. Oral and Written Transmission of Pharmacological Knowledge in Fifth- and Fourth-Century Greece* (Leiden and Boston: E.J. Brill, 2009 [*Studies in Ancient Medicine*, Vol. 34]). Of particular value is the "Index of Ingredients" (pp. 353–61) followed by "Key to Index 1: Scientific Names" (pp. 361–3), in turn followed by "Key to Index 2: Common Names" (pp. 363–6). The "Index" gives the Greek and the Linnaean names, the "Key to Index 1" reverses them (scientific terms, then the Greek), and "2" provides the 'common name' followed by the Greek. Totelin signals her cautions by "A Note on Identifications" (p. 353), and this paragraph in ten-point type includes a listing of "…studies [that complement] the LSJ."

IV. Theophrastus on herbals and herbal remedies

Completely supplanting the Loeb Classical Library edition and translation of Theophrastus' *Historia Plantarum* is Suzanne Amigues, ed., trans., with extended commentaries, *Théophraste: Recherches sur les plantes* (Paris: Les Belles Lettres, 1988–2006; 5 vols. [in the Budé series]). Amigues' commentaries include a huge collection of references to the secondary literature on botany, the state of scholarship on ancient plant lore, and the ever-present problems of identification of individual genera and species. By contrast, the edition of Sir Arthur Hort in the Loebs (unrevised since its first publication in 1916) carries the marks of Victorian prudery, e.g. some of the presumably offensive details on aphrodisiacs and anaphrodisiacs are blatantly omitted in both the Greek and English at *HP*, IX, 18.3; and the botanical identifications as provided by Sir William Thistelton-Dyer became notorious for their errors and obvious lack of specialized expertise.

The most accessible censure of Thiselton-Dyer's unfortunate influence on Anglophone scholarship on ancient botany is John Raven's "Unreliability of Some of Thistleton-Dyer's Identification of Greek Plant Names – Plants of Homer – Plants of Sappho," in Faith Raven, *et al.*, eds, *John Raven: Plants and Plant Lore in Ancient Greece* (Oxford: Leopard's Head Press, 2000), pp. 3–10. For a translation and discussion of the 'missing passages' in Hort's edition and translation of the *HP*, see esp. Anthony Preus, "Drugs and Psychic States in Theophrastus' *Historia plantarum* 9.8–20," in William W. Fortenbaugh and R.W. Sharples, eds, *Theophrastean Studies: On Natural Science, Physics and Metaphysics, Ethics, Religion and Rhetoric* (New Brunswick [New Jersey] and Oxford: Transaction Books, 1988 [*Studies in Classical Humanities*, Vol. III]), pp. 76–99, particularly "Drugs and Sex in HP 9: A Translation of Theophrastus HP 9.18.3–11," with commentary, pp. 88–91. Preus' study is, in many ways, a perceptive critique of my 1978 essay on Theophrastus; after some lengthy reflection, I have published a kind of reply and update in my "Drugs and Drug Lore in the Time of Theophrastus: Folklore, Magic, Botany, Philosophy and the Rootcutters," *Acta Classica,* 49 (2006), 1–29.

Now fundamental in Theophrastean scholarship is the vast collection of fragments (Greek, Latin, Arabic) with translations in William W. Fortenbaugh, Pamela M. Huby, Robert W. Sharples (Greek and Latin) and Dimitri Gutas (Arabic), eds, *Theophrastus of Eresus: Sources for his Life, Writings, Thought and Influence* (Leiden and New York: E.J. Brill, 1992; 2 vols). A series of commentaries has begun to emerge from Brill that take up particular aspects of Theophrastus' multifarious writings, and each carries the original titulature of the 1992 volumes (*Theophrastus of Eresus*, etc.) uniformly packaged in maroon bindings; these now include: Pamela Huby, *Logic*, Vol. 2 (2007); R. W. Sharples, *Sources on Biology*, Vol. 5 (1995); and William W. Fortenbaugh, *Sources on Rhetoric and Poetics*, Vol. 8 (2005). Also appearing from Brill are new editions, translations with commentaries (again uniformly bound in maroon), and among these are William W. Fortenbaugh, Robert W. Sharples, and Michael G. Sollenberger, *Theophrastus of Eresus On Sweat. On Dizziness, and On Fatigue* (2003), and David Sider and Carl Wolfram Brunschön, *Theophrastus of Eresus On Weather Signs* (2007). See also Robert W. Sharples, trans., brief commentary, "Theophrastus *On Fish*," in William W. Fortenbaugh and Dimitri Gutas, eds, *Theophrastus: His Psychological, Doxographical and Scientific Writings* (New Brunswick [New Jersey] and London: Transaction Pubs., 1992 [*Rutgers University Studies in Classical Humanities*, Vol. 5]), pp. 347–85, and Ulrich Eigler and Georg Wöhrle, eds, with trans. [German] and commentary, *Theophrast De odoribus* (Stuttgart: B. G. Teubner, 1993), which supersedes the Hort ed. and trans., 1916 (Loeb, Vol. 2), pp. 324–89.

V. Nicander's toxicology I: snakes

Remaining the standard edition (with translation and notes) of Nicander's *Theriaca* and *Alexipharmaca* is A.S.F. Gow and A.F. Scholfield, *Nicander. The Poems and Poetical Fragments* (Cambridge: University Press, 1953). The most recent edition, as ed. with trans. and commentary by Jean-Marie Jacques, *Nicandre. Oeuvres*, Tome II: *Les Thériaques. Fragments iologiques antérieurs à Nicandre* (Paris: Les Belles Lettres, 2002 [Budé series]) and *Nicandre. Oeuvres*, Tome III: *Les Alexipharmiques. Lieux parallèles du livre XIII des Iatrica d'Aétius* (same pub. and series, 2007) shrewdly solves a number of textual and philological problems – and there are many – in the poems, but Jacques does not do justice to the detailed zoology, botany, and toxicology characteristic of Hellenistic and later writers. Ignored is the deep lore on herpetology, entomology, and marine biology characteristic of Greek, Hellenistic, Roman, and Byzantine zoology.

Advancing considerably our understanding of ancient and Byzantine manuals on toxicology, and the methods followed in compilation, is Sibylle Ihm, ed., with critical commentary, *Der Traktat περὶ τῶν ἰοβόλων θηρίων καὶ δηλητηρίων φαρμάκων des sog. Aelius Promotus* (Wiesbaden: Ludwig Reichert, 1995 [*Serta Graeca*, Bd. 4]). Hieronymus Mercurialis in the 16th century provided the attribution of a poison lore tract "by" Aelius Promotus (2nd century AD), but Erwin Rohde (the last editor of the tract [1873 and 1901]) doubted such an authorship. Ihm determines that multiple sources underlie this anonymous work, ranging back to Nicander and forward to Aetius of Amida, esp. Book XIII of the *Tetrabiblon*. Ihm's Greek text incorporates many corrections, and her commentary elucidates the continuously adaptive quality of poison lore in antiquity. Turning her considerable abilities to some quandaries in Menander's use of medical terminologies, Ihm's sharply composed "Zu den medizinischen Szenen in Menanders *Aspis*," in Thorsten Fögen, ed., *Antike Fachtexte/Ancient Technical Texts* (Berlin and New York: Walter de Gruyter, 2005), pp. 91–105, delineates quite clearly that Menander knew rather well the abilities of some physicians in his own time, *c.* 310 B.C. The pun in the title of Menander's half-lost comedy (viz. *'aspis'* can mean either "shield" or "hoplite" or "cobra") suggests some expertise in toxicology by the fictional physician, who appears in the few lines from Act III recovered from a papyrus.

p. 4: line 31: I have recently suggested a much closer relationship between Attalus III and Nicander in my "Attalus III of Pergamon: Research Toxicologist," in Louise Cilliers, ed., *Asklepios: Studies on Ancient Medicine* (Bloemfontein: Classical Association of South Africa, 2008 [*Acta Classica Supplementum* II]), pp. 138–56. I do so on the basis of Attalus' research in toxicology – in particular on the sea hare – duly reported by Nicander and Galen as unique to the king among investigators in Hellenistic times.

VI. Nicander's toxicology II: spiders, scorpions, insects and myriapods

Two excellent monographs on ancient entomology are available as research tools: Malcolm Davies and Jeyaraney Kathirithamby, *Greek Insects* (London: Duckworth, 1986), and Ian C. Beavis, *Insects and Other Invertebrates in Classical Antiquity* (Exeter [England]: University of Exeter Press, 1988). Of special strength in *Greek Insects* is the accounting of bees and beekeeping, as well as a good survey of insect iconography in Greco-Roman antiquity; Beavis is comprehensive in his thorough catalogue, ranging as far forward as the Byzantine *Geoponica*, and his *Insects* takes its honored place next to D'Arcy Wentworth Thompson's *Glossary of Greek Birds* (London: Oxford University Press, 1936; rptd. Hildesheim: Georg Olms, 1966) and *Glossary of Greek Fishes* (London: Oxford University Press, 1947).

p. 6: lines 21–3: read: Aetius of Amida (reign of Justinian, AD 527–65) put together the bulky *Tetrabiblon*, quoting hundreds of earlier authorities,...

p. 6: lines 30–31: on Theophanes "Nonnus:" see Joseph A.M. Sonderkamp, *Untersuchungen zur Überlieferung der Schriften des Theophanes Chrysobalantes (sog. Theophanes Nonnos)* (Bonn: Rudolf Habelt, 1987 [*ΠΟΙΚΙΛΑ ΒΥΖΑΝΤΙΝΑ* 7]). Sonderkamp re-investigated the manuscripts, and determined that the "Nonnus" was a Renaissance misinterpretation. See also Faith Wallis, "Inventing Diagnosis: Theophilus' *De urinis* in the Classroom," *Dynamis* 20 (2000), 31–73.

p. 9: line 17: on Aemilius Macer: see Edward Courtney, "Aemilius Macer," in *The Fragmentary Latin Poets* (Oxford and New York: Oxford University Press, 1993), pp. 292–9, and Adrian S. Hollis, "Aemilius Macer," in *Fragments of Roman Poetry c. 60 BC–AD 20* (Oxford and New York: Oxford University Press, 2007), pp. 93–117; Hollis' commentary on the scrappy fragments is rather fuller than Courtney's; see esp. Hollis '54–66 *Theriaca*,' pp. 107–9. See also my "Attalus III Research Toxicologist" (as above under V), pp. 140–43 (on Pliny's use of Macer and Nicander).

p. 9: line 43: on Agatharcides: see Stanley M. Burstein, ed. and trans., *Agatharcides of Cnidus On the Erythraean Sea* (London: The Hakluyt Society, 1989); Burstein's notes and commentary are especially useful.

p. 18: line 25: I demonstrate that the *ioulos* is not a sowbug ("pillbug") but a millipede among *Spirobolidae* in "Nicander, *Theriaca*, 811," *Classical Philology* 75 (1980), 138–40.

p. 74: line 14: see my "Contraception in Antiquity: The Case of Pennyroyal," *Wisconsin Academy Review* 35, no. 2 (1989), 19–25. The commentary on Aristophanes *Lysistrata* by Jeffrey Henderson adds a few particulars not found in his 1975 (2nd ed., 1991) *The Maculate Muse: Obscene Language in Attic Comedy* (New York and Oxford: Oxford University Press), esp. p. 135 (No. 129). The pennyroyal here (*Lysistrata*, 88) is βλήχων or βληχώ, and is a pun on a Boeotian's girl's neatly trimmed pubic hair: κομψότατα τὴν βληχώ γε παρατετιλμένη, "with neatly clipped pennyroyal [garden] plots." See Henderson, ed., intro., comm., *Aristophanes' Lysistrata* (Oxford: Clarendon Press, 1987), p. 78, with refs. to methods used for depilation (both men and women): plucking or singeing, "Failure to do so could be considered slovenly" (*ibid.*). Martin Kilmer, however, argues that complete removal of *all* pubic hair is a modern misinterpretation in "Genital Phobia and Depilation," *Journal of Hellenic Studies* 102 (1982), 104–12; Kilmer's basic body of evidence is vase painting, which supports the casual references and allusions in Aristophanes, and both suggest the Athenian custom of "shaping" pubic hair according to current tastes and custom.

VII. The opium poppy in Hellenistic and Roman medicine

pp. 17–18: the pernicious myth that Marcus Aurelius was a drug addict continues to be assumed in the secondary literature, but an analysis by an experienced physician easily refutes this hypothesis. See François P. Retief, "Marcus Aurelius: Was He an Opium Addict?," in Louise Cilliers, ed., *Asklepios: Studies on Ancient Medicine* (Bloemfontein: Classical Association of South Africa, 2008 [*Acta Classica Supplementum* II]), pp. 131–7. "...Marcus Aurelius was not an opium addict. His daily opium ingestion by way of theriac was only a fraction of that necessary to cause addiction" (p. 135), *contra* the often-cited Thomas W. Africa, "The Opium Addiction of Marcus Aurelius," *Journal of the History of Ideas* 22 (1961), 97–102. Likewise to be dismissed is another proposed "addiction" (mandrake): "...that Marcus Aurelius was occasionally under the influence of another narcotic, mandragora, is almost certainly not to be taken seriously" (Retief, p. 135), *contra* E.C. Witke, "Marcus Aurelius and Mandragora," *Classical Philology* 60 (1965), 23–4.

VIII. Roman pharmacy and the eastern drug trade: some problems illustrated by the example of aloe

p. 135: line 3, with n. 1: in company with Raschke's extreme skepticism regarding the importation of "Indian" and "Asian" drugs into the Roman Empire, is Grant Parker, "Spices and Aromatics" in *The Making of Roman India* (Cambridge and New York: Cambridge University Press, 2008), pp. 150–54, considered as a section of "Contexts of a Discourse;" Parker rightly questions some of the botanical identifications and outrigger fantasies of J. Innes Miller's often-referenced *Spice Trade of the Roman Empire* (1969), but Parker indulges in some of the fancies advanced by the now-moribund theories of a debased structural anthropology, notably those of Marcel Detienne, in which spices and drugs float in a fluidly, un-historic and un-chronological limbo.

p. 138: 1st full parag., line 5: on Antyllus: this rather important – if obscured – surgeon and pharmacologist of the early 3rd century A.D. receives a brief and clear entry by Alain Touwiade ("Antullos [100–260 CE]") in Paul T. Keyser and Georgia Irby-Massie, eds, *The Encyclopedia of Ancient Natural Scientists: the Greek Tradition and its Many Heirs* (London and New York: Routledge, 2008), pp. 101–2. His works are extant only in fragments (Oribasius, Paul of Aegina, and the Pseudo-Galen *On Humors*), demonstrating that Antyllos was an innovative surgeon, performing laryngotomies, relieving abscesses in the head, and inventing some operations for the eye; and he was an acute observer of human preventive medicine, setting down a handbook on gymnastics. His pharmaceutical compilation, *Preparation of Medicines*, quoted many earlier authorities on pharmacy, ranging from Diocles of Carystos (a likely contemporary of Aristotle) to Rufus of Ephesus to Herodotus and Archigenes in the early 2nd century A.D. Still useful for a detailed account of Antyllus' surgery is "Antyllus" in E. Gurlt, *Geschichte der Chirurgie und ihrer Ausübung*, Vol. I (Berlin: August Hirschwald, 1898), pp. 474–86.

p. 140: line 6 with n. 73: the edition of H. Frisk (1927) *Le Périple de la mer Erythrée* has been magnificently superseded by Lionel Casson, ed., introd., trans., and commentary, *The Periplus Maris Erythraei* (Princeton: Princeton University Press, 1989). Casson's wealth of notes and commentary – and his use of "…experts in a wide variety of fields…" (p. x) – will lead any reader into any number of disparate topics, from how Hellenistic and Roman navigators exploited the monsoons to the spices and drugs brought from India and points further east into the Mediterranean world. Casson's expertise in sailing vessels, and their sometimes arcane terminologies and often archaic naval gear, detracts not a whit from his very readable style.

IX. Pharmacy in Pliny's *Natural History*: some observations on substances and sources

Pliny the Elder's opinions about medicine, Greek doctors, and medical folklore in his day, have often been the subject of analysis by modern scholars; some have challenged his caustic comments as a kind of super-patriotism, and thereby should be regarded with the proverbial "grain of salt," e.g. Vivian Nutton, "The Perils of Patriotism: Pliny and Roman Medicine," ch. 4 in the French and Greenaway, *Science in the Early Roman Empire* (1986), generally restated in his "Roman Medicine: Tradition, Confrontation, Assimilation," in Wolfgang Haase, ed., *Aufstieg und Niedergang der römischen Welt*, Teil II: *Principat*, Vol. 37, 1 (Berlin and New York: Walter de Gruyter, 1993), pp. 49–78, and ch. 11, "Rome and the Transplantation of Greek Medicine" in his *Ancient Medicine* (London and New York: Routledge, 2004). Other scholars, however, interpret much more positively Pliny's observations, seeking a nuanced understanding of Pliny's drug lore and views on medicine in the contexts of his own times, e.g Mary Beagon, "*Ars medicinae:* Man's Use of Nature in Medicine," ch. VI in *Roman Nature. The Thought of Pliny the Elder* (Oxford: Clarendon Press, 1992), esp. 'Herbal Medicine and Greek Theory,' 'Herbal Medicine: Pliny's Personal Interest,' and '*Humana salus*: Healing Herbs' (pp. 227–40); Beagon's ed., trans., with extended commentary, *The Elder Pliny on the Human Animal: Natural History Book 7* (Oxford: Clarendon, 2005), succinctly evinces the polymathic – if childlike – enthusiasm for exotic and homely tales, stuffed with animals and plants, occasionally given medical importance or derided as contrary to a Roman notion of practicality, e.g. the melding of witchcraft, snakes and their venoms, with cures from saliva, accompanied by tales of the evil eye, cannibalism, and reflections on Greek philosophy and religion (pp. 133–48: "13–20. Introd. *People with Uncanny Powers*").

Still useful for a broad synopsis is Ernst H.F. Meyer, "Cajus Plinius Secundus der ältere" in *Geschichte der Botanik*, Vol. 2 (Königsberg: Gebrüder Bornträger, 1855; rptd. Amsterdam: A. Asher, 1965), pp. 118–34, as is Edward Lee Greene's, "Caius Plinius Secundus," in Frank N. Edgerton, ed., *Landmarks of Botanical History: Edward Lee Greene* (Stanford [California]: Stanford University Press, 1983; 2 vols.), Vol. 1, pp. 225–8. The Budé edition of Pliny the Elder (each volume = a single book of the *Natural History*) usually incorporates detailed commentaries, so that one can track much of Pliny's botany and herbal lore by means of the notes to contemporary scholarship, e.g. Jacques André, ed., trans., comm., *Pline l'Ancien Histoire naturelle Livre XX* (Paris: Les Belles Lettres, 1965); André, ed., *Livre XXI* (1969); André, ed., *Livre XXII* (1970); André, ed., *Livre XXIII* (1971); André, ed., *Livre XXIV* (1972); André, ed., *Livre XXV* (1974); etc.

X. The pharmacy of Methodist medicine: the evidence of Soranus' *Gynecology*

pp. 204–5 passim: on the Methodists: the debate continues regarding the "origins"and presumed doctrines of the Methodist Sect. Our texts are often obscured, thanks to (especially) the normally vitriolic condemnation of the sect by Galen; and yet there is just enough evidence to suggest that Asclepiades of Bithynia and his "followers" espoused a kind of mechanical explanation for health and disease, perhaps to be linked with a rejection of Erasistratus' theories or a fuzzy adaptation of floating Epicurean "atomistic" notions, quite popular in the Late Roman Republic, as attested by the probable School of Philodemus at Herculaneum. For much of this, see J.T. Vallance, *The Lost Theory of Asclepiades of Bithynia* (Oxford: Clarendon Press, 1991); Vallance denies that Epicurean teachings had that much influence on Asclepiades, choosing instead the Platonist Heracleides of Heraclea Pontica, or Strato of Lampsacus, added to the refutation of Erasistratus, opinions stated clearly in Vallance's "The Medical System of Asclepiades of Bithynia," in Wolfgang Haase, ed., *Aufstieg und Niedergang der römischen Welt*, Teil II: *Principat*, 37, 1 (Berlin and New York: Walter de Gruyter, 1993), pp. 693–727. For Philodemus, see David Sider, "Philodemus and his Texts" in *The Library of the Villa dei Papiri at Herculaneum* (Los Angeles: J. Paul Getty Museum, 2005), pp. 78–95, and his "On the Bay of Naples" in *The Epigrams of Philodemos* (Oxford and New York: Oxford University Press, 1997), pp. 12–24. The collected papers in David Armstrong, *et al.* eds, *Vergil, Philodemus, and the Augustans* (Austin: University of Texas Press, 2004), document most lucidly the widespread vogue of Epicurean philosophy in the last years of the Roman Republic and the early reigns in the Roman Empire. See also my "Asklēpiadēs of Bithunia" in Paul T. Keyser and Georgia Irby-Massie, eds, *The Encyclopedia of Ancient Natural Scientists: the Greek Tradition and its Many Heirs* (London and New York: Routledge, 2008), pp. 170–71.

A convenient gathering of almost all the 'not-Soranus' Methodist remnants is Manuela Tecusan, ed. and trans., *The Fragments of the Methodists*, Vol. 1: *Methodism outside Soranus* (Leiden and Boston: E.J. Brill, 2004 [*Studies in Ancient Medicine*, Vol. 24.1]). Especially valuable is her 'Introduction" (pp. 1–43) in which Tecusan explains her method of analysis of the often obtuse fragmentary remains as contained in various texts, sometimes very hostile to the Methodists; and it is a boon to have the complete *Against Julian* by Galen in translation (Frg. No. 111 Tecusan [pp. 290–331]), neatly illustrating Galen's often vituperative criticisms of the Methodist Sect, a text easily given to students who wish to ascertain the difficulties of interpretation. Often founded on Tecusan's assembly, I contributed several essays on the "Asclepiadeans" to the Keyser and Irby-Massie, *Encyclopedia* (2008), including "Themisōn of Laodikeia," "Thessalos of Tralleis," "Eudēmos (Methodist)," and "Mnaseas (Methodist)," each equipped with a full and up-to-date bibliography.

p. 206: line 6 with n. 20: on the use of amulets among the Methodists: the prevalence of these medically powerful tokens in classical antiquity is demonstrated widely among archaeological sites, as well as literary references. See Ann Ellis Hanson, "Uterine Amulets and Greek Uterine Medicine," *Medicina nei Secoli, Arte e Scienza*, 7 (1995), 281–99.

p. 206: parag. 2, line 1: on Soranus of Ephesus: the most recent edited text with translation and commentary of Soranus' *Gynecology* is Paul Burguière, Danielle Gourevitch, and Yves Malinas, eds, etc., *Soranos d'Éphèse. Maladies des femmes* (Paris: Les Belles Lettres, 1988–2003; 4 vols [Budé series]). Although, in some respects, the French editors have improved the readings in the Greek manuscripts, as compared with the edition (1927) of J. Ilberg, but Burguière and colleagues make some very questionable "addenda" to the text from Book XVI of Aetius of Amida's *Tetrabiblon*, esp. to the famous tabulation of contraceptives and abortifacients in *Gynecology*, I, 60–63. Aetius' Justinianic era prescriptions are far more complicated than those found in Soranus' 2nd century account, so any scholar employing the new text and commentary in the Budé (esp. Vol. 1, pp. 61–7) must exercise due caution, not to assume these complex early Byzantine contraceptives are characteristic of the 2nd century.

A comprehensive account of Soranus, his times, and what can be discerned of his career and doctrines, is Ann Ellis Hanson and Monica Green, "Soranus of Ephesus: *Methodicorum princeps*," in Wolfgang Haase, ed., *Aufstieg und Niedergang der römischen Welt,* Teil II: *Principat*, 37, 2 (Berlin and New York: Walter de Gruyter, 1994), pp. 968–1075. See also my "Sōranos of Ephesos" in the Keyser and Irby-Massie, *Encyclopedia* (2008), pp. 749–51.

XI. Criton, physician to Trajan: historian and pharmacist

p. 389: parag. 3, lines 8 ff.: on Ctesias of Cnidus: now standard on this rather remarkable (if naive) doctor-traveler-(quasi)historian is Dominique Lenfant, ed., trans., voluminous introduction and commentary, *Ctésias de Cnide. La Perse. L'Inde. Autres fragments* (Paris: Les Belles Lettres, 2004 [Budé series]). As a Greek 'doctor at court' (to the Persian king, Artaxerxes II [405/4–359/8 B.C.]; Ctesias usually is dated to be in Persia *c.* 405–397

B.C.), Ctesias compiled his "History of Persia" likely "documented" by court gossip or perhaps oral traditions; his claim that he had consulted the royal archives has not been sustained by modern scholars. Ancients and moderns alike agree that Ctesias' tales have good entertainment value, but do not qualify as "history" in either era. Readers without French or Greek can sample Ctesias through Photius' rather lengthy summary of the *Persica* and *Indica* in J.H. Freese, trans., *The Library of Photius*, Vol. I [all that appeared] (New York: Macmillan, 1920), pp. 92–120, or N.G. Wilson, trans., *Photius: The Bibliotheca* (London: Duckworth, 1994), pp. 54–78. Of the 76 fragments assembled by Lenfant, only two (nos. 67 and 68) qualify as "medical": Galen mentions that Ctesias was one of the first to explicate Hippocratic "joint lore" (here hip joints) and Oribasius quotes Ctesias on the hellebore (Galen, *Commentary on Hippocrates' Joints*, IV, 40 [ed. Kühn, XVIII, pt. 1, p. 731], and Oribasius, *Medical Collection*, VIII, 8 [ed. Raeder, Vol. I, p. 261]).

See also my (with Alain Touwaide) "Kritōn of Hērakleia Salbakē, T. Statilius," in the Keyser and Irby-Massie, eds, *Encyclopedia of Ancient Natural Scientists* (2008), pp. 494–5.

XII. Pharmaceutical theory in Galen's commentaries on the Hippocratic epidemics: some observations on Roman views of Greek drug lore

With great diligence, fortitude, and an envied patience, Cajus Fabricius in his *Galens Exzerpte aus älteren Pharmakologen* (Berlin: Walter de Gruyter, 1972) quite successfully pulled apart many of the layers of quotations in Galen's massive collection of details on pharmacology and toxicology (Vols. XI–XIII – 2958 pages – in the Kühn edition are devoted to pharmacology, and pp. 1–294 in Vol. XIV are the texts [Greek in the top halves, a Latin translation at the bottom] of Galen's two books of the *Antidotes*). Anyone who labors on Galen's drug lore necessarily has at hand Fabricius, whose dissection of Galen's many authorities is a sure guide into the thickets of sources, quotations, personal opinions (quite frequently expressed in lengthy 'prefaces' or 'introductions' to his drug books), rearrangements and addenda on the huge numbers of pharmaceuticals in their often-replicated recipes of multiple ingredients. I use intentionally "layers of quotations" above in describing Fabricius' pioneering scholarship, since he determined that Galen likely consulted several, basic collections of authorities-and-substances, much as had Pliny the Elder in the mid-1st century; prominent for Galen (among 18 adduced) were Apollonius the Herophilean (*c.* 50 B.C. – A.D. 30), Heras of Cappadocia (*c.* 20 B.C. – A.D. 20), Andromachus the Younger (reign of Nero [A.D. 54–68]), Servilius Damocrates (*fl. c.* A.D. 70–80),

Criton (reign of Trajan [A.D. 98–117]), Asclepiadaes "The Pharmacist" (*fl. c.* A.D. 90–100), and Archigenes of Apamea (*fl. c.* A.D. 95–115).

Noteworthy in the collection of 14 essays in Armelle Debru, ed., *Galen on Pharmacology* (Leiden and New York: E. J. Brill, 1997 [*Studies in Ancient Medicine*, Vol. 16]) – some of which base conclusions on Fabricius – are Jean-Marie Jacques' "La méthode de Galien pharmacologue dans le traités sur les médicaments composés (Περὶ συνθέσεως φαρμάκον)," "Galen on Theriac: Problems of Authenticity" by Vivian Nutton, "Science and Magic in Galen's Recipes (Sympathy and Efficacy)" by Paul T. Keyser, Michael Stein's "La thériaque chez Galien: sa préparation et son usage thérapeutique," "Die Quellen der Giftkapital von Galens *De Antidotis* II" by Sibylle Ihm, and Alain Touwaide, "La thérapeutique médicamenteuse de Dioscoride à Galien: du *pharmaco-centrisme* au *medico-centrisme*." See also the more detailed analysis in Touwaide's "Galien et la toxicologie," in Wolfgang Haase, ed., *Aufstieg und Niedergang der römischen Welt*, Teil II: *Principat*, 37, 2 (Berlin and New York: Walter de Gruyter, 1994), pp. 1887–1986.

XIII. Early Byzantine pharmacology

p. 226: col. 2, lines 5 ff.: on Alexander of Tralles and drugs: see Owsei Temkin in *Hippocrates in a World of Pagans and Christians* (Baltimore and London: Johns Hopkins University Press, 1991), esp. pp. 232–6; Temkin's *World of Pagans* is one of the most important books, written in the late 20th century, to take up early Byzantine medicine.

p. 228: col. 1, line 1 (after quotation): on alchemical papyri and sources: now added to the 1981 *Les alchimistes grecs* Tome I: *Papyrus de Leyde, Papyrus de Stockholm, Fragments de recettes*, ed., trans., with comm. by Robert Halleux (Paris: Les Belles Lettres [Budé series]) are two further volumes in a projected dozen, that will encompass the Roman and Byzantine texts: Michèle Mertens, ed., trans., comm., *Les alchimistes grecs*, Tome IV, 1re partie: *Zosime de Panopolis: Mémoires authentiques* (Paris: Les Belles Lettres, 1995), and Andrée Colinet, ed., trans., comm., *Les alchimistes grecs*, Tome X: *L'Anonyme de Zuretti ou L'art sacré et divin de la Chrysopée par un anonyme* (Paris: Les Belles Lettres, 2002).

p. 228: col. 2, 2nd full parag., line 1: on Paul of Aegina: see now Peter E. Pormann, *The Oriental Tradition of Paul of Aegina's Pragmateia* (Leiden and Boston: E.J. Brill, 2004 [*Studies in Ancient Medicine*, Vol. 29])

Since 1985, there has been a slow, if steady, increase in the production of reliable texts (often with translations and commentaries) of Byzantine medical works. These now include:

Agnellus of Ravenna:

Nicoletta Palmieri, ed. [Latin], trans., and explanatory notes, *Agnellus de Ravenne: Lectures galéniques: le "De pulsibus ad tirones"*. St. Etienne: Université de Saint-Etienne, 2005 (Centre Jean Palerne, *Mémoires* XXVIII).

Alexander of Tralles:

D.R. Langslow, *The Latin Alexander Trallianus. The Text and Transmission of a Late Latin Medical Book*. London: Society for the Promotion of Roman Studies, 2006 (*Journal of Roman Studies*, Monograph 10). Ch. 5 includes "An Edition of the Latin Alexander on Coughing," with the text (Bk. 2, chs. 1–11), pp. 184–229.

St. Artemius:

Virgil S. Crisafulli and John W. Nesbitt, ed., trans., with commentary, *The Miracles of St. Artemios. A Collection of Miracle Stories by an Anonymous Author of Seventh-Century Byzantium*. Leiden and New York: E.J. Brill, 1997. St. Artemius' "specialty" was the healing of hernias, almost all men.

John of Alexandria:

John M. Duffy, ed., trans., notes, *John of Alexandria: Commentary on Hippocrates' Epidemics VI Fragments* and *Commentary of an Anonymous Author on Hippocrates' Epidemics VI Fragments* [with] T.A. Bell, D.P. Carpenter, D.W. Schmidt, M.N. Sham, G.L. Vardon, and L.G. Westerink, eds, and trans., *John of Alexandria: Commentary on Hippocrates' On the Nature of the Child*. Berlin: Akademie Verlag, 1997 (*Corpus Medicorum Graecorum* XI 1,4)

Oribasius:

Mark Grant, ed., trans., with commentary, *Dieting for an Emperor. A Translation of Books 1 and 4 of Oribasius' Medical Compilations*. Leiden and New York: E.J. Brill, 1997 (*Studies in Ancient Medicine*, Vol. 15).

Paul of Nicaea:

Anna Maria Ieraci Bio, ed., trans., and comm., *Paolo di Nicea: Manuale medico*. Naples: Bibliopolis, 1996 (*Hellenica et Byzantina Neapolitana Collana di Studi e Testi*, XVI)

Philagrius:

Rita Masullo, ed., trans., comm., *Filagrio: Frammenti*. Naples: Bibliopolis, 1999 (*Hellenica et Byzantina Neapolitana Collana di Studi e Testi* XVIII)

Stephanus of Athens/Alexandria:

Keith Dickson, ed., trans., and comm., *Stephanus the Philosopher and Physician: Commentary on Galen's Therapeutics to Glaucon*. Leiden and Boston: E.J. Brill, 1998 (*Studies in Ancient Medicine*, Vol. 19)

Leendert G. Westerink, ed. and trans., *Stephanus of Athens: Commentary on Hippocrates' Aphorisms*. Berlin: Akademie Verlag, 1985–1995; 3 vols (*Corpus Medicorum Graecorum* XI 1,3,1 – XI 1,3,3)

Translations of previously edited texts include:

Anthimus:

Mark Grant, ed., and trans., with commentary, *Anthimus De observatione ciborum. On the Observance of Foods*. Totnes [England]: Prospect Books, 1996; trans. from Eduard Liechtenhan, ed., and trans. [German], *Anthimi De observatione ciborum ad Theodoricum regem Francorum epistula* (Berlin: Akademie Verlag, 1963 [*Corpus Medicorum Latinorum* VIII 1]). See my "Anthimus (of Constantinople?) (*ca* 475–525 CE)" in the Keyser and Irby-Massie, *Encyclopedia of Ancient Natural Scientists* (2008), pp. 91–2.

Anonymous Dietary Manuals:

Andrew Dalby, trans., "The Eight Flavours," "Categories of Foods," "Humoral and Dietary Qualities of Foods," and "A Dietary Calendar," in Andrew Dalby, *Flavours of Byzantium* (Totnes [England]: Prospect Books, 2003), pp. 127–79. Translated from various sections in A. Delatte, ed., *Anecdota Atheniensia et alia*, Tome II: *Textes grecs relatifs à l'histoire des sciences* (Liège and Paris: Faculté de Philosophie et Lettres and Librarie E. Droz, 1939), pp. 455–79 (Delatte attributes the "Dietary Calendar" to Hierophilus). See also Andrew Dalby, "Some Byzantine Aromatics," in Leslie Brubaker and Kallirroe Linardou, eds, *Eat, Drink, and be Merry (Luke 12:19) – Food and Wine in Byzantium* (Aldershot [England] and Burlington [Vermont]:

Ashgate, 2007 [Society for the Promotion of Byzantine Studies *Publications* 13]), pp. 51–7. On water and wine, see Ewald Kislinger, "Being and Well-Being in Byzantium: The Case of Beverages," in Michael Grünbart, *et al.*, eds, *Material Culture and Well-Being in Byzantium (400–1453)* (Vienna: Verlag der Österreichischen Akademie der Wissenschaften, 2007 [*Veröffentlichungen zur Byzanzforschung*, Bd. XI]), pp. 147–58.

"Metrodora:"

Marie-Hélène Congourdeau, introd., trans., "'Mètrodôra' et son oeuvre," in Evelyne Patlagean, ed., *Maladie et société à Byzance* (Spoleto: Centro italiano de studi sull'Alto Medioevo, 1993), pp. 57–96. Translated (with addenda) from A. Kouzis, "Metrodora's Work 'On the Feminine Diseases of the Womb,' according to the Greek Codex 75, 3 of the Laurentian Library," Πρακτικὰ τῆς 'Ακαδεμίας 'Αθήνων, 20 (1945/pub. 1949), 46–8. See Holt N. Parker, "Mētrodōra," in the Keyser and Irby-Massie *Encyclopedia of Ancient Natural Scientists* (2008), pp. 552–3; Parker thinks little of the *editio princeps* by Kousis [Kuzes].

The *Typikon* of the Pantocrator Xenon:

Robert Jordan, trans., with introd. and bibliog., "28. *Pantokrator*: *Typikon* of the Emperor John II Komnenos for the Monastery of Christ *Pantokrator* in Constantinople," in John Thomas, Angela Constantinides Hero, and Giles Constable, eds, *Byzantine Monastic Foundation Documents: A Complete Translation of the Surviving Founders' Typika and Testaments*, Vol. 2 (Washington, D.C.: Dumbarton Oaks Research Library and Collection, 2000), pp. 725–81, esp. 757–68 [36–63: staff, provisions, etc. for the hospital]. Translated from Paul Gautier, ed., trans., with introd., "Le typikon du Christ Sauveur Pantocrator," *Revue des Études Byzantines*, 32 (1974), 1–145

Veterinary texts:

Robert G. Hoyland, "Theomnestus of Nicopolis, Ḥunayn ibn Isḥāq and the Beginnings of Islamic Veterinary Science, in Robert G. Hoyland and Philip F. Kennedy, eds, *Islamic Reflections Arabic Musings: Studies in Honour of Professor Alan Jones* (London: Gibb Memorial Trust, 2004), pp. 150–69; extended extracts in translation of Theomnestus' works as translated into Arabic.

Anne McCabe, "Anatolius," "Eumelus," "Apsytus," "Pelagonius," "Theomnestus," "Hierocles," "Hippocrates," in *A Byzantine Encyclopaedia of Horse Medicine: The Sources, Compilation, and Transmission of the*

Hippiatrica (Oxford and New York: Oxford University Press, 2007), pp. 71–258; extended blocks of Greek texts in translation, from the *Corpus hippiatricorm Graceorum,* the *Geoponica*, others; McCabe's book is the first to untangle the complicated chronology of the embedded authorities on veterinary medicine collected in the *CHG*, the *Geoponica*, and other Greek tracts on late Roman and Byzantine veterinary medicine. See my review in *Times Literary Supplement*, November 2, 2007, p. 31, and McCabe's "Apsurtos of Klazomenai," "Eumēlos of Thēbai," and "Theomnestos" in the Keyser and Irby-Massie *Encyclopedia of Ancient Natural Scientists* (2008), pp. 118–19, 318, and 792–3.

Since the publication of Timothy Miller, *The Birth of the Hospital in the Byzantine Empire* (Baltimore and London: Johns Hopkins University Press, 1985; new ed. 1997), the literature – and debate – on the "nature" of hospital care in the Byzantine Empire has engendered much interest among medievalists.

Illustrative are:

David Bennett, "Three Xenon Texts," *Medicina nei Secoli Arte e Scienza*, 11 (1999), 507–19. Bennett challenges the analysis of previous scholarship on hospitals, while augmenting our knowledge with some fragments surviving from listings of treatments and drugs in a Byzantine hospital (esp. the Mangana). It seems that hospital physicians grumbled about the lack of definitive texts, from which to teach students the elements of the art.

Peregrine Horden, "A Non-Natural Environment: Medicine without Doctors and the Medieval European Hospital," "Byzantine Hospital Manuals (*Iatrosophia*) as a Source for the Study of Therapeutics" by Alain Touwaide," and Piers D. Mitchell, "The Infirmaries of the Order of the Temple in the Medieval Kingdom of Jerusalem," in Barbara S. Powers, ed., *The Medieval Hospital and Medical Practice* (Aldershot [England] and Burlington [Vermont]: Ashgate, 2007 [*Avista Studies in the History of Medieval Technology, Science and Art*, Vol. 3]), pp. 133–45, 147–75, and 225–34. Each of these three scholars has further investigated the questions and problems attending texts and sources that reveal hospitals in their various guises:

In his collected articles (16), Horden's *Hospitals and Healing from Antiquity to the Later Middle Ages* (Ashgate/Variorum series CS 881 [2008]) provides a wider view of the controversies attending interpretations regarding what hospitals were, and were not, in antiquity and medieval times, including the Byzantine centuries, summarized in his "Health, Hygiene, and Healing" in Elizabeth Jeffreys, John Haldon, and Robin Cormack, eds, *The Oxford*

Handbook of Byzantine Studies (Oxford and New York: Oxford University Press, 2008), pp. 685–90.

Mitchell's *Medicine in the Crusades: Warfare, Wounds and the Medieval Surgeon* (Cambridge and New York: Cambridge University Press, 2004), along with a clear accounting of hospitals in the era of the crusades, incorporates anesthetic and other drugs in his pioneering account, and any student of the period will benefit from consulting esp. "Anaesthesia during Operations" (pp. 198–204).

Drugs and drug lore (hospital and otherwise) had an extremely long history of a heritage from classical antiquity, demonstrated succinctly by Touwaide in his "The Development of the Palaeologan Renaissance. An Analysis Based on Dioscorides' *De Materia Medica*," in M. Cacouros and M.-H. Congourdeau, eds, *Philosophie et sciences à Byzance de 1204 à 1453* (Leuven, Paris, and Dudley [Mass.]: Peeters, 2006 [*Orientalia Lovaniensia Analecta*, 146]), pp. 188–224. Likewise, Touwaide's "Les deux traités de toxicology attribués a Dioscoride" in Antonio Garzya, ed., *Tradizione e ecdotica dei testi medici tradoantichici e bizantini* (Naples: M. D'Auria, 1992), pp. 291–335, suggests how Byzantine copyists used (and altered) the pharmacology of the great Anazarban physician of the 1st century.

Timothy Miller himself published a response of sorts in his "Byzantine Physicians and their Hospitals," *Medicina nei Secoli Arte e Scienza*, 11 (1999), 323–35; the 'services' rendered by the doctors in the Byzantine hospitals were frequent, extended, and involved multiple expertise, including pharmaceuticals.

XIV. Herbs of the field and herbs of the garden in Byzantine medicinal pharmacy

Two other essays in the *Byzantine Garden Culture* collection, will be of interest to students of Byzantine botany, agriculture, and pharmacology:

Robert Rodgers, "Κηποποιΐα: Garden Making and Garden Culture in the *Geoponica*," pp. 159–75

Leslie Brubaker, "The Vienna Dioskorides and Anicia Juliana," pp. 189–214

Rodgers' essay is one of the very few that takes up the plants that are recorded for gardening purposes (and other uses as well) in the *Geoponica*. Of special interest will be the fresh translations that accompany Greek texts of *Geoponica* 11. 29 (ivy), 10. 83. 1–2 (To Make a Barren Tree Bear Fruit), 10.1. 1–4 (Florentinus on Making a Garden), and 12. 2.1–4 (another extract from Florentinus on how and why gardens are "essential for life" and the locales where it should be situated); added are the complex "literary traditions" (Table 1: a rough stemma) of the *Geoponica*, and Tables of Content for the full work as well as Tables of Content to the subsections of Books 10 through 12. One looks forward with pleasure to Rodgers' forthcoming edition and translation of the *Geoponica*.

Brubaker takes up the famous "Vienna Dioscorides" from the vantage of art history, and how the codex reflects the "life and times" of Anicia Juliana in the Byantium of the 6th century, and how the artists often "painted from life," and did not re-copy the illuminations in earlier papyrus-rolls or codices. One gains, too, an important analysis of the two "seven physicians" folios, as well as the initial depictions of the mandrake in the beginning folios (and mandrake is *not* pictured thereafter in the codex, suggesting its essential importance in the pharmacology of the day).

INDEX